Emergency Medicine

SECOND EDITION

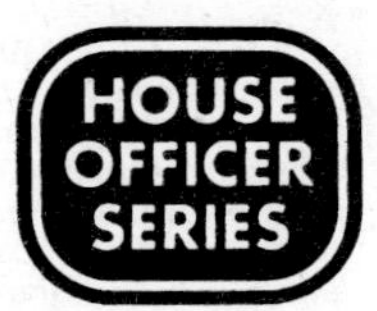

Emergency Medicine

SECOND EDITION

Lidia Pousada, MD, FACP

Chief, Division of Geriatrics and Gerontology
New Rochelle Hospital Medical Center
New Rochelle, New York
Associate Professor of Medicine
New York Medical College
Valhalla, New York

Harold H. Osborn, MD, FACEP, FACP, ACMT

Chairman, Department of Emergency Medicine
Professor of Emergency Medicine
New York Medical College
Valhalla, New York

David B. Levy, DO, FACEP

Residency Director, Program in Emergency Medicine
Temple University Medical School
Assistant Professor of Internal Medicine
Formerly Assistant Professor of Emergency Medicine
Medical College of Pennsylvania & Hahnemann University
Philadelphia, Pennsylvania

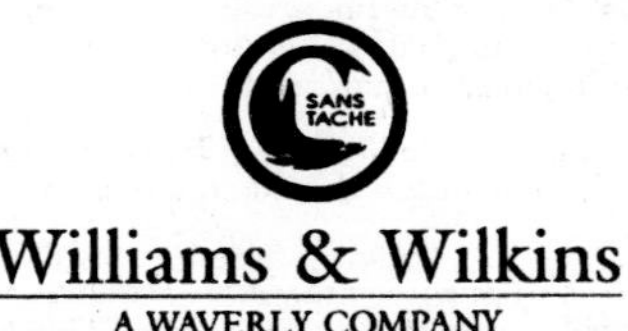

BALTIMORE • PHILADELPHIA • LONDON • PARIS • BANGKOK
BUENOS AIRES • HONG KONG • MUNICH • SYDNEY • TOKYO • WROCLAW

Editor: Charles W. Mitchell
Associate Managing Editor: Grace E. Miller
Production Coordinator: Linda C. Carlson
Copy Editor: Candace B. Levy, Ph.D.
Designer: Dan Pfisterer
Illustration Planner: Lorraine Wrzosek
Typesetter: Peirce Graphic Services, Inc.
Printer: Vicks Litho, Yorkville, NY

351 West Camden Street
Baltimore, Maryland 21201–2436 USA

Rose Tree Corporate Center
1400 North Providence Road
Building II, Suite 5025
Media, Pennsylvania 19063–2043 USA

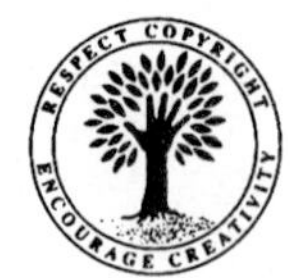

Accurate indications, adverse reactions and dosage schedules for drugs are provided in this book, but it is possible that they may change. The reader is urged to review the package information data of the manufacturers of the medications mentioned.

Printed in the United States of America

First Edition, 1986

Library of Congress Cataloging-in-Publication Data

Emergency medicine / [edited by] Lidia Pousada, Harold H. Osborn, David B. Levy.—2nd ed.
p. cm.—(House officer series)
Rev. ed. of: Emergency medicine for the house officer. c1986.
Includes bibliographical references and index.
ISBN 0-683-06963-2
1. Emergency medicine—Handbooks, manuals, etc. I. Pousada, Lidia. II. Osborn, Harold H. III. Levy, David B. IV. Emergency medicine for the house officer. V. Series.
[DNLM: 1. Emergencies—handbooks. 2. Emergency Medicine—handbooks. WB 39 E53 1994]
RC86.8.E535 1994
616.02′5—dc20
DNLM/DLC
for Library of Congress 93-47216
CIP

The publishers have made every effort to trace the copyright holders for borrowed material. If they have inadvertently overlooked any, they will be pleased to make the necessary arrangements at the first opportunity.

To purchase additional copies of this book, call our customer service department at **(800) 638–0672** or fax orders to **(800) 447–8438.** For other book services, including chapter reprints and large quantity sales, ask for the Special Sales department.

Canadian customers should call **(800) 268–4178,** or fax **(905) 470–6780.** For all other calls originating outside of the United States, please call **(410) 528–4223** or fax us at **(410) 528–8550.**

Visit Williams & Wilkins on the Internet: **http://www.wwilkins.com** or contact our customer service department at **custserv@wwilkins.com.** Williams & Wilkins customer service representatives are available from 8:30 am to 6:00 pm, EST, Monday through Friday, for telephone access.

96 97 98 99 00
1 2 3 4 5 6 7 8 9 10

Foreword

Emergency medicine is one of the fastest growing areas of health care in the United States. The volume of patient visits to emergency departments (EDs) across the country has more than doubled in the last two decades. There are now nearly 100 million patients seen in EDs yearly. Emergency medicine has served as the safety net for a faulty health care system for many years. ED patients typically receive care regardless of ability to pay. Although emergency physicians are trained to deliver acute care to patients with emergent needs, emergency physicians have also frequently provided general medical care.

Emergency medicine is practiced in urban, suburban, and rural communities. Although the practice approach may differ from hospital to hospital, the basic principles remain the same. Physicians who practice emergency medicine as a career typically possess strong interpersonal skills and a caring attitude toward patients of all backgrounds. Although the rewards of emergency medical practice are not always evident, the care delivered is appreciated by patients and families alike.

The field of emergency medicine has come a long way since the first residency programs were established in the United States in the early 1970s. Initially, the minimum training requirement for emergency medicine residents was 24 months, but that requirement has now expanded to a mandatory 36 months. There are still programs that require 48 months of training, and combined emergency medicine/internal medicine and emergency medicine/pediatrics residency programs are 60 months in length. Since their inception, the number of emergency medicine residency programs in the United States has increased from a mere handful to more than 100 programs.

As the American health care system undergoes reorganization in the 1990s, there may be fewer patients seen in the ED. It is to be hoped that patients with nonemergent illnesses will receive care in more appropriate settings, such as general medical clinics staffed by primary practitioners oriented toward general complaints and chronic illness. Critical to this goal is the provision of universal coverage for all Americans. In a system where health care is rationally planned, only truly acutely ill patients would present to the ED, where they would receive the most proficient emergency care. In the future, physicians working in the ED will be in the forefront of change, providing innovative care for geriatric patients, victims of violence, obstetric and gynecologic patients, trauma cases, patients with chest pain, pediatric patients, and many other individuals with emergency medical needs.

In the early years of emergency medicine training programs, there was little literature available for house officers and a paucity of textbooks dedicated to emergency medicine. Over the past 20 years, however, numerous textbooks have been published and several peer-reviewed journals have emerged. This body of literature has filled an important gap in our medical knowledge. The first edition of this emergency medicine text for house officers was one of the first of its kind. This updated and expanded second edition contains much valuable information concerning the treatment of emergency patients. It is a handy reference written especially for residents working in the ED, and it will serve you well as a ready source of emergency medicine information.

Marcus Martin, MD, FACP
Director, Division of Emergency Medicine
Allegheny General Hospital
Pittsburgh, Pennsylvania
Associate Professor of Emergency Medicine
Medical College of Pennsylvania & Hahnemann University
President, Council of Residency Directors/Society of Academic Emergency Medicine

Preface

The editors have been pleased to note the positive response to the first edition of *Emergency Medicine for the House Officer.* The material presented in this second edition is intended to update the information provided in the first edition. However, this text is not merely a revision of our previous work, as the scope of topics presented has been significantly broadened and the depth of each discussion enhanced. In addition, in the emergency department, patients do not present with a known diagnosis but instead embody a complex composite of clinical symptoms and signs, which the ED physician must analyze. This largely rewritten text thus serves to address this need and assist the house officer in the modern emergency department.

Thanks are due to our many contributors located throughout the country. The quality of their submissions and the scope of their credentials are a testimony to the multifaceted nature of emergency care.

Contributors

CARDIOLOGY

David B. Levy, D.O., F.A.C.E.P.
Residency Director
Program in Emergency Medicine
Temple University Medical School
Assistant Professor of Internal Medicine
Formerly Assistant Professor of Emergency Medicine
Medical College of Pennsylvania & Hahnemann University
Philadelphia, Pennsylvania

Timothy C. Evans, M.D., F.A.C.E.P.
Associate Professor of Emergency Medicine
Medical College of Pennsylvania—Allegheny Campus
Attending Physician, Division of Emergency Medicine
Allegheny General Hospital
Pittsburgh, Pennsylvania

Dennis P. Hanlon, M.D., F.A.C.E.P
Assistant Professor of Emergency Medicine
Medical College of Pennsylvania—Allegheny Campus
Department of Emergency Medicine
Allegheny General Hospital
Pittsburgh, Pennsylvania

Meta Podrazik, M.D.
Assistant Professor, Department of Emergency Medicine
Medical College of Pennsylvania & Hahnemann University
Attending Physician, Pediatric Emergency Medicine
St. Christopher's Hospital for Children
Philadelphia, Pennsylvania

PULMONOLOGY

B. Bryan Jordan, D.O.
Attending Physician, Department of Emergency Medicine
St. Barnabas Hospital
Bronx, New York

NEUROLOGY

Patricia A. Castillo, R.P.A.C.
Research Physician Assistant
Division of Geriatrics & Gerontology
New Rochelle Hospital Medical Center
New Rochelle, New York

TRAUMA

Robert Jones, D.O., F.A.C.E.P.
Assistant Professor, Department of Emergency Medicine
Wayne State University
Attending Physician
Grace Hospital
Detroit, Michigan

Anita Gage, M.D.
Medical Director, Department of Emergency Medicine
Detroit Receiving Hospital
Instructor of Emergency Medicine
Wayne State University
Detroit, Michigan

Peter Wachtel, D.O.
Attending, Department of Emergency Medicine
St. Barnabas Hospital
Bronx, New York

GASTROENTEROLOGY

Lidia Pousada, M.D., F.A.C.P.
Chief, Division of Geriatrics and Gerontology
New Rochelle Hospital Medical Center
New Rochelle, New York
Associate Professor of Clinical Medicine
New York Medical College
Valhalla, New York

Devang Dave, M.D.
Director, Dementia Treatment Center
Division of Geriatrics & Gerontology
New Rochelle Hospital Medical Center
New Rochelle, New York

METABOLISM

Lidia Pousada, M.D., F.A.C.P.

TOXICOLOGY

Fred Harchelroad, M.D., F.A.C.E.P., A.B.M.T.
Director, Medical Toxicology Treatment Center
Allegheny General Hospital
Associate Professor of Emergency Medicine
Medical College of Pennsylvania
Hahnemann University—Allegheny Campus
Pittsburgh, Pennsylvania

Richard F. Clark, M.D., F.A.C.E.P., A.B.M.T.
Assistant Professor of Clinical Medicine
Director, Division of Medical Toxicology
University of California at San Diego
San Diego, California

ALLERGY

James S. Cohen, M.D.
Attending Physician
Department of Emergency Medicine
Englewood Hospital and Medical Center
Englewood, New Jersey

Harold H. Osborn, M.D., F.A.C.E.P., F.A.C.P., A.C.M.T.
Professor & Chairman, Department of Emergency Medicine
New York Medical College
Valhalla, New York
Chief of Service
Lincoln Medical & Mental Health Center
Bronx, New York

INFECTIOUS DISEASE

Janet M. Williams, M.D.
Assistant Professor, Department of Emergency Medicine
Research Director, Center for Rural Emergency Medicine
West Virginia University School of Medicine
Morgantown, West Virginia

Dial Hewlett, M.D., F.A.C.P.
Chief, Infectious Diseases
Lincoln Medical & Mental Health Center
Bronx, New York
Associate Professor of Clinical Medicine
New York Medical College
Valhalla, New York

Harold H. Osborn, M.D., F.A.C.E.P., F.A.C.P., A.C.M.T.

OBSTETRICS AND GYNECOLOGY

Ted Gaeta, D.O., F.A.C.E.P.
Attending Physician, Department of Emergency Medicine
St. Barnabas Hospital
Bronx, New York
Assistant Professor of Emergency Medicine
New York College of Osteopathic Medicine
Old Westbury, New York

UROLOGY

Timothy C. Evans, M.D., F.A.C.E.P.

RENAL

Gerard Casey, M.D.
Assistant Professor and
Assistant Residency Director
Department of Emergency Medicine
State University of New York
Health Sciences Center at Brooklyn
Brooklyn, New York

HEMATOLOGY

Richard Lanoix
Assistant Professor and
Residency Director
Department of Emergency Medicine
New York Medical College
Valhalla, New York

Harold H. Osborn, M.D., F.A.C.E.P., F.A.C.P., A.C.M.T.

OPHTHALMOLOGY

David B. Levy, D.O., F.A.C.E.P.

EAR, NOSE, AND THROAT

David M. Chuirazzi, M.D.
Assistant Professor
The Medical College of Pennsylvania and
Hahnemann University—Allegheny Campus
Pittsburgh, Pennsylvania

Leonard Urbanski, D.O.
Attending, Department of Emergency Medicine
St. Francis Medical Center
Pittsburgh, Pennsylvania

BASIC ORTHOPEDICS

Dennis P. Hanlon, M.D., F.A.C.E.P.

PAIN CONTROL IN THE EMERGENCY DEPARTMENT

David B. Levy, D.O.

Harold H. Osborn, M.D., F.A.C.E.P., F.A.C.P., A.C.M.T.

ENVIRONMENTAL EMERGENCIES

Lidia Pousada, M.D., F.A.C.P.

Harold H. Osborn, M.D., F.A.C.E.P., F.A.C.P., A.C.M.T.

PSYCHIATRY

Frederick M. Schiavone, M.D., F.A.C.E.P.
Residency Director
University Hospital at Stony Brook
Assistant Professor of Emergency Medicine
State University of New York at Stony Brook
Stony Brook, New York

Harold H. Osborn, M.D., F.A.C.E.P., F.A.C.P., A.C.M.T.

Ann Lifflander, M.D.
Attending Physician
Bronx Lebanon Hospital
Bronx, New York

SOCIAL, LEGAL, AND ETHICAL ISSUES

Frederick M. Schiavone, M.D., F.A.C.E.P.

Robert Hamilton, M.D.
Assistant Professor of Emergency Medicine
Allegheny General Hospital
Pittsburgh, Pennsylvania

Vincent Pangalos, M.D.
Attending Emergency Medicine Physician
Qualified Emergency Specialists, Inc.
Cincinnati, Ohio

EMERGENCY PROCEDURES

Stan S. Rice, D.O.
Attending Physician
Department of Emergency Medicine
Brackenridge Hospital
Austin, Texas

Joseph J. Kuchinski, D.O., F.A.C.O.E.P.
Co-Director and Associate Emergency Medicine Residency Director
St. Barnabas Hospital
Bronx, New York

Harold H. Osborn, M.D., F.A.C.E.P., F.A.C.P., A.C.M.T.

Commonly Used Abbreviations

AAA	abdominal aortic aneurysm
ABG	arterial blood gas
ACE	angiotensin-converting enzyme
ACLS	advanced cardiac life support
A-fib	atrial fibrillation
AIDS	acquired immunodeficiency syndrome
AIVR	accelerated idioventricular rhythm
ALT	a serum transaminase (a.k.a. SGPT)
AMI	anterior myocardial infarction
AST	a serum transaminase (a.k.a. SGOT)
AVM	ateriovenous malformation
BLS	basic life support
BP	blood pressure
CABG	coronary artery bypass graft
CAD	coronary artery disease
CBC	complete blood count
CBF	cerebral blood flow
CCU	critical care unit
CHB	complete heart block
CHF	congestive heart failure
CK	creatine kinase
CK-MB	creatine kinase isoenzyme MB
CNS	central nervous system
CO	cardiac output
COPD	chronic obstructive pulmonary disease
CPAP	continuous positive airway pressure
CPB	cardiopulmonary bypass
CPK	creatine phosphokinase
CPP	cerebral perfusion pressure
CPR	cardiopulmonary resuscitation
CSF	cerebrospinal fluid
CSM	carotid sinus massage

CVA	cerebrovascular accident
CVP	central venous pressure
CVS	cardiovascular system
CXR	chest x-ray
DM	diabetes mellitus
DNR	do not resuscitate
DVT	deep venous thrombosis
ECC	emergency cardiac care
ECG	electrocardiography (a.k.a. EKG)
echo	echocardiography
ED	emergency department
EMD	electromechanical dissociation
ENT	ears, nose, and throat
epi	epinephrine
ETT	endotracheal tube
hCG	human chorionic gonadotropin
HEENT	head, eyes, ears, nose, and throat
HTN	hypertension
IABP	intraaortic balloon pump
IBD	inflammatory bowel disease
ICP	intracranial pressure
ICU	intensive care unit
IOP	intraocular pressure
IPG	impedance plethysmography
IVDA	intravenous drug abuser
JVD	jugular vein distention
LAH	left atrial hypertrophy
LAHB	left anterior hemiblock
LLQ	left lower quadrant
LR	lactated Ringer's
LUQ	left upper quadrant
LVEDP	left ventricular end-diastolic pressure
LVH	left ventricular hypertrophy
MAP	mean arterial pressure
MAST	military antishock trousers
MAT	multifocal atrial tachycardia
MI	myocardial infarction
MVP	mitral valve prolapse
NG	nasogastric
NS	normal saline

NSAID	nonsteroidal antiinflammatory drug
NSR	normal sinus rhythm
NTG	nitroglycerin
NVD	neck vein distention
OD	overdose
PACs	premature atrial contractions
PCWP	pulmonary capillary wedge pressure
PE	pulmonary embolism
PEA	pulseless electrical activity
PEEP	positive end-expiratory pressure
PEFR	peak expiratory flow rate
PMH	past medical history
PMNs	polymorphonuclear cells
PSVT	paroxysmal supraventricular
PTCA	percutaneous transluminal coronary angioplasty
PT	prothrombin time
PTT	partial thromboplastin time
PTX	pneumothorax
PVCs	premature ventricular contractions
PVD	peripheral vascular disease
RLQ	right lower quadrant
ROSC	return of spontaneous circulation
RUQ	right upper quadrant
SAH	subarachnoid hemorrhage
SL NTG	sublingual nitroglycerin
SMA	serum electrolytes
SNS	sympathetic nervous system
SOB	shortness of breath
SSS	sick sinus syndrome
STD	sexually transmitted disease
SVT	supraventricular tachycardia
TCP	transcutaneous pacing
TIAs	transient ischemic attacks
URI	upper respiratory infection
US	ultrasound
UTI	urinary tract infection
VF	ventricular fibrillation
VT	ventricular tachycardia
WBC	white blood cell count
WPW	Wolf-Parkinson-White syndrome

Contents

Chapter 1

Cardiology

1.1 CARDIOPULMONARY ARREST

Description

The goal of CPR and ACLS is to "save hearts too good to die" while preserving cerebral viability. Recommendations from the American Heart Association are merely guidelines and require emergency care providers to be flexible in their decision making. The recommendations herein reflect the consensus of the Fifth National Conference on CPR and ECC, held in 1992, and increase the emphasis on treating the patient rather than focusing on the cardiac tracing. Rapid decisions often become necessary, and little data may be available.

ACLS emphasizes the cardiac etiologies leading to cardiopulmonary arrest. Two-thirds of cardiac arrests stem from ischemic heart disease, with myocardial ischemia precipitating ventricular fibrillation (the most common lethal rhythm disturbance) followed by bradyasystole, pulseless electrical activity (previously referred to as electromechanical dissociation), and ventricular tachycardia.

History

Attempt to obtain a brief history from family, bystanders, and/or paramedics to determine the most likely etiology of the arrest and probability for successful resuscitation. Helpful information includes (1) preceding warning symptoms before arrest (e.g., chest pain, seizure, difficulty breathing, choking, headache, and trauma), (2) past medical history (e.g., cardiac disease, seizures, diabetes, renal disease, drug abuse, and use of any prescription or recreational drugs), (3) location and time of arrest (estimated length of "downtime"), (4) whether the arrest was witnessed, (5) whether bystander CPR was instituted, and (6) whether there was ever a return of spontaneous circulation. Ascertain interventions performed by the paramedics.

Physical Examination

Observe universal precautions during exposure to body secretions. After identification and treatment of the original rhythm disturbance, direct the primary examination toward the airway, breathing, and circulatory status. Only after stabilization of the patient or failure of initial measures should a secondary survey be completed.

Vital signs. Record respirations (look, listen, and feel), pulse (palpate the carotid artery for at least 10 sec), blood pressure, and temperature.

General. Is the patient cachectic (cancer or end-stage AIDS)? Inspect the skin for color (cyanosis), pallor (blood loss), petechiae (coagulation abnormality or infection), and ecchymosis (trauma, bleeding abnormality).

HEENT. Evaluate pupil for size and reactivity. Ensure airway patency. Leave dentures in place for bag-valve-mask ventilation, but extract them when intubating.

Neck. Regard neck vein distention (tension pneumothorax, cardiac tamponade, pulmonary embolus, cardiogenic shock). Flat neck veins may also accompany shock (septic, hypovolemic, or anaphylactic). Note tracheal position (deviated away from the midline in tension pneumothorax).

Chest. Auscultate breath sounds for symmetry along with inspecting and palpating the chest wall.

Heart. Note significant murmurs (ruptured intraventricular septum, papillary muscle rupture, aortic stenosis) or muffled heart sounds (cardiac tamponade).

Abdomen. Examine for distention, bruits, or a pulsatile mass.

Pelvis. Check for vaginal bleeding, uterine enlargement, and/or adnexal masses.

Extremities. Inspect for arteriovenous fistulas, track marks, bruising, and deformity (trauma) along with checking for pulse discrepancy.

Diagnostic Tests

Cardiac monitoring. Employ quick-look paddles. If initial defibrillation attempts are unsuccessful, begin continuous

ECG monitoring. Use more than one lead to verify asystole.

Fingerstick glucose. Obtain estimate of plasma glucose levels on any patient with an altered mental status (treat hypoglycemia, but avoid hyperglycemia).

ECG. Obtain a 12-lead ECG after ROSC.

CXR. Order a stat portable CXR after ROSC. **Remember:** *Tension pneumothorax should be a clinical rather than radiological diagnosis.*

ABG. Low priority in the early phase of resuscitation (correlates poorly with outcome).

CBC and serum electrolytes (SMAs). These tests are of limited importance during the initial resuscitation period. SMA values are occasionally helpful in cases of resistant dysrhythmias (e.g., hyperkalemia, hypokalemia, or hypomagnesemia).

End-tidal CO_2 monitoring ($Petco_2$). Provides a practical, noninvasive evaluation of the effectiveness of CPR. Increases in end-tidal CO_2 levels reflect improvement in lung perfusion and cardiac output (a level greater than 10 mm Hg is a positive predictor of ROSC).

Special Considerations

See algorithms in Figure 1.1*A–D*.

Withholding or Terminating CPR

Determine whether to initiate or withhold CPR on an individual basis. Specific contraindications to continuation of CPR include obvious death (decapitation, rigor mortis, dependent lividity, evidence of tissue decomposition), confirmed DNR orders, known terminal illness, or failure of prolonged prehospital resuscitation.

Informing the Family of a Sudden Death

The role of the health care provider does not end with the death of a patient. While it is difficult to be the bearer of bad news, it is the physician's responsibility to inform the family of a death, critical injury, or illness. Other duties do not relieve the physician of this responsibility. Enlisting the aid of clergy, social workers, and experienced nurses can be invaluable to both the family and physician. In addition, clergy may be requested to perform religious rites for the dead or dying.

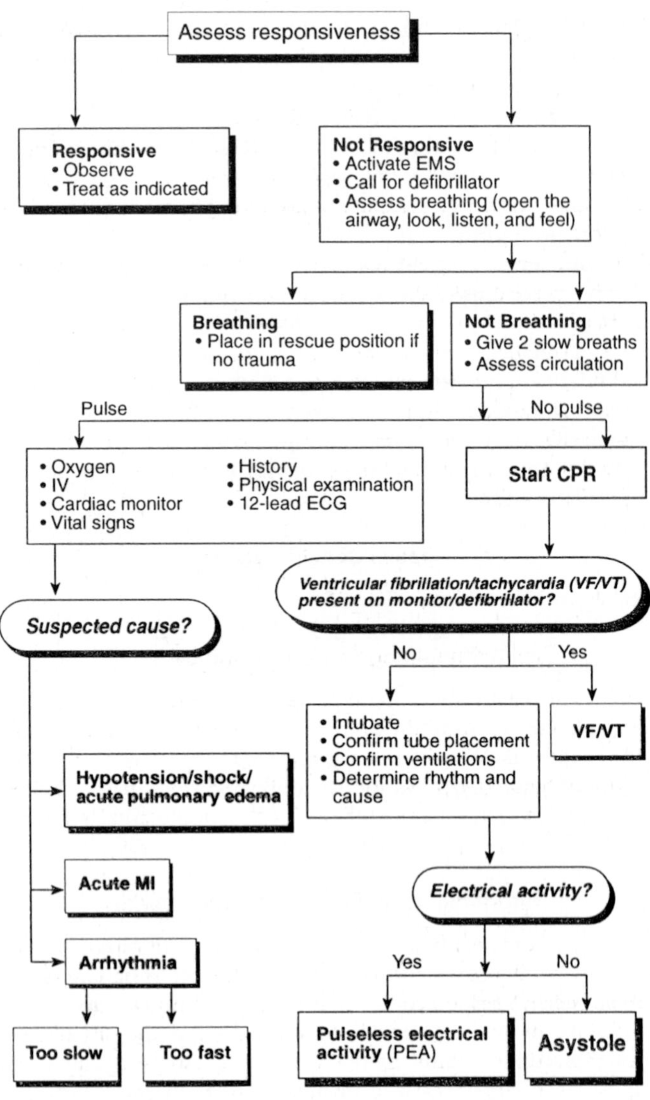

Figure 1.1.1 **A,** Universal algorithm for adult emergency cardiac care.

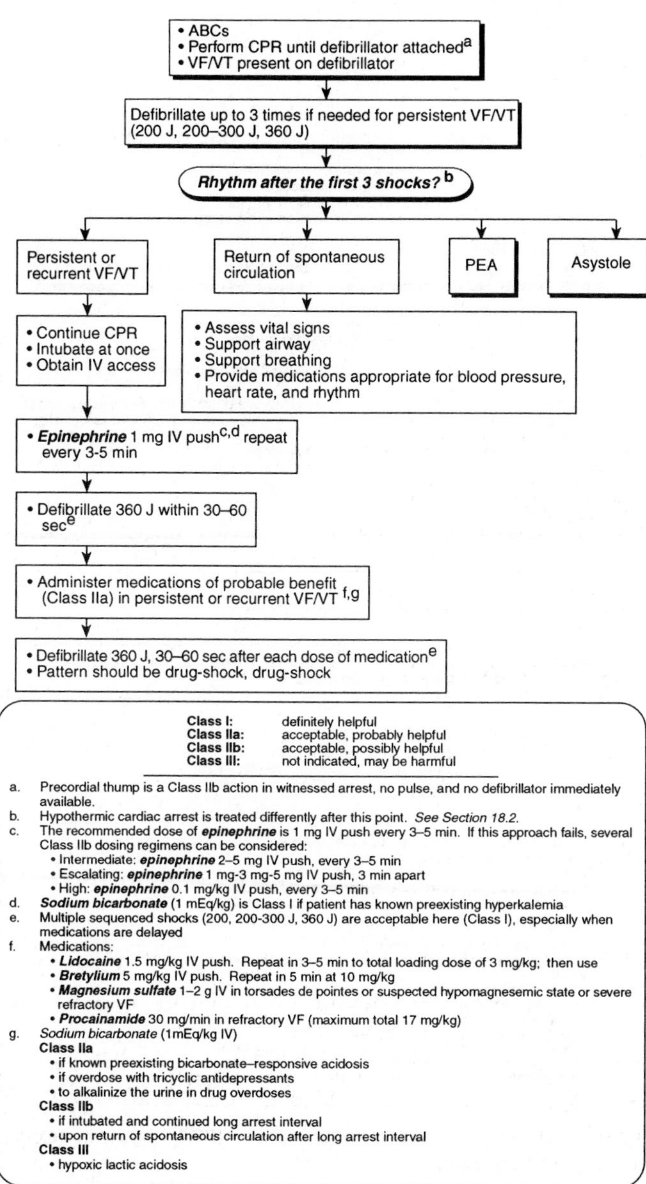

Figure 1.1.1 B, Ventricular fibrillation/pulseless ventricular tachycardia algorithm (VF/VT).

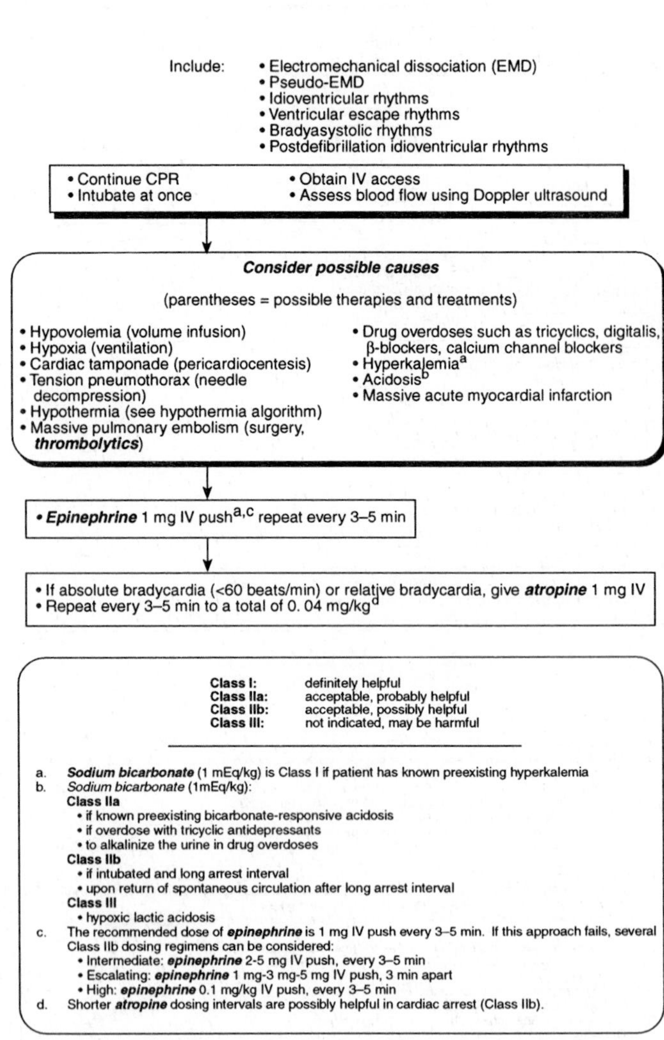

Figure 1.1.1 C, Pulseless electrical activity (PEA) algorithm (electromechanical dissociation).

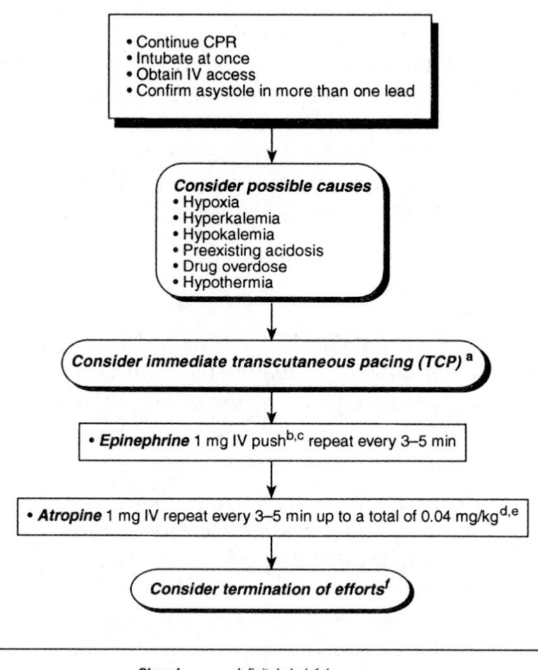

Class I: definitely helpful
Class IIa: acceptable, probably helpful
Class IIb: acceptable, possibly helpful
Class III: not indicated, may be harmful

---

a. TCP is a Class IIb intervention. Lack of success may be due to delays in pacing. To be effective TCP must be performed early, simultaneously with drugs. Evidence does not support routine use of TCP for asystole.

b. The recommended dose of ***epinephrine*** is 1 mg IV push every 3–5 min. If this approach fails, several Class IIb dosing regimens can be considered:
   - Intermediate: ***epinephrine*** 2–5 mg IV push, every 3–5 min
   - Escalating: ***epinephrine*** 1 mg-3 mg–5 mg IV push, 3 min apart
   - High: ***epinephrine*** 0.1 mg/kg IV push, every 3–5 min

c. ***Sodium bicarbonate*** 1mEq/kg is Class I if patient has known preexisting hyperkalemia

d. Shorter ***atropine*** dosing intervals are Class IIb in asystolic arrest

e. *Sodium bicarbonate* 1mEq/kg:
   Class IIa
   - if known preexisting bicarbonate-responsive acidosis
   - if overdose with tricyclic antidepressants
   - to alkalinize the urine in drug overdoses

   Class IIb
   - if intubated and continued long arrest interval
   - upon return of spontaneous circulation after long arrest interval

   Class III
   - hypoxic lactic acidosis

f. If patient remains in asystole or other agonal rhythms after successful intubation and initial medications and no reversible causes are identified, consider termination of resuscitative efforts by a physician. Consider interval since arrest.

Figure 1.1.1 D, Asystole treatment algorithm.

Treatment

The first priority in the ED management of any cardiac arrest is identification of the underlying rhythm disturbance. If ventricular fibrillation (VF) or unstable ventricular tachycardia (VT) is present, defibrillation takes precedence over all other actions: *VFIB* = DEFIB! Only after VF is successfully converted to a more stable rhythm, or three attempts at defibrillation are completed, should the practitioner consider airway, breathing, and circulatory interventions.

Precordial Thump

Precordial thump is indicated in a witnessed, pulseless, cardiac arrest when a defibrillator is unavailable. Deliver a single quick blow to the midsternum from a height of 8 to 12 inches.

Defibrillation

Rapid defibrillation is the major determinant of survival from cardiac arrest. Use a conductive substance with successive countershocks. For standard paddle placement, hold one paddle to the right of the proximal sternum (just underneath the right clavicle) and the other paddle lateral to the left nipple (aligned with the left midaxillary line). Use synchronized cardioversion for supraventricular tachycardia (SVT), atrial fibrillation, atrial flutter, and "stable" VT to avoid delivery of the shock during the vulnerable phase. Unsynchronized shocks are necessary in patients with VF, VT, and SVT associated with absent pulse, unconsciousness, hypotension, or pulmonary edema. **Note:** *The person delivering the countershock must ensure that no one else is in contact with the patient or the stretcher during cardioversion or defibrillation.*

Airway Management

Ensure a patent airway; remove any foreign bodies, secretions, or vomitus with a gloved finger or by suctioning. Ventilate with a face mask and Ambu bag attached to an oxygen source until the proper equipment and staff are available to intubate the patient. Injudicious attempts at intubation can make subsequent placement of the endotracheal tube (ETT) difficult if not impossible. Orotracheal intubation is preferred for patients who are potential thrombolytic candidates. See section 21.3 for additional information.

Routes for Drug and Fluid Administration

A central line (internal jugular or subclavian vein) is the preferred route if readily accessible. Advantages of a central line include faster drug delivery to sites of action and higher peak drug levels. Do not use distal wrist and hand veins (poor drug delivery to the central circulation). Avoid placing intravenous lines in the lower half of the body; if it is necessary to cannulate the femoral vein, use a catheter long enough to extend above the diaphragm. Give medications as a rapid IV bolus, followed by a 20 mL flush and elevation of the extremity. Use a femoral or antecubital vein preferentially if thrombolysis is contemplated.

Naloxone, atropine, Valium, epinephrine, and lidocaine (NAVEL) can be delivered through the ETT. Deliver 2 to 2.5 times the recommended IV dosage of the medication, diluted in 10 mL of normal saline, quickly spraying the contents down the ETT.

Pacemakers

Indications for emergency cardiac pacing include (1) bradyasystolic arrest, (2) hemodynamically unstable bradycardia, and (3) prophylaxis against complete heart block in the setting of acute MI. Transcutaneous pacing (TCP) is an optimal method of pacing in ED patients. See section 21.7.

Medications

- *Epinephrine* is a potent α-agent (vasoconstrictor, improves coronary and cerebral perfusion) and β-agonist (inotropic and chronotropic effects on the heart). The optimal dose of epinephrine is a source of controversy. Current ACLS recommendations call for administration of 1 mg IV of epinephrine q 3 to 5 min for VF, AS, and PEA.
- *Sodium bicarbonate* is no longer recommended for routine administration. Adequate ventilation and restoration of circulation are the mainstays to correct acid-base imbalances occurring with cardiac arrest. Restrict use to specific circumstances: preexisting metabolic acidosis, hyperkalemia, or overdoses (tricyclic antidepressants, phenobarbital, and salicylate). Give 1 mEq/kg IV push initially, followed by 0.5 mEq/L q 10 min until lab results return.
- *Lidocaine* is the antiarrhythmic of choice for treatment of ven-

tricular ectopy, VF, VT, and prophylaxis against recurrence of VF/VT. For VF, use only after failure of several attempts at defibrillation. Give an initial bolus of 1 to 1.5 mg/kg, with subsequent doses of 0.5 up to 3 mg/kg. Upon ROSC, start a lidocaine drip of 2 to 4 mg/kg (lower doses when congestive heart failure is present, age is more than 70 years, or liver dysfunction exists).

- *Procainamide* is an alternative to lidocaine and is especially useful when there is difficulty distinguishing the origin of a wide complex tachycardia. Dosing recommendations call for 20 mg/min until (1) the dysrhythmia is suppressed, (2) hypotension ensues, (3) the QRS complex is increased to more than 50% of its original width, or (4) a total of 17 mg/kg has been administered. Avoid the use of procainamide in patients with preexisting QT prolongation and/or torsades de pointes.
- *Bretylium* is used for refractory VF, refractory pulseless VT, or hemodynamically unstable VT and is generally given after defibrillation and lidocaine fail. Bretylium is the drug of choice in the presence of hypothermia. The recommended dose for VF arrest is a 5 mg/kg IV bolus (followed by electrical defibrillation). If VF arrest persists, give 10 mg/kg IV bolus q 15 min up to 30 to 35 mg/kg. A continuous IV infusion of 1 to 2 mg/min should be started upon ROSC. Consider an IV drip of 5 to 10 mg/kg of bretylium diluted in 50 mL NS or D_5W given over 5 to 10 min for resistant or recurring VT.
- *Atropine* is indicated for symptomatic bradycardia or asystole. Avoid use in patients with third-degree heart block accompanied by wide complex escape beats as well as Mobitz type II second-degree heart block. In addition, employ atropine cautiously in patients with myocardial ischemia, as it may worsen ischemia. For asystole, give 1.0 mg IV, repeating a 1.0 mg dose q 3 to 5 min prn, up to 3.0 mg total. Treat hemodynamically unstable bradycardia with a 0.5 mg IV bolus q 5 min, up to 2.0 mg. Doses of atropine < 0.5 mg IV may cause a paradoxical bradycardia and possibly precipitate VF.
- *Calcium chloride* use should be restricted to particular resuscitative situations: known hypocalcemia, hyperkalemia, and calcium channel blocker toxicity. The 10% calcium chloride solution is preferred in arrest scenarios and is given as a 0.1 mL/kg IV bolus. Exercise caution when giving calcium products to patients on digitalis therapy, especially when digitalis toxicity is suspected.

- *Magnesium* deficiency is capable of exacerbating cardiac dysrhythmias as well as complicating refractory VF and hindering replacement of intracellular potassium. For VF/VT, give 1 to 2 g magnesium sulfate in 100 mL of NS or D_5W over 1 to 2 min, and a similar dose over 5 min for torsades de pointes.
- *Adenosine* serves as effective therapy for narrow complex paroxysmal supraventricular (PSVT) dysrhythmias. Deliver the first dose as a 6 mg IV bolus through a large vein. Follow with a 20-mL saline flush. If there is no response within 5 min, give a second dose of 12 mg IV, similarly bolused. Side effects of adenosine include transient flushing, dyspnea, and chest pain (these effects resolve in 1 to 2 min). Higher doses of adenosine may be necessary in patients on theophylline therapy, whereas dipyridamole and carbamazepine may potentiate adenosine.

Internal Cardiac Compression

Internal cardiac compression (ICM) may be necessary in the following conditions: penetrating chest trauma, presence of an anatomic deformity of the chest precluding adequate external compression, severe hypothermia, ruptured aortic aneurysm or pericardial tamponade, and recent postoperative thoracotomy. Direct defibrillation of the heart requires specially designed paddles; place one electrode behind the left ventricle and the other on the anterior surface of the heart. Start at 5 J in the adult and gradually increase the energy level to a maximum of 50 J.

Cardiopulmonary Bypass

Cardiopulmonary bypass (CPB) has been successfully employed in hypothermic arrest victims. Limitations include the time required to cannulate the femoral artery and vena cava as well as limited availability of necessary equipment.

Selected Readings

Emergency Cardiac Care Committee and Subcommittees, American Heart Association: Guidelines for cardiopulmonary resuscitation and emergency cardiac care. JAMA 1992;268:2171–2288.

Kellerman AL, Hackman BB, Semes G: Predicting outcome of unsuccessful prehospital advanced cardiac life support. JAMA 1993;270: 1433–1436.

1.2 SHOCK

Description

Shock arises when the oxygen supply is insufficient to support vital organ function. The vital organs most at risk are the brain, heart, and kidneys. Adequate oxygen delivery depends on satisfactory blood flow. Any disturbance in the cardiovascular function can cause shock. A detailed discussion of the pathophysiology of shock is beyond the scope of this text, but it is important to understand the basis of blood flow:

$$\text{Blood pressure (BP)} = \text{Cardiac output (CO)} \times \text{Systemic vascular resistance (SVR)}$$

$$\text{Cardiac output (CO)} = \text{Stroke volume} \times \text{Heart rate}$$

Ineffective tissue perfusion leads to cellular anoxia and dysfunction and, if not rapidly corrected, death. The clinical presentation of shock depends on the underlying cause, time course of the illness, and the patient's physiologic reserve status.

History

The patient is often unable to provide a history. Alternative sources of information include family, friends, paramedics, old medical records, private physician, and Medic Alert badges. Focus on possible inciting events and the rapidity of progression of the illness. Initiation of supportive therapy must often precede the history. Specifically determine the following:

History of the present illness. Inquire about symptoms of heart disease (chest pain, shortness of breath, palpitations, and syncope), recent infection (fever, chills, dysuria, cough, headache, stiff neck, and altered mental state), insect bite or sting (possible anaphylactic reaction), and fluid loss (vomiting, diarrhea, melena, hematemesis, hematochezia, and polyuria).

Past medical history. Ask about previous history of cardiac disease, renal disease, diabetes, intravenous drug abuse, mental illness, and recent surgery.

Medications. Determine all current medications (particularly inquire about new medications), including over-the-counter medications, illicit drug use, and immunosuppressive therapy.

OB-GYN history. Determine last menstrual period and any abdominal pain or vaginal bleeding (possible ectopic pregnancy).

Allergies. Document allergies to drugs, foods, and/or insect bites.

Physical Examination

General. Findings are variable. Appearance ranges from normal to moribund. Mental status changes include agitation, restlessness, or coma.

Vital signs. The hallmark of shock is a decreased blood pressure. Check for orthostatic changes (presence of which implies a greater than 20% decrease in blood volume). Compensatory tachycardia and tachypnea frequently take place. A rectal temperature is mandatory.

Skin. May be cool, pale, and clammy in advanced shock; warm skin is associated with septic shock. Determine quality of skin turgor. Inspect for cyanosis, rashes, petechiae, ecchymosis, purpura, and urticaria.

HEENT. Record pupil size and reactivity. Examine the fundus for papilledema, preretinal or subhyloid hemorrhage, or Roth spots. Investigate for occult evidence of head trauma (hemotympanum, otorrhea, cerebrospinal fluid rhinorrhea), and inspect the oral cavity for laryngeal or uvular edema.

Neck. Check if the neck veins are flat or distended. Confirm the position of the trachea.

Chest. Auscultate for equality of breath sounds, and note the presence of adventitious sounds such as rales, wheezes, or stridor.

Heart. Determine if the heart rate is abnormally fast or slow. Listen for extra heart sounds, murmurs, and/or rubs.

Abdomen. Note the presence of distention, rigidity, guarding, masses, organomegaly, and/or bruits.

Rectal. Heme test the stool, and note the sphincter tone.

Pelvis. Examine for vaginal bleeding and/or adnexal masses.

Extremities. Check for adequacy of pulses, presence of edema, and capillary refill time (normal is < 2 sec).

Neurologic. Record any abnormal motor, sensory, or reflex findings.

Diagnostic Tests

Fingerstick glucose. Essential in any patient with an altered mental status.

CBC. The initial hematocrit may not reflect blood loss but does help to establish a baseline. White cell count may be elevated from stress or infection.

SMA. Electrolyte abnormalities may cause or result from shock.

In addition, electrolyte, BUN, and creatinine levels reflect hydration status and renal function.

Blood cultures. Order if sepsis is suspected.

Lumbar puncture. Do not perform on a hemodynamically unstable patient. Stabilize the patient first, administer antibiotics empirically, and obtain CSF studies once the patient is relatively stable.

Cardiac enzymes. Request if an AMI is suspected. Markedly elevated creatine phosphokinase (CPK) levels imply rhabdomyolysis (see section 12.2).

Lactic acid. Results from critical reduction in blood flow. A level greater than 5 mEq/L is abnormal and is associated with shock. The *normal* level is 0.5 to 5 mEq/L; greater than 8 mEq/L *may* be a poor prognosis, but could be due to a seizure.

PT/PTT, platelets. Check for coagulation abnormalities.

Type and cross-match (or screen). Hemorrhage is a frequent cause of shock, often requiring the use of blood products (see section 13.1).

Pulse oximetry. Provides rapid estimate of oxygenation status. Recognize its limitations (does not detect hypoventilation, carboxyhemoglobin, or modest changes in the PO_2).

ABG. Definitive measure of oxygenation, ventilation, and acid-base status.

Central venous pressure (CVP). Approximates fluid status. Trends are more significant than individual readings.

ECG. Examine for evidence of ischemia/infarction, conduction disturbances, and electrolyte abnormalities.

CXR. Obtain a stat portable (*never send an unstable patient to the radiology suite*). Review for evidence of pneumothorax, infiltrates, cardiomegaly, and free air under the diaphragm.

Ultrasound. Beneficial bedside test to detect cardiac tamponade, aortic aneurysm, dissection, and ectopic pregnancy.

Foley catheter. Monitor urine output and obtain specimen for urinalysis and culture.

Nasogastric tube. Insert to relieve gastric distention. It decreases risk of aspiration. Check for upper gastrointestinal bleeding.

Special Considerations

Traditionally, shock is classified into one of several broad categories: *cardiogenic* (myocardial infarction or ischemia, valvular disease, dysrhythmia, tamponade), *hypovolemic* (hemorrhage, burns, insensible fluid loss, diarrhea, vomiting, major fractures, intestinal obstruction), *septic* (infection), *neurogenic,* and *miscellaneous* (anaphylaxis, drug overdoses, etc.). Traumatic causes are discussed in chapter 4. A conceptual approach that views shock as a disturbance of the rate, volume, or pump mechanism improves both patient assessment and clinical decision making. These categories are not mutually exclusive, and in many cases, an overlap of mechanisms occurs as a clinical syndrome progresses.

Rate problems. The heart is either beating too fast or too slow to keep up with the body's demands. Rate problems are not synonymous with conduction disturbances, as conduction abnormalities can still generate a normal ventricular rate (see section 1.8).

Volume problems. Volume problems may be absolute (arising from actual fluid loss) or relative (due to vasodilation or redistribution of circulatory volume).

Pump problems. These are the consequence of a disorder in cardiac contractility. Pump problems may be primary (myocardial infarction, cardiomyopathies, myocarditis, ruptured chordae tendineae, acute papillary muscle dysfunction, ruptured intraventricular septum) or secondary (cardiac tamponade, pulmonary embolism, atrial myxomas, tension pneumothorax, aortic stenosis).

Treatment

Ensure that the airway is clear and ventilation and oxygenation is satisfactory. Provide supplemental oxygen to all patients in shock. **Remember:** *It is always better to intubate early rather than late.* Establish intravenous access and administer a fluid challenge of 500 mL of crystalloid (normal saline or lactated Ringer's), unless the patient is in overt congestive heart failure (see section 1.6). Place the patient flat, in a supine position (the value of the Trendelenburg position is questionable).

The treatment of rate problems is addressed in section 1.8. Generally, shock does not occur unless the heart rate is < 50 bpm or > 160 bpm.

Intravascular volume must be restored before vasopressors can be used. Critical decreases in the circulating blood volume are among the most prevalent types of shock seen in the ED. The choice of fluids for resuscitation is controversial. However, most ED physicians favor crystalloids (normal saline or lactated Ringer's) initially. A reasonable approach is to dispense fluid challenges in increments of 250 to 500 mL of crystalloid, up to 2000 mL, avoiding overhydration and iatrogenic CHF. Fluid rate is adjusted according to clinical parameters (mental status, blood pressure, lung sounds, urine output) and CVP readings (if available). Patients who remain hypotensive despite sufficient fluid administration may require vasopressors. Consider *norepinephrine* (Levophed), infused at a rate of 0.5 to 30 μg/min, or *dopamine,* administered as a drip at a rate of 5 to 20 μg/kg/min.

Pump dysfunction also diminishes cardiac output and may lead to shock. Specific therapy is contingent on the etiology. Dobutamine may be used in doses of 2.5 to 10 μg/kg/min IV. In addition, certain drug overdoses may depress myocardial contractility.

Early surgical consultation is essential when hemorrhagic shock is a consideration. If the patient remains unresponsive despite the aforementioned measures, *reevaluate the patient!* Consider alternative causes such as sepsis (see section 9.9), pneumothorax, anaphylaxis, unknown drug ingestion, Addison's disease, mesenteric ischemia, neurogenic shock, or irreversible shock.

Admission Criteria

All patients in shock require expeditious admission to the intensive care unit, while acute surgical problems (leaking abdominal aortic aneurysm, papillary muscle rupture, ventricular septal rupture, surgical abdomen) require immediate transport to the OR.

Selected Readings

Baraff L, Schriger DL: Orthostatic vital signs: variation with age, specificity, and sensitivity in detecting 450 mL blood loss. Am J Emerg Med 1992;10:99–103.

Bisonni RS, Holtgrave DR, Lawler F, et al.: Colloids versus crystalloids in fluid resuscitation: an analysis of randomized controlled trials. J Fam Pract 1991;32:387–390.

McGhie AI, Goldstein RA: Pathogenesis and management of acute heart failure and cardiogenic shock: role of inotropic therapy. Chest 1992;105:626S–632S.

1.3 SYNCOPE

Description

Syncope arises from a temporary impairment of cerebral perfusion, manifesting as a sudden loss of consciousness and postural tone. Symptoms spontaneously resolve. In *presyncope* or *near syncope* there is no actual loss of consciousness, but clinical findings, etiology, and "work-up" are similar. Both syncope and presyncope are common, with the scope of causes ranging from benign, self-limited illnesses to lethal conditions.

History

Obtain a complete history (from patient, family, medics, and witnesses) verifying a syncopal event truly happened (patients who state they were unconscious for a second or two most likely did not lose consciousness). Analyze prodromal symptoms, duration, findings while unconscious, and postsyncopal course. Specifically inquire about preceding events (stressful or painful situation, change in body or head position, coughing, micturating, exercising) as well as antecedent symptoms (chest pain, palpitations, dyspnea, nausea, anxiety, blurry vision, lightheadedness). For most syncope events, the patient begins in an upright position and then slumps to the floor. Myoclonic jerking may take place, confusing the event with a seizure. Generally, once the patient is supine or prone, consciousness is rapidly restored (seconds to minutes). Patients may remain dazed for a few minutes, but complete restoration of consciousness should occur.

Additional helpful information includes past medical history (similar episodes in the past, known heart disease, hypertension, neurologic disease, diabetes), medications (whether prescription, over-the-counter, or illicit drugs), and OB-GYN history, along with a focused review of systems.

Consider the possibility of trauma transpiring with syncope; injuries may occur during or after the loss of consciousness.

Physical Examination

General. Note the patient's overall appearance. Is the patient healthy, sickly, alert, or confused?

Vital signs. Check pulses in upper and lower extremities, and compare blood pressures in each arm. Test for orthostatic changes. Record respiratory rate and temperature.

HEENT. Verify pupil size and reactivity, inspect fundi (papilledema, hemorrhages) and tympanic membranes (hemotympanum, otorrhea), and look for evidence of trauma.

Neck. Inspect for tenderness, nuchal rigidity, and neck vein distention.

Lungs. Auscultate for breath sounds, rales, rhonchi, wheezes, and rubs.

Heart. Listen for murmurs (note any change with the Valsalva maneuver, suggesting mitral valve prolapse or hypertrophic cardiomyopathy), rubs, gallops, clicks, and the tumor "plop" of atrial myxomas.

Abdomen. Note distention, bowel sounds, masses, and peritoneal guarding or tenderness.

Rectal. Evaluate rectal tone, and test stool for gross or occult blood.

Pelvic. Examine for vaginal bleeding, adnexal masses, and/or tenderness.

Extremities. Investigate for venous insufficiency, cyanosis, clubbing, and edema.

Neurologic. Be particularly attentive for focal motor or sensory deficits as well as cerebellar signs.

Diagnostic Tests

Selectively order diagnostic tests. There is no "routine" syncope profile.

ECG. Order on all patients. Evaluate for evidence of myocardial ischemia, infarction, dysrhythmia, preexcitation syndrome, prolonged QT interval, and conduction disturbance. Patients with suspected dysrhythmias require prolonged cardiac monitoring.

Blood chemistries. Reserve for patients in whom a specific diagnosis is entertained. However, a lab stick for glucose is indicated in any patient with an altered level of consciousness, and a pregnancy test should be routine on females of child-bearing age presenting with syncope. Obtain ABG and cardiac enzymes as indicated.

CXR. Review for pulmonary pathology (e.g., pulmonary embolus) as well as enlargement of cardiac silhouette.

Special Considerations

Despite extensive testing, the cause of syncope remains unknown in more than 40% of cases. CT scanning is not helpful in the absence of neurologic findings on examination.

Cardiac Syncope

Cardiac syncope carries an ominous prognosis and transpires when the cardiac output declines to a level too low to maintain cerebral perfusion. Onset is rapid. Patients tend to be older and/or have a prior documented history of coronary artery disease. Etiologies include *tachydysrhythmias, bradydysrhythmias, left ventricular outflow-obstruction* (aortic stenosis, hypertrophic cardiomyopathy, atrial myxomas), *myocardial ischemia,* and *conduction disturbances* (prolonged QT syndrome, second- and third-degree blocks).

Vasovagal Syncope

Better known as "fainting," vasovagal syncope is by far the most common cause of syncope. Most prevalent in younger patients (< 40 years), it is incited by exposure to a stressful situation. A paradoxical bradycardia evolves, accompanied by prodromal symptoms (generalized warmth, blurring of vision, nausea, lightheadedness). Episodes are usually very brief.

Orthostatic Syncope

Orthostatic syncope customarily manifests when a patient tries to assume an upright position. Frequently there is an underlying problem (hemorrhage, gastrointestinal fluid losses, medications, autonomic disorders).

Carotid Sinus Hypersensitivity

Carotid sinus hypersensitivity is an exaggerated cardioinhibitory response resulting from innocuous neck pressure (shaving, wearing tight shirt collars). It is most common in elderly males with hypertension, diabetes, or vascular disease.

Neurologic Etiologies

Syncope may be misdiagnosed as either seizure disorder (see section 3.2) or cerebrovascular disease (see section 3.3). However, syncope is not a feature of transient ischemic attacks (TIAs). When compromise of the vertebrobasilar circulation does lead to syncope, it is generally part of a syndrome incorporating "the five D's": diplopia, dysarthria, dysphagia, dysesthesias, and dizziness. Subarachnoid hemorrhage (SAH) may also be associated with syncope.

Miscellaneous Causes

Miscellaneous causes include *psychogenic syncope, drug or alcohol intoxication, hypoxia, pulmonary embolus, hypoglycemia,* and *situational syncope* (coughing, micturition, defecation, Valsalva maneuver, swallowing).

Treatment

The main task of the ED physician is to ensure stabilization of the patient (the ABCs), determine etiology, treat reversible causes (hypoglycemia, rhythm disturbances), and identify secondary injuries.

Admission Criteria

Admit *all patients with a suspected cardiac etiology or a potentially life-threatening cause* (ectopic pregnancies or aortic aneurysms). Patients at high risk for morbidity and mortality include the following:

- Patients over age 55;
- Patients with a history of congestive heart failure, coronary artery disease, or ventricular ectopy;
- Patients with abnormal ECGs; and
- Patients with "worrisome" symptoms (sudden onset without warning; onset subsequent to exertion; or syncope associated with chest pain, dyspnea, palpitations, severe abdominal pain, or headache).

Selected Readings

Georgeson S: Acute cardiac ischemia in patients with syncope: importance of the initial electrocardiogram. J Gen Intern Med 1992;7:379–383.

Kapoor WN: Evaluation and management of the patient with syncope. JAMA 1992;268:2553–2560.

1.4 CHEST PAIN

Description

Chest pain is the primary complaint of almost 7% of all patients seeking medical attention in the ED. Life-threatening conditions mandating immediate diagnosis and treatment include *AMI, unstable angina, aortic dissection, pulmonary embolism, esophageal rupture,* and *tension pneumothorax.* Complicating the issue is the fact that the heart, aorta, lungs, esophagus, mediastinum, and upper abdominal viscera share interconnecting sensory fibers, making it difficult to distinguish myocardial ischemia from the more benign etiologies of chest pain. Any discomfort from the jaw to the upper abdomen should be viewed as a chest pain equivalent.

With few exceptions, a complaint of chest pain requires immediate triage to a monitored ED bed.

History

A thoughtfully elicited, guided history is the best method of determining the etiology of chest pain. While the history may not yield the exact diagnosis, it does narrow the possibilities considerably. Predictions of risk for serious disease are predicated on the patient's age, sex, past medical history, and description of the pain. However, patients experiencing cardiac ischemia may not perceive the sensation as true pain, so instead ask about any *discomfort or unusual sensation* in the chest. Be alert for atypical presentations, especially in *diabetics* and *elderly* patients. Obtain old records if possible, and speak to family members (some patients may be frightened by the thought of a "heart attack" and will minimize symptoms).

Specifically, investigate the following historical points.

Character and location of the pain. Descriptive terms applied to ischemic pain include pressure, heaviness, cramping, burning, or aching sensation in the chest or mid-epigastrium. Aortic dissection is often characterized as a tearing or ripping pain. A sticking or stabbing sensation exacerbated by respirations suggests a pleural or pericardial source of pain. Classically, ischemic chest pain is localized retrosternally, represented by a clenched fist over the sternum (Levine sign). Chest pain sites that can be depicted with one finger are unlikely to be ischemic in etiology. However, there are very few descriptive phrases that eliminate angina or AMI as a diagnostic possibility. In patients with a previous history of AMI and/or angina, the nature and location of the pain tend to duplicate earlier episodes of ischemia, even if the original description and location were atypical.

Radiation. Chest pain radiating to the arms or neck is more likely to characterize myocardial ischemia, while pain transmitted to the back implies a possibility of aortic dissection.

Onset. Rapid appearance of pain is seen with spontaneous pneumothorax, aortic dissection, pulmonary embolus, and esophageal rupture.

Timing and duration. Anginal chest pain generally lasts 3 to 15 min. Chest discomfort occurring for only a few seconds is unlikely to be ischemic. Anginal pain persisting > 20 min suggests AMI. Do not forget to ask the patient if he or she is currently experiencing pain.

Precipitating factors. Exclude trauma as a cause of chest pain. Anginal pain is often provoked by exertion, cold, postprandial, or emotional distress. Chest pain precipitated by swallowing or change in body position suggests esophagitis, pericarditis, chest wall disorder, or psychogenic etiology. Chest pain following forceful vomiting is suspicious for esophageal rupture.

Relieving factors. Anginal pain usually subsides within minutes of discontinuing the activity that precipitated the pain. Discomfort from pericarditis or pancreatitis is frequently relieved by sitting up and leaning forward. Do not exclude ischemia as a cause if the patient obtains relief with a "GI cocktail."

Associated symptoms. Diaphoresis, nausea, vomiting, syncope, or shortness of breath that accompanies chest pain increases the likelihood of myocardial ischemia. Hemoptysis associated with chest pain suggests lung infection or PE.

Risk factors. Documenting risk factors (male gender, diabetes, hypertension, smoking, history of CAD, family history of MI, hyperlipidemia, and advanced age) is important for epidemiological purposes; but from an individual diagnostic standpoint, the only risk factors with a strong positive predictive value are history of CAD, DM, and abuse of cocaine and/or amphetamines. More important, the absence of risk factors does not exclude the diagnosis of myocardial ischemia.

Past medical history. Ask about complicating medical illnesses (CAD, hypertension, diabetes, peripheral vascular disease, and cerebrovascular accidents). If thrombolytic therapy is considered, inquire about contraindications (see section 1.5).

Medications. A medication list assists in identifying current medical problems. Establish compliance. If the patient makes use of sublingual nitroglycerin (SL NTG), ensure potency of pills (burning sensation when placed under the tongue). Do not forget to ask about use of diet pills or illicit drugs (especially cocaine and amphetamines).

Allergies. Obtain a complete history of allergies.

Physical Examination

General. Often the most consequential component of the physical examination. Many patients with AMI appear pale and anxious. Patients suffering from aortic dissection are frequently restless and look as if they were in shock even when normotensive.

Vital signs. Compare pulses and blood pressures in arms and legs (discrepancy with aortic dissection). Hypotension can occur with AMI, massive PE, aortic dissection, and tension pneumothorax; but the blood pressure may be normotensive or hypertensive even in the presence of catastrophic illness. Tachypnea is a nonspecific sign, but rule out emergent conditions (early shock, PE, CHF) before attributing it to anxiety.

HEENT. Examine eyes and fundi for clues to atherosclerotic disease (xanthomas and arcus senilis as well as AV nicking and silver wiring).

Neck. Establish the midline position of the trachea (deviated with tension pneumothorax). Evaluate neck veins for distention or Kussmaul's sign (increase in venous distention with inspiration). Neck vein distension can be seen with PE, CHF, right ventricular MI, tension pneumothorax, and cardiac tamponade.

Lungs. Ensure equal, bilateral breath sounds. Auscultate for rales, rhonchi, and wheezes.

Chest. Inspect the chest wall for rashes or vesicles confined to a dermatome (herpes zoster). Palpate for subcutaneous air (esophageal rupture, pneumothorax) and tenderness (5% of MIs have associated reproducible pain!) as well as erythema and swelling (Tietze's syndrome).

Heart. Auscultation in the ED is often difficult at best, but try to listen for characteristic murmurs and heart sounds:

Condition	Comments
Aortic stenosis	Harsh crescendo-decrescendo systolic murmur over right upper sternal border
Hypertrophic subaortic stenosis	Valsalva maneuver augments intensity of systolic murmur (murmur of aortic stenosis decreases)
Aortic regurgitation	Early diastolic murmur associated with aortic dissection

Mitral valve prolapse	Hallmark is a midsystolic click and/or late systolic murmur
Findings	Classically triphasic; increase with Valsalva maneuver
Pericardial rub	Three parts; usually best heard with patient sitting up and leaning forward

Abdomen. Examine for guarding, tenderness, bruits, or masses.

Extremities. Assess for edema, pulses (presence as well as equality), cyanosis, clubbing, and calf tenderness or cords.

Neurologic. Check for focal weakness (focal findings accompanying chest pain imply aortic dissection).

Diagnostic Tests

ECG

Even though it is not 100% specific or sensitive for myocardial ischemia, the ECG assists in the diagnosis of myocardial ischemia (horizontal ST-segment depressions), AMI (new Q waves or ST-segment elevation), and pericarditis (see section 9.3). It also aids in determining the course of therapy for AMI (see section 1.5) and disposition (patients with nondiagnostic ECG changes can be admitted to a monitored step-down bed instead of a unit bed). If chest discomfort persists but the first ECG is nondiagnostic, repeat the ECG in 30 min. If the patient is felt to be at low risk (< 5% pretest probability based on historical data) and exhibits a normal ECG, there is < 1% chance of AMI. **However,** *never exclude the diagnosis of AMI or cardiac ischemia on the basis of a normal or nondiagnostic ECG alone!* Compare the ECG to old ECGs if available.

Cardiac Enzymes

Serial cardiac enzymes are the gold standard for diagnosing AMI, but technical problems limit their use in the ED (see section 1.5). Enzyme levels of conventional markers, CPK, and CPK isoenzyme MB (CPK-MB) are inclined to be normal early in the course of AMI. In addition, current serum markers fail to identify unstable angina. Single CPK and isoenzyme values may be helpful if positive, but they are insufficient to exclude AMI as a diagnosis. Investigation into alternative serum markers of myocardial injury (e.g., myoglobin, isoforms of CPK-MB, and troponin) may prove advantageous in early identification of AMI.

Other Tests

CXR. Review for noncardiac causes of chest pain (rib fracture, aortic dissection, pneumothorax, pneumonia, PE) as well as signs of CHF. Order a portable film in unstable patients.

CBC, SMA, serum amylase, or lipase. Attempt to be selective in requesting "routine" studies.

PT/PTT. Order when coagulopathy is suspected or to establish a baseline before anticoagulation therapy.

Special Considerations

See Table 1.4.1.

Admission Criteria

Patients requiring admission to an ICU bed: those who need aggressive resuscitation or who are strongly suspected of having a life-threatening disorder (e.g., unstable angina, acute MI, aortic dissection, pulmonary embolus, and esophageal rupture).

Patients requiring admission (usually to a monitored or step-down bed): those diagnosed with pericarditis or pneumothorax and those with a significant risk for MI but atypical presentation with normal or equivocal ECG findings.

Patients who generally do not require admission: those with stable angina, those who are at low-risk with normal ancillary findings, and those who are at low-risk with clinical findings that suggest benign disorders.

Note: *It is important to arrange appropriate follow-up for all patients with chest pain discharged from the ED, often within the next 24 hr.* Always err on the side of caution.

Selected Readings

ACEP Standards Task Force: Clinical policy for management of adult patients presenting with a chief complaint of chest pain and no history of trauma. Dallas: American College of Emergency Physicians, 1991.

Howell JM, Hedges JR: Differential diagnosis of chest discomfort and general approach to myocardial decision making. Am J Emerg Med 1991;9(6):571–579.

Karlson B, Wiklund I, Bengston A, et al.: Prognosis and symptoms one year after discharge from the emergency department in patients with acute chest pain. Chest 1994;105:1442–1447.

Table 1.4.1
Special Considerations

Condition	Type of Pain	Associated Symptoms	Physical Signs	Diagnostic Tests	Treatment
Cardiovascular					
Stable angina pectoris	Episodic; often described as tightness, heaviness, burning. Lasts $>$ 1 min but $<$ 15 min. Usually occurs retrosternally but discomfort can occur in throat, epigastrium, interscapular, shoulder, or arm.	Minimal	No characteristic findings	ECG may be normal or show transient ST-T wave changes	NTG 0.4 mg SL; peak action within 2 min; if no relief, repeat in 5 min up to 2 times
Variant angina (Prinzmetal's angina)	Similar to pain of stable angina but occurs during rest or upon awakening. Related to vasospasm.	Syncope, dizziness; prone to dysrhythmias	No specific physical signs	Reversible ST-segment elevation on ECG	Initial treatment with SL NTG; calcium channel blockers may provide prophylaxis
Unstable angina[a]	New-onset angina, increasing frequency of anginal pain, or pain at rest. Recurrence of anginal pain 4 weeks post-MI or -PTCA considered unstable angina.	Nausea, dyspnea, diaphoresis	S_4 or apical systolic murmur with symptoms	Transient ST-T wave changes	Titrate IV NTG (5–200 mg/min); heparinize (5000 unit bolus followed by 500–1000 units/hr); give aspirin (325 mg PO)

Acute myocardial infarction[a] *(see section 1.5)*					
Pericarditis *(see section 9.3)*					
Mitral valve prolapse (Barlow's syndrome)	Usually nonexertional, sharp, and felt near apex.	Palpitations, hyperventilation, anxious	Midsystolic click, late systolic murmur	CXR and ECG generally normal	Acute therapy usually not needed; β-blockers may help long term
Aortic stenosis	Angina-like pain provoked by exertion.	Syncope, dyspnea	Harsh midsystolic murmur with delayed or diminished carotid upstroke	Presence of bundle branch block or left ventricular hypertrophy (LVH)	Exercise caution when prescribing preload reducing agents, including NTG
Dissecting aortic aneurysm *(see section 1.9)*					
Pulmonary					
Spontaneous pneumothorax or tension pneumothorax[a] *(see section 2.6)*					

Table 1.4.1—*Continued*

Condition	Type of Pain	Associated Symptoms	Physical Signs	Diagnostic Tests	Treatment
Pulmonary embolus *(see section 2.4)*					
Pleurisy	Sudden onset of pleuritic chest pain.	Dyspnea	Low-grade fever; pleural friction rub	CXR may reveal an infiltrate or pleural effusion	Analgesic antibiotics
GI					
Esophageal rupture[a] (Boerhaave's syndrome)	Sudden onset of severe, persistent, left-sided chest pain after vomiting or instrumentation of esophagus.	Dysphagia; pain increases with neck flexion	Fever, tachycardia, tachypnea, and hypotension along with SQ air base of neck and Hamman's sign (crunching sound of heart)	On CXR may see pneumomediastinum and/or left-sided pleural effusion	Definitive treatment is surgical; while waiting for surgeon, aggressively hydrate (LR or NS), keep patient NPO, and start broad-spectrum antibiotics
Pancreatitis, cholecystitis, peptic ulcer disease *(see Chapter 5)*					

Musculoskeletal					
Chest wall syndromes (costochondritis or Tietze's syndrome, xyphodalgia, and cervical or thoracic spine disease)	Refers pain to the chest; often dull ache at rest, exacerbated with deep breathing and changes in body position. Pain is of variable duration, lasting from seconds to hours.	Coughing and splinting of respirations	Observe and palpate chest wall for bruising, masses, tenderness, or swelling; pain often localized with one finger	Various maneuvers can be used to elicit pain, including bending forward at the waist, scissors maneuver (each arm adducted across chest), and hedge clipper maneuver (pressing palms together with elbows flexed)	Provide reassurance, local heat or cold, and short-term course of NSAIDs; avoid precipitating activities
Herpes zoster	Sharp, unilateral burning pain, more pronounced in posterior thorax; usually confined to one or two intercostal spaces.	Rash and hypesthesia of affected area; pain may precede rash by 3–10 days	Exanthem begins as erythematous plaque in a dermatomal distribution and then evolves into umbilicated vesicles on red base	Tzanck smear or culture	Oral acyclovir (800 mg 5 times/day); use of prednisone is controversial; supplement all pain relief with oral narcotic analgesics

Table 1.4.1—*Continued*

Condition	Type of Pain	Associated Symptoms	Physical Signs	Diagnostic Tests	Treatment
Miscellaneous					
Hyperventilation panic attacks, cardiac neurosis	Habitually described as constant diffuse pain over left mediastinum or left precordium. Pain may last for only seconds to days, weeks, or months. "All-or-none" phenomenon—either everything precipitates pain or nothing will.	Dyspnea, palpitations, fatigue, circumoral numbness, tingling of fingers and toes	No characteristic findings	Suspect the diagnosis in young and otherwise healthy patients who have already undergone extensive workup; provide reassurance and psychiatric referral; remember that the presence of psychosomatic pain does not exclude organic disease	

[a]An immediately life-threatening disorder.

1.5 MYOCARDIAL INFARCTION

Description

Acute myocardial infarction (AMI) is a medical emergency depicted by irreversible ischemia leading to death of the myocardium. Most AMIs arise from occlusion of a coronary artery. Less common causes of myocardial infarction (MI) include dissection, vasculitis, vasospasm, and embolic involvement of the coronary arteries. MI also occurs when myocardial oxygen demand exceeds supply (carbon monoxide poisoning, hypotension, profound anemia). *Transmural MI* implies necrosis of the entire thickness of the myocardial wall (usually the left ventricle), while in *subendocardial infarctions* damage is limited to the innermost portion of myocardium. Generally, thrombosis of the left anterior descending artery gives rise to an anterior infarction, and blockage of the right coronary artery causes infarction of the inferior portions of the left ventricle with possible extension to the right ventricle. The size and anatomic location of the infarction, along with the patient's underlying cardiac status, determine the clinical picture (see "Cardiac Enzymes" on page 33).

Because "time is muscle," it is crucial that patients with suspected MIs are rapidly identified and treated. Delays from the time of presentation to the ED (whether by ambulance or walk-in) to evaluation and treatment must be kept to a minimum.

History

There are no pathognomonic symptoms characterizing an acute MI. Customarily, the principal complaint is chest pain. Descriptions of the chest discomfort range from a crushing tightness to a dull pressure or a squeezing sensation that is constant and unaffected by respirations or movement. Pain frequently radiates to the neck, jaw, teeth, shoulder, arm, or back. Patients with known coronary artery disease may describe the pain as similar to their usual anginal pain, but more severe and persistent and unrelieved with nitroglycerin. The onset of MI may occur during rest (as opposed to stable angina, which usually occurs with exertion), and most often in the early morning hours. However, almost half of the patients with MI present with *atypical symptoms* (burning pain in the epigastrium, shortness of breath, syncope, weakness, or exacerbation of congestive heart failure). Painless MI is seen in almost 25% of patients, especially in the elderly and diabetics. Other non–chest pain symptoms associated with AMI include dyspnea, diaphoresis, and nausea. In terms of therapy, establish the time of onset of the AMI; this is not always clear-cut, as some patients cannot explicitly state when their symptoms began or may relate a stuttering course.

Physical Examination

Note: *The physical exam is highly variable in patients with AMI, with no clinical sign being particular for AMI.* Specific findings are determined by the extent and location of myocardial damage, ranging from a normal examination to frank pulmonary edema and/or cardiogenic shock (which indicates > 40% damage to the left ventricle). The physical exam is better in verifying nonischemic causes of chest pain than in diagnosing ischemia.

General. Patients sustaining extensive MIs often appear anxious, pale, and diaphoretic.

Vital signs. Pulse and blood pressure findings rest on the balance between parasympathetic and sympathetic stimulation. Typically with early anterior infarctions, sympathetic stimulation predominates, resulting in tachycardia and hypertension; whereas inferior infarctions are characterized by increased parasympathetic tone with ensuing bradycardia and hypotension. Profound hypotension takes place with ventricular dysfunction (left or right), dysrhythmias, hypovolemia, or medications (nitrates, morphine, antiarrhythmics). Tachypnea may be secondary to pain and anxiety of infarction, or respiratory distress may be secondary to left ventricular failure. A low-grade fever (38 to 39°C) may accompany early MI.

Neck. Examine for jugular venous distention (CHF or right ventricular infarction).

Lungs. Listen for rales or wheezes (CHF).

Heart. Auscultate for heart sounds and murmurs (a new systolic murmur can signify papillary muscle dysfunction or rupture or herald ventricular septal rupture).

Rectal. Check stool for occult blood, especially if thrombolytic or anticoagulant therapy is considered.

Extremities. Note color, temperature, pulses, edema, and cyanosis (cool and clammy with decreased capillary refill in the shocky patient).

Diagnostic Tests

ECG

The ECG is the best test for the early diagnosis of acute MI. Patients presenting with acute chest pain associated with new Q waves or ST-segment elevation have a high probability of AMI. However, particularly early in the course of AMI, the ECG may be nondiagnostic or even normal. A normal or minimally abnormal ECG does not exclude the diagnosis of AMI in patients whose history is highly suggestive for ischemic heart disease. If the initial ECG is nondiagnostic and the patient is still experiencing symptoms, repeat the ECG in 30 min. Patients with inferior wall changes in the ECG (II, III, AVF) should have right ventricular leads (V3R and V4R) performed. The location of the MI is determined by the leads that indicate characteristic changes. ECG changes diagnostic of AMI can be mimicked by nonischemic conditions (pericarditis, early repolarization, ventricular aneurysm, left bundle branch block (LBBB), left ventricular hypertrophy, hypothermia, and intracerebral catastrophes) or masked by the presence of a paced rhythm or LBBB. In addition, a previous MI, lead misplacement, tricyclic overdose, type IA antiarrhythmics, and Wolf-Parkinson-White syndrome may all confuse the diagnosis or suggest an incorrect anatomic location of the AMI.

Cardiac Enzymes

CPK and CPK-MB tend to be normal early in the course of AMI. LDH levels peak later and can remain elevated for a week or longer post-MI. Determination of LDH values (an LDH_1:LDH_2 ratio > 1 is specific for the diagnosis of AMI) may be worthwhile in the patient who presents more than 24 hr after the onset of symptoms. Several other serum markers and methods of measurement of myocardial injury hold promise: myoglobin, CPK-MM isoforms, troponin, and rapid CPK-MB assays.

Enzyme	Rise	Peak	Normalize
CPK	6–8 hr	12–24 hr	1–4 days
CPK-MB	3–4 hr	12–24 hr	1–3 days
LDH	8–24 hr	48–96 hr	7–14 days

Note: *Serial cardiac enzymes are the gold standard for diagnosing MI and a single normal sample of cardiac enzymes does not exclude the diagnosis.*

Other Tests

CBC. Leukocytosis of 15,000 cells/mm^3 or greater is not uncommon with MI. Check the hematocrit to ensure anemia is not a contributing factor to myocardial ischemia.

SMA. Hyperglycemia may accompany an AMI, especially in diabetics, possibly leading to diabetic ketoacidosis or nonketotic hyperosmolar coma. Check electrolyte values to ensure that they are not contributing to myocardial irritability (hypokalemia, hypomagnesemia).

Sedimentation rate. Often elevated in the first 24 to 48 hr of infarction.

ABG. Avoid in patients being considered for thrombolytic therapy.

Coagulation studies. Determine baseline values before thrombolytic therapy.

Type and cross-match. Have blood products available in case bleeding complications develop.

CXR. Evaluate heart size. CHF findings may become visible radiographically before clinical signs.

Echocardiography. Helpful in recognizing wall motion abnormalities and complications of AMI (tamponade, mitral regurgitation, ventricular septal rupture).

Treatment

Immediate Therapy

Give supplemental oxygen (4–6 L/min via nasal cannula), establish intravenous access, and place the patient on continuous cardiac monitoring. If thrombolytic therapy is considered, initiate a second line and minimize invasive procedures. Furnish SL NTG to patients experiencing ischemic chest pain, unless the systolic blood pressure is < 90 mm Hg or the patient is markedly bradycardic or tachycardic.

Analgesics

If sublingual nitroglycerin fails to relieve the pain, consider dispensing an opioid analgesic. *Morphine* is still the drug of choice, combining potent analgesic effects with beneficial hemodynamic actions. Inject 2 to 4 mg IV, repeated every 5 to 10 min until the pain is controlled or serious side effects develop (hypotension, respiratory depression). If respiratory depression becomes severe, counteract with *naloxone* (in 0.4 mg IV doses).

Thrombolytic Therapy

Thrombolytic agents cause activation of plasminogen to plasmin, resulting in fibrinolysis of the clot. They are most effective when administered in the first 1 to 2 hr postinfarction (however, current protocols allow administration in first 6 hr).

Indications

Indications include presence of chest pain or chest pain equivalent consistent with AMI for more than 30 min accompanied by ECG findings of > 1 mm ST elevation in two or more limb leads; > 2 mm ST elevation in two or more contiguous precordial leads; or ST depression with a prominent R wave in V_2, $_{V3}$, representing a posterior AMI.

Absolute Contraindications

Absolute contraindications include active internal bleeding, major trauma or surgery in the past 6 weeks; cerebrovascular accident (CVA) within the previous 6 months; intracranial or intraspinal surgery within the past 2 months; known allergy to thrombolytic agents; known or suspect aortic dissection; history of intracranial turmor, aneurysm, or AVM; and severe hypertension (systolic > 200 mm Hg; diastolic > 120 mm Hg) resistant to treatment.

Relative Contraindications

Relative contraindications include traumatic or prolonged CPR (> 10 min), noncompressible puncture sites, major malignant disorder, bleeding disorder, pregnancy, and history of CVA for > 6 months.

Agents

1. *Streptokinase.* Administer 1.5 million units over 1 hr as a constant infusion. Advantages include lower cost and lack of proven superiority of competitive agents. Disadvantages involve potential for allergic reactions and higher incidence of hypotension when compared with other agents.
2. *Tissue plasminogen activator (tPA).* Give as a 10 mg IV bolus, followed by 50 mg over the 1st hr and 20 mg/hr for the next 2 hr. Advantages are that it rarely causes allergic reactions, is more clot specific, and is better tolerated in hemody-

namically unstable patients. The main disadvantage is its cost, almost 10 times that of streptokinase.

3. *Anisoylated plasminogen streptokinase activator (APSAC)*. Infuse a 30 unit bolus IV over 5 min. The primary advantage is its ease of administration. Disadvantages include the increased rate of allergic reactions and its high cost relative to streptokinase.

Complications

The most common problem associated with thrombolytic therapy is bleeding, with the greatest risk being in elderly females with either underlying hypertension or diabetes. The complication of greatest concern is intracerebral hemorrhage, which can occur in up to 1% of cases.

Indicators or Reperfusion

Although not highly specific, reperfusion may be clinically indicated by relief of chest pain, occurrence of dysrhythmias (particularly accelerated idioventricular rhythm), rapid evolution of Q waves, resolution of ST segment elevation, and early peaking of CPK values.

Percutaneous Transluminal Coronary Angioplasty

Preliminary studies indicate PTCA is superior to thrombolytic therapy. Benefits include angiographically confirmed opening of the occluded artery and its applicability to patients in whom thrombolytic therapy may not be indicated or may have failed (cardiogenic shock, symptoms compatible with AMI but a nondefinitive ECG, elderly patients, recent postoperative patients, or presence of active bleeding). The major drawbacks are limited availability (only a minority of hospitals offer angioplasty, and a smaller number on a 24-hr basis) and cost.

Heparin

Because of the high rate of reocclusion, anticoagulant therapy with heparin is started in most patients who have received thrombolytic agents. It is given as a 5000 unit IV bolus, followed by a 1000 unit/hr infusion. Adjust the infusion to keep the activated partial thromboplastin time between 1.5 and 2.0 times the control. Heparin by itself is able to reduce the rate of mortality from MI.

Aspirin

Aspirin reduces long-term mortality and has an additive effect on reduction of short-term mortality when given with thrombolytic agents. Recommended doses range from 80 to 325 mg PO daily. Give the first dose as soon as possible in the setting of AMI.

Beta-Blockers

Beta-blockers reduce morbidity and mortality post-MI by decreasing the work load of the heart and raising the threshold for VF. They are particularly useful in patients who are tachycardiac and hypertensive. Contraindications to β-blockers include presence of CHF, bradydysrhythmias (heart rate < 50/min), hypotension (systolic pressure < 100 mm Hg), asthma, and heart block (PR interval > 0.22, types I and II AV block, or complete heart block).

- *Metoprolol.* Initially, three doses of 5 mg given IV at 5-min intervals. Follow by oral dosing (30 to 60 min after last IV dose) of 50 mg q 6 hr for 2 days, then 100 mg PO BID.
- *Propranolol.* A total of 0.1 mg/kg divided into three doses given at 5-min intervals IV. At 30 min after the last IV dose, give 20 to 80 mg q 6 hr.

Intravenous Nitroglycerin

Intravenous nitroglycerin reduces myocardial ischemia by decreasing preload, afterload, and coronary spasm as well as increasing coronary blood flow. Start the infusion rate at 10 mg/min and increase every 10 min in 5 to 10 mg increments until chest discomfort is relieved, while maintaining the systolic blood pressure > 100 mm Hg. Exercise caution when administering nitroglycerin to patients with an inferior MI who may have concomitant right ventricular involvement.

Lidocaine

Do not use lidocaine prophylactically in AMI (see section 1.1).

Magnesium

Magnesium (1 to 2 g mixed in 50 to 100 mL of D5W over 30 min) has been used, but the results of the latest large series fail to demonstrate a benefit in AMI.

Angiotensin-Converting Enzyme Inhibitors

Angiotensin-converting enzyme inhibitors (ACE-Is), especially when started within 24 hr of AMI, may improve ventricular wall remodeling and decrease mortality.

Special Considerations

Dysrhythmias

Dysrhythmias are most common in the first 24 hr postinfarction and range from uniform PVCs (which generally require no treatment) to life threatening VT and VF. Accelerated idioventricular rhythm (AIVR) is associated with reperfusion therapy but is generally benign and does not require treatment. Determine the cause of sinus tachycardia (heart failure, hypoxia, hypovolemia, fever, pain).

Conduction Disturbances

Heart block accompanying an inferior MI is usually transient. Therapy ranges from observation in the stable patient to the use of atropine (0.5 mg IV up to 2.0 mg), and/or transcutaneous pacing in the unstable patient. Conduction disturbances associated with anterior MIs imply extensive damage and can abruptly degenerate into complete heart block (CHB). A pacemaker is generally indicated in the setting of MI for the patient with CHB, type 2 second-degree block, new LBBB, and symptomatic bradycardia not responsive to medications.

Pump Failure

Pump failure can range from mild CHF to cardiogenic shock (implies > 40% damage of the left ventricle). Patients with severe CHF or cardiogenic shock normally require invasive hemodynamic monitoring. Treatment ranges from fluids to vasopressors or intraaortic balloon pump. The *Killip Classification* can be used to predict prognosis:

Classification	Signs	Mortality
I	No signs of heart failure or shock	5%
II	Mild to moderate CHF; rales < ½ lung fields	15–20%
III	Frank pulmonary edema, > ½ lung fields with rales	40%

IV	Cardiogenic shock, systolic BP < 90 mm Hg, signs of systemic hypoperfusion	80%

Right Ventricular Infarction

Right ventricular infarction is almost always associated with inferior MIs. It can present with hypotension, distended neck veins, and clear lung fields. The diagnosis is suggested by ST-segment elevation in the right ventricular leads (V_{3R} and V_{4R}). Treatment includes aggressive volume resuscitation (1 L or more of crystalloid) and inotropic support (dobutamine or dopamine).

Mechanical Complications

Complications usually occur more than 24 hr postinfarction. They include ruptured papillary muscle, ventricular septal rupture, and cardiac rupture.

Admission Criteria

All patients suspected of having an MI require admission to a monitored bed. *Patients who are actively infarcting* require a unit bed without delay, while those *patients at risk* of a myocardial infarction who have a normal or nondiagnostic ECG and are hemodynamically stable may be admitted to a step-down or telemetry unit.

Selected Readings

Herr CH: The diagnosis of acute myocardial infarction in the emergency department. J Emerg Med 1992;10:455–461, 591–599.

National Heart Attack Alert Program Coordinating Committee, 60 Minutes to Treatment Working Group: Emergency department: rapid identification and treatment of patients with acute myocardial infarction. Ann Emerg Med 1994;23:311–329.

1.6 CONGESTIVE HEART FAILURE

Description

Congestive heart failure (CHF) is the inability of the heart to pump blood commensurate with the metabolic needs of the body. Appropriate acute care depends on determining the underlying disorder leading to CHF and the precipitating event exacerbating CHF. Various classification schemes describe subsets of patients with heart failure. Clinically, heart failure is often categorized by the ventricle most affected. The clinical picture of *left-sided failure* is one of low cardiac output and pulmonary congestion, whereas for *right-sided failure* signs of fluid retention predominate. However, most patients exhibit symptoms and signs of both right- and left-sided failure. In fact, the most common cause of right-sided failure is left-sided failure. When right-sided heart failure predominates, consider disorders affecting the pulmonary circulation, (pulmonary hypertension, pulmonary embolus, COPD) or right ventricle compliance (mitral stenosis, right ventricular infarction). CHF can occur acutely (after a cardiac dysrhythmia or AMI) or follow a more chronic and progressive course (dilated cardiomyopathy secondary to ethanol abuse). There are four primary determinants of cardiac function: *preload, afterload, myocardial contractility,* and *heart rate.* A disturbance in any one of these functions is capable of causing congestive heart failure.

The vast majority of disorders linked to CHF result in low cardiac output. A less common situation occurs when the heart is functioning at normal or supernormal levels but cannot keep pace with the metabolic demands of the body. This is termed high-output heart failure and occurs in pregnancy and severe anemia as well as arteriovenous fistula, thyrotoxicosis, beriberi, pheochromocytoma, and Paget's disease of the bone. In addition, cocaine or amphetamine abuse can precipitate CHF by causing an increased metabolic state and elevated afterload.

History

Specifically inquire about events surrounding the *history of present illness.* The chief complaint of *dyspnea on exertion* is frequently the initial symptom of CHF. Quantify changes in activity. Certain patients subconsciously restrict activity on their own; therefore, ask patients how far they can walk now or how many stairs they can climb compared with an earlier time. Additional significant historical clues to CHF include *orthopnea* (dyspnea on recumbency) and paroxysmal *nocturnal dyspnea* (episodes of "air hunger," which usually occur during the night and cause the patient to sit up), a nocturnal cough, and nocturnal angina. Constitutional complaints reflecting decreased cardiac output include fatigue;

generalized weakness; and particularly in the elderly, neurologic symptoms such as depression, confusion, insomnia, and even psychosis with hallucinations due to decreased cerebral perfusion. Patients with predominantly right-sided failure complain of swelling of the lower extremities, weight gain, abdominal bloating or fullness, anorexia, nausea, vomiting, right upper quadrant pain (due to congestive hepatomegaly), and nocturia (increased renal perfusion in the recumbent position). Patients with acute pulmonary edema classically manifest "the three S's"—sitting up (unable to lie down), sputum production (frothy and red tinged), and sweating (hyperadrenergic output)—along with pronounced air hunger.

Review the *medical history* for clues to the etiology of CHF, including a detailed cardiac history (previous MIs, coronary artery disease, hypertension, valvular heart disease). Also inquire about a history of connective tissue or HIV infection (cardiomyopathies) and the presence of any diseases that may simulate heart failure (pulmonary disease, cirrhosis, renal disease, or diabetic ketoacidosis).

Apart from the standard questions about medications, ask about any changes in dosages (whether instructed by the physician or done by the patient) as well as recently added medications (particularly negative inotropes such as β-blockers, including those in eye drops, as well as medications capable of causing fluid retention such as steroids, estrogens, and nonsteroidal antiinflammatories). If the patient is taking digitalis, note possible signs and symptoms of digitalis toxicity (e.g., anorexia, nausea, vomiting, lethargy, and supraventricular tachycardia with block).

Do not forget to ask about dietary sodium intake, intravenous drug abuse (along with other risk factors for HIV), alcohol intake, cocaine use, smoking, and any unusual toxic exposures (anthracycline, cobalt, lead). In females, determine the date of the last menstrual period or recent pregnancy (postpartum cardiomyopathy). Note any family history of heart disease, especially history of any sudden death at a young age (asymmetric septal hypertrophy) or systemic diseases that can affect the heart (amyloidosis).

Finally, when covering *review of systems,* try to determine the precipitating event: cardiovascular (chest pain, palpitations, syncope), pulmonary (prolonged bed rest, surgery, hospitalization, lower extremity trauma, or other risk factors for pulmonary embolus), endocrine (thyroid disease, diabetes mellitus), hematologic (anemia, blood loss), infectious (myocarditis), or renal.

Physical Examination

Physical findings depend on the ventricle(s) affected as well as on the stage of cardiac dysfunction. *Do not depend solely on physical signs to determine cardiac output.*

General. Does the patient appear chronically ill? Note position (most patients in CHF need to sit up), level of distress (can speak in sentences, phrases, words), and level of consciousness (confused, lethargic).

Vital signs. Check heart rate (regular versus irregular; tachycardia, bradycardia), respiratory rate for tachypnea or Cheyne-Stokes (alternating phases of apnea and hyperventilation, most prevalent in elderly patients with CHF), and blood pressure (hypotension may be due to myocardial failure, medications, or dysrhythmias). Note temperature (infection).

Skin. Inspect for diaphoresis, pallor, and peripheral cyanosis.

Neck. Note jugular venous distention along with carotid upstroke. Check for thyroid enlargement.

Chest. Listen carefully for rales (may be fine and confined to the bases in moderate failure or prominent and diffuse with severe failure) and wheezing (cardiac asthma versus pulmonary disease).

Cardiovascular. Palpate for precordial heave or thrill. An S_3, heard in early diastole, is reasonably specific for failure in middle-aged and older adults; an S_4 occurs in late diastole and implies a noncompliant ventricle, with lower specificity than an S_3. Note murmurs and the presence and quality of pulses (delayed carotid upstroke = aortic stenosis, water-hammer pulse or pistol-shot pulse = aortic regurgitation, and pulsus alternans = severe myocardial dysfunction).

Abdomen. Examine for hepatomegaly (may be tender) and splenomegaly as well as ascites.

Extremities. Note edema (symmetrical with CHF). In bedridden patients, look for sacral edema.

Diagnostic Tests

CXR. Note cardiomegaly (cardiac silhouette greater than one-half transthoracic diameter). A normal size heart with CHF suggests AMI, constrictive pericarditis, or mitral stenosis. CXR findings commonly correlate with pulmonary capillary wedge pressure (PCWP).

PCWP	CXR
> 18 mm Hg	Increased vessel markings appear in the apices
20–25 mm Hg	Interstitial edema, Kerley A and B lines, and possibly pleural effusions
> 25 mm Hg	Alveolar edema with bilateral hilar infiltrates in a "bat wing" or "butterfly" distribution

Peak expiratory flow rate (PEFR). May help distinguish early CHF from COPD; PEFR > 150 L/min suggests acute CHF, whereas a PEFR < 150 L/min implies COPD.

ECG. Analyze for both acute (AMI, dysrhythmia, pulmonary embolism) and chronic changes (LVH, evidence of old AMI).

ABG. Mild hypoxia, hypocarbia, and respiratory alkalosis occur early in CHF. Worsening PaO_2 accompanied by a developing metabolic acidosis implies critical CHF.

Pulse oximetry. Provides noninvasive estimate of oxygen saturation (optimal levels > 92%).

CBC. Check the hematocrit (anemia) and white cell count (elevated with both infection and stress).

SMA. Note electrolytes. Especially be alert for dilutional hyponatremia (may suggest poorer prognosis as well as guide treatment), hypokalemia (diuretics), and hyperkalemia (renal insufficiency, concomitant use of potassium-sparing diuretics and ACE inhibitors). Obtain liver function tests (transaminases elevated with CHF).

Miscellaneous laboratory tests. Additional studies guided by the patient's clinical findings may be called for (e.g., cardiac isoenzymes, thyroid studies, ESR, digitalis level).

Echocardiography. Extremely useful tool for evaluating etiology of CHF (aortic stenosis, asymmetric septal hypertrophy) as well as extent (chamber size, ejection fraction, wall motion abnormalities) and complications (cardiac tamponade).

Treatment

Initially, focus on improving oxygenation (nasal cannula 4 to 6 L/min, high-flow mask, Venturi mask) and ventilation (elevate head of bed). Secure IV access, and place patient on a monitor.

Search for reversible causes (acutely ruptured aortic valve, acute MI, dysrhythmia). Further treatment decisions are based on acuity of symptoms, degree of respiratory distress, underlying etiology, and identifying precipitating cause of CHF.

Supplemental measures include the following.

Morphine

Morphine is a modest venodilator and also reduces anxiety. Employ the smallest effective dose to minimize the side effects, while restricting use to patients with a systolic blood pressure > 100 mm Hg. Generally, the initial dose is 2 to 4 mg IV, with 2 mg IV increments being given every 5 min until the desired effect is obtained, as long as the patient is hemodynamically stable. Naloxone (0.4 mg IV) can be used to reverse respiratory depression.

Diuretics

Diuretics decrease preload in fluid overloaded patients. Loop diuretics (furosemide and bumetanide) should be given intravenously in the acute setting (avoid oral and intramuscular routes because of variable absorption). *Avoid overdiuresis,* which may reduce preload, provoking a decrease in cardiac output. Confine use to patients with a systolic pressure greater than 100 mm Hg. Exercise extreme caution before giving diuretics with the following (many of these conditions are preload dependent): (1) aortic stenosis, (2) hypertrophic cardiomyopathy, (3) constrictive pericarditis or cardiac tamponade, and (4) acute CHF secondary to an acute MI.

- *Furosemide.* The starting dose is 20 to 40 mg IV (unless the patient is already taking furosemide). If no improvement occurs within 15 to 30 min, double the initial dose; if still no improvement occurs in another 30 min, quadruple the initial dose. Patients with renal failure commonly require higher doses. Do not exceed 150 mg IV and do not administer more quickly than 20 mg/min. The initial effect is seen in 5 to 15 min with peak diuretic action occurring in 30 min.
- *Bumetanide.* The initial dose is 0.5 to 1.0 mg IV (bumetanide is 40 times more potent than furosemide). Double the first dose if there is no response in 30 min and double it again in another 30 min (1 hr after initial dose) if there is still no response.

Vasodilators

Vasodilators counteract increased preload and/or afterload occurring with CHF. They are classified into those agents acting mainly on the venous system (venodilators), those whose primary action is on the arterial side (arterial dilators), and those with an equal effect on both systems (balanced dilators). The two agents employed in the acute care of CHF are

- *Nitrates.* Principally a venodilator (preload reduction). Routes of delivery include sublingual (0.4 mg) or buccal spray (rapid onset, 30 to 60 sec), topical (0.5 to 2.0 inches, which can be wiped off if adverse effects occur), and intravenous (10 to 200 mg/min, titratable). Preferred therapy in patients with CHF and ischemic heart disease.
- *Sodium nitroprusside.* Combination venodilator and arterial dilator; most effective when hypertension accompanies CHF. Initiate at 0.5 mg/kg/min IV, and slowly titrate to achieve the desired level. Do not exceed 10 mg/kg/min or let systolic pressure fall below 100 mm Hg. Sodium nitroprusside may worsen myocardial ischemia (steal syndrome from coronary arteries). Thiocyanate toxicity is usually not a problem in the ED.

ACE Inhibitors

ACE inhibitors are ideal agents in the chronic setting (improve hemodynamics, enhance diuresis, reduce symptoms, and prolong survival). Such agents include captopril, enalapril, and lisinopril. They also have a potential role in the acute therapy of CHF, particularly CHF accompanied by hypertension. Give enalapril (1.25 mg IV) or captopril (12.5 mg tablet crushed and administered SL). Adverse effects include hypotension, skin rash, cough (up to 5% of patients), and impaired renal function. Avoid use in patients with intrinsic renal disease or bilateral renal artery stenosis.

Inotropic Agents

It is best to use inotropic agents under invasive hemodynamic guidance. Reserve for CHF with concomitant cardiogenic shock (see section 1.2).

- *Dopamine.* Preferred in the setting of hypotension (systolic pressure $<$ 90 mm Hg) and oliguria. Low-dose dopamine (1 to

2 μg/kg/min) dilates renal arteries. High doses (2 to 5 μg/kg/min) improve heart rate and cardiac output, while even higher doses (> 5 μg/kg/min) cause vasoconstriction.

- *Norepinephrine.* Employ when hypotension is severe (systolic pressure <70 mm Hg). Start dosing at 2 to 5 μg/min, and increase as necessary to elevate systolic pressure to the 90 mm Hg range.
- *Dobutamine.* Improves cardiac output. Use when blood pressure is stabilized and systolic pressure is > 90 mm Hg. Initiate dosing at 2 μg/kg/min IV, titrating up to 15 μg/kg/min.
- *Digoxin.* A weak inotrope with a high potential for toxicity. Its principal value is for managing atrial dysrhythmias (atrial fibrillation with rapid ventricular response) in the ED and as part of a long-term therapeutic regimen for chronic CHF.

Continuous Positive Airway Pressure

Continuous positive airway pressure (CPAP) improves PO_2 and may help avoid mechanical ventilation in patients with CHF and elevated PCWP. Mask or nasal CPAP is started at 10 cm H_2O.

Intubation

If adequate oxygenation cannot be accomplished with supplemental oxygen delivery systems (Venturi mask, oxygen-reservoir mask, CPAP) or if the patient's overall state declines (e.g., lethargy, inability to maintain respiratory rate, inability to protect airway), then *intubate!* Do not rely on ABG parameters alone. Judge the patient's overall clinical status. **Remember:** *It is always better to intubate early than late.*

Special Considerations

Pulmonary edema. Necessitates immediate attention and intervention. As always, support the ABCs. Initial therapy is the same as with CHF but is executed with greater urgency.

Pulmonary edema and renal failure. The definitive treatment for this condition is dialysis. Temporizing measures include CPAP, high-dose furosemide (even if the patient does not make urine), intravenous nitroglycerin, judicious use of phlebotomy, nebulized bronchodilators (β-agonists), and oral sorbitol (50 g given twice at 30-min intervals to induce diarrhea and fluid shift into the bowel).

Cardiogenic shock. This is the most catastrophic manifestation of CHF, where fluid overload of the lungs accompanies systemic hypotension. AMI is the most frequent cause. In addition, rule out potential surgically correctable problems early (prosthetic valve malfunction, ventricular septal rupture). See section 1.2 for a more detailed discussion.

Admission Criteria

Patients with mild failure who have a benign, identifiable precipitating cause of CHF (medication noncompliance, dietary indiscretion) and rapidly respond to diuretic therapy may be managed as outpatients as long as timely follow up and explicit instructions are given.

Patients with new-onset, acute CHF require admission to rule out serious underlying disease.

Patients in acute pulmonary edema require ICU admission as does any patient with CHF associated with hypotension, need for intubation or CPR, life-threatening dysrhythmia (other than uncontrolled chronic atrial fibrillation), significant digitalis toxicity, or AMI.

Selected Readings

Baker DW, Konstam MA, Bottorff M, et al.: Management of heart failure. JAMA 1994;272:1361–1366.

Marantz PR, Kaplan MC, Alderman MH: Clinical diagnosis of congestive heart failure in patients with acute dyspnea. Chest 1990;97:776–781.

McNamara RM, Ciorni DJ: Utility of the peak expiratory flow rate in the differentiation of acute dyspnea: cardiac vs. pulmonary origin. Chest 1992;101(1):129–132.

1.7 HYPERTENSION

Description

Hypertension (HTN) in adults is defined as a blood pressure > 180/90 mm Hg, recorded on at least two occasions. *Isolated systolic hypertension* reflects a systolic pressure > 160 mm Hg, with diastolic pressure remaining < 90 mm Hg. Classically, in *severe HTN* or a *hypertensive urgency* the diastolic blood pressure is > 115 mm Hg, but clinical findings reflecting end organ damage are lacking. In both *accelerated* and *malignant HTN,* the diastolic pressure again tends to be > 115 mm Hg; however, in this scenario, elevations are accompanied by characteristic funduscopic changes—flame hemorrhages and/or soft exudates occur with accelerated HTN (grade III retinopathy), while papilledema takes place with malignant HTN (grade IV). A *hypertensive emergency* is not predicated on surpassing some critical number, rather this crisis describes a condition whereby an inappropriately elevated blood pressure provokes damage to essential end organs, such as the *central nervous system* (hypertensive encephalopathy, intracranial hemorrhage), the *cardiovascular system* (aortic dissection, AMI, unstable angina, pulmonary edema), and/or the *kidneys* (acute renal failure). While no specific number defines a hypertensive emergency, typically the blood pressure is > 220/130 mm Hg.

Table 1.7.1 lists various etiologies of hypertension. The vast majority of hypertensive patients (> 90%) are classified as having *essential hypertension,* though secondary causes of hypertension (especially underlying renovascular disease) account for 50% of hypertensive emergencies.

History

Chief Complaint

The detection of hypertension is commonly an incidental finding. In the ED, it is essential to identify patients at "immediate" risk for complications arising from an elevated blood pressure. Therefore, determine if the presenting symptoms relate to the appearance of hypertension, specifically *CNS complaints* (headache, vertigo, dizziness, seizures, focal neurologic complaint), *CVS complications* (chest and/or back pain, dyspnea, claudication), *eye problems* (blurred vision, scotoma), and *renal difficulties* (hematuria, oliguria). Establish the onset, time course, and description of all symptoms.

Past Medical History

Inquire about prior history of hypertension, especially age of onset and level of control. Also, ask about complicating illnesses (CAD, CVA, DM, renal insufficiency). Document any diseases that may influence choice of therapeutic agents, including asthma (prohibits β-blockers) and depression (must be alert for possible interactions with MAO inhibitors).

Table 1.7.1
Etiologies of Hypertension

Cardiovascular
Arteriosclerosis
Aortic regurgitation
Patent ductus arteriosus
Increased stroke volume due to fever
Aortic coarctation
Aortic dissection
Renal
Glomerulonephritis
Pyelonephritis
Polycystic renal disease
Renovascular stenosis
Diabetic nephropathy
Arteriolar nephrosclerosis
Endocrine
Oral contraceptives
Pheochromocytoma
Thyrotoxicosis
Myxedema
Cushing's disease and syndrome
Neurogenic
Psychogenic
Polyneuritis
Acute increased intracranial pressure
Acute spinal cord injury
Toxicologic
Drug withdrawal states
Sympathomimetic intoxication
Unknown etiology

Medications

Note use of prescription (birth control pills, thyroid replacement extracts) and nonprescription medications (cold preparations, nasal sprays, diet pills). Also verify compliance, as abrupt cessation of β-blockers or clonidine may precipitate hypertensive crisis.

Social History

Document alcohol use (withdrawal), drug abuse (amphetamines, cocaine), and diet (beware of complications arising from coingestion of MAO inhibitors and tyramine-rich foods).

Obstetric History

Suspect *preeclampsia/eclampsia* in any pregnant female with HTN and associated proteinuria and edema who is beyond 20 weeks gestation (see "Preeclampsia/Eclampsia" on page 52).

Physical Examination

General. Note level of consciousness, presence of respiratory distress, and body habitus (particularly stigmata of Marfan's or Cushing's syndrome).

Vital signs. Ensure use of proper cuff size when measuring blood pressure. Check pressure in each extremity in the sitting position (if possible). If pressure is elevated, repeat after the patient has been given a chance to rest (after about 10 min). Elderly patients frequently demonstrate *pseudohypertension* (stiffening of blood vessels falsely elevates blood pressure readings).

HEENT. Funduscopic examination affords direct evaluation of blood vessels affected by hypertension.

Neck. Inspect for jugular venous distention and thyromegaly.

Lungs. Listen for rales.

Heart. Note increased size (displaced point maximal impulse), S_3, S_4, or murmurs.

Abdomen. Auscultate for flank and abdominal bruits (renal artery stenosis, abdominal aneurysm). Examine for masses (gravid uterus, aortic aneurysm, enlarged kidneys).

Extremities. Note edema, radial-femoral pulse delay (coarctation of the aorta), or discrepancy of pulses (aortic dissection).

Neurologic. Check mental status, reflexes, and cerebellar function; look for any focal neurologic abnormalities.

Diagnostic Tests

CBC. Check hematocrit and peripheral smear (microangiopathic hemolytic anemia seen with hypertensive emergencies).

SMA. Note elevated glucose (diabetes), BUN and creatinine (renal function), and electrolyte abnormalities (hypokalemia can imply hyperaldosteronism).

Urinalysis. Note presence of blood and/or protein (hematuria and proteinuria can reflect renal damage), red cell casts (glomerulonephritis), and white cell casts (pyelonephritis).

ECG. Check for evidence of ischemia, infarct, or left ventricular hypertrophy (long-standing HTN). Presence of prolonged PR interval or other conduction abnormalities may preclude use of β-blockers.

CXR. Note heart and aorta size, evidence of pulmonary edema, and rib notching (coarctation of the aorta).

CT scan of the head. Indicated with severe hypertension and altered mental status (e.g., hypertensive encephalopathy, cerebrovascular accident, intracerebral hemorrhage), severe headache (subarachnoid hemorrhage or posterior fossa hemorrhage), or focal neurologic abnormalities.

Miscellaneous tests. Selectively order additional studies based on history and clinical findings. Examples include drug screens (cocaine, amphetamines, or related drugs), serum calcium (endocrine problem), urinary vanillylmandelic acid (pheochromocytoma), and angiography or CT scan of chest (aortic dissection).

Treatment

The need for emergent blood pressure reduction depends on the etiology and the type of presentation (form of end organ damage). Hypertensive emergencies generally oblige parenteral therapy to achieve both an immediate and a controlled reduction in blood pressure. *Do not* delay therapy for test results. A rational approach to hypertensive emergencies calls for a gradual lowering of the blood pressure, attempting to avoid lowering the *mean arterial pressure* (MAP) no more than 20% in the first hour. A precipitous drop in pressure risks impairment of cerebral blood flow.

$$\text{MAP} = \frac{\text{Systolic BP} + (2 \times \text{Diastolic BP})}{3}$$

The treatment of a *hypertensive urgency* remains controversial. Although some authorities advocate initiating treatment in the ED with oral agents (clonidine, nifedipine), an alternative viewpoint cautions against the rapid reduction of blood pressure because of the inherent risk of inducing hypoperfusion to the brain and heart, possibly causing a CVA or AMI. The specifics of medications currently used in ED therapy of hypertension are listed in Table 1.7.2.

Special Considerations

Hypertensive Encephalopathy

Hypertensive encephalopathy is an uncommon, but reversible condition, taking place when the blood pressure elevation exceeds the ability of cerebral autoregulation to control the cerebral blood flow. This leads to increased vascular permeability, spasm, and cerebral edema. Initial symptoms may be subtle (headache, blurred vision, drowsiness), but eventually signs of cerebral dysfunction (confusion, obtundation, seizures) will prevail. If untreated, hypertensive encephalopathy rapidly progresses to coma and death.

Preeclampsia/Eclampsia

Also known as *pregnancy-induced hypertension,* preeclampsia is a disease unique to pregnancy, seen from the 20th week of gestation to the 6th week postpartum. Preeclampsia is defined by blood pressure recordings > 140/90 mm Hg or an increase of more than 30 mm Hg in systolic or more than 15 mm Hg in diastolic pressure from pregestational levels. The etiology is unclear, but preeclampsia is most prevalent in nulliparous women, especially those at the extremes of reproductive life (adolescents and women > 35 years old). In multiparous females, elevations in blood pressure are more inclined to occur in multiple gestation pregnancies, molar pregnancies, and diabetics as well as in women with a family history of preeclampsia or with coexisting renal disease.

Preeclampsia is considered *mild* or *moderate* when the patient has few complaints, other than the triad of hypertension, edema, and proteinuria together with a relative absence of laboratory abnormalities. *Severe* preeclampsia manifests as a headache, visual disturbances, right upper quadrant abdominal pain (due to hepatic edema), hyperreflexia (including clonus), and oliguria (if suspected, insert a Foley catheter to monitor urine output) together with a rise in serum creatinine, an elevation in liver en-

Table 1.7.2
Medications Used in Treatment of Hypertensive Emergencies

Drug	Brand Name(s)	Major Action	Dose	Clinical Considerations	Indications
			Vasodilators		
Nitroprusside	Nipride	Arterial and venous vasodilator	Start infusion at 0.25–1.0 μg/kg/min (average effective dose is 3 μg/kg/min)	Route: IV Requires ICU admission and continuous cardiac and BP monitoring Watch for hypotension and toxic thiocyanate levels Unstable in uv light, therefore cover IV bag Not safe in pregnancy	Hypertensive encephalopathy Malignant hypertension Aortic dissection (use β-blocker first, then start Nipride infusion)
Nitroglycerin	Tridil Nitrodur Nitrostat Nitrobid Transderm Nitroglycerin	Arterial and venous vasodilator Coronary artery vasodilator	Start infusion at 10 mg/min Increase 5–10 μg/min every 10 min until therapeutic effect achieved	Route: IV, PO, SL, topical Side effects: HA, nausea, vomiting Watch for hypotension	Unstable angina Acute MI Pulmonary edema
Diazoxide	Hyperstat	Arterial vasodilator	50-mg bolus every 5–10 min *or*	Route: IV Contraindications include CAD, aortic coarctation,	Hypertensive encephalopathy Malignant hypertension

Table 1.7.2—*Continued*

Drug	Brand Name(s)	Major Action	Dose	Clinical Considerations	Indications
			15–30 mg/min infusion, for a max. of 58 mg/kg or until therapeutic effect achieved	aortic dissection, ICH, and pulmonary edema because of reflex tachycardia, increased myocardial oxygen consumption, and sodium and water retention	
Hydralazine	Apresoline	Arterial vasodilator	10–20 mg IV, IM Repeat dose in 30 min as needed	Route: IV, IM, PO As with diazoxide, avoid use in patients with CAD or aortic dissection Side effects: lethargy, HA, nausea, postural hypotension Lupus-like syndrome with chronic oral use	Pregnancy-induced hypertension (eclampsia)
Nifedipine	Procardia	Coronary and peripheral arterial vasodilator	10–20 mg PO up to 3 times daily	Route: PO, SL, rectal Pill should be punctured; then patient should bite, chew, and swallow	Hypertensive urgencies Aortic dissection (use with β-blocker)

Minoxidil	Loniten	Arterial vasodilator blocks calcium uptake through cell membrane	10–20 mg PO Repeat dose in 4 hr as needed	Route: PO Contraindicated in recent MI, CHF, pheochromocytoma due to fluid retention and tachycardia Safe in renal insufficiency Hirsutism with chronic use	Hypertensive urgencies
Phentolamine	Regitine	Blocks α-receptors Arterial and venous vasodilator	5 mg IV, IM	Route: IV, IM Reported cases of MI, CVA, arrhythmias, death Side effects: weakness, dizziness, flushing, nausea, vomiting, diarrhea	Pheochromocytoma
Prazosin	Minipress	Arterial vasodilator	1 mg PO	Route: PO May cause orthostatic hypotension	Hypertensive urgencies
			Beta-Blockers		
Propranolol	Inderal	Nonselective β-blocker	1–10 mg IV Repeat in 4 hr as needed	Route: IV, PO Watch for heart block, bradycardia, hypotension, impaired adrenergic response to hypoglycemia, bronchospasm, and heart failure Sudden withdrawal of drug can precipitate angina or MI	Catecholamine excess Aortic dissection

Table 1.7.2—*Continued*

Drug	Brand Name(s)	Major Action	Dose	Clinical Considerations	Indications
Labetolol	Trandate Normodyne	Selective α-1-blocker Nonselective β-blocker	20 mg IV over 2 min Repeat every 10 min as needed in increments of 20, 40, or 80 mg until a maximal dose of 300 mg is reached	Route: IV, PO Contraindication: pheochromocytoma The same cautions for propranolol apply here Good transition to oral therapy	Hypertensive Encephalopathy Malignant hypertension Intracranial hemorrhage
Esmolol	Brevibloc	Selective β-1 blocker	Loading dose: 500 μg/kg/min for 1 min, then 50 μg/kg/min for 4 min If adequate therapeutic effect, continue infusion Otherwise, repeat loading dose and then infuse 100 μg/kg/min for 4 min Continue titrating infusion every 5 min, repeating the loading	Route: IV Very short (9 min) elimination half-life Side effects: hypotension, dizziness, nausea	Myocardial ischemia IHSS Aortic dissection Pheochromocytoma

			dose for 1 min and increasing the infusion rate by 50 μg/kg/min When approaching the desired blood pressure and pulse, the loading dose may be omitted from the titration procedure Titrate to a max. of 300 μg/kg/min		
			Diuretics		
Furosemide	Lasix	Inhibits Na^+ resorption in the ascending limb of Henle's loop	20–200 mg	Route: PO, IV Watch for hypokalemia and hyperuricemia	Pulmonary edema Newly diagnosed hypertension
Bumetanide	Bumex	Same as for furosemide	0.5–2 mg PO daily 0.5–1 mg/IV, may be repeated in 23 hr for a maximum of 10 mg per day	Route: PO, IV 1-mg dose has a diuretic potency equivalent to approximately 40 mg of furosemide	Same as for furosemide
			ACE Inhibitor		
Captopril	Capoten	Angiotensin-converting enzyme inhibitor	25 mg PO 2–3 times daily	Route: PO Effective in CHF Renal insufficiency results in increased plasma levels	Hypertensive urgencies, pulmonary edema

Table 1.7.2—*Continued*

Drug	Brand Name(s)	Major Action	Dose	Clinical Considerations	Indications
				Side effects with chronic use: cough, rash, loss of taste, angioedema	
Enalapril	Vasotec	Angiotensin-converting enzyme inhibitor	1.25 mg IV over 5 min, 2.5 mg PO	Route: PO, IV; same as above	Hypertensive urgencies, pulmonary edema
			Centrally Acting Agents		
Methyldopa	Aldomet	Alpha-adrenergic antagonist	250 mg–1.0 g every 6 hr	Route: IV, PO Side effects: sedation, postural hypotension, fluid retention, impotence Avoid in hypertensive encephalopathy	Hypertensive urgencies
Trimethaphan	Arfonad	Ganglionic blocker	0.3–3 mg/min	Route: IV Elevate head of bed Side effects: ileus,	Aortic dissection Pulmonary edema

				bladder and gastric atony; cycloplegia, postural hypotension Tachyphylaxis seen	
Clonidine	Catapres	Potent α-2-agonist	Loading dose: 0.2 mg PO 0.1 mg PO q 1 hr until desired therapeutic effect or until max. dose of 0.7 mg is reached	Route: PO, topical No postural hypotension seen Safe in renal failure	Syndromes of catecholamine excess, especially clonidine/narcotic withdrawal Hypertensive urgencies

zymes, and thrombocytopenia (< 100,000 /μL). The *HELLP* syndrome (hemolysis, elevation of liver enzymes, low platelets) is a form of severe preeclampsia. Eclampsia is diagnosed when seizures develop in a female with preeclampsia.

Fetal evaluation (nonstress or stress testing) is an integral part of the emergency assessment of women suspected for preeclampsia/eclampsia. Delivery is the definitive therapy for both preeclampsia and eclampsia. Generally, the decision to start antihypertensive therapy is made by the consultant, since lowering the blood pressure too much may induce placental insufficiency. Avoid diuretics. However, *hydralazine* (5 to 10 mg IV increments q 20 min) is indicated for a diastolic pressure > 110 mm Hg, with the goal being to lower the diastolic pressure to 90 to 100 mm Hg. *Magnesium sulfate* is reserved for severe preeclampsia or eclampsia. Administer a 4 g bolus (IV over 10 min) followed by a continuous infusion of 3 g/hr. Exercise caution when using in patients with compromised renal function. Monitor deep tendon reflexes, respiratory rate and depth, and urine output.

Pheochromocytoma

The presence of "the four P's"—spells of palpitations, perspiration, pounding headache, and pallor—provides clues to diagnosis, as do tremor and nervousness. The diagnosis is made on the basis of 24-hour metanephrine levels or urinary VMA. Treatment is begun with phentolamine (5 mg IV).

Admission Criteria

All hypertensive emergencies mandate ICU admission.

Suspected cases of secondary hypertension (pheochromocytoma, acute nephritis, clonidine withdrawal, MAO inhibitor interaction) should be discussed with the consultant regarding appropriate disposition (most of these patients require admission).

Consultation is essential in all *women with pregnancy-induced hypertension,* with hospitalization mandated for women with moderate or severe preeclampsia as well as those with an unreliable home situation.

Selected Readings

Cunningham FG, Lindheimer MD: Hypertension in pregnancy. N Engl J Med 1992;326:927–932.

Gifford RW: Management of hypertensive crisis. JAMA 1991;266:829–835.

Zeller KR, Kuhnert LV, Matthews C. Rapid reduction of severe asymptomatic hypertension. Arch Int Med 1989;149:2186–2189.

1.8 DYSRHYTHMIAS AND CONDUCTION DISTURBANCES

Description

Cardiac rhythm and conduction disturbances range from innocuous ECG to life-threatening clinical syndromes. Tolerance to a rhythm disorder depends on the degree of heart rate disruption, duration of the dysrhythmia, and severity of underlying heart disease. Dysrhythmias and conduction disturbances become dangerous when they compromise cardiac output; interfere with blood flow to the heart and/or brain; or deteriorate into a nonperfusing lethal rhythm such as VT, VF, or asystole. *Ischemia, hypoxia, electrolyte imbalances* (hypokalemia, hyperkalemia, hypomagnesemia, hypocalcemia, hypercalcemia), *acid-base disorders,* and certain *drugs* (antiarrhythmics, antipsychotics, antidepressants, sympathomimetics) increase the predilection for cardiac rhythm and conduction disturbances.

History

Patients employ a variety of expressions to describe an irregular heart rate: *palpitations, racing, pounding, fluttering,* and *skipping* as well as conveying a general feeling of uneasiness or a sense that "something's not right." Determine the onset and duration of the current episode along with associated symptoms suggesting compromised cardiac output (chest pain, dyspnea, dizziness, weakness, confusion, lightheadedness, or syncope), similar previous episodes (frequency, mode of termination), past medical history (presence of CHF, angina, MI, dysrhythmia, pulmonary, or thyroid disease), medications (especially cardiac medications such as β-blockers, calcium channel blockers, antiarrhythmics, digitalis, α-methyldopa, clonidine, diuretics, and antiarrhythmics), family history of sudden death or dysrhythmias (congenital prolonged QT syndrome), and social history (use of alcohol, caffeine, cocaine, amphetamines, or other stimulants).

If the patient has a *pacemaker,* inquire about the type as well as the time of implantation (problems in the first 6 months usually implicate the electrodes, whereas later failures are more often related to the battery) and when the pacemaker was last checked.

Physical Examination

General. Determine the patient's level of alertness and hemodynamic status. Note if the patient is clammy, ashen, anxious, or confused.

Vital signs. Confirm the pulse for at least 1 min to determine presence and regularity. Carefully check blood pressure, being aware of possible beat-to-beat variation in systolic pressure.

Neck. Inspect for Cannon a waves (suggest AV dissociation). Palpate thyroid for size and nodularity.

Lungs. Auscultate for rales, wheezes, or rhonchi.

Heart. When listening, focus on first heart sound intensity: variability in intensity suggests AV dissociation, a soft S_1 implies PR prolongation (first-degree block), and a prominent S_1 is associated with shortened PR intervals (hyperdynamic states, mitral valve disease). Listen for clicks (mitral valve prolapse), murmurs (aortic or mitral disease), and rubs (pericarditis).

Extremities. Evaluate for edema (CHF), tenderness, warmth, or erythema (DVT).

Neurologic. Note evidence of focal neurologic deficit, aphasia, or presence of seizures (atrial fibrillation, anterior MI, and mitral valve disease all predispose to embolic stroke).

Note: *Always focus on treating the patient and not the monitor.*

Diagnostic Tests

ECG. Systematically review each ECG for *rhythm, rate, intervals, axis,* and *waveforms.* Specifically, clarify the following questions:

- What is the ventricular rate?
- Is the QRS narrow (< 0.10 sec) or wide (> 0.10 sec)? (Check more than one lead.)
- Is the ventricular rate regular or irregular?
- Is atrial activity present? (Under normal circumstances, the P waves are best seen in leads aVF and V_1 and should be upright in lead II and inverted in aVR.)
- What is the morphology of the P waves—regular P waves, fibrillatory waves, or flutter (F) waves?
- What is the relationship between the P waves and the QRS complexes? Are they "married" or do they turn up independently?

Are there more P waves than QRS complexes? Is the PR interval constant or changing?

Special leads may be assembled to accentuate atrial activity. A bipolar lead can be created by placing the standard left arm lead (coded black) over the apex of the heart, and using the right arm lead (coded white) to explore the precordium while recording in lead I.

CXR. Inspect for cardiomegaly or CHF. If a pacemaker is noted, confirm position of the electrode (on an AP projection, a normally implanted RV lead is directed leftward and anteriorly; if the tip of the electrode extends beyond the lateral heart border, suspect perforation).

Serum chemistries. Assess electrolytes (especially K^+). If indicated, order calcium and magnesium levels. Dysrhythmias (atrial and ventricular premature contractions) are associated with hypoglycemia.

Drug levels. Check levels of antiarrhythmics (quinidine, procainamide), digitalis, and theophylline as indicated. Obtain a drug screen (urine or blood) if recreational drug use (cocaine, amphetamines, PCP, or hallucinogens) is suspected.

ABG, cardiac enzymes, and thyroid function tests. Order selectively, guided by the history and examination.

Vagal maneuvers. Stimulate the vagus nerve, increasing parasympathetic tone, and thereby slowing conduction through the AV node. Vagal maneuvers include coughing, gag reflex, Valsalva maneuver (bearing down like a bowel movement), and the diving reflex (immersion of the face in ice cold water). Vagal maneuvers facilitate identification of atrial activity during supraventricular tachycardias (SVTs).

Carotid sinus massage (CSM). Also stimulates the vagus nerve. Avoid use on patients with a history of CVA or TIA or on patients who are noted to have bruits on auscultation of the carotid arteries. There is a risk of precipitating a life-threatening dysrhythmia when CSM is performed; therefore, place patients on a cardiac monitor, obtain IV access, and ensure that emergency cardiac medications are readily available when performing CSM. Apply firm pressure with the index, middle, and ring fingers (enough to indent a tennis ball) over the point of maximal pulsation of the carotid artery for 10 to 20 sec. **Caution:** *Never compress both carotid arteries simultaneously!* CSM may terminate paroxysmal supraventricular tachycardia (PSVT), decrease the ventricular rate in atrial fibrillation and atrial flutter (increases AV block), and slow sinus tachycardia (resumes once CSM stopped) but has no effect on VT.

Treatment

Note: *If the patient is tachycardic (rate > 150 bpm) and unstable, do not waste time attempting to determine the origin of the rhythm disturbance—cardiovert the patient, starting at 100 J!*

Patients who are hemodynamically stable without serious clinical findings (chest pain, shortness of breath, decreased level of consciousness, pulmonary congestion, congestive heart failure, or evidence of acute myocardial infarction) may be given a brief trial of medications as outlined in Figure 1.8.1. For stable narrow complex SVT, give *adenosine* (6 mg as a rapid IVp) (Fig. 1.8.2). If unsuccessful, administer a second 12 mg dose. If the second dose fails or SVT recurs, consider *verapamil* (2.5 to 5.0 mg IVp over 2 min). Concomitant use of calcium gluconate (as little as a 100 mg IV bolus) often blunts the hypotensive effect of verapamil. **Caution:** *DO NOT use verapamil in patients with wide complex tachydysrhythmias.*

Alternatives to verapamil for SVT include the β-blocker *esmolol* (500 μg/kg given over 1 min followed by 50 to 200 μg/kg/min), *digoxin* (0.5 to 1.0 mg IV followed by 0.25 mg q 2 to 4 hr up to 1.5 mg/24 hr), or *diltiazem* (loading dose of 0.25 mg/kg IV with a second bolus of 0.35 mg/kg IV 15 min later if necessary, followed by an infusion of 5 to 15 mg/hr). **Note:** *Calcium channel blockers and β-blockers can worsen CHF. Avoid using any of the calcium channel blockers or digitalis if ventricular rates are more than 250 bpm or the QRS is widened (potential to precipitate VT or VF).*

Procainamide is an effective drug for both VT and SVT and for prolonging the refractory period of accessory tracts. Dosing is 20 to 30 mg/min up to 17 mg/kg, as long as the patient remains normotensive and the QRS does not widen by more than 50%.

Follow the approach outlined in section 1.1 for VT. *Lidocaine* (1 to 1.5 mg/kg initial IV bolus, repeating up to total of 3.0 mg/kg IV, followed by a maintenance infusion of 2 to 4 mg/min; reduce dosages for patients with CHF, shock, hepatic dysfunction, or age > 70 years) may be effective in *stable* patients with *sustained VT.*

When treating *torsades,* avoid class IA agents. Correct any electrolyte abnormalities. Reserve cardioversion for unstable pa-

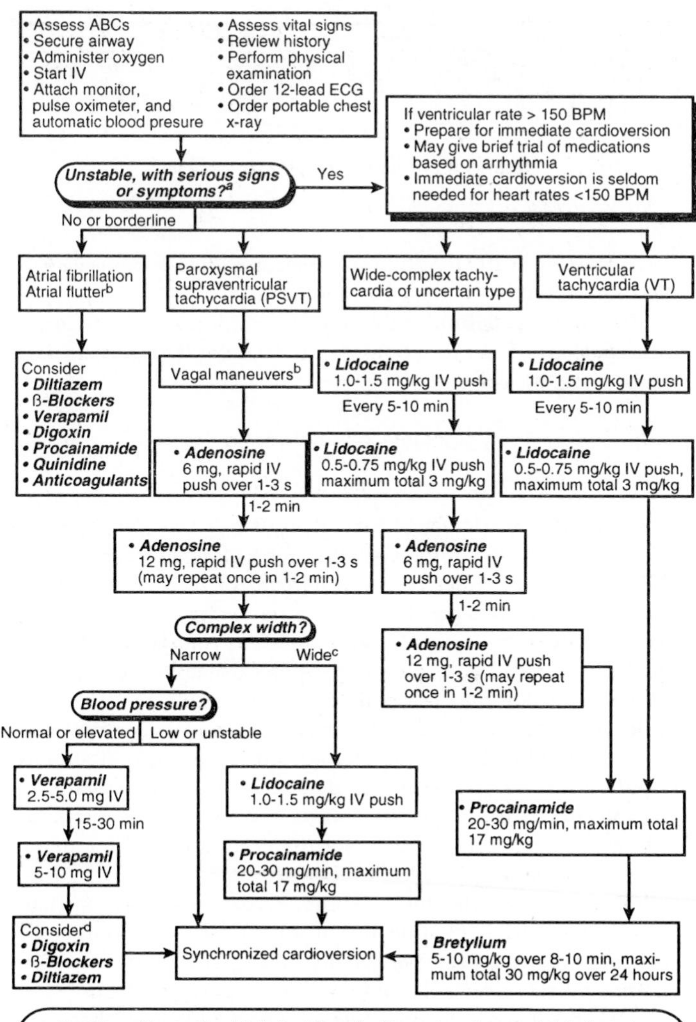

Figure 1.8.1 Tachycardia algorithm.

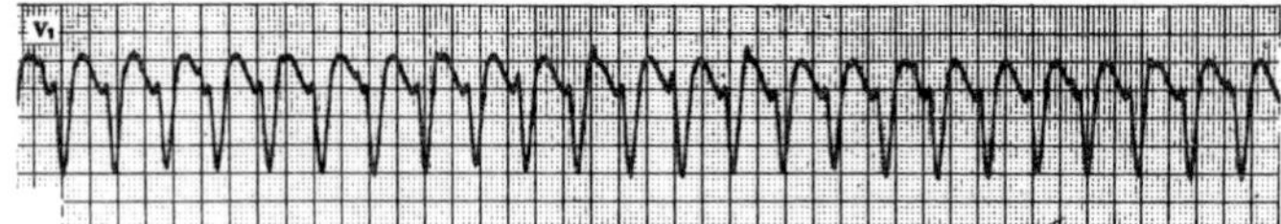

Figure 1.8.2 Narrow complex tachycardia.

tients, starting at 200 J. Additional measures include *overdrive pacing* and *magnesium* (1 to 2 g IV over 2 min).

Pacing is the definitive therapy for symptomatic bradycardia with *atropine* (0.5 mg IV q 5 min up to 0.03 mg/kg), serving as a temporizing measure.

Special Considerations

Supraventricular Tachycardias

SVTs are characterized by a heart rate usually > 160 bpm together with a narrow QRS complex (< 0.10 sec width). Fundamentally, SVT results from either reentrant circuits or by increased automaticity of abnormal pacer cells. *AV nodal reentry* accounts for the vast majority of cases of SVT (also known as *paroxysmal supraventricular tachycardia*) and takes place when cardiac conduction employs both a slow and fast pathway incorporating the AV node while bypassing the sinus node. During AV nodal reentry, a retrograde impulse depolarizes the atrium, while a simultaneous impulse evokes a QRS complex that buries the P wave, causing difficulty in distinguishing the P wave. The AV nodal reentry also displays a sudden onset and an abrupt termination, with individual episodes lasting hours. The ECG reveals a regular rhythm, with rates between 130 and 240 bpm. Paroxysmal supraventricular tachycardia (PSVT) appears in normal hearts and occurs with rheumatic heart disease, pericarditis, myocardial infarction or ischemia, mitral valve prolapse (MVP), or hyperthyroidism.

SVTs mediated by *accessory pathways* (Wolf-Parkinson-White syndrome) also demonstrate reentry, but here the AV node constitutes one of the two pathways between the atrium and ventricles, with an accessory pathway connecting the atrium and ventricles directly, bypassing the AV node. If the sinus impulse is first transmitted over the normal route, via the AV node (*orthodromic* conduction), a narrow complex tachycardia results. When initial impulse conduction travels through the bypass tract (*antidromic* conduction), a wide QRS complex occurs. The resting ECG between bouts of tachycardia may show a QRS with a slurred or notched upstroke (δ wave) and/or a shortened PR interval (< 0.12 sec) appears. Hemodynamic instability may occur when a patient with WPW and associated antidromic conduction develops a-fib.

Sinus node reentrant tachycardia mimics sinus tachycardia but has an abrupt onset and ending. This is a rare form of SVT in which the P waves appear normal.

Unifocal atrial tachycardia arises from an ectopic focus in the atrium and accounts for approximately 15% of SVTs. Aberrant atrial pacemakers may turn up in normal hearts, be harbingers of drug toxicity (digitalis, theophylline, caffeine, alcohol), reflect organic heart disease (myocardial ischemia, infarction, myocarditis), or accompany pulmonary or metabolic diseases. The P-wave complex exhibits a configuration and PR interval that are distinct from those seen with normal sinus P waves. Vagal maneuvers tend to be ineffective.

Multifocal Atrial Tachycardia

MAT is an irregular atrial tachycardia (rate typically 100 to 200 bpm), characterized by at least three distinct P waves (nonsinus) in the same lead along with varying PR intervals. MAT is most prevalent in the elderly, particularly those with COPD or CHF, and may signal underlying digitalis toxicity, theophylline toxicity, or sepsis. Treatment is directed toward the underlying condition.

Atrial Fibrillation

A-fib depicts rapid, chaotic, depolarization of the atrium, with an ensuing loss of effective atrial contraction. The consequence is an irregularly irregular pattern of QRS complexes. Despite atrial rates > 300 impulses/min, the ventricular response remains limited by the refractory period of the AV node (with no set ratio of P waves:QRS complexes). In the absence of cardiac disease and drug therapy, the ventricular rate ranges from 120 to 180 bpm. Discrete P waves do not occur. Instead undulations of the base line, called *fibrillatory waves* (best seen in lead V_1) appear between QRS intervals. The QRS complexes in a-fib are usually narrow (< 0.10 sec) but may widen when rapid heart rates prompt aberrant conduction.

A-fib may take place as a paroxysmal episode, lasting from hours to days, or may occur as a chronic dysrhythmia. Conditions commonly associated with paroxysmal a-fib include alcohol ingestion *(holiday heart)*, pericarditis, chest trauma, pulmonary embolism, MI, and preexcitation syndromes. Chronic a-fib usually results from hypertension, atherosclerosis, rheumatic heart disease, or thyrotoxicosis (HART). Chronic a-fib with a slow or regular ventricular response implies digitalis toxicity. Complications resulting from a-fib include CHF, myocardial ischemia, and arterial emboli (especially embolic CVA).

Atrial Flutter

Atrial flutter results from rapid atrial contractions (usually 280 to 320 per min) with variable AV conduction (2:1 ratio of atrial to ventricular beats most common). Characteristic sawtooth-shaped P waves appear in leads II, III, and aVF. Atrial flutter is relatively uncommon, usually degenerating into a-fib, and is almost always associated with an underlying illness (CAD, rheumatic heart disease, atrial septal defect, pericarditis, pulmonary embolus, alcohol abuse).

Wide Complex Tachycardia

Wide complex tachycardia takes place when a ventricular rate > 100 bpm is accompanied by widened QRS complexes (> 0.12 sec). There are four primary causes of wide complex tachycardia:

1. Functional or rate-related bundle branch block (known as aberrant conduction);
2. Preexisting bundle branch block;
3. Accessory pathways (Wolf-Parkinson-White syndrome); and
4. Ventricular tachycardia.

Two variants of ventricular tachycardia are *torsades de pointes* and *accelerated idioventricular rhythm.* Misdiagnosis of wide complex tachycardia can lead to therapeutic misadventures with disastrous consequences. Determining the answer to two questions helps distinguish VT from SVT with aberrance: (1) Have you ever had a heart attack, and if so, (2) Did your heart start beating fast after the heart attack? If the answer to both questions is yes, the diagnosis is almost always VT.

Look for evidence of AV dissociation (present in 50% of cases of VT), including Cannon a waves in jugular venous pulsations, varying intensity of the first heart sound, and beat-to-beat changes in systolic blood pressure. The hemodynamic stability of the patient is *not* a distinguishing feature between VT and SVT with aberrancy.

Review the ECG for clues to the origin of the tachycardia; the leads that best determine the origin of a wide complex beat are V_1 and V_6. ECG findings favoring VT include markedly widened QRS complexes (> 0.14 sec), presence of capture or fusion beats, AV dissociation (independent P waves), and a totally negative or positive precordial QRS pattern (concordance). ECG findings supporting SVT with aberrancy include appearance of a triphasic rSR′ pattern in lead V_1 (where R′ > r), a QRS right bundle branch block pattern in lead V_6, and a slowing or termination of rhythm with CSM.

Ventricular Tachycardia

VT is characterized by three or more PVCs in succession, with rates ranging from 100 to 240 bpm. The QRS complex is widened > 0.12 sec, while accompanying ST segments and T waves display discordant polarity. *Sustained VT* is arbitrarily defined as lasting longer than 30 sec and should be treated as a life-threatening dysrhythmia. Appearance of sustained VT implies underlying heart pathology (ischemic heart affliction, cardiomyopathy, valvular heart disease).

Torsades de Pointes

Torsades de pointes is an unusual variant of VT that features polymorphic QRS complexes that appear to "twist" around an isoelectric line (changing its axis). Most episodes are paroxysmal and self-limited, with rates of 160 to 300 bpm. Occasionally, torsades degenerates into VF and sudden death. The basic prerequisite for torsades de pointes is a *prolonged QT interval.* The degree of QT prolongation that heralds torsades is unknown; but in most cases, the corrected QT is > 0.6 sec (normal upper limit is 0.46 in males and 0.47 in females). There are numerous causes of a prolonged QT segment, including *congenital etiologies* (Romano-Ward, Lange-Nielsen), *drugs* (class IA, 1C, and 3 antidysrhythmics; phenothiazines; and tricyclic antidepressants), *drug interactions* (coingestion of erythromycin, ketoconazole, or itraconazole with the H1 antagonists terfenadine and astemizole as well as the combination of pentamidine with erythromycin or ketoconazole), *electrolyte imbalances* (hypomagnesemia, hypokalemia, hypocalcemia), and underlying *cardiac ischemic disease.*

Accelerated Idioventricular Rhythm

AIVR depicts a wide QRS complex rhythm, occurring at a rate of 50 to 100 bpm, typically emerging in the setting of acute MI (especially following thrombolytic therapy). It generally follows a benign course.

Bradycardia

Bradycardia covers a variety of conditions that display a heart rate < 60 bpm. A slow heart rate may occur as a normal variant (the well-conditioned athlete) or may arise from abnormal autonomic influences or conduction disturbances. Drugs and metabolic abnormalities also are capable of inducing bradycardia.

Sick Sinus Syndrome

SSS is a designation describing an assortment of rhythm disturbances: *persistent sinus bradycardia, sinus arrest,* and *sinoatrial block.* Frequently, episodes of bradycardia are punctuated by episodes of SVT, especially paroxysmal a-fib and a-flutter. SSS can remain clinically silent for a long time. Symptoms range from generalized weakness to dizziness to syncope. The two most common causes of SSS are progressive fibrosis/degeneration of the conduction system and CAD.

Heart Block

Also known as *atrioventricular (AV) block,* heart block is characterized as either incomplete or complete. Incomplete AV blocks are divided into *first-degree* (PR interval > 0.20 sec, where every P wave proceeds to a QRS complex) and *second-degree* (intermittent failure of atrial conduction). Second-degree blocks are further subdivided into *Mobitz type I (Wenckebach),* which displays a progressive lengthening of the PR interval until one of the P waves fails to conduct ("group" beating), and *Mobitz type II,* distinguished by regularly occurring P waves (PR interval remains consistent) that are not always accompanied by a QRS complex. Mobitz type I blocks are generally the result of a conduction disturbance in the AV node, whereas Mobitz type II blocks are usually due to disorders in the His bundle system. In *third-degree atrioventricular block (complete heart block)* there is a complete absence of atrial conduction to the ventricles. Syncope may follow sudden onset of a complete heart block *(Stokes-Adams attack)*.

Pacemakers

Pacemakers are battery-powered devices designed to stimulate the heart electrically when the patient's heart rate is inadequate to maintain normal perfusion. There are two major components: a battery that provides the power and a wire electrode that is implanted in the chamber being stimulated (usually the right ventricle). *Threshold* is the amount of energy needed to capture the atrium and/or ventricles (expressed in milliamps).

The ECG is the most important tool for diagnosing pacemaker problems. A paced heart displays a vertical line preceding each QRS complex (pacemaker spike), a widened QRS complex (usually LBBB morphology), and ST-T wave abnormalities. Compare the current tracing to prior tracings, looking for any alteration in QRS axis or morphology. Specially designed magnets will turn off the sensing mechanism of the pacemaker when placed over the generator. The result is continuous pacing, allowing documentation of capture.

Complications associated with pacemakers include the following:

- *Absence of pacemaker spikes despite an excessively slow heart rate.* Due to oversensing pacemaker, lead fracture or displacement, or battery depletion.
- *Failure to capture—pacemaker spikes appear without subsequent QRS complexes.* Causes include dislodgment of the pacemaker wire, lead or insulation fracture, battery depletion, or alteration of threshold stimulation
- *Failure to sense—pacemaker spikes appear despite adequate intrinsic rate of patient.* Usually consequence of dislodgment of the pacemaker wire, inadequate signals (undersensing), or excessive fibrosis around the tip of the pacing wire.
- *Pacemaker-mediated tachycardia.* Occurs in patients with DDD pacemakers.

- *Myocardial perforation.* Occurs when pacing electrode perforates the ventricular wall.
- *Thrombosis and pulmonary embolism.* Evidence of mild thrombosis is reported in up to 30% of pacemaker patients; rarely, a superior vena cava syndrome results from thrombosis extension.
- *Infection.* Early or late complication, with endocarditis as a possible outcome.

Admission Criteria

Base all admission decisions on the patient's clinical status as well as potential for serious complications.

For SVT, admit the patient to a monitored bed if the episode was complicated by chest pain, prolonged hypotension, or CHF. Any patient suspected of harboring a serious underlying illness, such as AMI, ischemia, or pulmonary embolus, should be admitted. Patients requiring electrocardioversion or overdrive pacing warrant admission to a monitored bed. A previously healthy, young patient whose episode of SVT easily responded to vagal maneuvers, adenosine, or a single dose of verapamil and remained stable throughout the event, can be followed up on an outpatient basis. Maintain a lower threshold for admitting elderly patients.

Generally, admit *all patients with new onset atrial fibrillation.* While a-fib may be benign, potentially serious etiologies (e.g., AMI) can be the cause. Any patient with rapid a-fib who became unstable in the ED (pulmonary edema, hypotension) warrants admission to a critical care bed. Patients with uncomplicated chronic a-fib whose rate was easily controlled in the ED (80 to 110 bpm) may be followed on a close outpatient basis.

When WPW occurs as an incidental finding in an asymptomatic patient, future management decisions may be deferred to the outpatient setting (discuss with consultant). Patients requiring cardioversion or exhibiting ominous signs or symptoms (prolonged chest pain, CHF, ischemia, hypotension) necessitate admission—regardless if the associated tachycardia appears wide or narrow. All patients with concomitant WPW and a-fib require direct admission to a monitored bed (high risk for VF or sudden death).

Patients experiencing PVCs require admission only if the PVCs are signaling the presence of a serious disorder that would otherwise warrant admission (e.g., AMI, CHF, digitalis toxicity). Patients displaying *sustained VT* call for stabilization in the ED before transfer to the ICU/CCU.

Admit *all patients with new-onset or acquired CHB* to a monitored bed. An exception for mandatory admission and pacemaker placement are patients with congenital CHB who are asymptomatic and maintain an adequate ventricular rate (> 50/min). Patients with new onset type II second-degree AV block require admission to a monitored bed. First-degree and Mobitz type I blocks require admission only if the underlying condition dictates it.

Patients suspected of a pacemaker complication should be admitted to a monitored bed. Only experienced personnel should reprogram the pacemaker.

Selected Readings

Ganz IL, Friedman PL: Medical Progress—supraventricular tachycardia. N Engl J Med 1995;332:162–173.

Garratt CJ, Griffith MJ, Young G: Value of physical signs in the diagnosis of ventricular tachycardia. Circulation 1994;90:3103–3107.

Wellens HJJ, Conover MB: The ECG in emergency decision making. Philadelphia: WB Saunders, 1992.

1.9 AORTIC CATASTROPHES

Description

Dissection of the aorta is the most prevalent of the aortic disasters (three times more common than ruptured abdominal aneurysms). An aortic dissection entails cleavage of the intima from the media and adventitia, whereas a true aneurysm involves dilation of all three layers of the arterial wall. Aortic dissections occur in the setting of long-standing hypertension, Marfan's syndrome, Ehlers-Danlos syndrome, pregnancy (more than half the cases occurring in females under age 40 occur during pregnancy, usually during the third trimester), congenital heart disease, coarctation of the aorta, Turner's syndrome, trauma (see section 4.4), and iatrogenic complications (cardiac surgery or catheterization).

Aortic dissections are classified by the location of the dissecting process. The DeBakey classification identifies three types: type I involves both the ascending and the descending aorta; type II is limited to the ascending aorta and does not involve the arch;

and type III dissections are confined to the descending aorta, usually beginning just distal to the left subclavian artery. The Stanford classification combines type I and type II dissections into one group proximal (type A) and distal (type B) similar to DeBakey type III. Two-thirds of patients suffer type A dissections.

Aortic aneurysms develop in all portions of the aorta, but are most prevalent in the abdominal section. *Abdominal aortic aneurysms* (AAA) affect 2% of the population over age 50 and primarily result from atherosclerotic disease. Other predisposing factors are age over 60, a history of cigarette smoking, hypertension, coronary artery disease, and male sex. All but 1 to 2% of AAA are infrarenal. Thoracic aneurysms are most common in the descending aorta, tend to enlarge more slowly than abdominal aneurysms, and rupture less often.

History

In aortic dissection, patients customarily experience a sudden onset of excruciating pain (described as ripping or shearing), frequently maximal at onset. Location of the discomfort tends to reflect the position of the dissection, with migration of the pain corresponding with progression of the dissection. Neurologic deficits (cerebrovascular accidents, spinal cord ischemia, peripheral nerve ischemia) occur if the blood supply to these locations is interrupted. Syncope is the principal complaint in 5% of patients with aortic dissection. Dyspnea may result from aortic insufficiency or rupture of the dissection into the pleural space.

Thoracic or abdominal aneurysms also cause chest or abdominal pain, either from expansion of the wall of the aneurysm or by pressure exerted on neighboring structures. Thoracic aneurysms may also produce dysphagia (from esophageal compression), hoarseness (from compression of the recurrent laryngeal nerve causing vocal cord paralysis), superior vena cava syndrome (secondary to compression of the superior vena cava), cough or dyspnea (from tracheal or pulmonary artery compression), or shock (resulting from rupture of the aneurysm). Less common presenting symptoms are hemoptysis (from erosion of the aneurysm into the pulmonary parenchyma or rupture into the bronchus) and gastrointestinal bleeding (from rupture of the aneurysm into the intestinal tract or formation of an aortoenteric fistula—higher incidence in patients with previous abdominal surgery, especially aortic surgery). *Suspect AAA in any patient over the age of 50 with the sudden onset of severe abdominal, back, flank, or pelvic pain.* Radicular pain to the scrotum, perineum, or thighs arises from compression of the surrounding nerves by an expanding hematoma. Blood loss may precipitate syncope.

Physical Examination

General. Note if patient appears acutely ill, anxious, pale, and/or diaphoretic. Patients with aortic dissection may appear shocky even when the blood pressure is normal or increased. Look for signs of Marfan's syndrome (arachnodactyly, tall stature, high arched palate, and kyphoscoliosis).

Vital signs. Patients can be hypertensive, normotensive, or hypotensive (hypotension suggests the possibility of cardiac tamponade, external rupture, or hypovolemia). Check blood pressure in both upper extremities and compare upper and lower extremity pressures in suspected dissection (systolic pressure differential > 15 mm Hg is considered significant).

HEENT. Check for signs of Horner's syndrome (ipsilateral ptosis, miosis, anhidrosis, and enophthalmos) and vocal cord paralysis.

Neck. Examine for tracheal deviation or swelling of the neck as well as presence of jugular venous distention

Chest. Inspect for pulsations of the right sternoclavicular joint, dilation of veins of the upper chest, or visible and palpable pulsations of the anterior chest wall. Listen for rales.

Cardiac. Auscultate for aortic insufficiency murmur (high-pitched blowing diastolic murmur) as well as muffled heart tones (tamponade).

Abdomen. Note mottling of the flanks. Palpate for an expansive mass in the periumbilical area between the xiphoid process and umbilicus, often to the left of the midline (this may be difficult in obese and muscular patients). A normal aorta is palpable in an anterior-posterior (AP) plane, while an aneurysmal dilation transmits impulses in both the AP and transverse planes. The diameter of the abdominal aorta is considered normal when < 3 cm. Suprarenal aneurysms are generally nonpalpable. Listen for abdominal systolic bruit (AAA).

Neurologic. Positive neurologic findings with chest pain suggest aortic dissection.

Extremities. Check for presence and strength of pulses (especially note pressure differences) as well as reduplication of pulses (presence of a palpable pulse without evidence of a ventricular contraction). Pulse deficits are frequently transient. Document signs of arterial insufficiency of the legs (pale, cool, painful).

Diagnostic Tests

If the diagnosis of ruptured AAA is apparent on history and physical examination, no further diagnostic evaluation is needed. In such circumstances, the patient needs immediate surgical intervention. Any action that delays surgical intervention may prove fatal.

Blood tests. Routine blood work does not help make the diagnosis but establishes a baseline. Parameters affected include the hematocrit, BUN and creatinine (involvement of renal arteries), and PT/PTT (DIC can occur). *Type and cross-match* blood for surgery (when surgery is emergent, order type-specific blood). Consider testing for syphilis in older patients with thoracic aneurysms, along with blood cultures in febrile patients with suspected aneurysm (mycotic aneurysm).

CXR. Abnormal in up to 90% of cases of aortic dissection. The most common abnormality is a widened mediastinum. Other radiographic findings consistent with aortic dissection include a change in configuration of the aortic knob compared to prior films, obliteration of the aortic knob, displacement of the trachea or a nasogastric tube to the right, increased distance of the aortic intimal calcification to the outer shadow (> 1 cm), and left-sided pleural effusion.

Abdominal x-rays. Abdominal aneurysms may be detected on more than 50% of AP and lateral roentgenograms (look for calcification of aorta). Rupture into the retroperitoneal region may cause loss of the psoas shadow.

ECG. Findings are typically nonspecific and may reflect longstanding hypertension (left ventricular hypertrophy, nonspecific ST-T changes). Sinus tachycardia is frequently seen. Absence of ECG findings in a patient who appears to be having an MI should heighten the suspicion for aortic dissection.

Angiography. Remains the gold standard for diagnosing aortic dissection, with approximately 90% accuracy. An angiogram also delineates the site of origin of the dissection, the extent of the dissection, and the integrity of the arteries originating directly from the aorta.

CT scan. Indicated when aortic dissection is a possibility but not likely (does not define site of origin of dissection) or for the hemodynamically stable patient with suspected abdominal aortic aneurysm.

Ultrasonography. Can be done at the bedside and is both sensitive and specific in detecting abdominal aneurysms. Its main drawback is that it may not be able to detect a leak.

Transesophageal echocardiography. Holds promise as a screening tool. The transducer is placed directly posterior to the heart and adjacent structures via the esophagus. Potential disadvantages are that the test is user dependent and usually requires sedation.

MRI. Offers high sensitivity and specificity for aortic dissection. Drawbacks include the length of time required for the study and incompatibility with life-support devices.

Treatment

Aortic Dissection

Initiate treatment for aortic dissection before radiological confirmation in the hemodynamically stable patient. After securing the ABCs, supplying supplemental oxygen, and placing the patient on a monitor, administer a narcotic analgesic for patient comfort. Next, simultaneously lower the blood pressure while reducing the pulse pressure. Unless contraindicated (bradycardia, asthma, hypotension, CHF), administer a β-blocker. Traditionally, *propranolol* has been used, with an initial dose of 0.5 mg IV, followed by 1 mg IV q 5 min (for a total of 0.15 mg/kg). Strive for a target heart rate of 60 to 80 bpm. *Esmolol,* a cardioselective β-blocker with a rapid onset and short duration of action, is also effective; the loading dose is 500 μg/kg/min IV bolus over 1 min, followed by a 4-min infusion of 50 μg/kg/min. If an adequate effect is not seen within 5 min, repeat the loading dose followed by a 4-min infusion of 100 μg/kg/min. Once adequate β-blockade is obtained, lower the systolic pressure to 90 to 110 mm Hg. *Nitroprusside* displays a rapid onset of action (1 to 2 min) and is readily titratable (see section 1.7 for dosing information).

If β-blockers are contraindicated or nitroprusside is poorly tolerated, employ *trimethaphan* (500 mg in 500 mL D_5W starting at 1 mg/min). Trimethaphan is a ganglionic blocker, and its main side effects are orthostatic hypotension, somnolence, urinary retention, and ileus. A third regimen uses *labetalol,* a combined selective α-antagonist and nonselective β-blocker. The initial dose is 20 mg IV bolus, with subsequent doses of 20 to 80 mg IV q 10 min (to a maximum of 300 mg), until adequate control is achieved.

For unstable patients, or symptomatic patients with type A dissection, emergent surgical consultation is warranted while the evaluation is initiated. If cardiac surgery is not at hand, transport the patient in the most expedient manner to a hospital that provides cardiac surgery. Although surgical intervention is recognized as the treatment of choice for type A dissections, the treatment of type B dissections is usually medical.

Abdominal Aortic Aneurysms

Successful management of abdominal aortic aneurysms depends on timely recognition—even before the onset of symptoms (the mortality of an elective resection of an abdominal aneurysm is 2 to 5%; it is 25 to 50% if the aneurysm is ruptured). The critical size at which repair of the abdominal aorta is deemed necessary is 5 cm. Almost 75% of ruptured AAAs are retroperitoneal, allowing a tamponade effect to contain the bleeding. Unstable patients require immediate transport to the OR (the benefit of aggressive fluid resuscitation is controversial).

Admission Criteria

All patients with suspected aortic dissections require admission to an ICU bed. Those patients who are unstable with a proximal (type A) dissection should be prepared for immediate surgery. Distal (type B) dissections proceed to the ICU for medical stabilization.

Patients with a suspected ruptured AAA should be transferred directly to the OR if possible, even without ED stabilization. Asymptomatic patients discovered to have an aneurysm larger than 4 cm need to be referred to an appropriate surgeon for elective repair.

Selected Readings

Cigarroa JE, Isselbacher EM, DeSanctis RW, et al.: Diagnostic imaging in the evaluation of suspected aortic dissection. N Engl J Med 1993; 328(1):31–43.

Ernst CB: Abdominal aortic aneurysm. N Engl J Med 1993;328:1167–1172.

Marston WA, Ahlquist R, Johnson G, et al.: Misdiagnosis of ruptured abdominal aortic aneurysms. J Vasc Surg 1992;16:17–22.

1.10 DEEP VENOUS THROMBOSIS

Description

Deep venous thrombosis (DVT) occurs from deposits of fibrin, RBCs, platelets, and WBCs in the venous channels, resulting in obstruction of venous outflow and/or inflammation of the vessel walls. The precipitating events are customarily components of *Virchow's triad:* (1) damage to the lining of the vessel wall, (2) diminished flow of blood or stasis, and/or (3) a hypercoagulable state. Venous thrombosis is most prevalent in the lower extremities or pelvic veins but can occur in the upper extremities. The clinical manifestations of DVT depend on the degree of obstruction and inflammation of the venous vessels. Often, the first manifestation of DVT is pulmonary embolus (see section 2.4).

History

History of Present Illness

Pain (present in 50% of cases) and swelling (found in 75% of patients) are usually the initial two complaints. Inquire about previous episodes of DVT. A strong family or personal history of DVT or PE before age 40 is particularly suggestive of protein C deficiency.

Risk Factors

Inquire about previous history of DVT or PE, recent catheter placement (particularly central venous catheters resulting in upper extremity DVT), intravenous drug abuse, heart disease (MI, CHF), CVA, cancer (pancreatic, lymphoma, prostate cancer), collagen-vascular disorders (lupus procoagulant), hematopoietic disorders (sickle cell disease; polycythemia; deficiency of antithrombin III, protein S, or protein C), nephrotic syndrome, recent trauma to the pelvis or lower extremities, obesity, prolonged immobilization (whether involuntary from stroke or illness or voluntary as in a long car or airplane trip), estrogen therapy or oral contraceptive use, pregnancy or postpartum state (hypercoagulable states are most common in the third trimester and may continue for 3 months postpartum), recent surgery (gastrointestinal, genitourinary, or orthopedic), and age over 40. In addition, repetitive motion of the upper extremities (hyperabduction or extension rotation of the shoulder as seen in tennis, baseball, and swimming) can cause spontaneous thrombosis of the subclavian vein.

Review of Systems

Inquire about possible symptoms related to PE such as chest pain, shortness of breath, cough, hemoptysis, palpitations, or syncope.

Physical Examination

The physical signs of DVT are neither sensitive nor specific. Thrombosis is not always complete, which accounts for the variability of the clinical picture.

General. Is the patient in distress? Note the patient's habitus (obese, cachectic).
Vital signs. Check all vital signs, including temperature.
Chest. Auscultate for rales and rhonchi (signs of CHF, pneumonia, PE).
Abdomen. Check for hepatosplenomegaly.
Skin. Look for petechiae and purpura (bleeding dyscrasia).
Extremities. Confirm pulses and normal capillary refill to all extremities and digits. Examine for erythema, cords (inflammation of veins), warmth (secondary to inflammation), and localized areas of discoloration or ulceration. Inspect and palpate the lower extremity for tenderness (particularly the calf, popliteal fossa, and inguinal region). Swelling is not always obvious; if in doubt, measure the maximal circumference of thighs and calves. Unilateral, nonpitting edema may be the only sign of DVT of the upper extremity. *Homans's sign* (tenderness of the calf muscles on forced dorsiflexion of the foot) and *Pratt's sign* (tenderness on compression of the calf against the leg) are at best 50% sensitive and specific. Extremity findings for DVT are usually isolated to one extremity.

Diagnostic Tests

When the history and physical examination suggest DVT or the diagnosis cannot be excluded, further testing will be required. *Clinical history and physical examination are at best 50% reliable.*

CBC, PT/PTT, SMA, platelets. Establish baselines. Thrombocytosis and polycythemia predispose to DVT.
CXR. Generally normal unless patient has developed a PE or has underlying heart disease.
ECG. Normal unless associated cardiac disease or PE present.

ABG. While a normal ABG does not exclude the diagnosis of PE, an abnormal PCO_2 or PO_2 should heighten suspicion for occult PE.

Duplex ultrasound. Excellent screening tool for detecting thrombosis of the veins; noninvasive and can be repeated periodically to assess changes in the venous system. DVT is suggested when the venous walls do not easily compress or echogenic thrombi are seen.

Impedance plethysmography (IPG). Useful for detecting proximal vein thrombosis or recurrent DVT but has a low sensitivity for calf DVT or partially obstructive DVT. False-positive results are seen in patients with CHF or postoperative leg swelling.

Venogram. Considered the gold standard. A positive diagnosis is made if a filling defect is demonstrated. However, it is an invasive procedure, and injection of the contrast agent may itself cause inflammation of the vein and DVT.

Treatment

Thrombosis localized to only the calf veins usually requires no treatment. However, in 20 to 30% of cases, extension into the popliteal veins occurs. Therefore, patients in whom lower leg DVT is suspected but IPG or duplex ultrasound is negative should undergo repeat testing in 2 to 5 days.

Proximal DVT of the lower extremity (above the calf) or DVT of the upper extremity should be treated with *heparin.* In addition, initiate therapy if suspicion is high for DVT (and no absolute contraindications) but testing is negative or equivocal. The initial loading dose is usually 5000 units IV followed by a drip of 1000 units/hr. The goal of therapy is to increase the PTT from a normal of 30 to 40 sec to 60 to 80 sec (1.5 to 2.0 times the control value). Check PTT 4 to 6 hr after initiation of therapy. The main complication of ED therapy is bleeding and necrosis of the skin if the heparin extravasates. Contraindications to heparin therapy include a source of active bleeding, recent eye or central nervous system (CNS) surgery, thrombocytopenia, and CNS tumors or hemorrhages. Recently, *low molecular weight heparin* and *heparinoids* have been used to treat DVT (these agents have a longer half-life and are given once daily subcutaneously). The role of thrombolytics is controversial.

Patients with contraindications to heparin or who develop a

PE despite adequate anticoagulation require placement of a percutaneous inferior vena cava filter.

Special Considerations

Pulmonary emboli. See section 2.4.

Phlegmasia alba dolens. Also known as *white* or *milk leg*—characterized by thrombosis of the iliofemoral vessels and usually occurs in the immediate postpartum period.

Phlegmasia cerulea dolens. Also known as *blue leg*—occurs when thrombosis of the veins and collaterals of the lower extremity lead to massive venous occlusion.

Both *phlegmasia alba dolens* and *phlegmasia cerulea dolens* are medical emergencies that require emergent treatment with broad-spectrum antibiotics and anticoagulants as well as possible surgical intervention (debridement, vena caval ligation).

Admission Criteria

All patients with proximal vein DVT (involvement of the popliteal, femoral, and/or iliac vessels) need admission with initiation of heparin.

Patients with massive venous occlusion (phlegmasia alba and cerulea dolens) require ICU admission.

Patients with DVT of only calf veins who are reliable and have an adequate living situation can be discharged home with instructions for bed rest, elevation of the involved extremity, and applications of moist warm heat to the affected area. Prescribe a nonsteroidal antiinflammatory agent if not contraindicated (aspirin is adequate) and schedule a return appointment in 24 to 48 hr for repeat testing to exclude proximal propagation of the clot. These patients will need careful instructions to return immediately if pain or swelling worsens or if they develop fever or dyspnea. Unreliable patients may require admission to ensure compliance with repeat testing.

Patients in whom initial testing is negative can be discharged with close follow up.

Selected Readings

Dodson TF. Recognition and management of deep vein thrombosis. Heart Dis Stroke 1993;2(3):231–234.

O'Meara JJ, McNutt RA, Evans AT, et al.: A decision analysis of streptokinase plus heparin as compared to heparin alone for deep-vein thrombosis. N Engl J Med 1994;330:1864–1869.

Chapter 2

Pulmonary

2.1 UPPER AIRWAY OBSTRUCTION

Description

Upper airway obstruction (UAO) is a dire emergency that requires rapid establishment of the diagnosis along with virtually instantaneous treatment. The upper airway is considered to extend from the oropharynx to the carina and exhibits two consistent areas of narrowing: at the *base of the tongue* and at the *level of the vocal and false cords.*

Causes of *acute UAO* are diverse and include *infection* (epiglottitis, tracheitis, retropharyngeal or peritonsillar abscess, severe pharyngitis, Ludwig's angina), *foreign body aspiration* (food, medication), *trauma* (facial trauma with posterior displacement of tongue, fracture of larynx), *anaphylaxis* (angioedema, Steven's-Johnson syndrome), *poisonings and toxic inhalation* (caustic burns secondary to acid or alkali ingestion, smoke, and thermal injury), and *iatrogenesis* (hematoma of neck from central line insertion). In addition, large foreign bodies in the proximal esophagus may lead to findings of UAO.

Subacute or chronic etiologies of UAO include *infection* (tonsillar hypertrophy), *posttraumatic strictures* (previous trauma, tracheostomy, or long-term intubation), *neoplastic or fibrous growth* (expansion of local laryngeal, tracheal, or esophageal tumor; metastatic extension; vascular rings; and pulmonary slings), *external masses* (lymphadenopathy, goiter), and *miscellaneous* causes (Pickwickian/sleep apnea syndromes, morbid obesity, Ehlers-Danlos syndrome, Wegener's granulomatosis).

History

Classically, UAO is preceded by a *choking episode*, usually on food that has been incompletely chewed and lodged in airway or aspirated *(café coronary)*. Presentation depends on whether the obstruction is incomplete or complete (with the patient losing consciousness in 2 to 3 min). If the patient's clinical status permits, attempt to establish onset (abrupt, insidious) and duration (seconds, minutes, hours, weeks) of symptoms, antecedent events (eating, trauma, recent upper respiratory infection, insect sting), associated symptoms (fever, coughing, hoarseness or change in voice, dyspnea, dysphagia for liquids and/or solids), PMH (chronic throat infections, recent intubation, pulmonary disease, cancer, AIDS, thyroid disease), and allergy history (medications, foods, insects).

Physical Examination

General. Note general signs of significant UAO (agitation, choking, paroxysmal coughing, noisy respirations, universal distress signal of clutching throat between thumb and forefinger, venous engorgement of head and neck, cyanosis) along with the position of the patient (sitting up, tripod, supine, prone). Most important, if the patient is conscious, determine if he or she is able to phonate (aphonia implies complete obstruction); if the patient can speak, note the character of the voice (supraglottic disorder is associated with muffled or "hot potato" voice, and glottic pathology produces coarse or scratchy speech).

Vital signs. Elevation of heart rate and blood pressure appear early; but as the patient deteriorates, respirations become depressed and pulse and blood pressure may fall. Check temperature if time allows.

HEENT. Assess the oropharynx for foreign bodies (including dentures), erythema, edema, mass, or exudate along with deviation or swelling of the tongue or uvula. Check for trismus, dental infection, singed nasal hairs, carbonaceous sputum, and asymmetry of face. Observe how the patient is handling his or her secretions (drooling). **Note:** *Exercise caution if you suspect epiglottitis.*

Neck. Palpate and inspect for subcutaneous air, masses, and thyroid enlargement or irregularity. Check the position of the trachea. Listen carefully for *stridor,* a cardinal sign of upper airway obstruction. Also determine if the stridor is *inspiratory* alone (supraglottic or glottic obstruction) or inspiratory and expiratory (subglottic or tracheal problem).

Lungs. Observe not only respiratory rate but respiratory effort (intercostal retractions, nasal flaring) and adequacy of breathing (presence and equality of breath sounds, wheezing).

Diagnostic Tests

Note: *In serious UAO, do not delay treatment for ancillary studies.*

Pulse oximetry. Allows for rapid, noninvasive measurement of oxygen saturation.

ABG. Accurately measures oxygenation, carbon dioxide, and pH.

X-rays. If possible, obtain beside portable PA and lateral films of the neck (soft tissue penetration) and chest. *Do not* send a patient in distress unaccompanied to x-ray. Consider inspiratory/expiratory CXR or a lateral decubitus film to aid in detecting radiolucent foreign bodies.

Treatment

Encourage the UAO patient who is *conscious, alert, and can still speak* to clear his or her own airway (natural cough produces optimum increases in intrathoracic pressure). If the patient appears unable to open the airway or proceeds to an unconscious state, render upper abdominal thrusts *(Heimlich maneuver)* for potential *foreign body obstruction. Chest compression* is substituted for women in the later stages of pregnancy or those patients who are morbidly obese. In the *unconscious patient,* initially attempt to ventilate the patient (try repositioning airway with a *jaw thrust* and, if trauma is excluded, a *chin* or *neck lift*). If this is unsuccessful, perform five manual thrusts and reattempt ventilation. If these measures are still ineffectual, *suction* the oropharynx with large-tip device (Yankauer or use the end of the suction tube itself), while visualizing the upper airway with a direct laryngoscope. Removal of foreign bodies can be undertaken with McGill forceps. Failure to locate or remove a foreign body with persistent UAO necessitates an artificial airway, either *endotracheal intubation* or, if the obstruction is irresolvable, *percutaneous transtracheal catheter ventilation* (PTCV), *guided retrograde transcricoid intubation,* or *cricothyrotomy.* In rare cases (laryngeal trauma) a tracheostomy is required.

Additional measures include supplemental oxygen and treatment for anaphylaxis (see Chapter 8), bronchospasm (see section 2.5), and infection (see section 15.4). In cases of a suspected deeply situated foreign body or a partial airway obstruction not amenable to ED treatment, urgent consultation for indirect or fiberoptic laryngoscopy, bronchoscopy, and/or endoscopy is essential.

Admission Criteria

Patients with acute upper airway obstruction ordinarily mandate admission. *Patients exhibiting signs or symptoms of extreme respiratory distress* warrant ICU admission. Even if a patient readily responds to treatment, observe the patient for 4 to 6 hr before determining final disposition.

Suggested Readings

Brink LW: Transport of the critically ill patient with upper airway obstruction. Critical Care Clin 1992;8(3):633–647.

Jacobson S: Upper airway obstruction. Emerg Med Clin North Am 1989; 7:205–217.

2.2 ACUTE RESPIRATORY FAILURE

Description

Acute respiratory failure (ARF) is the inability to supply sufficient *oxygenation* to the arterial blood with or without adequate elimination of carbon dioxide. ARF may arise from various primary or secondary disturbances of the airway, lung parenchyma, chest wall, and/or neural regulation of breathing. Although no rigid criteria can be applied to all patients, it is generally accepted that respiratory failure is present when the arterial oxygen tension (PaO_2) < 50 mm Hg *(hypoxia)* and/or arterial carbon dioxide ($PaCO_2$) > 45 mm Hg *(hypercarbia)*.

Hypoxemia may result from nonpulmonary conditions (right-to-left intracardiac shunt, low inspired oxygen), and tissue hypoxia can be caused by a multitude of conditions (anemia, reduced cardiac output, carbon monoxide or cyanide poisoning) not due to failure of the respiratory system. The most prevalent pulmonary conditions leading to acute respiratory failure are *asthma* (see section 2.5), *COPD* (see section 2.3), and *pneumonia* (see section 9.2). *Adult respiratory distress syndrome* (ARDS) is another cause of acute respiratory failure and is associated with a variety of clinical disorders (e.g., major trauma, aspiration of gastric contents, and systemic infection). While there are no distinctive features of ARDS, dyspnea and tachypnea soon lead to hypoxia that is unresponsive to oxygen and finally to acute respiratory failure.

History

Cardinal symptoms suggestive of *hypoxia* include disorientation, restlessness, agitation, and dyspnea. *Hypercapnia* presents more commonly as a productive cough, wheezing, or a headache, along with increasing somnolence or stupor.

The history is directed toward trying to determine the etiology for respiratory compromise. Possible inciting causes include *infection, pulmonary disease* (COPD, asthma, toxic inhalations), *heart disease* (hypertensive heart disease, myocardial infarction, congestive heart failure), *trauma* (pulmonary contusions, flail chest, pneumothorax, fat embolism), *inhalation exposures* (smoke, ammonia, chlorine, nitrous oxide, phosgene), *drug ingestion* (heroin, methadone, aspirin, propoxyphene), and *miscellaneous* causes (high-altitude illness, preeclampsia, pancreatitis).

Physical Examination

Physical findings and ancillary studies of ARF can be extremely subtle.

General. Assess general demeanor (comfortable, agitated, stuporous, coma). Determine if the patient is able to communicate verbally. **Remember:** *In a supine comatose patient, the tongue can fall against the posterior pharyngeal wall, blocking respiration.*

Vital signs. Obtain rectal temperature. Early hypoxia is associated with an increase in sympathetic discharge (hypertension, tachycardia, peripheral vasoconstriction), while hypercapnia tends to cause peripheral vasodilation, diaphoresis, hypertension, and tachycardia.

Skin. Examine the skin for rashes, ecchymosis, cyanosis, urticaria, or petechiae. Cyanosis appears when $PaO_2 < 40$ mm Hg and at least 5 g/100 mL of reduced hemoglobin is present.

HEENT. Document any signs of trauma. Examine for evidence of facial burns (singed nasal hairs, carbonaceous sputum). Drooling signifies upper airway obstruction.

Neck. Listen for stridor. Look for swelling of the submandibular glands (Ludwig's angina) and adenopathy; note the trachea's position and any neck vein distention.

Lungs. Note the quality of air movement and the type of muscle use. Listen for adventitious breath sounds, wheezing (inspiratory versus expiratory), rales, rhonchi, pleural rubs, asymmetry, or absent breath sounds. Percuss for hyperresonance, dullness, and fremitus.

Heart. Listen for murmurs, clicks, or gallops.

Abdomen. Massive ascites and obesity can compromise respiratory function.

Extremities. Check for edema, clubbing, track marks, venous insufficiency, calf tenderness (Homans's sign), and symmetry of pulses.

Neurologic. Document and follow the mental status and check for deficits and/or weakness.

Diagnostic Tests

Arterial blood gas. Obtain initially on room air (if possible) and then 15 min after any changes are made (FIO_2, intubation, change in ventilator setting). The *alveolar-arterial* gradient ($PAO_2 - PaO_2$) is approximated by the formula $150 - PaO_2 - (PaCO_2 \times 1.25)$. Normally the gradient is 10 to 20 mm Hg but may reach up to 30 mm Hg in the elderly (a good rule of thumb is that the gradient should equal one-third the patient's age). Higher gradients appear in smokers. An abnormal gradient suggests intrinsic pulmonary pathology. Acutely, the pH may be a more sensitive indicator of ARF than the $PaCO_2$. Suspect a shunt when there is no improvement in oxygenation following administration of 100% oxygen.

CBC. Check the hemoglobin and hematocrit, white cell count, and differential.

SMA. Review the serum bicarbonate to analyze presence of acute or chronic metabolic or respiratory acid-base imbalance.

CXR. Look for infiltrates, pulmonary edema, pneumothorax, foreign bodies, or skeletal abnormalities. **Remember:** *The severity of hypoxemia does not always correspond to the degree of lung pathology.*

Pulse oximetry. A noninvasive method of assessing oxygen saturation. (Cannot detect poisoning with carbon monoxide or methemoglobin.)

ECG. Rule out underlying cardiac ischemia, infarct, and rhythm disturbances.

Treatment

Definitive therapy depends on the etiology, but the immediate goals of airway management are to ensure an unobstructed upper airway, provide adequate oxygen, and ensure that ventilation is effective in eliminating any excess in PCO_2, while maintaining normal pH.

Patients with chronic respiratory failure can frequently maintain a lower PaO_2 and a higher $PaCO_2$ than those patients with acute respiratory failure. When deciding to initiate intubation and mechanical ventilation, the emergency specialist needs to take into account the patient's clinical appearance as well as the results of the blood gas analysis. Determine if the cause of the ARF is readily correctable (opioid ingestion can be reversed by naloxone), if supplemental oxygen will be sufficient, or if an artificial airway will be necessary (endotracheal intubation, surgical airway).

Intubated patients with unresponsive hypoxia or progressive hypoventilation accompanied by hypercapnia and respiratory acidosis frequently require *mechanical ventilatory support.* Although the ventilator is often set up by a respiratory therapist, the emergency specialist needs to know how to operate and control it. The first decision that must be made involves what type of ventilator to use: *volume-cycled ventilators* (deliver a predetermined tidal volume) or *pressure-cycled ventilators* (discharge gas flow at a preset pressure, with tidal volume being the dependent variable). The pressure necessary to deliver a preset tidal volume is termed the *peak airway pressure.* A large increase in peak pressure signals problems in the lung parenchyma or chest wall (worsening of pulmonary edema, tension pneumothorax, mainstem intubation, large region of atelectasis) or airway problems (kinking of the endotracheal tube, mucous plugs, bronchospasm).

There are also two types of ventilatory control of respirations. *Intermittent mandatory ventilation* (IMV) permits the patient to breathe at his or her own rate and tidal volume, supplemented by the ventilator, which adds a predetermined number of breaths at a preset tidal volume each minute. In *controlled mechanical ventilation* (CMV), the ventilator provides each breath. In *assist control ventilation* (ACV), the patient's inspiratory effort triggers a fixed volume breath from the ventilator. If the patient does not initiate respirations, the ventilator then discharges at a preset rate. Additional settings determined by the physician are FIO_2 and the *tidal volume* (8 to 12 mL/kg). Few aspects of ventilator management are more controversial than *positive end expiratory pressure* (PEEP; a technique that prevents end-expiratory pressures from falling below a set value, keeping distal airways open). PEEP is the treatment of choice for patients with ARDS who are refractory to high FIO_2. When PEEP values are greater than 15 mm Hg, there is an increased risk of compromising cardiac output and barotrauma.

Continuous positive airway pressure (CPAP) provided with a nasal mask has been used recently to treat respiratory failure due to COPD, CHF, pulmonary infections, and trauma. With CPAP, oxygen is administered under pressure to maintain alveolar patency, similar to PEEP in intubated patients. CPAP can be administered using a face mask and a mechanical ventilator to provide continuous positive airway pressure in inspiration and expiration.

Admission Criteria

The *majority of patients with acute respiratory failure* will require admission, and most will require an intensive care bed. *Patients with upper airway obstruction due to a foreign body* aspiration that is relieved in the ED may not require admission.

Suggested Readings

Hee MK: Intubation of critically ill patients. Mayo Clinic Proc 1992;67: 569–576.

Tobin MJ: Mechanical ventilation. N Engl J Med 1994;330:1056–1061.

2.3 CHRONIC OBSTRUCTIVE PULMONARY DISEASE

Description

Chronic obstructive pulmonary disease (COPD) is a group of disorders distinguished by both chronic and irreversible obstructions of expiratory airflow. The two most common causes of COPD are *chronic bronchitis,* which is characterized by hypersecretion of mucus, a cough productive of sputum for at least 3 months a year for a minimum of 2 years, and structural changes in the bronchi; and *emphysema,* which is a destructive process involving the lung parenchyma. Chronic bronchitis and emphysema may occur together, arising from a common etiology (cigarette smoking), and clinically it is often difficult to distinguish the two.

History

A chronic productive cough and a persistent and progressive exertional dyspnea are the hallmarks of COPD. Patients with chronic bronchitis may also present with wheezing (mimicking asthma). Attempt to determine the reason for exacerbation of the disease. Clarify the following points, allowing the patient to reply with simple nods, if necessary:

- History of intubation, hospitalizations, and steroid dependence;
- Onset and duration of present exacerbation;
- Comparison of severity with previous attacks;
- Cough with or without sputum production;
- Color of sputum (including presence of hemoptysis);
- Associated symptoms (fever, chest pain, alteration in mood or agitation);
- Medications and compliance;
- Prior cardiopulmonary disease; and
- Smoking, work, and family history.

Note: *A sudden onset of symptoms accompanied by chest pain suggests alternative diagnosis such as pulmonary embolism, pneumothorax, or myocardial ischemia.* Old records can help establish trends in oxygenation, hypercapnia, and pulmonary function tests.

Physical Examination

General. Note the general appearance of the patient ("pink puffer" is characteristic of emphysema, while "blue bloater" is associated with chronic bronchitis) and level of alertness (agitated, in extremis, or alert and able to communicate orally). Sweating implies severe distress.

Vital signs. Pay strict attention to all vital signs, including temperature (rectal is best).

HEENT. Observe for pursed-lip breathing.

Neck. Examine for neck vein distention, suprasternal retractions, and position of the trachea. Listen for upper airway stridor.

Lungs. Inspect the chest configuration (barrel shaped). Assess for the use of accessory muscles, paradoxical abdominal breathing, and evidence of hyperinflation. Percuss all lung fields. Palpate for tactile fremitus and subcutaneous emphysema. Auscultate for asymmetry of breath sounds, inspiratory and expiratory wheezes, rales (COPD, CHF), and/or rhonchi.

Heart. Auscultate for murmurs, rubs, or gallops. Listen for signs of *pulmonary hypertension* (wide split S_2, a loud P_2, tricuspid insufficiency murmur).

Abdomen. Palpate for hepatosplenomegaly (cor pulmonale) or pulsatile liver (tricuspid insufficiency).
Extremities. Inspect for cyanosis, clubbing (not typical of COPD), and edema as well as symmetry and quality of pulses.

Diagnostic Tests

Arterial blood gas. Significant hypoxia, hypercapnia, and acidosis need to be identified and treated. Determine the primary acid-base disturbances.
Pulse oximetry. A quick and noninvasive monitoring tool. A reading less than 93% correlates with a PO_2 of less than 70 mm Hg.
CBC. Check hemoglobin and hematocrit for underlying anemia or a compensatory erythrocytosis. Elevation of WBC count may result from medications (steroids, β-agonists), stress, or infection. A left shift in the differential favors infection.
SMA. Electrolytes (serum bicarbonate in particular) help diagnose an acid-base disturbance. Hypokalemia may follow β-adrenergic therapy.
Sputum Gram stain. May help detect infection (see section 9.2).
Theophylline level. Check levels in patients on theophylline or if toxicity is suspected.
CXR. Rule out infiltrates, pneumothorax, or asymmetric hyperaeration of lung fields. Radiographic abnormalities associated with COPD include flattened diaphragms and an increase in the retrosternal air space. The cardiac silhouette typically appears tall and narrow in patients with emphysema and normal to enlarged in patients with chronic bronchitis. Bullae are also characteristic for emphysema.
ECG. Look for signs of ischemia and arrhythmia as well as right ventricular hypertrophy or strain *(cor pulmonale)*.

Treatment

Oxygenation

Patients with COPD who appear ill should be given supplemental oxygen (hypoxia, with or without hypercapnia, is prevalent in COPD), placed on a cardiac monitor, and have intravenous access secured. The goal is to increase the PO_2 to approximately 60 mm Hg (oxygen saturation about 90%). Employ either a nasal cannula (2 to 4 L/min) or a *Venturi* mask (delivers a fixed oxygen concentration of 24 to 50%). Excessive oxygen in chronic carbon dioxide retainers may actually worsen hypercapnia and acidosis, because of a blunting of the hypoxic stimulus; but *treatment of hypoxia is primary.*

Bronchospasm

Although chronic bronchitis and emphysema are diseases of fixed airflow obstruction (in contradistinction to asthma), a trial of *bronchodilators* is reasonable. The bronchodilators used in COPD are the same as those employed in the management of asthma (see section 2.5), with the exception that the *anticholinergics* appear more effective for both chronic bronchitis and emphysema than for asthma. *Ipratropium bromide* (Atrovent) is the preferred inhaled anticholinergic (fewer side effects) and is available as an inhalation solution (500 μg in 2.5 mL of normal saline; maximal effect in 1 to 2 hr, lasting for 6 to 12 hr) and a metered dose inhaler (MDI). Ipratropium can be given with β-agonists, possibly conferring a synergistic benefit.

Corticosteroids

Use of corticosteroids in COPD is controversial. However, there is a subset of patients who improve from both short- and long-term use, but they cannot be easily identified. If the patient has a history of current steroid use or exhibits severe symptoms of COPD on presentation, give steroids early (methylprednisolone 125 mg IVp).

Methylxanthines

The use of *theophylline* and *aminophylline* in the acute setting of an exacerbation of COPD is widely debated. If used, try to achieve a serum concentration in the therapeutic range (10 to 20 μg/mL). Side effects of aminophylline (nausea, vomiting, anxiety, tachycardia, hypokalemia) appear more frequently with toxic serum levels, but they can occur within the therapeutic range. Aminophylline interacts with many other medications (erythromycin, cimetidine, ranitidine, phenytoin, ciprofloxacin). The loading dose is 6 mg/kg IV or PO liquid (based on lean body weight). The maintenance dose is 0.5 to 0.9 mg/kg/hr; smokers exhibit a faster metabolism and require a higher maintenance dose, while metabolism is decreased in patients with hepatic dysfunction, CHF, and severe COPD.

Antibiotics

Unlike asthmatics, patients with COPD often have exacerbations provoked by bacterial infections and may benefit from antibiotic administration for acute episodes.

Intubation

The decision to intubate a patient with COPD requires a modification of the normal criteria (see section 2.2); hence, predicate the decision on clinical parameters (patient with inadequate respiratory effort, altered mental status, inability to protect airway). Keep in mind that patients with COPD chronically function with a compensated hypoxemia and/or hypercarbia.

Admission Criteria

All patients with COPD and pneumonia. Patients with significant deterioration of baseline blood gas. Patients who do not respond clinically to 4 hr of aggressive ED therapy or who state they do not feel subjectively improved at this time. Patients can be safely discharged only if they respond quickly to therapy, have no serious underlying illness (pneumonia, CHF), and have vital signs and respiratory parameters that reach baseline status. Close follow-up is essential.

Suggested Readings

Fei RH, Murata GH: Contemporary management of the patient with chronic obstructive pulmonary disease. Comp Ther 1994;20:277–281.

Fergusen GT, Cherniack RM: Management of chronic obstructive pulmonary disease. N Engl J Med 1993;328:1017–1022.

2.4 PULMONARY EMBOLUS

Description

Pulmonary embolus (PE) is an obstruction of the pulmonary arteries, usually originating from a thrombus in the deep venous system. Greater than 90% of pulmonary emboli develop from *deep vein thrombosis* of the proximal legs. However, less than 33% of patients display evidence of phlebitis. Emboli may also arise from the pelvic veins, right side of the heart, or the upper extremities (intravenous drug use, upper extremity trauma). PE is difficult to diagnose on the basis of history or physical examination alone, with the presentation being contingent on the degree of occlusion of the pulmonary arterial system as well as the patient's underlying cardiopulmonary status. One must have a high index of suspicion, as more than 75% of the deaths from PE occur within the first few hours.

History

The symptoms of PE tend to be nonspecific. However, PE must be considered in any patient complaining of sudden onset of *dyspnea* (85%) or *pleuritic chest pain* (75%). Other symptoms include *agitation* or *apprehension* (60%), *cough* (50%), *hemoptysis* (35%), *palpitations* (30%), and *syncope* (10%). While patients with massive PE may present in cardiovascular collapse, previously healthy patients with small PEs may remain asymptomatic (occult PE occurs in approximately 50% of patients with DVT). Risk factors (immobilization, surgery in past 3 months, previous PE, history of malignancy, CHF, COPD, antithrombin III or protein C or S deficiency, recent or current pregnancy, estrogen use, lower extremity or hip trauma) are readily identified in almost 90% of patients with confirmed PE. Lack of a precipitating cause, repeated chest pain in the same location, and recurrent hemoptysis make the diagnosis of PE less likely. The differential diagnosis includes all diseases that are capable of inducing sudden chest pain or shortness of breath (see section 1.4). PE is known as the great impostor and must be considered when patients present atypically.

Physical Examination

General. Note the general mental status (especially if patient anxious or agitated).

Vital signs. Tachypnea is seen in 90% of patients and tachycardia in 50%. Fever may be seen with pulmonary infarction, although generally $\leq$ 38°C. Hypotension can accompany massive PE.

Neck. Look for distended neck veins or carotid bruits.

Heart. Auscultate for extra heart sounds (S_3, S_4), a pericardial rub, and accentuated P_2.

Lungs. Listen for asymmetric breath sounds, wheezes, rhonchi, and/or pleural friction rub.

Abdomen. Examine for abdominal or pelvic masses.

Extremities. Check for any evidence of phlebitis or thrombosis (see section 1.10).

Diagnostic Tests

ABG. The prevailing findings are *hypoxemia* (85% of patients with a PE will have a $PaO_2 < 80$ mm Hg on room air), *hypocarbia* and/or *respiratory alkalosis,* and a widened alveolar-arterial gradient (PAO_2–PaO_2). Hyperventilation may increase the PaO_2 but can widen the alveolar-arterial gradient (see section 2.2). Patients with a normal PaO_2 along with a normal PAO_2–PaO_2 have less than a 5% chance of experiencing a PE.

CXR. A normal CXR in a severely dyspneic patient strongly suggests a PE, although most patients with PE do exhibit some abnormality on CXR *(elevated hemidiaphragm, unilateral pleural effusion, atelectasis, region of oligemia, parenchymal infiltrate). Hampton's hump* (an area of density or lung consolidation with a rounded border pointing to the hilum) and *Westermark's sign* (a dilated pulmonary outflow tract on the side of embolization with a distal area of decreased perfusion) are uncommon findings but are specific for PE.

ECG. The most important use is to eliminate cardiac ischemia or pericarditis as the etiology of dyspnea or chest pain. *Sinus tachycardia* and *nonspecific ST-T wave* changes are the most common associated findings. Patients with massive PE may show signs of acute right ventricular strain manifested by either a new *S_1, Q_3, T_3 pattern, right axis deviation, a new right bundle branch block,* or *right ventricular ischemia.*

Blood studies. If anticoagulant or thrombolytic therapy is a consideration, order baseline blood work (CBC platelet count, PT, PTT, T+S).

Lung scan ($\dot{V}/\dot{Q}$ scans). $\dot{V}/\dot{Q}$ scans compare the blood perfusion with the ventilation of the lungs; the outcome is classified into one of four subsets: *normal, low probability, intermediate probability,* and *high probability.* A high-probability $\dot{V}/\dot{Q}$ scan implies presence of a PE, while a normal $\dot{V}/\dot{Q}$ scan is strong evidence against PE (although it is still a remote possibility). A low- or intermediate-probability scan combined with a high clinical suspicion still indicates an almost 33% chance of PE. In addition, *the majority of patients with PE will fall into the low or intermediate probability categories.*

Angiography. The definitive test for PE. Although it is an invasive procedure, pulmonary angiography is less dangerous than a missed PE.

Miscellaneous tests. Alternative diagnostic modalities include *impedance plethysmography* (IPG) or *duplex ultrasound* of the legs, D-dimer testing (a degradation product of endogenous fibrinolysis), *echocardiography* (visualization of the right atrium, right ventricle, and proximal pulmonary artery for a thrombus and/or right ventricular overload), *MRI,* and *spiral CT* of the chest.

Treatment

Thrombolysis

Thrombolytic therapy actively dissolves the thrombus causing a PE, rather than depending on the body's slow, natural fibrinolytic process. While once reserved for patients who were hemodynamically unstable, a growing body of evidence supports its use in many patients with a PE. Current FDA-approved thrombolytic regimens for PE include *streptokinase* (250,000 units IV loading dose over 30 min followed by 100,000 units/hr IV for 24 hr), *urokinase* (2000 units IV loading dose over 10 min followed by 200 units/hr IV for 12 to 24 hr), and *TPA* (100 mg continuous IV infusion over 2 hr).

Anticoagulation

Use of such agents as heparin is directed at new clot formation but has little effect on a performed clot. Those patients *without* absolute contraindications for anticoagulation (bleeding ulcer, recent surgery, recent CVA) should be started on heparin (5000 units or 80 units/kg IVp, followed by a constant infusion of 1000 to 1600 units/hr or 18 units/kg/hr). The aim is to prolong the activated PTT to 1.5 to 2.0 times the control. Heparin may also be used following thrombolysis.

Surgical Procedure

Patients with contraindications to anticoagulation or thrombolysis may require surgical interruption of the inferior vena cava, with placement of a mechanical filter to prevent the passage of emboli. Embolectomy is a heroic measure but requires availability of cardiopulmonary bypass.

Admission Criteria

Protocols should be in place for evaluation, disposition, and treatment of *patients with significant risk factors,* suggestive histories, and compatible blood gases in whom a lung scan cannot be obtained immediately. If there is any doubt, consultation with a pulmonologist is warranted. *All patients with low, intermediate, and high probability lung scans* require hospitalization for further testing (angiography) and treatment.

Suggested Readings

Goldhaber SZ, Marpurgo M: Diagnosis, treatment and prevention of pulmonary embolism. Report of the WHO/International Society and Federation of Cardiology Task Force. JAMA 1992;268(13):1727–1733.

Stein PD, Saltzman HA, Weg J: Clinical characteristics of patients with acute pulmonary embolism. Am J Cardiol 1991;68:1723–1724.

2.5 ASTHMA

Description

Asthma is defined as a respiratory disease characterized by airway hyperresponsiveness to a variety of stimuli (inhaled allergens, environmental irritants, respiratory infections, aspirin, cold air, exercise, emotional distress), manifesting in airway obstruction. Airway narrowing arises from a number of causes, including a reduction in airway caliber by bronchial smooth muscle contraction, mucus plugging, and inflammatory-mediated airway and mucosal edema. The prevalence, morbidity, and mortality of asthma in the United States and other industrialized nations have risen sharply over the past 20 years (see Table 2.5.1).

History

The classic triad of asthma is *wheezing, coughing,* and *dyspnea.* Chest tightness is also a frequent complaint. Nevertheless, remember "all that wheezes is not asthma, and all asthma does not wheeze" (coughing and dyspnea may occur without wheezing). Consider other conditions that may present with wheezing as the principal complaint (CHF, pulmonary embolus, allergic reaction, foreign body obstruction), especially in patients with a new onset of wheezing who have no prior history of asthma. Symptoms tend to be worse at night. A history focused on the airway disease should be elicited as patients are being treated, trying to

Table 2.5.1
Emergency Department Indices of Severe Asthma in Adults

Symptoms and historical data	Severe breathlessness
	Difficulty walking > 100 feet
	Speech fragmented by rapid breathing
	Syncope or near syncope
Physical findings	Accessory muscle recruitment
	Diaphoresis
	Inability to lay supine
	Heart rate > 130 bpm
	Respiratory rate > 30 breaths/min
PEFR	Initial < 30% of predicted or personal best
	Failure to improve at least 15% after initial treatment
Oxygenation	$Pao_2 < 60$ mm Hg
	Pao_2 saturation < 90%
Ventilation	$Paco_2 \geq 40$ mm Hg

allow the patient to answer questions with nods and head movements. Points to cover include the following.

- Previous history of intubation;
- Steroid use or dependency;
- Present medications and compliance;
- Onset and duration of the current attack;
- Comparison to previous attacks (is this attack like the patient's worst attack?);
- Recent patterns of ED visits and hospitalizations;
- Precipitating factors, upper respiratory symptoms, fever, cough, smoke or chemical exposure, or change in the weather (especially abrupt changes in temperature and humidity);
- The patient's best or normal peak flow; and
- Other contributing past medical history (cardiac, neurologic, immune system status) as well as history of allergies.

Physical Examination

General. Note the general appearance and positioning of the patient (alert, agitated, in extremis). Establish the patient's ability to speak (sentences, phrases, words, or unable to talk). Sweating implies severe distress.

Vital signs. Obtain a full set, including temperature (rectal is best) and pulsus paradoxus. Tachypnea may precede wheezing. Tachycardia (> 130 bpm) in adults signals a severe asthma attack. Patients with moderate to severe asthma may experience transient hypertension (hypotension is ominous).

HEENT. Check the oropharynx and sinuses for infection.

Neck. Listen for stridor and observe for accessory muscle recruitment (supraclavicular, sternocleidomastoid). Confirm the position of the trachea and document any neck vein distention. Palpate the neck area for crepitus.

Lungs. Examine for labored breathing patterns—particularly paradoxical movement of abdominal musculature characterized by a rocking or an alternating breathing pattern between the chest and abdominal musculature (paradoxical movement)—respiratory rate, amount of air entry, expiratory:inspiratory ratio, and use of intercostal muscles. Note any asymmetry of breath sounds (atelectasis, pneumothorax). Determine the presence, location, and severity of wheezing. Remember, tight asthmatics may be too constricted to move enough air to cause audible wheezing *("beware the silent chest")*.

Heart. Note changes in rate and rhythm, murmurs, and gallops.

Abdomen. Look for use of abdominal muscles.

Extremities. Check for cyanosis, clubbing, or edema.

Diagnostic Tests

Peak expiratory flow rate measurement (PEFR). Pulmonary function is best measured with spirometry; however, it is often unavailable in the ED. PEFR provides a simple, quantitative, reproducible assessment of airway obstruction. The major drawback to PEFR is that it is effort dependent. While expected normal values are contingent on gender, age, and height, PEFRs of < 120 L/min, or < 30% of predicted value, imply a severe asthmatic episode. Check PEFR after every treatment; a 15% increase represents a significant improvement.

Pulse oximetry. Readings below 94% require supplemental oxygen and arterial blood gas analysis.

ABG. Indicated in patients with mental status changes, signs of severe asthma, saturation < 94% on pulse oximetry, and/or lack of improvement after 30 to 60 min of aggressive therapy. While not a sensitive indicator of severity of airway obstruction, ABGs do provide the an optimum gauge of severity of hypercapnia, hypoxemia, and acid-base status. A normal or elevated

$PaCO_2$ along with a falling pH implies that the patient is tiring and may signal impending respiratory collapse.

CBC. WBC count may be elevated from stress, medications (steroids, β-agonists), or infection (look for left shift). Eosinophilia is associated with allergic disorders.

ECG. Obtain in older patients or those asthmatics with a heart rate > 130 bpm, irregular pulse, chest pain, or a history of cardiac disease.

CXR. Not indicated unless asthma is severe or an underlying disorder (pneumothorax, CHF, foreign body, pneumonia) is suspected.

Sputum Gram stain. May be helpful in assessing for bacterial infection (see section 9.2). Characteristic findings for asthma include presence of *Curshmann's spirals, Charcot-Leyden crystals,* and eosinophils.

Theophylline level. Order after bolus loading or before administering additional theophylline to patients claiming to take theophylline.

Special Considerations

Pregnancy

Asthma is one of the most common illnesses complicating pregnancy. Occurrence and severity of attacks in asthma may increase (33%), decrease (33%), or continue unchanged (33%). However, all asthma attacks in pregnancy must be treated aggressively to prevent both maternal and fetal complications. Generally, "what is good for the mother is good for the fetus." It is essential to maintain the mother's normal oxygenation (keep the oxygen saturation > 95%), since slight decreases in maternal PaO_2 can profoundly alter fetal oxygen saturation (the fetus functions as a built-in pulse oximeter); and fetal monitoring may be necessary during severe exacerbations. The preferred pharmacologic regimen is β-agonists (inhalation delivers the drug directly to the airway in high concentrations, while minimizing systemic side effects), especially terbutaline. Use systemic corticosteroids (studies demonstrate relative safety in pregnancy) when inhaled medications are not sufficient. Theophylline is generally considered safe in pregnancy and may be beneficial for controlling nocturnal asthma. Employ a lower threshold for admission when caring for pregnant asthmatics and consult with OB-GYN.

Status Asthmaticus

Asthmatics who deteriorate (worsening mental status, cyanosis, apnea, exhaustion) despite aggressive treatment and reveal a rising $PaCO_2$ ($\geq$ 50 mm Hg) obligate *intubation* with *mechanical ventilation.* Prepare for problems when attempting to intubate and ventilate this group of patients. Orotracheal intubation is the preferred route (allows use of a larger endotracheal tube); have pharmacologic agents at hand to perform *rapid sequence induction,* if necessary (see section 21.8). However, do not administer sedatives or hypnotics to acute asthmatics who are not intubated. *Ketamine* (1 to 2 mg/kg) is favored by some specialists as an induction agent for intubation, because of its bronchodilating properties and lack of effect on blood pressure. Intubated patients may become agitated and unable to cooperate with assisted ventilation, forcing use of paralytics (*succinylcholine,* 1.5 mg/kg; *pancuronium,* 0.10 mg/kg; or *vecuronium,* 0.8 to 0.1 mg/kg). A continuous infusion of vecuronium (1 μg/kg/min) or pancuronium (1 μg/kg/min) may be necessary.

Mechanically ventilated asthmatics are susceptible to barotrauma (high peak airway pressures) as well as to the development of auto-PEEP (air trapping). Employ the concept of "mechanically controlled hypoventilation" (permissive hypercapnia), using a *volume-cycled ventilator,* together with slower than normal rates (6 to 10 ventilation/min), lower tidal volumes, longer expiratory times, and peak airway pressures < 50 cm H_2O. The goal of mechanical ventilation is not to restore a normal arterial $PaCO_2$ immediately but instead to allow the $PaCO_2$ to correct gradually as underlying airflow obstruction resolves. If necessary, sodium bicarbonate can be given intravenously to correct the acidosis. Beta-agonists can be nebulized in line into the inspiratory circuit of the ventilator. Close monitoring (heart rate, blood pressure, oxygenation) is mandatory in the intubated asthmatic.

Treatment

Patients with a history of intubation, steroid dependence, labile asthma, recent increase in ED visits, or persistent attacks despite compliance with medications are at high risk for severe decompensation and should be *treated aggressively, observed closely,* and *admitted early.* The goal of treatment of an acute exacerbation of asthma is to reverse bronchospasm, remove airway obstruction, improve the flow of air, and correct significant hypoxia. Comprehensive therapy frequently requires treatment with multiple medications, depending on the severity of the asthma and the response to initial therapy. Moreover, aggressive recognition and management of complications (pneumothorax, pneumomediastinum, subcutaneous emphysema, electrolyte abnormalities, dehydration, dysrhythmias, theophylline toxicity) are imperative.

Primary or first-line agents in the treatment of asthma include *oxygen, inhaled* β-agonists, and *corticosteroids*. Supplemental therapy includes *parenteral* β-agonists, methylxanthines, magnesium, anticholinergics, and *intubation*.

Oxygen

Ensuring adequate oxygenation is the highest priority in asthma. Not only is oxygen beneficial in severe asthma because of likely accompanying hypoxia but β-agonists may exacerbate $\dot{V}/\dot{Q}$ mismatches and cause an aggravation of hypoxia.

Inhaled Beta-Agonists

Beta-agonists are the medication of choice for acute exacerbations of asthma. Onset of action is usually within 5 min. Continuous nebulizer treatments may be given until a clinical response or improvement in peak flow values is seen. If the cardiac (tachycardia, dysrhythmias), gastrointestinal (nausea, vomiting), or neurologic (tremor) side effects become intolerable, the nebulizer treatments can be diluted or spaced at greater intervals. Typical dosages are *albuterol* (2.5 mg or 0.5 mL in 2.5 mL NS) or *metaproterenol* (15 mg or 0.3 mL in 2.5 mL NS q 20 min). An MDI with a spacer (1 puff q 1 to 5 min) and proper instruction may be just as effective as nebulized treatments.

Corticosteroids

Recent guidelines encourage more liberal use of corticosteroids —potent medications in the treatment of asthma (especially for patients with a long duration of symptoms before presentation, history of chronic steroid use or recent suspension of steroid therapy, frequent ED visits, and patients requiring intubation in the past). Although aerosolized steroids are effective in the outpatient setting, intravenous or oral steroids ought to be used for acute exacerbations. In patients with severe asthma, give methylprednisolone 125 mg IV initially followed by 60 to 80 mg q 6 hr IV. In patients with less severe symptoms, give 60 mg PO of prednisone and follow it with a 7- to 10-day course.

Parenteral Beta-Agonists

Subcutaneous epinephrine may be given as 0.3 mL of 1:1000 solution SQ q 20 min to a total of three doses accompanied by constant monitoring of blood pressure and cardiac rhythm. Although general safety has been established, use subcutaneous epinephrine cautiously in elderly patients and those with a history of CAD. *Subcutaneous terbutaline* is administered in a dose of 0.25 mg q 45 min.

Inhaled Anticholinergics

While not as effective in patients with asthma as in those with COPD, anticholinergic agents may provide additional bronchodilation when combined with nebulized β-agonists. *Ipratropium* (500 μg via nebulizer or 2 puffs via a MDI) is the preferred anticholinergic, with *atropine* (1 mg nebulized) and *glycopyrrolate* (0.2 mg nebulized) serving as possible alternatives.

Methylzanthines

Once a mainstay in the treatment of asthma, the use of methylxanthines *(aminophylline, theophylline)* for acute asthma is now being contested, and these are no longer considered to be primary drugs. The loading dose is 6 mg/kg IV or PO based on lean body weight, with maintenance infusions of 0.5 to 0.9 μg/kg/hr. Attempt to achieve a serum concentration in range of 10 to 20 mg/mL.

Magnesium

Both aerosolized magnesium (100 to 200 mg nebulized) and intravenous magnesium (2 g over 20 min) may provide transient, additional bronchodilation, especially in patients with severe attacks. The main side effects are hypotension, malaise, and a feeling of warmth.

Intravenous Fluids

Routine use of intravenous fluids is not recommended unless there are clinical signs of dehydration or the patient cannot take orally. Overzealous hydration can be detrimental.

Admission Criteria

Disposition decisions for asthma patients need to be individualized and based on a patient's past medical history and response to therapy. The ED physician should have a lower threshold for admission of pregnant asthmatics, patients on chronic steroid therapy, patients with a history of intubation or CO_2 retention, and the elderly. *The following patients ought to be admitted:*

- Patients treated aggressively for 4 hr without clinical improvement;
- Failure of PEFRs to reach 70% of predicted or normal baseline values;
- Patients with a $P_{CO_2} > 40$ mm Hg who do not chronically retain CO_2;
- Recent increase in frequency of ED visits for asthma;
- Recent discharge from hospital for asthma;
- Patients with angina, arrhythmias, or ischemia on ECG;
- Theophylline toxicity; and
- Patients with such complications as pneumonia, pneumothorax, atelectasis.

Suggested Readings

National Asthma Education Program: Management of asthma during pregnancy, Publication no. 93–3279A. Bethesda, MD: National Institutes of Health, 1993.

National Heart, Lung, and Blood Institute: International consensus report on diagnosis and treatment of asthma, Publication no. 92–3091. Bethesda, MD: National Institutes of Health, 1992.

Rudnitsky GS, Eberlein RS, Schoffstall JM, et al.: Comparison of intermittent and continuously nebulized albuterol for treatment of asthma in an urban emergency department. Ann Emerg Med 1993;22: 1842–1846.

2.6 SPONTANEOUS PNEUMOTHORAX

Description

A pneumothorax arises from accumulation of air in the pleural space and is designated as either *spontaneous* or *traumatic* (see section 4.4). Spontaneous pneumothorax can be further classified into *primary* (occurs in the absence of underlying disease and is five times more common in males) or *secondary* (a complication of preexisting disorder). A *tension pneumothorax* (pressure in the pleural space exceeds lung pressure leading to hemodynamic and respiratory compromise) is more frequently associated with a traumatic pneumothorax. There is a 50% recurrence rate of spontaneous pneumothorax (usually on the ipsilateral side).

Consider the possibility of a pneumothorax in any critically ill patient who suddenly develops dyspnea, chest pain, and/or hypoxia (especially patients on mechanical ventilators).

History

Dyspnea and *chest pain* are the most common symptoms, usually localized to the affected side. Patients may be acutely ill or may not seek medical attention for days. It is important to obtain a history of previous pneumothorax, respiratory disorders (asthma, COPD, cystic fibrosis, TB, pneumocystosis pneumonia), smoking, and menstrual history (catamenial pneumothorax).

Physical Examination

Note: *If the pneumothorax is small, physical findings may be unimpressive.*

General. Patients of thin, tall body habitus are more prone to spontaneous pneumothorax.

Vital signs. Check for tachycardia, tachypnea, and hypotension.

Neck. Examine for tracheal deviation (tension pneumothorax), distended neck veins, and tactile fremitus.

Lungs. Inspect the chest wall. Palpate for local tenderness or crepitus (rib fractures). The collapsed side will have diminished breath sounds, decreased tactile fremitus, and increased percussion resonance (especially with large or tension pneumothorax). In hydropneumothorax, a succussion splash may be elicited.

Diagnostic Tests

X-rays. A CRX should always be obtained if lung collapse is suspected. End-expiratory films are advantageous in detecting a small pneumothorax (visceral-pleural line). In the supine patient, look for abnormally radiolucent costophrenic sulcus (deep sulcus sign).

ABG. Due to ventilation/perfusion mismatching, patients with pneumothorax will initially demonstrate some degree of hypoxia on blood gas. After several hours, perfusion of the affected lung decreases, which leads to improvement in the ventilation:perfusion ratio and some resolution of hypoxia.

Treatment

The treatment of a spontaneous pneumothorax depends on its magnitude, the presence of underlying disorders, and the history of previous pneumothorax. In stable patients tolerating a spontaneous pneumothorax that is < 25% of the apparent lung volume, hospitalization for bed rest and serial chest films may be sufficient. About 1% of the normal lung volume will be reabsorbed daily. Supplemental oxygen may be of value (decreases alveolar nitrogen concentration gradient).

Tube thoracostomy is the treatment of choice in patients with pulmonary or other serious disease, pneumothoraces that are > 25%, recurrent pneumothorax, pneumothoraces associated with trauma, and pneumothoraces occurring in mechanically ventilated patients (advance to tension pneumothorax may be swift in positive-pressure ventilated patients). Small size chest tubes (approximately 16 gauge) are usually as effective as larger tubes in the treatment of uncomplicated pneumothoraces and allow ambulation when combined with a Heimlich valve.

Surgery or *chemical pleurodesis* may be indicated for recurrent spontaneous pneumothorax.

Suspicion of a *tension pneumothorax* mandates emergent treatment: the insertion of a large-bore needle or catheter into the pleural cavity of the affected side in the second intercostal space along the midclavicular line to relieve the pressure. Subsequent management requires a chest tube thoracostomy (see section 21.2).

Admission Criteria

Virtually all *patients with pneumothorax* should be admitted after appropriate therapy is instituted in the emergency department. *Healthy patients with small pneumothoraces* usually require observation for a day or two in the hospital. Order repeat chest films after treatment to follow resolution.

Suggested Readings

Engdahl O, Toft T, Boe J: Chest radiograph—a poor method for determining the size of a pneumothorax. Chest 1993;103(1):26–29.

Light RW: Management of spontaneous pneumothorax. Am Rev Respir Dis 1993;148:245–248.

Chapter 3

Neurology

3.1 COMA AND ALTERED MENTAL STATUS

Description

A diminished level of consciousness occurs when either both cerebral hemispheres are affected or there is a suppression of the brainstem reticular activating system (RAS). *Mental status* is the most sensitive barometer of a CNS disturbance. It is important to use universally understood terminology when describing the degree of unresponsiveness: *Coma* represents the most extreme deviation from a "normal" state of consciousness and is characterized by a state of unresponsiveness to both verbal and physical stimuli. *Stupor* refers to a condition in which the patient responds to noxious physical stimuli but not to verbal stimuli; speech should elicit a reply from a *drowsy* patient; while a patient who is *alert and oriented* is aware of himself or herself and interacts appropriately with the environment.

Coma and altered mental state can result from many etiologies. A simplified approach is to divide the causes into those that are due to *structural disease* (hemorrhage, infarct, tumor) and those that are of *metabolic* or *toxin* origin. A focal neurologic deficit arises from a structural disorder, which can be further subdivided into *supratentorial* and *subtentorial* disturbances. Supratentorial focal lesions (subdural hematomas, epidural hematomas, subdural empyema, cerebral neoplasm, CVA) can deteriorate in an orderly rostral-caudal fashion, where pressure placed on the cortex is directed to the brainstem or temporal lobe, resulting in a *central* or *uncal herniation*. Clinically, a third nerve palsy appears on the side of the lesion, followed by ptosis and pupillary dilation. Next, depression in the level of consciousness ensues, accompanied by either a contralateral (the classical scenario) or ipsilateral (10% of cases) hemiplegia. Subtentorial compression arises from disorders that directly affect the brainstem (brainstem tumors, pontine hemorrhage) or from lesions that place pressure on the brainstem (acute cerebellar hemorrhage). Subtentorial compression tends to exhibit an abrupt onset, accompanied by symmetric neurologic deficits and either pinpoint pupils or conjugate deviation of gaze.

In the ED, toxins or metabolic disorders account for the majority of cases (more than two-thirds) of coma and altered mental state. Typically, toxins and metabolic disorders display a gradual onset, while preserving normal pupil reactivity.

Although there is an exhaustive differential diagnosis for causes of coma and altered mental state, the following mnemonic may help: "TIPPS on vowels."

TIPPS
T = Trauma, Tumor, Temperature
I = Infection (both CNS and systemic)
P = Psychiatric, Porphyria
P = Poison
S = Space occupying lesions, Stroke, Shock, Subarachnoid hemorrhage, Seizure

Vowels
A = Alcohol
E = Endocrine, Exocrine, Electrolytes
I = Insulin (diabetes)
O = Oxygen (lack of), Opiates
U = Uremia (renal disease)

History

The history often must be obtained from sources other than the patient (ambulance personnel, bystanders, family members, friends, coworkers). Find out the particulars preceding the change in mental state. How was the patient behaving before arrival? Did the patient express any recent symptoms or worries? Were there any abnormal motor movements? Does anyone else at home have a similar problem? When was the patient last seen in his or her usual state of health? Did this alteration in mental state happen abruptly or has there been a gradual decline (an altered mental state secondary to a vascular insult occurs almost instantaneously [seconds to minutes], whereas coma secondary to metabolic causes takes place over minutes to hours and that from infection or tumor transpires over days to weeks)? Specific inquiries should also cover any history of trauma, recent illness, depression, medication usage, possible food or drug ingestion, and the environmental conditions in which the patient was found. Ask about preexisting conditions that might explain the patient's current mental state (diabetes, renal failure, chronic liver disease, seizure disorder, alcohol, other substance abuse) and whether this has happened before. Also inquire about presence of systemic symptoms—fever, chills, chest pain, nausea or vomiting, and weight loss. Additional sources of information include a patient's personal effects, such as a Medic Alert bracelet, wallet, suicide note, and/or pill containers. Old medical records should be obtained if possible.

Physical Examination

Note: *History, physical exam, and treatment are frequently performed simultaneously.*

General. Determine if the patient looks well, distressed, or critical.

Vital signs. Respiration, pulse, and blood pressure are regulated by the medulla, hence check all vital signs carefully. Assess core temperature to rule out hyperthermia or hypothermia.

Skin. Note skin turgor and presence of cyanosis, rashes, or jaundice.

HEENT. Examine for skull and facial trauma. Check extraocular movements (Table 3.1.1) and pupil size and reactivity (if pupils remain equal and reactive midbrain is intact).

Neck. Check for stiffness, thyroid size, and jugular venous distention.

Lungs. Listen for equality of breath sounds and for presence of rales, wheezes, and rhonchi.

Heart. Auscultate for rhythm, rate, and occurrence of murmurs or gallops.

Abdomen. Listen for bowel sounds and note distention, rigidity, organomegaly, ascites, or presence of a pulsatile mass.

Rectal. Check for rectal tone. Test stool for occult blood.

Extremities. Note edema, bruising, or track marks.

Neurologic. Search for focal neurologic findings (including asymmetric deep tendon reflexes, unilateral flaccidity, spasticity, or weakness) and upper motor signs (Babinski's reflex).

Table 3.1.1
Extraocular Movements in Coma[a]

Doll's head phenomenon	
Eyes gaze ahead despite head turning	Cortical dysfunction
No eye movement	Brainstem dysfunction
Roving gaze	Suggests metabolic cause
Oculovestibular calorics (cold water instilled into one ear canal with head raised 30°)	
Eyes deviate toward side of stimulation	Brainstem intact
With corrective nystagmus	Cortex intact
Without corrective nystagmus	Cortex depressed

[a]Adapted from Edwards FJ: Evaluation and management of coma. AAPA Recertification Update 1992;3(2):11.

Examination must be repeated frequently to detect any change or deterioration. The Glasgow Coma Scale can be valuable in this setting (see section 4.2). Note presence or absence of spontaneous movements as well as *decorticate posturing* (arms and elbows flexed, legs extended) or *decerebrate posturing* (arms and legs extended, teeth clenched).

Diagnostic Tests

Fingerstick glucose. Obtain immediately to rule out hypoglycemic coma.

SMA. Obtain serum electrolytes, calcium, magnesium, blood urea nitrogen, creatinine, blood glucose, and liver function tests when indicated.

CBC. Check the hematocrit, white blood cell count with differential, and platelet count.

Urinalysis. Check for glucose, ketones, and blood.

ABG. Assess oxygenation and ventilation. Check for hypoxia, hypercapnia, or acid-base disorder.

PT/PTT. Obtain to rule out coagulopathy.

Cultures of blood and urine. Indicated when infection or sepsis is suspected.

Serum alcohol and drug levels. Toxicology screen and specific drug levels (e.g., digoxin, phenytoin, phenobarbital, salicylates, and acetaminophen) should be obtained as indicated.

ECG. May reflect metabolic abnormalities or display nonspecific changes occurring with intracranial disorders or ischemia.

Pulse oximetry. Quickly assesses oxygen saturation.

CT scan or MRI of the head. For identification of intracranial hemorrhage, infarct, abscess, edema, or tumor.

Lumbar puncture. A lumbar puncture is necessary to make the diagnosis of meningitis and may confirm the diagnosis of hemorrhage. **Warning:** *Contraindicated when the intracranial pressure is elevated.* In this situation, obtain a CT scan of the head before performing the LP. If meningitis is suspected, obtain blood cultures and administer antibiotics before obtaining the CT scan.

Treatment

Whatever the origin of coma or altered mental status, the initial management goals is the same—stabilization, identification of reversible causes, and prevention of further brain injury. Treatment often takes place concurrently with assessment, starting with the standard *ABC* approach: securing the airway and ensuring adequate breathing (ventilation) and cardiac output, and protecting against potential cervical spine (C-spine) injury (see section 4.3). For the patient with an altered mental status or who is comatose the mnemonic *ABC* can be supplemented with *DEFG:* *d*isrobe and look for *d*isabilities or *d*eficits and *e*xamine *f*or *g*lucose. When blood sugar levels cannot be rapidly determined, give dextrose empirically.

Thiamine (100 mg IVp) should be provided for patients prone to malnourishment, such as alcoholics, anorectics, and cancer patients. Empiric naloxone administration is indicated in cases suspicious for narcotic overdose. Timely neurosurgical consultation is essential for any patient suspected of harboring a structural lesion. Once the patient is stabilized, definitive specific therapy is based on postulated etiology.

Admission Criteria

Patients who present with coma generally require admission. Possible exceptions include psychogenic coma patients (after evaluation by a psychiatrist), stable insulin-dependent diabetics with hypoglycemia that rapidly responds to therapy, postictal patients with known seizure disorder (see section 3.2), and certain opiate ODs (see section 7.2).

Suggested Readings

Alguire PC: Rapid evaluation of comatose patients. Postgrad Med 1990; 87(6):223–230.

Bates D: The management of medical coma. J Neurol Neurosurg Psych 1993;56:589–601.

3.2 SEIZURES

Description

A seizure is a paroxysmal alteration in neurologic function due to a sudden, excessive, and temporary discharge of cerebral neurons. *Epilepsy* is a syndrome of unprovoked, recurrent seizures. Seizures may be idiopathic or associated with a precipitating factor.

Seizures are classified as either *generalized* or p*artial* (affecting only part of the brain), based on the clinical and EEG localization of seizure activity. In primary generalized seizures, both cerebral hemispheres display a lack of focal activity and there is an absence of a prodromal aura. Types of generalized seizures include *absence* (petit mal), *myoclonic, tonic, atonic, generalized tonic-clonic,* and *grand mal.* Grand mal seizures are characterized by a loss of consciousness that is preceded by tonic rigidity, apnea, and cyanosis, which progress to clonic jerking, tongue biting, eye deviation, and urinary incontinence. Generalized tonic-clonic seizures culminate with flaccidity and coma, which may be accompanied by Babinski's sign and dilated pupils. Postictally, the patient experiences confusion, headache, and sleepiness.

Manifestations of *partial* (focal) seizures are contingent on the area of the brain involved. They are preceded by an *aura* and comprise focal motor symptoms that may spread or "march" (Jacksonian); in other instances, the patient may display psychic (déjà vu, dreamy states, structured hallucinations), autonomic (pallor, sweating, flushing), or somatosensory (epigastric sensations, tingling, light flashes) symptoms. Complex partial seizures are accompanied by an altered sensorium; while in simple partial seizures, consciousness is not impaired. Most grand mal seizures in adults result from a partial seizure that undergoes secondary generalization. Partial seizures are often due to local pathology (trauma, tumor, vascular lesions, congenital abnormalities) but can occur with a metabolic imbalance (hypoglycemia, hyperglycemia, uremia, hepatic failure).

Seizures that start in adolescence are usually idiopathic, but may arise from trauma or drugs. First-time seizures in young adulthood are probably due to trauma, alcohol or drug use, metabolic disorders, or neoplasm. Seizures that begin in middle age are often due to neoplasm, alcohol use, vascular disease, or trauma. Late life seizures tend to originate from cerebrovascular disease, neoplasm, or trauma.

History

Find a witness who is able to describe the seizure activity—laypersons' ideas of what constitutes a seizure are remarkably divergent. Significant historical information includes the behavior preceding the onset of the seizure (automatisms such as blank smiling, lip smacking), the appearance of focal features (deviation of the eyes and head), a fall in which the patient struck his or her head, an episode of loss of consciousness, any ensuing incontinence, and the duration of the seizure activity. Also ask if there was more than one seizure.

Try to establish if there is a prior history of seizures. For first-time seizures, determine if the patient has experienced new neurologic disturbances (headaches, disorders of vision, gait, hearing, sensory, or motor function), neurologic insults (trauma, CVA), or infectious illnesses. Consider the possibility of intoxication with prescription drugs (tricyclic, theophylline, isoniazid, phenothiazines, oral hypoglycemics, lithium), drug interactions, allergic reactions, and illicit use of drugs (cocaine, amphetamines, heroin cut with strychnine) as well as the cessation from alcohol or drug use. Ask about recent environmental stresses (sleep deprivation, heat stroke). Seek clues to disorders that could precipitate or mimic seizure activity—cardiac disease, endocrine and metabolic disorders (particularly diabetes), renal disease, history of cancer or AIDS, and in females consider the possibility of eclampsia.

If there is a known seizure history, verify age of onset, type and frequency of seizures, previous workup, and current medications (note compliance and dosages) as well as change in pattern of seizure activity.

Physical Examination

Note: *There are two reasons for the physical examination: (1) to help determine the etiology of the seizure and (2) to learn if any secondary injury has occurred.*

General. Note level of consciousness. Check for urinary or fecal incontinence. Remark about any developmental asymmetries.

Vital signs. Note temperature (low-grade fever may occur with seizures but usually resolves within 4 hr). Both tachycardia and blood pressure elevations are common with seizure activity.

Skin. Check for lesions associated with neurocutaneous disorders (Lisch nodules, café au lait spots, etc.) as well as presence of jaundice, cyanosis, ecchymosis, diaphoresis, petechiae/purpura, or track marks.

HEENT. Examine for signs of head trauma. Document pupil size and reactivity as well as the sharpness of the optic disk margins, presence of venous pulsations, and fullness of extraocular movements. Check the oral cavity for tongue lacerations and gingival hypertrophy (phenytoin).

Neck. Immobilize the C-spine if neck trauma is being considered. After the C-spine has been cleared, examine for meningeal irritation.

Lungs. Auscultate for rales, rhonchi, and rubs (aspiration is a common complication of seizures).

Heart. Listen for irregularity (dysrhythmias), murmurs, and gallops.

Extremities. Examine for musculoskeletal swelling, ecchymosis, deformity, tenderness and crepitus. *Seizures are the most common cause of posterior dislocations of the shoulder.*

Neurologic. Check for focal neurologic deficits. Transitory (lasting minutes to hours), localized weakness and/or paralysis may take place immediately after a seizure *(Todd's paralysis)*. Documentation is vital to detect changes over time.

Differential Diagnosis

Complicated migraine headaches;
Hyperventilation syndrome;
Vertigo;
Syncope (cardiogenic, vasovagal);
Cardiac dysrhythmias; and
Pseudo-seizures.

Diagnostic Tests

Note: *Diagnostic tests are used to support the diagnosis and exclude complications and should be guided by the medical history and physical find-*

ings. Routine ordering of laboratory studies has a low yield, particularly in patients with a prior history of seizures. Patients who are noncompliant with medications may need only a measurement of anticonvulsant levels and a fingerstick glucose.

Fingerstick glucose. Obtain immediately.

SMA. Note serum sodium (hyponatremia) and calcium (hypocalcemia). An anion gap acidosis may accompany generalized seizures. Check for hyperglycemia.

CBC. Check the WBC count when infection is suspected (an elevated white count can occur with a generalized seizure, but a left shift suggests infection).

ABG. Indicated if clinical hypoxia, carbon monoxide exposure, or a metabolic disturbance is suspected.

Toxicologies. When appropriate, check for cocaine and additional specific drug levels as indicated.

Anticonvulsant drug levels. Check drug levels when the patient has a known seizure disorder and is on medication.

CT scan or MRI. Should be done as soon as possible for first-time seizures, evidence of focal neurologic findings, or signs of increased intracranial pressure.

ECG and/or monitor. Necessary when underlying ischemia, dysrhythmia, or hemodynamic instability is considered.

X-rays. The need for a chest x-ray, cervical spine films, and extremity radiographs is determined by the history and physical examination.

Lumbar puncture. Indicated if infection or subarachnoid hemorrhage is suspected and there is no evidence of increased intracranial pressure.

Special Considerations

Status epilepticus (SE) is defined as greater than 30 min of seizure activity, either a single continuous seizure or two or more sequential seizures without a full recovery of consciousness between seizures. Beyond 30 min, damage to neurons begins. Repetitive generalized convulsive status epilepticus is the most prevalent and most serious form of status epilepticus.

Treatment

For patients no longer seizing, immediate medications are not required. Patients ought to be placed in the left lateral decubitus position, protected against self-injury (keep the side rails up, remove constrictive clothing and dentures); suctioned; and given supplemental oxygen as needed. One should refrain from "jamming" objects in a patient's mouth if the patient can protect his or her airway. Generally, it is a good idea to establish intravenous access (a "life line"). Most grand mal seizures last only 2 to 5 min. Specific therapy is predicated on the clinical situation. Life-threatening causes of seizure that mandate immediate action include *hypoglycemia, hypoxia, cardiac dysrhythmia, toxicological overdoses, meningitis, encephalitis, sepsis,* and *eclampsia.*

For patients in status epilepticus, first ensure an adequate airway (insert a *nasal* or *oral airway* if necessary) and provide supplemental oxygen (mask or bag-valve-mask ventilator). If respiratory difficulty persists, consider endotracheal intubation. It may be necessary to administer an anticonvulsant drug to facilitate intubation (a benzodiazepine like lorazepam or diazepam is the drug of choice). Gain intravenous access and administer thiamine (100 mg IV), followed by 1 amp of D_{50} IVp for hypoglycemic, alcoholic, malnourished patients or for patients in whom a rapid glucose level cannot be determined within 5 min. Place the patient on a cardiac monitor and frequently assess the vital signs (especially after infusion of medications).

No single medication possesses all the desired properties necessary to treat SE. Since time is of the essence, *benzodiazepines* are the conventional first choice. *Diazepam* is administered at 5 mg/min IV, up to 0.2 mg/kg. *Lorazepam* (0.1 mg/kg IV at 2 mg/min up to 8 mg), a benzodiazepine with a longer duration of action, is an alternative. Finally, *midazolam* (0.1 to 0.3 mg/kg IV bolus) may be employed.

If seizures fail to terminate within 20 min of benzodiazepine therapy, give *phenytoin* (which is incompatible with glucose-containing solutions). Some physicians elect to administer phenytoin concomitantly with diazepam therapy through a separate line to prevent recurrent status. The initial loading dose of phenytoin is 18 mg/kg, at a rate *not* to exceed 50 mg/min. Give cautiously, as phenytoin may precipitate hypotension, especially in older patients and those with preexisting cardiac disease. Repeated infusions can be given up to a maximum of 30 mg/kg.

If the aforementioned regimen fails to control seizures, intubation is mandated (if not already accomplished). Next, employ a trial of *phenobarbital,* infused at a rate not to exceed 100 mg/min to a total of 20 mg/kg.

If seizures still persist, options include more *phenobarbital, pentobarbital,* continuous *midazolam* infusion (0.9 to 11.0 μg/kg/hr), *lidocaine* (1 mg/kg IV followed by an infusion of 2 to 4 mg/min), or other modes of *general anesthesia.* At this point, the patient has been in status for more than 1 hr, so a neurologist, anesthesiologist, and/or intensivist ought to be involved in the patient's care. The patient requires continual EEG monitoring at this stage.

Admission Criteria

Patients generally obligating admission include *those in status epilepticus, patients with persistent fever or disorientation, patients whose seizure results from serious illness or head injury, and seizures that are a consequence of drug ingestion or withdrawal.* Discuss the care of the first-time seizure patient with a consultant (admission is often based on the patient's age, reliability, and support systems).

Note: *Any patient discharged should be cautioned about ongoing physical activities;* patients with seizures potentially present a risk to themselves and to others. All states have prerequisites regarding driving privileges for patients with seizures.

Suggested Readings

American College of Emergency Physicians: Clinical policy for the initial approach to patients presenting with a chief complaint of seizures who are not in status epilepticus. Ann Emerg Med 1993;22:875–883.

Henneman PL, DeRoss F, Lewis RJ: Determining the need for admission in patients with new-onset seizures. Ann Emerg Med 1994;24:1108–1114.

Working Group on Status Epilepticus: Treatment of convulsive status epilepticus. JAMA 1993;270:854–859.

3.3 CEREBROVASCULAR DISEASE

Description

Cerebrovascular disease is the third leading cause of death in the United States and arises from either occlusion or hemorrhage of the cerebral circulation. "Brain attacks" may cause a temporary focal neurologic disturbance—*transient ischemic attacks* (TIAs)—that resolves within 24 hr (usually lasting < 1 to 2 hr) or result in permanent disability, in which case they are referred to as a *cerebrovascular accident* (CVA) or *stroke.* The four major types of strokes are *thrombotic, embolic, lacunar,* and *hemorrhagic.* Cerebral infarction results from occlusion of an intracerebral blood vessel or blockage of blood flow by an embolus arising outside the CNS and accounts for 80% of CVAs. Hemorrhagic strokes are a consequence of an *intracerebral hemorrhage* or *subarachnoid hemorrhage* (SAH).

A *stroke in evolution* refers to a CVA that progresses over hours to days. A *completed stroke* implies presence of an irreversible, pale, nonhemorrhagic infarct.

Expeditious evaluation is imperative to prevent complications and extension of injury. *Only one-third of stroke patients present in the first 24 hr!*

History

Consider the possibility of TIA or CVA in any patient presenting with an acute neurologic deficit or altered mental status. The exact clinical profile is highly variable and depends on both the type of stroke (*thrombotic* versus *hemorrhagic*) and area of brain affected. Hemiparesis, aphasia, and cognitive impairment suggest involvement of the internal carotid artery and its branches, while findings associated with disturbances of the vertebrobasilar circulation include "the five D's": dysarthria, dysphagia, dysesthesia, diplopia, and dizziness (vertigo). Headache is more common with large vessel occlusion and cerebral hemorrhage. Abruptness and time of onset assist in distinguishing the type of stroke. In addition, ask about antecedent warning symptoms (headache, TIA, visual disturbance).

The single strongest risk factor for stroke is age (70% of strokes occur after the age of 65), followed by hypertension. However, especially in younger adults with a CVA, pursue risk factors such as alcohol, smoking, drug abuse (particularly cocaine and amphetamines), use of oral contraceptives or anticoagulants, history of MI, mitral valve disease (including mitral valve prolapse), atrial fibrillation, patent foramen ovale (paradoxical embolism), blood dyscrasias (sickle cell disease, lupus anticoagulant, factor deficiencies), medical disorders (liver disease, polycystic kidney disease), and neck trauma or manipulation (carotid arterial dissection).

Physical Examination

Note: *Physical findings are contingent on the region of brain affected and type of stroke.*

General. Determine the level of consciousness and degree of distress.

Vital signs. Hypertension is a common finding early in the course of a CVA. Bradycardia may signal an increase in intracranial pressure (ICP). Respirations are variable; a sudden change in pattern may warn of impending herniation. An elevated temperature suggests a possible infection.

HEENT. Inspect for trauma. Examine the fundi for hemorrhages, exudates, cholesterol emboli (*Hollenhorst* plaques), and papilledema (increased ICP). Table 3.3.1 lists eye signs that indicate the site of the intracerebral hemorrhage.

Neck. Auscultate for bruits (atherosclerosis) and meningeal signs (infection, SAH).

Lungs. Listen for rales or wheezes, suggesting possible aspiration.

Heart. Note rate and rhythm (a-fib) as well as murmurs (valvular disease), gallops, or clicks.

Neurologic. Assess mental status, cranial nerve function (note abnormalities ipsilateral or contralateral to body weakness/numbness), and cerebellar function (nystagmus, ataxia, past-pointing). Also check for motor (compare arms to legs) and sensory (pain, touch, proprioception) deficits, presence of deep tendon reflexes (hyporeflexia with flaccidity occurs early in the course of CVA, while hyperreflexia is a later finding), and Babinski's signs.

Diagnostic Tests

Bedside glucose. Should be part of the initial assessment (both hyperglycemia and hypoglycemia are potentially harmful).

Table 3.3.1
Eye Signs of Intracerebral Hemorrhage

Site of Bleed	Eye Findings
Putaminal hemorrhage	Eyes deviate to the side of the lesion; pupils remain normal size and reactive
Thalamic hemorrhage	Eyes focus on nose with limitation of upward gaze; pupils appear small and nonreactive
Pontine hemorrhage	Eyes fixed in midline; pinpoint pupils
Cerebellar hemorrhage	Eyes diverge away from side of lesion; pupils remain normal size and reactive

Serum chemistries. Routinely order for potential stroke patients to assess baseline status, identify risk factors, and detect complications.

CBC. An abnormally high hematocrit or platelet count suggests a hypercoagulable state.

PT/PTT. Prolonged PT/PTT may offer a clue to the presence of antiphospholipid antibody or an abnormality in clotting factors (antithrombin III, protein C, or protein S).

ABG. Often necessary to assess respiratory function, which can be compromised with a CVA.

Urinalysis. Presence of hematuria suggests a bacterial endocarditis etiology to an embolic stroke.

CXR. Examine for increased heart size and look for evidence of aspiration, infection, or unsuspected malignancy.

ECG. Inspect for evidence of dysrhythmia (particularly a-fib), recent MI or current ischemia, and atrial or ventricular enlargement.

CT scan. Generally is more readily accessible, can be done more quickly, and requires less patient cooperation than MRI. CT of the head can differentiate hemorrhagic from nonhemorrhagic stroke, identify shifts of intracranial contents (increased intracranial pressure), and detect conditions that may clinically mimic a stroke (subdural hematomas, abscess, brain tumors). A new bleed produces an area of increased density (whiteness) on the CT scan, while an infarction often appears as an area of decreased density (darkness). Although sensitive for intracerebral hemorrhage and most cases of subarachnoid hemorrhage, a CT scan of the head does not always detect a new infarct, especially if the infarct is small, located in the brainstem, or less than 24 hr old.

MRI. Increasingly important in the diagnosis and management of CVAs. MRI is superior to CT for detection of lesions in the posterior fossa (brainstem, cerebellum) and of lacunar infarcts (especially those < 1 cm). Contrast-enhanced MRI assists in the diagnosis of AVMs and carotid dissection.

LP. Warranted if the CT is negative and SAH or CNS infection is being considered.

Arteriography. Identifies surgically correctable lesions (intracranial aneurysms, AVMs, carotid artery stenosis). Both conventional and digital methods are used.

Special Considerations

TIAs

TIA represents reversible CNS ischemia. Presentation of a TIA varies markedly among individuals, but the symptoms in a given patient tend to be consistent. Onset is inclined to be abrupt and without warning. TIAs occurring in the carotid distribution may exhibit a transient monocular blindness (amaurosis fugax), temporary aphasia, or numbness or weakness of the contralateral arm or leg. Vertebrobasilar TIAs may present as ataxia, dizziness, abnormalities of eye movement, and unilateral or bilateral sensory and motor findings. Isolated vertigo, dizziness, or nausea is seldom caused by TIA; and syncope is never due to TIA.

Thrombotic Stroke

Typically resulting from atherosclerosis, thrombotic stroke is characterized by a gradual, stepwise onset and progression, often occurring during sleep or noted when the patient awakens in morning with loss of function. Generally, some sort of warning heralds a thrombotic stroke. Disruption of blood flow to the *middle cerebral artery* results in hemiparesis (face > arm > leg), aphasia (if the dominant side is involved), sensory loss (face > arm > leg), and a homonymous hemianopsia. Disturbances of *anterior cerebral artery* display a motor and sensory loss of the lower extremities only, occasionally accompanied by incontinence. Occlusion of the *posterior cerebral artery* manifests as a homonymous hemianopsia (which may be the sole finding) along with a prominent sensory loss (but minimal or no motor weakness). The most common brainstem affliction is *lateral medullary (Wallenberg's) syndrome,* which presents as a facial numbness, limb ataxia, *Horner's syndrome* (miosis, ptosis, anhidrosis) ipsilateral to the side of the lesion together with a contralateral sensory loss of the arm and leg, vertigo, nausea, hiccups, dysarthria, and/or diplopia.

Embolic Stroke

Embolic stroke may arise from the heart or originate from plaque in a diseased artery. Predisposing factors for cardiac emboli include mural thrombus following MI, mitral valve disease, and atrial fibrillation. Additional risk factors for embolic strokes include prosthetic valves, endocarditis, atrial myxomas, and cardiomyopathies. Embolic strokes tend to occur without warning, producing a maximal deficit at onset and often appearing during waking hours. Seizures may accompany an embolic stroke.

Lacunar Stroke

Most prevalent in patients with hypertension, lacunar strokes tend to take place during periods of sleep or inactivity. They represent infarction of a limited area of the brain and manifest as either pure motor or pure sensory deficits.

Hemorrhagic Stroke

Intracranial hemorrhages ordinarily transpire during waking hours in patients with long-standing hypertension or with coagulopathies and those taking anticoagulants; they affect deep brain tissue. The most common site of intracerebral hemorrhage is the putamen region, presenting as a headache, contralateral hemiplegia, and eye deviation to the side of hemorrhage. Hemorrhage into the pons is ordinarily fatal, manifesting as coma with pinpoint pupils, quadriparesis, and Babinski's sign. *Cerebellar hemorrhage* is a surgical emergency and is characterized by a sudden onset of headache (customarily occipital), vomiting, and ataxia. Additional findings associated with cerebellar hemorrhage and infarct include gaze paresis (inability to look toward the side of lesion), nystagmus, ipsilateral facial numbness, hiccups, dysphagia, dysarthria, and limb ataxia. The cardinal feature of a *SAH* is sudden onset of an oppressive headache, often occurring during or immediately after a period of physical exertion (see section 3.5).

Treatment

The initial goal of emergency management of the stroke patient is stabilization. A CVA may limit the patient's ability to maintain and protect his or her airway, risking hypoxia, hypoventilation (hypercapnia), and aspiration. In addition, adequate oxygenation is essential to prevent further hypoxic insult to the brain. Intubation becomes necessary in patients who are unable to maintain oxygenation and ventilation status by other means, patients who cannot protect their airway, and those with signs of ICP. Rapid deterioration in suspected stroke patients is usually due to elevated ICP, resulting from cerebral edema or hemorrhage.

A particular area of concern is the *blood pressure.* Any intervention affecting the blood pressure must be executed with extreme caution. A disruption of cerebral autoregulation occurs early in the course of a CVA, causing the brain to be more susceptible to hypotension. An elevation in blood pressure might actually be an important compensatory mechanism. Overzealous lowering of blood pressure in patients with ischemic strokes can be disastrous. Initially elevated pressures tend to subside spontaneously in the first 12 to 72 hr (see section 1.7 for specific recommendations for blood pressure control). Generally, observation and sedation if the patient is agitated is all that is required. One exception is SAH, where the blood pressure should be lowered (diastolic pressure < 100 mm Hg) if significantly elevated.

Institute cardiac monitoring to safeguard against onset of dysrhythmias (common early in the course of a CVA).

Cerebellar hemorrhage is a neurosurgical emergency requiring intervention without delay. The decision on the timing and necessity for surgery is the domain of the neurosurgeon, and prompt consultation is strongly advised.

Seizures occur in 5 to 7% of CVA patients. Treat according to the protocols outlined in section 3.2.

The *definitive management of ischemic strokes* is an evolving area of medicine. Unfortunately, other than general supportive measures, little can be done for *completed strokes. Anticoagulant* therapy *(heparin)* is possibly beneficial in the early management of crescendo TIAs, strokes in evolution, and cardioembolic strokes but should *not* be undertaken until *after* a CT or MRI is obtained, and then only in conjunction with neurology or neurosurgery consultation. *Antiplatelet* drugs may confer protection against recurrent TIAs and CVA. *Aspirin* is normally the initial choice, with *dipyridamole* and *ticlopidine* being reserved for patients who cannot tolerate aspirin or who develop subsequent TIAs or CVAs despite aspirin therapy. The role of thrombolytic therapy is currently under investigation.

Admission Criteria

All patients diagnosed with a suspected acute CVA or TIA require admission to a monitored bed. Admission to the appropriate service depends on the etiology of the stroke. It is essential to be aggressive in pursuit of the diagnosis of a TIA, since early identification of cerebrovascular disease provides an opportunity to prevent a stroke (about 50% of patients who develop a stroke have a history of a prior TIA).

Suggested Readings

Goldstein LB, Matchar DB: Clinical assessment of stroke. JAMA 1994;271: 1114–1120.

Gress DR: Stroke: revolution in therapy. West J Med 1994;161:288–291.

National Stroke Association: Consensus statement: stroke: the first 6 hours: emergency evaluation and treatment. J Stroke Cerebrovasc Dis 1993;3:133–144.

3.4 SPINAL CORD COMPRESSION

Description

Spinal cord compression is a neurosurgical emergency requiring rapid diagnosis and treatment to avoid permanent complications. The corticospinal tracts, posterior spinal columns, and spinal cerebellar tracts are most vulnerable to cord compression. Causes of spinal cord compression can be anatomically separated into those originating inside (intramedullary) or outside the spinal cord (extramedullary and intradural) versus those emanating from the surrounding meninges (epidural). The thoracic spine is the most common site of epidural metastasis (approximately 60% of cases).

Location	Etiologies
Intramedullary	Primary cord neoplasms, syringomyelia, AVM
Extramedullary/intradural	Meningioma, neurofibroma
Epidural	Metastatic tumor (especially from lung and breast), epidural abscess or hematoma, multiple myeloma, lymphoma, disk protrusion (central cord syndrome), spondylosis or spondylolisthesis, atlantoaxial subluxation (most common with rheumatoid arthritis)

History

Consider spinal cord compression in all patients with central spinal pain, especially when accompanied by bilateral extremity motor or sensory disturbances (numbness, paresthesias, weakness), ataxia, and autonomic dysfunction (bowel, bladder). However, back or neck pain may be the sole complaint, either localizing to the site of involved vertebra or manifesting as radicular pain due to spinal nerve root compression. A gradual onset is commonly followed by an insidious course (days to weeks to months). Once neurologic symptoms other than pain emerge, progression is rapid. Paraplegia and bowel or bladder disorders (constipation; urinary hesitancy, retention, or incontinence) are typically late findings, except in *conus medullaris syndrome,* where sphincter dysfunction and saddle anesthesia turn up early. Back or neck discomfort in a patient with cancer (especially breast, lung, prostate, kidney, myeloma, or lymphoma) should alert the clinician to the possibility of spinal metastasis.

Additional historical clues suggesting serious pathology include age greater than 50 years; pain unrelieved with rest or recumbency; unrelenting progressive pain (especially if > 1 month); appearance of fever, chills, weight loss, anorexia, or fatigue; history of immunocompromising illness (AIDS, DM); use of parenteral drugs, anticoagulants, or immunosuppressive agents; and recent major trauma (fall, MVA), surgery (particularly spinal surgery), or genitourinary manipulation.

Physical Examination

General. Look for evidence of systemic illness (cachexia). Observe casual movements of patient.

Vital signs. Only 50% of patients with an epidural abscess will exhibit a fever.

Skin. Inspect for abscesses, tract marks, petechiae, or purpura.

HEENT. Observe for trauma. Presence of iritis implies possible inflammatory arthritis (ankylosing spondylitis).

Neck. Examine for masses, adenopathy, and meningismus. *Lhermitte's sign* occurs when neck flexion leads to electric shock–like sensations that radiate down the spine to the arms, legs, and buttocks and indicates intrinsic or extrinsic cervical spinal cord pathology.

Breast. Check for masses and axillary nodes.

Back. Palpate along the spinous processes for localized tenderness and document presence of swelling or erythema.

Abdomen. Assess for tenderness, organomegaly, masses, and bladder distention.

Rectal. Determine sphincter tone and sensation. Examine the prostate.

Neurologic. Deficits are determined by the level of the spinal cord affected. Spasticity; hyperreflexia (lower extremity reflexes tend to exhibit greater hyperreflexia than upper extremities); and loss of pinprick, temperature, position, and vibration sensations appear early in the course. Later signs include defined muscle weakness, clear demarcation of sensory disruption, bilateral Babinski's sign, and loss of anal sphincter tone and bulbocavernous reflexes. Straight leg raising that causes contralateral leg pain (pain that radiates down the nonaffected leg when the painful leg is elevated) strongly suggests cord compression. **Note:** *Patients with spinal cord compression may have a normal neurologic exam.*

Diagnostic Studies

Laboratory studies are generally not helpful in establishing the diagnosis (although marked elevation in sedimentation rate implies presence of infection or inflammation). Confirm the postvoid urinary residual (> 300 mL is significant) when bladder disturbance is considered. *MRI* is the imaging study of choice for presumed cord compression, precisely distinguishing soft tissue abnormalities. If the patient cannot tolerate an MRI or MRI is unavailable, order a CT myelogram. A lumbar puncture is contraindicated in the setting of spinal cord compression (there is a risk of seeding an abscess).

Treatment

Outcome is determined by pretreatment functional status—once neurologic deficits appear, they often are irreversible (if paralysis is present, less than half of patients will regain neurologic function). Therefore *stat* consultation with the appropriate consultant (neurosurgeon, radiation oncologist) is essential. Temporizing measures (give before radiological studies) include administration of dexamethasone (10 to 50 mg IV) to control spinal cord edema and suitable antibiotic coverage (cover both *Staphylococcus* and Gram negatives) if *epidural abscess* or infection is suspected.

Admission Criteria

Suspicion of spinal cord compression mandates admission.

Suggested Readings

Byrne TN: Spinal cord compression from epidural metastasis. N Engl J Med 1992;27:614–619.

Schmidt RD, Markovchick V: Nontraumatic spinal cord compression. J Emerg Med 1992;10:189–199.

3.5 HEADACHE

Description

Headache is a symptom, not a disease, caused by irritation of pain-sensitive structures in the head, face, or neck. People with headaches come to the ED for two reasons: (1) the headache is new, different, or very severe or (2) the headache is their customary type, but they have exhausted self-treatment options. Most headaches result from a harmless cause, but the emergency caregiver must always exclude serious etiologies that could account for the pain: *subarachnoid hemorrhage (SAH), intracerebral hemorrhage, subdural hematoma, brain tumor, brain abscess, meningitis, temporal arteritis, hypertensive encephalopathy,* and *glaucoma.*

History

The history is often the most indispensable part of the diagnostic work-up. However, since the information is being obtained from a patient experiencing severe discomfort, diligent and specific inquiries are necessary (see Table 3.5.1). Fundamental questions include severity (SAH is often associated with comments such as the "worst headache of my life") and quality (sharp, dull, pulsating) of pain, rapidity of onset (sudden versus gradual), location (unilateral, occipital, frontotemporal, facial, neck), course (worsening, improving, stable), duration (minutes, hours, days), alleviating and exacerbating factors (provoked by exertion, straining, or ingestion of alcohol or drug), previous history of headaches (ask patient to compare earlier incidents to the current episode), antecedent head trauma, infection (numerous infectious states are associated with a headache, including CNS infections), toxic exposure (carbon monoxide), presence of underlying illness (hypertension, AIDS, cancer), medications (including headache medications already employed, anticoagulants, and illicit drugs such as cocaine or amphetamines), and associated symptoms (prodromal auras, visual disturbances, fever, nausea, vomiting, confusion or mental cloudiness, jaw claudication, gait or neurologic dysfunction).

Table 3.5.1
Clinical Clues to Serious Etiology of Headache

First or worst headache ever
Sudden "thunderclap" onset
Precipitated by or following exertion
Aggravated by bowel movement or coughing
Altered mental status
Fever
Meningeal signs
Neurologic deficits

Physical Examination

General. Observe the overall appearance (Does the patient look sick?) and level of consciousness.

Vital signs. Pay special attention to temperature (fever) and blood pressure (diastolic pressure > 120 mm Hg suggests hypertensive encephalopathy).

HEENT. Inspect for evidence of trauma. Palpate the temporal arteries, sinuses, and temporomandibular joint for tenderness. Perform an attentive ocular examination: determine translucency of the cornea (a steamy cornea is seen with glaucoma), pupil size and reactivity, extraocular movements (third nerve palsy), and appearance of the fundus (especially looking for papilledema and retinal hemorrhages).

Neck. Check for nuchal rigidity.

Neurologic. Carry out a careful neurologic examination, concentrating on mental status, cerebellar function, and deep tendon reflexes. Note peripheral motor or sensory deficits.

Diagnostic Tests

CBC and serum chemistries. Useful when infectious, metabolic, or toxic illness is suspected. Check electrolytes, BUN, and creatinine if dehydration is suspected or if the patient has taken an excessive amount of analgesics. In addition, order specific studies when the history suggests a specific condition (blood lead, carbon monoxide level).

Sedimentation rate. Obtain if temporal arteritis is considered.

Imaging studies. A CT scan or MRI is mandated when focal neurologic deficits or signs of increased intracranial pressure

(ICP) are evident. Generally, the CT scan is preferred in the acute setting of headache (especially if related to trauma), while MRI is superior in patients with more chronic conditions or those with signs and symptoms of increased ICP or suspected posterior fossa lesions.

Lumbar puncture. CT scans fail to detect SAH in 5 to 10% of cases, thus an LP is required if a diagnosis of SAH is strongly suspected based on clinical findings. A lumbar puncture should also be performed if meningitis considered (see section 9.1). **Warning:** *Patients with suspected subarachnoid hemorrhage, mass lesion, or stroke should have a CT scan before a spinal tap.*

Ocular pressure. Perform when glaucoma is part of the differential diagnosis (see section 14.2).

Special Considerations

Emergent Etiologies

Specific causes that require immediate attention include *subarachnoid hemorrhage* (SAH), *subdural or epidural hemorrhage* (see section 4.2), *CVAs* (see section 3.3), *meningitis* (see section 9.1), *hypertensive encephalopathy* (see section 1.7), and disorders inducing an increase in intracranial pressure with impending herniation. Rapid recognition of SAH is essential; if left undiagnosed, the outcome can be disastrous. Most SAHs arise from the rupture of a saccular aneurysm, although AV malformations may occur in younger patients. The diagnosis of SAH is not difficult in the patient with a "thunderclap" onset of an excruciating headache accompanied by nuchal rigidity and focal neurologic deficits that soon advance to stupor or coma. However, headaches produced by small leaks (sentinel bleed) may appear benign but can progress to a full-blown SAH followed by death in hours to days. Be suspicious of headaches in patients who always experience a "migraine" on the same side of the head.

Urgent Etiologies

Brain tumors, abscesses, or other *space-occupying lesions* are suggested by deep, dull headaches that appear upon awakening, are located in the occipital or frontal region of the head, and are aggravated by coughing or straining during a bowel movement. *Temporal arteritis* occurs in older patients (see section 14.3). Headache may also be the cardinal complaint in patients with *acute narrow-angle glaucoma* (see section 14.2). *Purulent sinusitis* obligates prompt diagnosis to avoid complications (see section 15.2).

Less Urgent Etiologies

Less urgent etiologies include the more innocuous causes as well as chronic or previously diagnosed recurrent problems. *Migraine* accounts for many ED visits for headache. Typically, symptoms begin in the late teens and persist to middle age. It is now postulated that migraines arise from disturbances in neurochemical mediators and can be aborted by serotonin agonists. Onset of headache is generally gradual. Approximately, one-third of migraine patients experience an "aura" preceding their migraine; these episodes are designated as *classical migraines.* The aura may display visual or sensory disturbances. Visual disturbances include the appearance of bright lights, zigzag lines (fortification scotoma), wavy lines, and frank hemianopsia, while sensory disorders are confined mostly to the face and upper extremities. After 30 min, prodromal symptoms resolve and a throbbing, pulsatile headache appears. The headaches may be global, hemicranial, or focal. However, migraines usually cross the midline and are rarely confined to the same side with each attack.

A *common migraine* lacks antecedent warning and is triggered by a variety of events (e.g., birth control pills, wine, and chocolate).

Migraines in females may be triggered by birth control pills. Key clinical features in all types of migraines are photo and sound sensitivity, nausea, vomiting, irritability, and pallor.

Rarer forms of migraines include *basilar migraine* (associated with vertigo, tinnitus, visual disturbances, and ataxia), *ophthalmoplegic migraine* (mimics carotid aneurysm and presents as a unilateral headache with ipsilateral paralysis), and *hemiplegic migraine* (hemiplegia, aphasia, and/or confusion before the headache). *Status migrainous* is a term reserved for a refractory and continuous migraine, usually $>$ 48 hr in duration.

Tension headache (due to muscle contraction) is a dull persistent pain described as a band-like constriction about the head. The headache lasts from minutes to days.

Cluster headaches tend to affect males between 20 and 45 years of age and manifest as severe orbital pain associated with nasal discharge, tearing, and ipsilateral lid or pupillary abnormalities. As noted by the name, the headaches occur in "clusters," lasting from 15 min to 4 hr and commonly awakening the patient without warning. They are repetitious over weeks to months.

Miscellaneous Etiologies

Miscellaneous etiologies of headaches presenting to the ED include *spinal tap headaches,* which start 48 hr after an LP. The cardinal feature is a headache that is worse when the patient is upright and improves when he or she lies flat. *Pseudotumor cerebri* occur in obese females with menstrual irregularities. Small slit-like ventricles are seen on CT. *Drug withdrawal headaches,* or rebound headaches, result from excessive use of analgesics or antimigraine agents.

Treatment

The primary task of the emergency physician is to rule out life-threatening causes of headache while securing the vital signs. Presence of a life-threatening etiology necessitates immediate action. Timing of surgery for SAH is determined by the neurosurgeon. *Nimodipine* is administered to prevent vasospasm secondary to SAH; the dosage is 60 mg PO q 4 hr for 3 weeks (if the patient cannot swallow, give the crushed pill via an NG tube).

It is usually not critical in the ED to differentiate between *migraine* and *tension* headaches; they probably represent the ends of a continuum and often respond to similar therapy. Furthermore, there is no difference in approach to the treatment of common or classic migraines. Consider treating all migraine and tension headaches first with a serotonin receptor blocker rather than with a narcotic. Two medications with selective "abortive" properties are *Sumatriptan* (6 mg SQ) and *dihydroergotamine* (DHE) (0.5 to 1 mg IM or IV). Sumatriptan is *contraindicated* in patients with a history of coronary artery disease (CAD) or uncontrolled hypertension and *should not* be used concurrently with MAO inhibitors or DHE. DHE is associated with a high incidence of GI side effects and is *contraindicated* in pregnancy and in patients with CAD, renal, hepatic, or peripheral vascular disease. DHE is best dispensed in combination with an antiemetic, such as *prochlorperazine* (Compazine, 10 mg IV) or metoclopramide (Reglan 10 mg IV) Other routes of administration of DHE (intranasal, subcutaneous) are generally not as efficacious as the intravenous or intramuscular route. Furthermore, both prochlorperazine and metoclopramide are effective as sole agents in treating migraine-type headaches and demonstrate exceptional safety profiles.

Salvage medications that may be effective if the above medications fail include *nonsteroidal antiinflammatories* (ketorolac 30 to 60 mg IM), *corticosteroids* (hydrocortisone 100 mg IV; or prednisone taper starting at 80 mg PO), and *narcotics* (morphine 5 to 10 mg IV, IM, or SQ; or Demerol 1 mg/kg IV or IM). Migraine prophylaxis should be initiated by the consultant.

Cluster headaches can be frustrating to both the patient and the treating physician. DHE (1 mg IM or IV), Sumatriptan (6 mg SQ), inhalation of 100% oxygen (6 to 8 L/min flow for 10 to 15 min), and intranasal installation of 1 mL of 4% lidocaine (local anesthesia of sphenopalatine fossa) have resulted in varying success. Prophylactic regimens (corticosteroids, lithium, cyproheptadine) should be discussed with the consultant. Narcotics should be reserved for patients for whom the other regimens have failed.

Postspinal tap headaches are treated with analgesics (oral narcotics if tolerated), adequate hydration, and caffeine sodium benzoate (500 mg caffeine solution in 1 L NS, infused over 1 hr). When all else fails, an epidural blood patch may be placed by an experienced anesthesiologist.

Admission Criteria

All patients with emergent or urgent etiologies require admission for definitive care along with appropriate consultation. In addition, *patients with less urgent etiologies who do not respond to ED measures, display intractable vomiting, or suffer persistent neurologic deficits* obligate admission and consultation with a neurologist. All discharged patients need clear instructions (return if the headache becomes worse, if the mental status changes, or if neurologic deficits develop) and appropriate follow-up.

Suggested Readings

Couch JR: Headache to worry about. Med Clin North Am 1993;77:141–167.

Thomas SH, Stone CK: Emergency department treatment of migraine, tension, and mixed-type headache. J Emerg Med 1994;12:657–664.

Chapter 4

Trauma

4.1 MULTIPLE TRAUMA

Description

Trauma is the leading cause of death and disability in people under the age of 40. Three time intervals constitute trauma mortality: (1) immediate death (first few minutes), (2) death within minutes to hours, and (3) death ensuing in days to weeks. Instantaneous death generally results from exsanguinating great vessel hemorrhage or massive CNS injury, and only a very small percentage of these patients is successfully resuscitated. It is during the second time frame (the so-called golden hour), in which a wide range of problems may occur in the multiply injured patient (airway compromise, the number one cause of preventable early trauma-related death; traumatic exsanguination; CNS bleeds; chest trauma; intraabdominal injuries), that emergent intervention is critical to survival. Successful management of the trauma patient, as recommended by the American College of Surgeons and endorsed by the American College of Emergency Physicians, calls for adherence to an established "order of priority" in the initial assessment and management, while minimizing time delays for definitive treatment.

History

The initial assessment begins with a concise history that attempts to identify life-threatening injuries. However, *it is essential to simultaneously identify and treat any potentially mortal injuries.* The patient's ability to relate the course of events may be compromised by head injury, hysteria, or intoxicants. Attempt to obtain the following information (often provided by the EMT or paramedic).

Nature and Mechanism of Injury

Awareness of the mechanism of injury is frequently helpful in anticipating existing injuries as well as deciding subsequent management strategies. For *penetrating trauma,* ascertain the type of weapon used. If *stab wounds* are discovered, try to obtain a description of the object used (length, width).

The potential severity of *gunshot wounds (GSWs)* is determined by the amount of kinetic injury dissipated to the wound (the kinetic injury of a missile is proportional to its mass times its velocity squared). GSWs are classified into low-velocity, high-velocity, and shotgun-type wounds. Low-velocity missiles account for most civilian bullet wounds; injury is generally restricted to the path and residual cavity of the bullet. However, additional injuries can occur when external articles (clothing) are driven into the wound or when there is bone fragmentation. Shotgun wounds can be devastating, especially when administered at close range, and create large soft-tissue defects. High-velocity missile wounds (military, hunting rifles) are capable of causing extensive damage to areas remote from the missile track. High-velocity wounds are also associated with small entrance wounds and large exit wounds. Additional information that can be helpful in the management of GSWs includes the estimated number of shots fired (as a general rule, the number of bullet holes plus the number of bullets seen on the radiograph should add up to an even number—if not bullet embolization or previous GSW should be suspected) and the distance between the firearm and victim.

For *blunt trauma* determine the type and magnitude of force absorbed. Injuries associated with falls from heights and motor vehicle accidents (MVAs) produce both direct injury and more subtle injuries secondary to rapid deceleration forces; as the body rapidly decelerates, the momentum of the internal organs persists forward. Heavy organs susceptible to deceleration injuries include the liver, spleen, blood-filled thoracic aorta, and fluid-filled loops of bowel. Additional damage may also occur when the still moving, mobile portion of the viscus is torn from the tethered section, pulling blood vessels and tissues from their points of attachment. Low-velocity compression injuries to the body (pedestrian hit by motor vehicle; injury from a punch, kick, or bat) may cause damage to the solid parenchymal organs (liver, spleen) or crush syndromes of an extremity (see section 16.4).

Obtain a *report of the MVA,* including the estimated speed of the vehicles on impact, the orientation of the vehicles, and the position of patient in the vehicle (driver or front- or rear-seated passenger). Determine if the patient was ejected from the vehicle. Other information includes any *damage to the structures surrounding the patient in the vehicle* (steering wheel or column deformation, windshield damage) and any *mitigating circumstances.* For victims of MVA, inquire if the patient was restrained and/or if airbag devices employed; for motorcycle or bicycle-related accidents find out if victim was wearing a helmet. Further questions about the accident cover the presence of a fire or explosion, extraction time, and the ambient temperature.

Other Information

Time of injury.

Character of any pain. Determine onset, severity, quality, constancy, location, and radiation.

Concurrent complaints and symptoms. Ask about loss of consciousness at the scene and check for shortness of breath, numbness, and weakness.

Blood loss. Determine the amount (if any) of blood loss at the scene.

Events preceding the injury. Determine if there were any prior symptoms.

Prehospital course and treatment.

Additional important historical data are the patient's *last oral intake, prior illnesses, injuries, surgeries, current medications, allergies* (especially antibiotics and contrast medium), *previous immunizations, and recent alcohol or drug use.* If the patient is female, determine the date of the *last menstrual period* (LMP) and whether she is *pregnant.* A useful mnemonic is to take an *AMPLE* history:

A = allergies;
M = medications;
P = past medical history;
L = last meal; and
E = events preceding injury.

Physical Examination

The physical examination begins with an expedient primary survey designed to immediately identify and treat any life-threatening injuries. Once this is accomplished and the patient is stabilized, move on to a secondary survey with appropriate investigations. In the severely ill patient, the secondary survey is omitted or shortened when lifesaving definitive care is required (surgery).

Primary Survey: ABCDE

The ABCDE mnemonic is recommended by the American College of Surgeons as an initial approach to the trauma patient:

A = airway management with protection of the cervical spine;
B = breathing;
C = circulation with hemorrhage control;
D = disability (look for neuro deficits); and
E = exposure (completely undress the patient).

A = Airway Management. Airway obstruction is generally recognized as the most rapidly fatal problem complicating the course of the multiple trauma patient and must be dealt with as such. Airway compromise may be sudden and complete or insidious and partial. Significant facial injuries (particularly mandibular or midfacial), foreign bodies, blood, vomitus, and the tongue are all capable of provoking airway obstruction. Situations dictating a need for emergent airway management include (1) securing the airway in an unresponsive patient, (2) protecting against aspiration, (3) preventing hypoxia, and (4) hyperventilating a patient with severe head injury.

Assess the airway quickly; talk to the patient, striving to stimulate an oral response. If he or she replies in a normal voice and gives reasonable answers to your questions, then assume the airway is patent and the brain is being perfused. Look, listen, and feel for objective signs of airway compromise (changes in mental status, cyanosis, retractions and use of accessory muscles, abnormal or noisy breath sounds, movement of air with expiratory effort, position of trachea).

Extreme caution must be exercised when examining the head and neck, during intubation attempts, and when transporting the patient. Any multiple trauma patient who has sustained an injury above the clavicles (especially if a concurrent head injury is impairing consciousness) and/or a patient with high-risk mechanisms (unrestrained or intoxicated driver involved in a head-on collision) requires cervical spine precautions. An intact neurologic status *does not* exclude cervical spine injury. Spinal immobilization dictates keeping the patient's head and neck in a neutral position. A typical way to accomplish this is to place a standard hard collar around the neck, securing the patient to a long backboard, and supplementing by either placing sandbags on both sides of the patient's head and neck, taping the patient's head to the backboard, or applying manual in-line stabilization. A soft cervical collar alone *does not* provide adequate immobilization.

Airway maintenance techniques include *chin lift, jaw thrust, artificial airway placement,* and *suctioning.* In a patient with a diminished level of consciousness, the tongue is the most common cause of airway obstruction (it moves backward). This can usually be corrected with a jaw thrust maneuver. If the jaw thrust maneuver does not correct the obstruction, the patient's oropharynx should be checked for the presence of foreign bodies. An oropharyngeal airway can be temporarily employed to maintain the airway patency in the unconscious patient. However, an oropharyngeal airway should not be used in a conscious patient with an intact gag reflex; instead use a nasopharyngeal airway (less likely to induce gagging, better tolerated). In addition, *always provide supplemental oxygen to the multiple trauma patient.*

Intubation provides a definitive airway and is indicated in *apnea, inability to protect the airway, impending or potential compromise of airway* (inhalation injury, facial fractures), *closed head injury requiring hyperventilation,* and *inability to maintain adequate oxygenation and ventilation by face mask.* Various intubation options exist, and the route chosen (orotracheal or nasotracheal intubation) is dictated by the urgency of the situation, the circumstances surrounding the need for airway intervention, and the skill of the performer. A surgical airway should be performed if the airway cannot be secured via orotracheal or nasotracheal intubation.

B* = *Breathing. Immediately after the airway has been secured, ensure that both sides of the chest are being ventilated. If the patient was intubated or underwent a surgical airway, auscultate the chest for bilateral breath sounds (listen closely in the axilla) and observe for symmetrical chest expansion. If unable to hear breath sounds, listen over the stomach to ensure an esophageal intubation has not taken place. Inadequate ventilation following intubation generally arises from misplacement of the endotracheal tube into the esophagus, main-stem bronchus intubation (most often in the right main bronchus), or underlying tension or hemothorax. Carefully examine the chest for the presence of sucking wounds, subcutaneous air, and areas of paradoxical motion.

C = Circulation. Once satisfactory ventilation and oxygenation are established, proceed rapidly to the next phase of resuscitation, namely ensuring adequate tissue perfusion and circulation. A quick assessment of circulatory status includes determining the *character and presence of pulses* (presence of a carotid pulse corresponds to a blood pressure of at least 60 mm Hg, a palpable femoral pulse implies blood pressure ≥ 70 mm Hg, and a radial pulse suggests a pressure ≥ 80 mm Hg), *skin color, capillary refill* (squeeze a nail bed, normal capillary refill is < 2 sec, or less than the time it takes to say "capillary refill"), and *blood pressure.* Trauma patients are frequently young and able to initially compensate for blood loss, but rapid deterioration may take place once compensatory mechanisms are exceeded. Note that elderly patients do not tolerate hypotension well.

Control external hemorrhage with direct pressure; tourniquets are rarely if ever required, and blind clamping of vessels is to be condemned. Insert two large-bore (14- to 16-gauge) peripheral lines and obtain blood samples for typing and other studies. The use of central lines (8.5 French or 10 gauge) during the initial resuscitation is controversial but may be beneficial in guiding fluid therapy (follow trends in CVP measurements). Establish intravenous access above and below the diaphragm in cases of penetrating trauma to the chest or abdomen. If a pneumothorax is present, place the central line on the affected side. However, when a major vascular injury is suspected, establish the central line on the opposite side.

Fluid resuscitation, both type and amount, is a controversial issue. Recent work has focused on the merits of aggressive fluid resuscitation in patients with penetrating torso trauma; some experts argue that increasing blood pressure to normotensive levels may worsen bleeding and homeostasis. When fluids are necessary, crystalloids (normal saline, lactated Ringer's) remain the first choice. Preliminary work with hypertonic saline suggests it may restore intravascular volume more rapidly than isotonic crystalloid. If the patient remains hypotensive after 2 L crystalloid, administer packed red blood cells (see section 13.1). Typed and cross-matched blood is not necessary and may require 1 hr of laboratory time. The critically ill patient should be given type-specific blood, which is customarily available within 10 min. O negative blood (the universal donor) is usually obtainable immediately and should be given to exsanguinating patients unable to provide a blood sample. Blood will flow more quickly when warmed, mixed with normal saline to reduce viscosity, and infused under pressure through large-bore tubing. Rapid volume infusion machines are now available that will perform all these functions.

Military antishock trousers (MAST) are controversial but may be used in select hypotensive trauma patients (those with pelvic fracture or fractures at risk for retroperitoneal hemorrhage). Contraindications to MAST include pulmonary edema, myocardial infarction, diaphragmatic rupture, and uncontrolled hemorrhage outside the confines of the garment (thorax, upper extremities, scalp, face, neck injury).

Shock (see section 1.2) is a hypotensive syndrome that results in cellular hypoperfusion. Classes of shock are determined by volume of blood loss (Table 4.1.1). *Do not depend on blood pressure alone to make the diagnosis of shock.* Constantly reevaluate the patient, the vital signs, and the response to fluid challenges.

Table 4.1.1
Classes of Shock

Class I
- Loss of up to 15% of blood volume (normal adult = 70 mL/kg)
- Clinical symptoms are minimal

Class II
- Loss of 15–30% blood volume
- Narrow pulse pressure, tachycardia, tachypnea, apprehension, and decreased capillary refill

Class III
- Loss of 30–40% blood volume
- Decreased systolic blood pressure, tachycardia, altered mental status, and decreased urine output

Class IV
- Greater than 40% blood volume loss
- Marked hypotension, marked tachycardia and tachypnea, decreased level of consciousness, and mottled skin loss.

Following a fluid challenge of 1 L, one of the following scenarios happens:

- The vital signs return to normal; usually < 20% of the blood volume has been lost.
- The vital signs improve initially, but then deteriorate; usually > 20% of blood volume has been lost. Active bleeding may be transpiring, necessitating transfusion of blood products.
- No improvement of vital signs; either hypovolemia is not the cause of shock or a significant blood loss has occurred. The history, mechanism of injury, physical exam, and central venous pressure help differentiate these two possibilities.

The definitive treatment for ongoing hemorrhage is customarily surgical, and ED to OR turnaround time should be minimized.

D = Deficits of Neurologic Function. Perform a brief neurologic examination to assess motor and sensory functions, pupil size and reactivity, and level of consciousness. Avoid confusing terminology (see section 3.1) by employing objective descriptions such as "responds to tactile stimuli but not to oral stimuli." Serial assessments of the Glasgow Coma Scale (GCS) are essential (see Table 4.2.1). Consider reversible causes of altered level of consciousness (hypoglycemia, drug overdose, Wernicke's encephalopathy, hypoxia, hypoperfusion).

E = Exposure. Completely undress all trauma patients and search for occult injuries. Be sure to log roll the patient to examine the back. Minimize patient movement. Cut clothing, if necessary. Avoid iatrogenic hypothermia by maintaining a warm resuscitation room and providing adequate covers for the patient when he or she is not being examined.

Secondary Survey: Physical Examination

After securing the airway and ventilation, protecting against further C-spine damage, and identifying and treating potential causes of shock, a secondary head-to-toe survey is performed. Place third-trimester pregnant females in the left lateral decubitus position to avoid the supine hypotensive syndrome (due to the compression of the inferior vena cava by the gravid uterus).

Table 4.2.1
The Glasgow Coma Scale

1. Eye opening response	
Spontaneous	_____ (4)
To voice	_____ (3)
To pain	_____ (2)
None	_____ (1)
2. Best verbal response	
Oriented	_____ (5)
Confused	_____ (4)
Inappropriate words	_____ (3)
Incomprehensible sounds	_____ (2)
None	_____ (1)
3. Best motor response	
Obeys commands	_____ (6)
Localizes (pain)	_____ (5)
Withdraws (pain)	_____ (4)
Flexion (pain)	_____ (3)
Extension (pain)	_____ (2)
None	_____ (1)
Total GCS points (1 + 2 + 3)	_____

HEENT. Palpate the scalp and face for lacerations and/or fractures. Check the eyes for pupil reactivity, extraocular function, and visual acuity. Inspect the ears for tympanic membrane rupture, hemotympanum, and CSF otorrhea. Search for CSF rhinorrhea, epistaxis, and septal hematoma. Examine for loose or missing teeth, malocclusion, and mobility of the maxilla.

Neck. Examine for tenderness, spinous process deformities, neck vein distention, hematomas, wounds, and tracheal deviation.

Chest. Inspect for evidence of sucking wounds, flail chest, and asymmetrical movements. Bruising of the chest wall often suggests underlying injury. Palpate for crepitus and tenderness (underlying rib fractures). Auscultate for evidence of diminished air entry (suggesting a possible hemothorax or pneumothorax).

Abdomen. Examine the abdomen for any evidence of blunt (distention, ecchymosis) or penetrating injury. Palpate to determine if tenderness is present. Auscultate for bowel sounds.

Pelvis. Evaluate for tenderness or instability upon palpation and compression (pelvic rock).

Genitourinary. Inspect for blood at the urinary meatus; presence of priapism, perineal hematomas, or wounds (consider possible open pelvic fracture); and vaginal bleeding.

Rectal. Assess rectal tone and integrity of rectal wall and bony pelvis. Check for gross blood and high-riding prostate.

Back. Log roll the patient and assess for ecchymosis, wounds, deformity, or tenderness.

Extremities. Assess neurovascular status, deformities (both fractures and dislocations), contusions, and wounds.

Diagnostic Tests

Nasogastric tube and Foley catheter. Gastric dilation is frequently present in the trauma patient and can lead to vomiting with subsequent aspiration. However, avoid placing a nasogastric (NG) tube in patients with suspected basilar skull fracture or significant maxillofacial trauma. Bladder decompression with a Foley catheter allows one to assess the urine for hematuria and to monitor urinary output constantly. Nevertheless, blood at the urethral meatus, gross hematuria, pelvic fractures, a nonpalpable prostate, or perineal hematomas preclude immediate insertion of a transurethral catheter.

X-rays. *Never delay trauma resuscitation care for an x-ray order.* Initial trauma films should be taken in the trauma resuscitation area. Radiographic assessment of the cervical spine, chest (AP), and pelvis is performed as early as possible, usually in conjunction with the secondary survey. Additional films can be taken as required, after all life-threatening injuries are identified and treated. It is probably unwise to order any films beyond the C-spine, chest, and pelvis in patients who require transfer.

Blood tests. Include CBC, SMA, fingerstick glucose, PT/PTT, ABG, mixed venous gas, and type and cross-match. Toxicology screens and drug levels may also be indicated.

Note: *Additional diagnostic studies are discussed in the sections pertaining to specific organ-related trauma.*

Disposition

Trauma is a surgical disease, and the surgical consultant ought to be involved early in the care of the patient. Proper transport and triage of patients to an appropriate trauma center (level I when available) are essential when the patient's condition or trauma score dictates a higher level of care.

Selected References

American College of Surgeons: Advanced trauma life support instructors manual, 5th edition. Chicago: ACS, 1993.

Bickell WH, Wall MJ, Pepe PE, et al.: Immediate versus delayed fluid resuscitation for hypotensive patients with penetrating torso injuries. N Engl J Med 1994;331:1105–1109.

Trunkey D: Initial treatment of patients with extensive trauma. N Engl J Med 1991;324:1259–1263.

4.2 HEAD TRAUMA

Description

Head trauma is a frequent challenge to the emergency physician. Approximately 50% of all trauma deaths are due to head trauma. Proper management is essential to prevent subsequent brain damage through control of intracranial pressure and correction of hypovolemia and hypoxia. Head trauma may be divided into *penetrating* and *nonpenetrating (closed head)* injuries. Penetrating injuries may be caused by missiles (bullets, metallic fragments) or by severe direct trauma, resulting in fracture and intrusion of bone or foreign bodies into the cranial vault. Nonpenetrating injuries include both impact trauma (direct tissue deformation) and injuries arising from sudden acceleration or deceleration forces accompanied by rotational stress (nonimpact trauma).

Alteration of consciousness is the paramount sign of brain injury. There are two categories of brain injury: *primary* and *secondary.* Primary brain injury occurs at the time of impact and is associated with a wide variety of disorders, ranging from trivial to life threatening. Secondary brain injury displays a delayed onset, following initial intracranial damage sustained at impact. Most primary brain injuries are not amenable to treatment, but secondary brain injury can often be prevented or reduced by controlling *intracranial pressure* (ICP) and by maximizing *cerebral perfusion pressure* (CPP).

$$\text{CPP} = \text{Mean arterial pressure (MAP)} - \text{ICP}$$

ICP (normally < 15 mm Hg) is defined by the relationship among the volumes of CSF, blood, and brain, all of which are enclosed in the fixed space of the cranial vault. Cerebral autoregulation attempts to maintain blood flow to the brain by inducing a compensatory rise in MAP whenever there is an increase in ICP.

However, rapid increases in ICP that result from cerebral edema or hematoma formation quickly exhaust physiologic reserves in severe head injury. In addition, serious head injuries impair cerebral autoregulation. The result is a decrease in CPP, which places the brain at risk for further damage from ischemia.

History

Head trauma is frequently a component of multisystem trauma. The same orderly approach outlined for multiple trauma (see section 4.1) needs to be followed for head trauma. By establishing the mechanism of injury, it is possible to determine the scope of the injury—head injury associated with a fall greater than 15 feet has a fourfold greater chance of intracranial pathology than a MVA. Ascertain the mental status immediately following the accident (question prehospital personnel and other observers); try to determine if the patient is improving or deteriorating. Establish the duration of the stupor or coma and whether a lucid interval took place. In patients who are awake and responsive, verify the appearance of *posttraumatic retrograde or anterograde amnesia.* Headache is a nonspecific symptom as are nausea and dizziness. Inquire about use of alcohol or other drugs. When reviewing the patient's past medical history, ask about illnesses that may have precipitated the event (DM, cardiac disease, seizures) as well as medications and allergies.

Physical Examination

Note: *The physical examination always begins with an initial assessment and stabilization of the ABCs* (see section 4.1). The rapid and safe establishment of an adequate airway is essential in the management of the head injured patient. Care must be taken to ensure adequate immobilization of the neck until cervical spine injury has been excluded. Hypotension should never be attributed to a head injury until other causes are ruled out. Once life-threatening injuries are identified and addressed, a systematic approach to the rest of the physical examination is followed. Special attention is given to the neurologic and head examinations.

Vital signs. Frequent assessment of the pulse, blood pressure, and respirations is essential. Bradycardia accompanied by hypotension and irregular breathing (Cushing's response) is a *late* finding of increased ICP. Hypertension may occur early in serious head injury to compensate for increased ICP. Hypotension and bradycardia together imply an injury to the cervical spine (spinal shock).

HEENT. The head and scalp need to be carefully inspected and palpated for wounds (use a sterile glove when palpating). Any drainage from the ears or nose requires evaluation for a possible CSF leak that is secondary to a skull fracture with a dural tear. Look for a double halo (appearance of two circles) sign by placing a small amount of drainage on filter paper, permitting the blood to separate from the CSF, and check fluid for glucose. Additional clues to a possible basilar skull fracture include ecchymosis behind the ears *(Battle's sign),* hemotympanum, extensive subconjunctival hemorrhage that is unlimited posteriorly, bilateral periorbital hematomas *(raccoon eyes),* and deafness. Test for pupillary size, equality, and reflexes. Establish presence or absence of gag reflex.

Neck. Examine for C-spine tenderness, step-off, and/or crepitus.

Neurologic examination. The extent is dictated by the patient's condition. Mental status is the single most important indicator of serious head injury. Examine for focal neurologic deficits. *Decorticate* and *decerebrate* posturing signal an increased ICP with possible herniation. *Serial exams must be performed in all patients to document changes.* The Glasgow Coma Scale (GCS) is an objective measure of brain dysfunction that can be performed by all levels of health care workers (Table 4.2.1). The GCS addresses three separate responses: (1) eye opening, (2) verbal response, and (3) motor response. *Mild head injury* is defined as a GCS score of 13 to 15. *Moderate head injury* is defined as a GCS score of 9 to 12. *Severe head injury* is defined as a GCS score less than 8.

Prognosis

Stratifying patients according to risk for serious head injury not only is helpful in determining the need for subsequent diagnostic studies but also assists management. Presence of any single criterion from a higher risk group warrants assignment of the patient to the highest risk group applicable.

Low-risk criteria. Asymptomatic, mild headache or dizziness, minor scalp wounds (abrasions, lacerations, contusions, and hematomas), and absence of moderate- or high-risk criteria.

Moderate-risk criteria. Altered level of consciousness at time of injury or later, progressive headache, alcohol or drug intoxication, vomiting, posttraumatic seizure, posttraumatic amnesia (> 5 min), multisystem trauma, serious facial injury, signs of basilar skull fracture, chance of skull penetration or depressed skull, and unreliable or inadequate history.

High-risk criteria. Coma not clearly due to alcohol, drugs, or other causes (e.g., metabolic or postictal state), focal neurologic signs, decreasing level of consciousness, and evidence of penetrating skull injury or palpable depressed fracture.

Note: *Never assume a head injured patient with alcohol on the breath is simply drunk without documenting an alcohol level and excluding intracranial pathology first.*

Diagnostic Studies

Skull x-ray. Plain radiographs have little use in the evaluation of the patient with closed head trauma because of the limited information provided. While there is a higher incidence of associated intracranial hemorrhage in patients with skull fractures, the converse *is not* true; it is possible to sustain serious brain damage without a fracture.

CT scan. The diagnostic procedure of choice in the evaluation of the acutely head injured patient. CT studies are generally advocated for any head injured patient with a *GCS score* < 15, *presence of focal neurologic signs,* or patients with an *abnormal mental status not clearly attributable to alcohol, drugs, or other known causes.* Some trauma centers are promoting liberal use of CT as a screening tool, even in patients with low-risk criteria. In the acute setting, CT scans are performed without contrast material.

MRI. Despite its superiority to CT imaging in detecting cerebral contusions and small collections of blood, its use is limited by availability, cost, the time required to complete the study, and incompatibility with certain metal objects.

Cervical spine x-rays. A high index of suspicion for cervical spine injury is mandatory for all patients with head injury and altered level of consciousness. C-spine x-rays are not needed in conscious patients without distracting injuries who deny pain or tenderness to palpation.

Serum chemistries, WBC, T&C, blood alcohol, and drug screens. Usefulness is determined by clinical findings.

ABG. Indicated when hypoxia is suspected or to help guide hyperventilation therapy after intubation.

Special Considerations

Scalp lacerations. The scalp consists of five layers (the mnemonic is SCALP: skin, cutaneous tissue, aponeurosis, loose connective tissue, and pericranium). Scalp lacerations tend to bleed profusely because the vessels do not retract. Despite their often dramatic appearance, these wounds undergo satisfactory healing as long as basic wound management principles are followed. Generally, only a single-layer closure is required, except when the galea is violated, which is closed as a separate layer.

Penetrating and missile injuries. Treatment includes surgical débridement, antibiotics, and controlling ICP.

Basilar skull fracture. Usually appears in the petrous portion of the temporal bone although it may occur anywhere along the base of the skull. Clinical findings include hemotympanum, CSF rhinorrhea or otorrhea, periorbital ecchymosis, and postauricular hematomas. Diagnose clinically or radiographically by using CT or skull films. Use of antibiotics is controversial (discuss with consultant).

Depressed skull fractures. Concomitant intracranial pathology is common. Clinically, palpate the wound with a sterile glove (though the absence of scalp soft tissue injury does not always rule out skull fracture). Use CT bone windows or skull films to detect radiographically. Prompt neurosurgical attention is essential.

Concussion. Implies a head injury without a significant brain lesion. Temporary loss of consciousness occurs, as does amnesia (retrograde and anterograde). Additional transient symptoms include headache, dizziness, or nausea, but the neurologic exam should not reveal any deficits or localizing findings. The CT scan will be negative.

Contusion. Characterized by a focal area of petechial hemorrhage and/or cerebral edema, most commonly affecting the frontal and temporal lobes (especially along their undersurface). The contusion may occur at the site of impact *(coup)* or directly across the brain from the site *(contrecoup)*. Therapy is directed at controlling the ICP. Patients require admission for observation at the minimum.

Diffuse axonal injuries (DAIs). Preferentially involve the subcortical white matter at the gray matter–white matter interface and at the corpus callosum and brainstem. Typically occur after acceleration-deceleration-type injuries (often without direct impact). Patients may be comatose despite the absence of significant findings on CT. MRI is much more sensitive than CT in detecting DAI.

Epidural hematoma (EDH). Customarily arises from a tear in the middle meningeal artery, with blood collecting between the dura and cranial vault. Classically, a loss of consciousness immediately follows the incident and is followed by a lucid interval. Transtentorial herniation and rapid neurologic deterioration may occur if not promptly treated (stat neurosurgical consultation is mandated). EDHs are most commonly found in the temporal region and typically appear as a biconvex (lenticular) hyperdensity (density limited by cranial sutures) on CT.

Subdural hematoma (SDH). Results from tears of the veins bridging the cerebral cortices and dural sinuses. Predisposed patients include individuals with brain atrophy (elderly, alcoholics) and patients taking anticoagulants. Symptoms tend to be nonspecific. Onset can be rapid or insidious. CT scanning reveals a crescent-shaped density that conforms to the convexity of the cerebral hemisphere and can cross cranial suture sites. SDHs are classified by time frame and presentation on CT (CT attenuation characteristics depend, for the most part, on age of the injury but can be affected by the patient's hematocrit): *acute* (hyperdense on CT) presents in first 3 days postinjury, *subacute* (isodense on CT) manifests in 3 to 20 days, and *chronic* (hypodense on CT) appears more than 20 days after trauma. Morbidity and mortality are often due to associated intraparenchymal damage. Prompt neurosurgical consultation is called for.

Subarachnoid hemorrhage. Most prevalent form of intracranial hemorrhage following head trauma.

Intracerebral hemorrhage. Usually follows acceleration-deceleration-type injury. Seen as a small, round, or oval focus of high attenuation on CT (although delayed hemorrhage may not be seen on initial scan).

Treatment

After initial stabilization measures, the primary question for the ED physician is deciding which patients require *emergent* or *urgent neurosurgical* intervention. Time is of the essence and may influence transfer decisions. Patients requiring prompt surgical evaluation are those with *massive, depressed,* or *open skull fractures* along with those who exhibit large focal lesions on CT. Three factors are beneficial in estimating the need for neurosurgical intervention: (1) presence of coma, (2) altered mental status resulting from nonvehicular trauma, and (3) unequal motor strength. *However, a nonfocal neurologic examination and absence of LOC do not exclude an intracranial injury.*

Temporizing measures focus on maintaining CPP and controlling the ICP to prevent or lessen secondary insults to the brain parenchyma. Emergency treatment includes the following.

1. Provide the brain with adequate substrates of metabolism, mainly oxygen and glucose. Blood glucose concentration is typically not a problem in the trauma patient. Recent work has implied that hyperglycemia needs to be avoided as well as hypoglycemia. Satisfactory oxygenation depends on arterial hemoglobin and oxygen concentrations. Keep the $PaO_2 >$ 80 mm Hg. Blood transfusion may be necessary to ensure normal oxygen-carrying capacity.
2. CPP relies on both the systemic arterial pressure and the arterial $PaCO_2$. Strive to adjust the blood pressure to the patient's normal levels while maintaining the $PaCO < 40$ mm Hg. If the $PaCO_2$ rises too high, it can aggravate ICP.
3. A rapid rise in the $PaCO_2$ not only affects the cerebral circulation (causing cerebral vasodilation) but also aggravates the ICP. Although controversial, *hyperventilation* to a $PaCO_2$ of 26 to 28 mm Hg has been used to reduce ICP. Hyperventilation usually requires *rapid sequence intubation* followed by mechanical ventilation. Monitor blood gases closely. Judicious use of sedatives and paralyzing agents may be needed to prevent the increases in ICP seen with agitation or straining.
4. Diuretics may be beneficial in regulating ICP. *Mannitol* is an osmotically active agent that shifts water from brain tissue to the blood, shrinking brain volume and lowering ICP. For the average patient, the recommended dose is 1 g/kg IV (as a 20% solution over 20 min). However, exercise caution when using mannitol, as azotemia, electrolyte imbalances, and CHF may result. Generally, administer mannitol only after consultation with a neurosurgeon, because a rebound phenomenon may occur. Some neurosurgeons advocate supplementing

mannitol with furosemide (40 to 80 mg IV for adults) to control ICP.

5. Seizures increase the ICP and oxygen consumption and must be aggressively treated in the head injured patient (see section 3.3). The prophylactic administration of phenytoin (18 mg/kg IV as 50 mg/min) may be helpful.
6. Protect the patient from overhydration, which worsens cerebral edema. Monitor blood pressure and urine output frequently.
7. Guard against hyperthermia, as this also increases the risk for additional damage.
8. It may help to elevate the head of the bed to a 30° angle (with appropriate C-spine precautions).
9. Steroids are currently not recommended for head trauma patients.
10. The role of barbiturates is not clearly defined. After discussion with the neurosurgical consultant, consider pentobarbital in severely head injured patients who are unresponsive to standard therapy.
11. Restrict the use of *burr holes* (trephination) to dire circumstances, such as when the patient continues to deteriorate despite all other appropriate interventions and definitive neurosurgical care is not immediately available (e.g., neurosurgeon is many miles or hours away). Burr holes *should not* be done in patients who have shown evidence of brainstem dysfunction from the moment of injury. If CT scanning is not available, neurosurgeons recommend that the burr hole should be placed in the temporal region ipsilateral to the dilated pupil in comatose patients with decerebrate or decorticate posturing that is unresponsive to hyperventilation and mannitol. It is important to receive prior proper training in this procedure.
12. Methods of measuring ICP include *intraventricular catheter, subarachnoid screw,* and *epidural transducer.* Try to keep the ICP $<$ 15 mm Hg.

Admission Criteria

Any patient with an initially abnormal neurologic examination, depressed or worsening level of consciousness, skull fracture, or an abnormal CT scan requires hospitalization and neurosurgical consultation. If there is any question, neurosurgical consultation is warranted.

Patients who remain at a GCS score of 15, with no reported LOC, no signs of intoxication, and no evidence of skull fracture; *and* who maintain a normal level of alertness during observation (4 to 6 hr); *and* who have reliable observation at home may be safely discharged with a head instruction sheet and clear arrangements for follow-up. Some trauma centers advocate routine CT scanning on all head injury patients, especially those with reported LOC or posttraumatic amnesia.

Suggested Readings

Duus BR, Lind B, Christensen H, et al.: The role of neuroimaging in the initial management of patients with minor head injury. Ann Emerg Med 1994;23:1279–1283.

Fessler RD, Diaz FG: The management of cerebral perfusion pressure and intracranial pressure after severe head injury. Ann Emerg Med 1993;22:998–1003.

Walls RM: Rapid-sequence intubation in head trauma. Ann Emerg Med 1993;22:1008–1013.

4.3 SPINE AND SPINAL CORD TRAUMA

Description

Spinal injuries range from ligament sprain to minor avulsions of the spinous processes to complete cord transection. Motor vehicle accidents account for a majority of these injuries, with other common mechanisms being falls and sporting injuries (penetrating injuries are uncommon). The cervical spine accounts for more than half of spinal injuries. Patients with one spinal injury are at greater risk for additional spinal injuries. Be aware that vertebral injuries may present without indication of spinal cord injury. However, inadequate immobilization or injudicious movement or manipulation of the patient may cause a spinal cord injury or worsen a patient's prognosis.

History

Spine and spinal cord injuries are frequently sequelae of multisystem trauma. The orderly approach outlined for multiple trauma (see section 4.1) must be followed for spinal trauma. It is essential to try to establish what the patient's neurologic condition was before the current trauma. Descriptions of mechanism of injury are important in determining the potential for spinal trauma and the presence of other injuries. A conscious patient with paralysis should be capable of indicating the site of injury, because a loss of sensation occurs below this level.

Physical Examination

Note: *In many patients, spinal trauma is but one component of multiple injuries; therefore, the physical examination always begins with an initial assessment and stabilization of the ABCs* (see section 4.1). As long as the patient is properly immobilized, clearance of the spine can be safely delayed until adequate breathing and hemodynamic stability is ensured.

General. For the multiple trauma patient, ensure complete immobilization, maintaining the cervical spine in a neutral position, until roentgenograms are obtained and vertebral injury is excluded. Clinical signs of *cervical cord injury* in the *unconscious patient* include flaccid areflexia, apnea (lesion at C2–3), diaphragmatic breathing (lesion at or below C4–5), ability to flex but not extend arm at elbow, response to pain only above the clavicles, priapism, and hypotension along with bradycardia in the absence of hypovolemia.

Spine. Examine the entire spine (from the occiput to the sacrum). Log roll the patient, using people: one to maintain in-line immobilization of the head and neck, one to secure the torso, one for the legs, and a team leader to direct the maneuver and remove the spinal board as necessary. Assess spine for localized pain, tenderness, deformity (step-off), edema, ecchymosis, and muscle spasm. Also check the anterior neck for tracheal deviation, tenderness, and hematoma.

Neurologic exam. An attentive examination is essential. Check for motor strength and weakness, sensory deficits, and variations in reflexes; assess the rectal sphincter tone and bulbocavernosus reflex (these may be only signs of neurologic function, implying sacral sparing and improving the prognosis). *A negative neurologic examination does not confirm absence of injury to the spine or spinal cord.*

Diagnostic Tests

Cervical spine x-rays. Obtain an adequate cross-table roentgenogram of the cervical spine (identify all seven cervical vertebra as well as C-7 on T-1) in all patients at risk for cervical spine injury, once life-threatening problems are recognized and controlled. A cross-table lateral x-ray discloses only 80 to 90% of the injuries. If lower cervical vertebra cannot be adequately visualized, a swimmer's view or supplemental studies are obligatory (CT scan, tomograms). A three-view series is considered routine and includes an open-mouth (odontoid), AP and lateral views. All three films need to be reviewed scrupulously by a qualified physician and checked for the *ABCs:* alignment and angulation of the vertebral bodies and spinous processes, the bony contour and integrity, the cartilage, and the soft tissue and interspinous spaces. Flexion-extension films may be indicated in patients with persistent neck pain who remain neurologically intact but lack radiographic abnormalities; however, *these studies may be dangerous and should only be done under the direct supervision of a knowledgeable physician.* See Table 4.3.1 for radiological criteria that suggest an unstable cervical spine injury. Currently, studies are under way to identify high-risk criteria, which will allow more selective ordering of cervical spine x-rays. For now, complete cervical spine roentgenograms are indicated in all victims of major multiple trauma, trauma patients with manifestations of cervical spine injury (posttraumatic neck pain, neurologic deficits), and patients with conditions that may interfere with clinical evaluation (head injury, alcohol or drug use, painful distracting injury).

CT or MRI. Further investigation is needed anytime spinal injury cannot be excluded by plain roentgenograms or there is a suspicion that a bone or disk fragment is encroaching on the spinal cord.

Table 4.3.1
Radiological Criteria That Suggest Unstable Cervical Spine Injury

Vertebral body compression $> 25\%$
Angulation between vertebral bodies $> 12°$
Vertebral override of superior on inferior vertebra $> 25\%$
Teardrop fracture of anteroinferior margin of cervical vertebra
Lateral masses of C-1 displaced laterally (Jefferson fracture)
Bilateral pedicle fractures of C-2 (Hangman's fracture)
Soft tissue space between the posterior aspect of C-2 and the anterior margin of the odontoid > 3 mm (Odontoid fracture)

Thoracolumbar spine. Cross-table lateral and AP views of the thoracolumbar spine are generally obtained as part of secondary radiographic survey when indicated (back pain, neurologic deficit, mechanism of injury). The incidence of thoracic and lumbar spine fractures is increasing. Unlike a cervical hematoma, a paravertebral hematoma in the thoracolumbar region is best seen on the AP view. Maintain immobilization of the entire spine until the radiographic evaluation has been completed and the spine cleared.

Special Considerations

Complete Cord Syndrome

In complete cord syndrome, the patient exhibits loss of all neurologic function below the level of injury. The chance of recovery in these patients is very poor. Complete disruption of the cervical or upper thoracic spinal cord may induce vasodilation, bradycardia, and hypotension (due to interruption of autonomic innervation). This state is known as *neurogenic or spinal shock.*

Incomplete Spinal Cord Lesions

In incomplete spinal cord lesions, the patient retains some neurologic function after the time of injury. Examine such patients carefully, because the presence of any motor or sensory response (sacral sparing) greatly improves the prognosis. Examples of incomplete cord injuries include the following:

- *Central cord syndrome* is usually caused by hyperextension injuries and is characterized by a disproportionately greater weakness and sensory loss of the upper than of the lower extremities; bladder dysfunction also occurs.
- *Brown-Sequard syndrome* involves a hemisection of the spinal cord following penetrating trauma and manifests as loss of power and fine sensation on the side of the injury along with a contralateral loss of pain and temperature below the level of the lesion.
- *Anterior cord syndrome* is produced by flexion injuries whereby bony fragments or the intervertebral disk protrudes onto the spinal cord, resulting in complete paralysis and loss of pain and temperature sensation below the level of the injury while retaining light touch and vibratory sensation.

Treatment

Heed the basic tenets outlined in section 4.1, especially those that pertain to securing and sustaining the airway. Remember that patients with C-spine injuries are at risk of partial or total loss of respiratory function. *Until proven otherwise, the spine should be considered unstable, placing the cord at risk for further injury.* Continuous immobilization is essential until a spinal and/or spinal cord injury can be conclusively ruled out; if necessary, maintain immobilization until the patient can be seen by an appropriate consultant (multisystem trauma patients who are being transferred to a trauma center also require immobilization of the entire spine). Skull traction, employing Gardner-Wells tongs to correct alignment of the spine, may be necessary and mandates a call to the neurosurgeon.

Corticosteroids may lessen the degree of neurologic injury in a certain subset of patients with blunt spinal cord injuries. Current protocols call for a 30 mg/kg bolus of *methylprednisolone* administered within 8 hr of injury, followed by a 5.4 mg/kg/hr infusion for 23 hr.

Always attempt to identify life-threatening bleeding that may explain shock before attributing findings to *neurogenic shock.* Fluid therapy is provided to obtain a systolic blood pressure > 90 mm Hg. If pressure cannot be elevated despite adequate fluid restoration, pressors such as dopamine may be warranted. Also, early use of an NG tube and Foley catheter are recommended to avoid distention of the stomach and bladder.

Admission Criteria

All patients with spinal or spinal cord injury must be admitted for further evaluation and treatment. In addition, neurosurgery needs to be involved in the early care of spinal cord injury patients.

Suggested Readings

Bracken MB, et al.: Methylprednisolone or naloxone treatment after acute spinal cord injury: 1-year follow-up data. Results of the Second National Acute Spinal Cord Injury Study. J Neurosurg 1992; 76(1): 23–31.

Hoffman JR, Schriger DL, Mower W, et al.: Cervical spine radiography in blunt trauma: a prospective study. Ann Emerg Med 1992;21: 1454–1460.

Pal JM, Mulder DS, Brown RA, et al.: Assessing multiple trauma: is the cervical spine enough? J Trauma 1988;28:1282–1286.

4.4 CHEST TRAUMA

Description

Chest injuries account for 25% of the trauma deaths in the United States, yet less than 15% of thoracic trauma victims require surgery. Both penetrating (knife wounds, gunshot wounds, sharp objects) and blunt (compression or crush type injury, deceleration event) chest trauma are capable of causing severe damage to the chest wall, lungs, trachea, major bronchi, esophagus, thoracic duct, heart, diaphragm, mediastinal vessels, and spinal cord. Any combination of these injuries may occur. Immediately perceptible life-threatening injuries include *airway obstruction, tension pneumothorax, open pneumothorax, massive hemothorax, flail chest,* and *cardiac tamponade.* Subtler injuries detected during the secondary survey include *pulmonary contusion, myocardial contusion, aortic disruption, traumatic diaphragmatic rupture, tracheobronchial disruption,* and *esophageal rupture.*

History

Quickly determine the mechanism and severity of the injury, complying with the principles outlined in section 4.1.

Physical Examination

Note: *Significant intrathoracic injury can occur without apparent external chest wall damage.*

General. Abide by the principles of the primary survey. Verify that the airway is clear of blood, secretions, and vomitus. Determine the "degree of extremis" as well as the initial blood pressure, heart rate, and respiratory rate.

Neck. Check the position of the trachea (deviated away from the side of tension pneumothorax) and decide if neck veins are distended or collapsed. Palpate for swelling, tenderness, and subcutaneous emphysema in addition to the carotid pulses.

Chest. Inspect the chest wall for wounds, bruising, and seat-belt marks and observe the motion of the chest wall (intercostal retractions, splinting, paradoxical motion). Auscultate for symmetry of breath sounds and palpate for tenderness and crepitus.

Abdomen. Diaphragmatic rupture with herniation of the abdominal contents into the chest cavity may present with a scaphoid abdomen (see section 4.5).

Diagnostic Tests

Follow the suggestions given in section 4.1 for ordering diagnostic adjuncts. Specific studies that may be beneficial in identifying and managing chest trauma include the following.

CXR. Obtain immediately after stabilization measures and cervical spine films. An erect film is best, if feasible; supine radiographs may conceal a hemothorax or pneumothorax and can mimic the findings of traumatic disruption of the aorta. **Note:** *Tension pneumothorax is a clinical diagnosis; life-saving maneuvers must be performed before the CXR is taken.*

ABG. Hypoxia may be deceptive with chest injuries.

ECG. Indicated in patients with blunt chest trauma to rule out a myocardial contusion.

Bronchoscopy. Aids in the diagnosis of tracheal or bronchial rupture.

Special Considerations

Rib and Sternal Fractures

Rib and sternal fractures are the products of blunt trauma to the chest wall, crush injuries (seat belt), and blast injuries. Clinically, patients with chest wall injuries experience pain (exacerbated with deep breathing), tenderness or crepitus on palpation, and bruising. The foremost concern with rib and sternal fractures (especially with damage to the first or second rib) is the possibility of concomitant intrathoracic injury. Rib fractures customarily occur at the point of impact or the posterior lateral angle. A chest x-ray may or may not reveal the fracture, but it is indicated to rule out more significant intrathoracic injuries. Therapy is directed at pain control and maintenance of adequate ventilation. Elderly patients, patients with multiple rib fractures, and patients with preexisting lung disease are more prone to complications (atelectasis, pneumonia, respiratory failure); thus it is prudent to hospitalize these patients for pain control and pulmonary toilet.

Flail Chest

Flail chest is characterized by multiple (more than three) rib fractures in two or more places, resulting in a free-floating segment of the chest wall. Classically, paradoxical movement (sucked in during inspiration) of the flail segment appears. However, a flail chest is not always obvious because of muscle splinting. Therefore, careful inspection and palpation of the chest wall are essential to detect subtle findings. The majority of patients who harbor a flail chest also display serious intrathoracic injuries, which might compromise breathing. While a flail segment itself does not mandate mechanical ventilation, endotracheal intubation is generally required for patients with an altered mental status, shock, multisystem trauma, and history of chronic lung disease. Intubation is also required for elderly victims (> 65 years) and patients for whom the PaO_2 cannot be adequately maintained despite 100% oxygenation via face mask. All victims of a flail chest should be admitted to the ICU for monitoring, pulmonary toilet, and satisfactory pain control (parenteral analgesics, intercostal and epidural nerve blocks).

Simple Pneumothorax

Simple pneumothorax may follow blunt or penetrating trauma. The presence of air within the pleural space causes collapse of the lung and ventilation problems that may ultimately compromise oxygenation. Patients complain of dyspnea and severe chest pain, while exhibiting tachypnea, decreased breath sounds, hyperresonance on the affected side, and presence of subcutaneous air. Treatment consists of lung reexpansion with a large-bore chest tube (see section 21.2).

Tension Pneumothorax

Tension pneumothorax results from the development of a one-way valvularair leak (allowing air to enter the chest cavity but not to escape). Eventually, collapse of the lung occurs, followed by displacement of the mediastinum and trachea to the contralateral side. It culminates in the distortion of the vasculature, with diminished venous return to the heart, compression of the contralateral lung, and cardiovascular collapse. Tension pneumothorax should be diagnosed clinically, not radiographically, and manifests as tachypnea, hypotension, tracheal deviation, jugular venous distention, and diminished breath sounds on the affected side. Treatment consists of immediate decompression via needle thoracostomy followed by the placement of a chest tube.

Hemothorax

Although more common with a penetrating injury, hemothorax can arise from blunt trauma. Blood loss into the chest cavity can jeopardize cardiac output and impair ventilation by compressing the lung. Findings on physical exam include shock, respiratory distress, decreased breath sounds, and dullness to percussion on the affected side. Treatment involves tube thoracostomy and restoration of volume deficits. A *massive hemothorax* is defined as >1500 mL of fluid drained initially or a continuing blood loss greater than 200 mL/hr for 3 to 4 hr and requires surgical consultation for an open thoracotomy. Consider autotransfusion if the appropriate collecting device is available.

Open Pneumothorax

While most penetrating wounds to the chest seal spontaneously, a few remain open, creating a sucking chest wound. If the defect is more than two-thirds the diameter of the trachea, air is preferentially drawn through the chest defect than through the trachea, causing a tension pneumothorax scenario (discussed above). ED management consists of inserting a chest tube (*not* through the wound) and dressing the defect with a sterile occlusive dressing large enough to cover the wound.

Pulmonary Contusions and Lacerations

A consequence of blunt or penetrating trauma is bruising or lacerations of the lung. Pulmonary parenchymal injuries can proceed to interstitial edema and hemorrhage, provoking pulmonary shunting with subsequent hypoxia. Associated rib fractures or flail chest is common. A nonsegmental pulmonary infiltrate emerges on the chest x-ray, although radiological findings may not become apparent for 6 to 8 hr. ABGs reveal hypoxia and an increased alveolar-arterial gradient (see section 2.2). Treatment is similar to that for a flail chest: maintain adequate ventilation and oxygenation, avoid fluid overload, and supply adequate analgesia.

Myocardial Contusion

Myocardial contusion can occur with blunt chest trauma, typically following an MVA when the chest strikes the steering wheel. Cardiac contusion, if clinically significant, may provoke dysrhythmias, ventricular failure, conduction blocks, or myocardial ischemia (the right ventricle is most frequently affected because of its proximity to the chest wall). The ECG is generally nonspecific, usually exhibiting tachycardia or nonspecific ST-T wave changes; but it may reveal evidence of ischemia, conduction blocks, or arrhythmias. The best method of diagnosing cardiac contusion is controversial, with most authors advocating echocardiogram when the diagnosis is considered. Cardiac enzymes tend to be nonspecific.

Cardiac Tamponade

Although the most common cause is penetrating injury, blunt trauma may also result in a tamponade. Classical findings *(Beck's triad)* include neck vein distention, muffled heart tones, and hypotension. In reality, some of these findings are often absent. The neck veins may be flat because of hypovolemia, while heart sounds can be difficult to assess in a noisy ED. A central venous line and CVP measurement may assist in the diagnosis. Electrical alternans may appear on the ECG. Signs and symptoms are similar to those of a tension pneumothorax. Initial therapy is directed to ensuring adequate oxygenation and providing sufficient fluid to try to improve cardiac output. Pericardiocentesis (see section 21.2) may be lifesaving for the patient in extremis. However, this is not a definitive procedure and needs to be followed by a thoracotomy.

Traumatic Aortic Rupture

TAR accompanies severe decelerating injuries (automobile collision, fall from great height) and is usually instantaneously fatal. The injury normally occurs at the junction of the fixed and mobile portions of the aorta, just distal to the subclavian artery. Survival is possible if the transection is not complete and the hematoma is contained (false aneurysm). Rapid diagnosis and treatment are essential if patients are to be salvaged. A high index of suspicion is mandatory, as there may be no external evidence of trauma. Manifestations include retrosternal or interscapular pain, hoarseness, upper extremity hypertension (coarctation), harsh systolic murmur, and frank shock. Chest x-rays do not reveal aortic transection directly, but certain signs imply possible aortic injury: widened mediastinum ($>$ 8 cm), ill-defined aortic knob, left apical cap, downward displacement of left bronchus, tracheal deviation to the right, NG tube deviation to the right, widened paraspinal stripes, and fracture of first or second rib. Although CT scan or transesophageal echocardiography is a useful diagnostic adjunct, aortography remains the gold standard and should not be delayed in cases highly suspicious for TAR.

Esophageal and Major Tracheobronchial Injuries

Esophageal and major tracheobronchial injuries are uncommon, but if they are not diagnosed, they may be lethal. Consider the diagnosis in patients who exhibit unique features, such as pneumomediastinum, particulate matter in thoracostomy drainage, or a massive air leak in the chest. Hints to diaphragmatic rupture on chest x-ray include irregularity of diaphragmatic contour or elevation of diaphragm, gas collections in the hemithorax, a contralateral mediastinal shift, and lower lobe opacification. If the diagnosis remains unclear, a Gastrografin or dilute barium swallow may confirm an esophageal leak.

Treatment

Comply with the basic tenets outlined in section 4.1, recalling that hypoxia is the gravest initial threat to life. Therefore, establish a reliable airway and restore the mechanics of breathing. Resuscitate the cardiovascular system as necessary. See "Special Considerations" on page 158 for specific recommendations. Guidelines for the use of needle and tube thoracostomy are in section 21.2. Resuscitative thoracotomy is generally reserved for victims of penetrating trauma who show some signs of life (see section 21.2) but is of little clinical use for victims of blunt trauma.

Suggested Readings

Biff WL, Moore FA, Moore EE, et al.: Cardiac enzymes are irrelevant in the patient with suspected myocardial contusion. Am J Surg 1994; 168:523–528.

Groskin SA: Selected topics in chest trauma. Radiology 1992;183:605–617.

Ivatury RR, Kazigo J, Rohman M, et al.: "Directed" emergency room thoracotomy: a prognostic prerequisite for survival. J Trauma 1991;31: 1076–1082.

4.5 ABDOMINAL TRAUMA

Description

Abdominal injuries may be subtle or overt. Several factors account for the difficulty in assessing abdominal trauma: (1) a wide spectrum of injuries is possible because of the number of organs that can be involved, (2) initial physical findings are frequently unreliable as 20% of patients with acute hemoperitoneum exhibit a benign abdominal exam, and (3) many patients manifest a diminished perception to pain secondary to head injury or drug or alcohol intoxication.

The abdomen extends from the nipples (fifth intercostal space) to the gluteal creases, encompassing three distinct anatomical compartments: the *peritoneum* (incorporates the portion of the abdomen covered by the bony thorax and the anterior abdominal segment), the *retroperitoneum* (difficult to evaluate; includes the aorta, vena cava, pancreas, kidneys, ureters, and portions of the colon and duodenum), and the *pelvis* (includes the rectum, bladder, iliac vessels, uterus, and ovaries). Customarily, abdominal trauma is classified as penetrating or blunt, but the initial ED assessment and resuscitation are similar. **Remember:** *Penetrating chest trauma may damage abdominal organs.*

History

Abdominal trauma is frequently accompanied by injury to other organ systems. Follow the approach summarized in section 4.1. Specifically note the particulars of the accident to estimate the forces involved. While any abdominal discomfort after trauma is significant, especially when accompanied by shoulder tip pain (Kehr's sign; blood irritating the diaphragm), absence of pain does not exclude serious abdominal injury. Any woman beyond 20 weeks of pregnancy is at high risk for injury to herself and the baby.

Physical Examination

Note: *In any trauma patient, always start by conducting a primary survey to identify and treat life-threatening injuries.*

General. Note any altered level of consciousness, obvious intoxication, or obtundation from shock. Ensure the patient is completely exposed by removing all clothing.

Vital signs. Tachycardia is often the only sign of hemorrhage. Although uncommon, some patients with significant abdominal trauma may be bradycardic (vagal effect). Observe how the abdomen moves with respiration.

Chest. Abdominal viscera are concurrently injured in a significant portion of patients with penetrating or blunt chest trauma. Scrupulously inspect the chest wall and ensure equality and presence of breath sounds. Thoracic bowel sounds imply a diaphragmatic injury.

Abdomen. Systematically inspect the abdomen, including all anterior structures, flanks, and posterior structures (back, buttocks, and perineum) for signs of penetrating injury (entrance and exit wounds), bruising, abrasions, lacerations, seat-belt marks or impressions, distention, and scars. Absent bowel sounds frequently accompany intraperitoneal injury, but the lack of bowel sounds is not definite for intraabdominal injury. Palpate, both superficially and deeply, all abdominal structures. Note if the tenderness is localized (particularly over the liver and spleen) or diffuse, although a false-positive outcome may occur secondary to abdominal wall injury. Involuntary guarding and rebound tenderness imply peritoneal irritation. Signs of intestinal rupture (especially the small bowel) may be slow to develop, necessitating *serial abdominal examinations* (best if done by same observer).

Rectal. Note the presence of bruising, penetrating injury, blood within the bowel lumen, rectal wall tears, abnormal prostate position, or lack of sphincter tone.

Genitourinary. Observe for priapism (suggests spinal cord injury). Check for meatal blood in males and vaginal bleeding in females.

Back. After taking the necessary precautions for possible spinal injury, log roll the patient to examine the flank and back to rule out unsuspected injury. Palpate the entire spine.

Diagnostic Tests

Laboratory tests. Order appropriate blood studies (as delineated in section 4.1) to establish baseline values along with type and cross-matching. Amylase levels may be elevated with duodenal or pancreatic trauma (although serum levels lack both sensitivity and specificity and are not useful as screening tools).

Plain abdominal films. Of limited value in the acute situation. An erect chest x-ray is preferable to a supine abdominal film when looking for free intraperitoneal air.

Abdominal CT scan. A scan with double contrast (oral and intravenous) is very helpful in assessing the hemodynamically stable abdominal trauma patient and allows simultaneous evaluation of the intraperitoneal and retroperitoneal spaces. CT scans are also used to stage parenchymal injuries (spleen, liver). Hollow viscus and pancreatic injuries bear the greatest risk of a false-negative result, although the use of both oral and intravenous contrasts increases the sensitivity. The timing of the intravenous contrast administration is important; the head CT should be done before administering the intravenous contrast.

Abdominal ultrasound. Ultrasound holds much promise since it can be easily done at the bedside of the trauma patient; is safe and inexpensive; provides another means of detecting subcapsular, intraparenchymal, and intramesenterial hematomas; and supplies information about retroperitoneal structures (bladder, kidneys, aorta). Nevertheless, hollow viscus injuries are difficult to detect, and the sensitivity of the test is operator dependent.

Diagnostic peritoneal lavage (DPL). Permits a rapid evaluation of the abdominal cavity for significant intraabdominal injury (as little as 5 mL of free intraperitoneal blood can be detected). It does not provide organ-specific information, may fail to detect diaphragmatic ruptures, and may miss injuries to the retroperitoneal organs (pancreas, duodenum, kidneys, bladder, ureter). Relatively insignificant injuries (minor liver laceration) may yield positive results, prompting unnecessary surgery. Performance of a DPL significantly alters the subsequent physical findings of the abdomen and should be done in conjunction with the surgical consultant. An NG tube and Foley catheter must be inserted before performing the DPL. The only absolute contraindication is the need for immediate laparotomy, while relative contraindications include multiple previous surgeries, massive obesity, presence of bleeding diathesis, and pelvic fractures.

Wound exploration. A gunshot wound that penetrates the peritoneum requires an exploratory laparotomy. Stab wounds may be managed selectively with local wound exploration; determine if the rectus fascia is intact or violated.

Treatment

Heed the principles summarized in section 4.1 for initial management of both penetrating and blunt abdominal trauma. A nasogastric tube is inserted for therapeutic and diagnostic purposes. Removal of the stomach contents decreases the risk of aspiration, and the presence of blood in the gastric drainage implies an injury to the GI tract. If there are severe facial fractures, insert the NG tube through the mouth. Insertion of a Foley catheter decompresses the bladder, evaluates for hematuria, and permits more accurate fluid monitoring. Contraindications to Foley insertion include a high-riding prostate, scrotal hematoma, and blood at the meatus. Notify the surgical consultant or trauma team the moment a significant abdominal injury is suspected.

Admission Criteria

Immediate laparotomy (do not squander time with a DPL or radiological studies) is indicated when abdominal bleeding progresses to profound shock, major vasculature injuries are prominent, a retroperitoneal hematoma is expanding, peritoneal findings are unequivocal, abdominal wall disruption is apparent, the bowel is eviscerated, the peritoneum has been punctured, the bladder or diaphragm is ruptured, a gunshot wound is not clearly tangential and superficial, or free air is present on the chest film. *Patients with an equivocal history or physical findings* necessitate serial examinations, and further diagnostic procedures (CT, DPL). The order of priority of diagnostic studies for patients with combined head and abdominal injuries is determined by the surgical consultant. S*table patients with a negative DPL and/or CT scan* require close observation for a minimum of 12 to 24 hr. Trauma victims who arrive in a hospital not equipped to deal with significant trauma should undergo stabilization and should be transferred as soon as possible via paramedic vehicle or air transport.

Suggested Readings

American College of Emergency Physicians: Clinical policy for the initial approach to patients presenting with acute blunt trauma. Ann Emerg Med 1993;22:1101–1113.

Liu M, Lee, CH, P'eng FK: Prospective comparison of diagnostic peritoneal lavage, computed tomographic scanning, and ultrasonography for the diagnosis of blunt abdominal trauma. J Trauma 1993;35: 267–270.

Wisner DH, Victor NS, Holcroft JW: Priorities in the management of multiple trauma: intracranial versus intraabdominal injury. J Trauma 1993;35:271–278.

4.6 PELVIC AND UROLOGIC TRAUMA

Description

In the general evaluation of the trauma patient, a pelvic fracture underscores the magnitude of disruptive energy at the time of injury. The pelvis is well vascularized, as are the surrounding muscles. Consequently, victims of severe pelvic disruptions are at risk of life-threatening exsanguination and of sustaining a concomitant genitourinary (GU) injury. A wide spectrum of injuries is associated with GU trauma, with injuries being classified as upper (kidney, ureter) or lower (bladder, prostate, urethra, genitalia). Anyone with trauma to the genitalia, back, abdomen, flank, pelvis, or perineum is at risk for GU trauma. Isolated GU system injury is rare, and while few GU injuries necessitate immediate intervention, missed GU injuries may result in significant morbidity and mortality. Optimal management depends on prompt and accurate diagnosis of injuries.

History

Establish the mechanism of trauma (blunt versus penetrating). A preponderance of severe pelvic injuries arises from auto-pedestrian, motor cycle, or high fall accidents. Signs and symptoms of GU trauma are often obscured by concomitant injuries. Meaningful data from the past medical history include congenital abnormalities of the GU tract, coagulopathies, and renal disease. In women, determine the date of the last menstrual period and the possibility of pregnancy.

Physical Examination

General. Completely undress the patient so the chest, abdomen, and perineum are completely exposed.

Vital signs. Hypotension in the pelvic trauma victim may arise from hemorrhage associated with the fracture of the pelvic bones, intraabdominal injuries, or retroperitoneal or pelvic vasculature damage.

Back. Log roll the patient to inspect for contusions, hematomas, or ecchymosis. Palpate for tenderness, masses, and swelling.

Check for localized flank tenderness; a flattening of the flank together with a flank mass implies the presence of a perinephric hematoma.

Abdomen. Refer to section 4.5.

Bony pelvis. The integrity of the pelvic ring can be grossly tested by gentle lateral compression and distraction of the iliac crests, gentle inward compression of the symphysis pubis, and hip flexion. Do this carefully to prevent further displacement of unstable fractures.

Gastrourinary. Spread the legs apart to adequately visualize the perineum. Inspect for evidence of penetrating trauma, and note any swelling or bruising. Examine the penis for direct trauma or blood at the meatus. **Note:** *Do not introduce a Foley catheter if any of these signs is present.*

Rectum. Evaluate for sphincter tone, position of the prostate, presence of presacral hematoma, impression of bony integrity, and appearance of frank blood.

Vagina. Blood in the vagina suggests either a penetrating wound or compound pelvic fracture (open fracture). If the patient is pregnant, blood appearing at the cervical os may signify abruption of the placenta (see section 10.6). Amniotic fluid in the vaginal vault suggests rupture of membranes.

Extremities. Note gross leg length discrepancy. Check for the presence and quality of the pulses symmetrically. Verify sensation, strength, and deep tendon reflexes.

Diagnostic Tests

Urinalysis. If the patient is conscious, determine if he or she can void spontaneously. An adequate urinary specimen is an essential screening test in all patients with suspected GU injury. The degree of hematuria is not indicative of severity or extent of injury; indeed life-threatening pedicle avulsion can occur in the absence of hematuria. Consequential hematuria is characterized by gross hematuria accompanying blunt trauma, presence of any degree of hematuria (including microscopic hematuria) secondary to penetrating trauma, or microscopic hematuria with shock (blood pressure < 90 mm Hg) and blunt trauma.

Foley catheter. If the patient is unconscious, in shock, or cannot micturate and if there are no contraindications (see Table 4.6.1), a Foley catheter is inserted to sample the urine and

Table 4.6.1
Contraindications to Urinary Catherization

Perineal bruising
Blood at the meatus
Scrotal hematoma
High-riding prostate
Severe pelvic fracture
Bladder perforation

monitor resuscitation. *Always perform a careful rectal/genital exam before inserting a Foley catheter.*

Plain films. Pelvic x-rays are part of the initial radiological screening process in multiple trauma patients. Sometimes, abdominal films are helpful (loss of psoas shadow implies retroperitoneal injury). Presence of lower posterior rib fractures or fractures of the lumbar transverse processes suggests possible renal or ureter injury.

Ultrasound. May be useful in patients without significant hematuria to rule out renal trauma.

Contrast studies. Execute a *urethrogram* before inserting a Foley catheter when a urethral tear is suspected. A *cystogram* is performed to demonstrate the integrity of the bladder. An *intravenous pyelogram* (IVP) may be beneficial in patients with suspected renal trauma or isolated ureteral injury. In the stable patient, many trauma centers now prefer CT with double contrast to IVP when there is suspicion of concomitant intraabdominal and/or retroperitoneal injuries. Intravenous contrast studies are unreliable in the hypotensive patient.

Renal arteriography. Indicated when there is suspicion for major kidney injury or involvement of the renal pedicle. CT scanning has decreased the need for arteriography in assessing renal artery injuries.

Diagnostic peritoneal lavage (DPL). In the patient with suspected pelvic fracture, DPL must be performed above the umbilicus. While the presence of the free flow of gross blood obligates a celiotomy (laparotomy), a positive diagnostic lavage by RBC count must be interpreted cautiously (RBCs may represent retroperitoneal leakage instead of intraabdominal injury).

Special Considerations

Pelvic fractures. The Kane classification helps estimate the severity of pelvic damage and the probability of associated injuries (see Table 4.6.2).

Table 4.6.2
Fracture Types and Associated Injuries

Type	Description	Associated Injuries	Examples
I	Fracture of individual bones without a break in the continuity of the pelvic ring; represents 33% of pelvic fractures	Rare	Avulsion fractures of anterior superior iliac spine, ischial tuberosity, or antero-inferior iliac spine; fractures of pubis or ischium; fracture of the wing of the ilium; fracture of the sacrum or coccyx
II	Single break in the pelvic ring; generally stable if < 5 mm of displacement is present; be sure not to overlook a less obvious second fracture	Intrapelvic visceral injuries may occur in up to 25% of cases	Fracture of two ipsilateral rami; minimal subluxation or fracture of sacroiliac joint; minimal subluxation or fracture of pubic symphysis
III	Double vertical breaks in the pelvic ring; commonly severe and unstable	Resultant hemorrhage may be life-threatening; serious GU, intraabdominal, and neurologic injuries may occur	Malgaigne (double break in hemipelvis); bilateral pubic rami and ischial rami fractures (straddle fractures); sprung pelvis (wide separation of pubic symphysis and one or both sacroiliac joints)
IV	Acetabular fractures with or without hip dislocation	Extremity fractures appear in 50% of cases; nerve injuries (e.g., sciatic) seen in up to 20% of patients	Rim fracture; central acetabular fracture-dislocation; ischioacetabular fracture

Renal injuries. Classified as *minor, major,* or *critical.* Minor injuries (contusions, lacerations) consist of minor bruising or tearing of the renal parenchyma, but the renal capsule remains intact, and there is no calyceal disruption. Major injuries include deep lacerations of the kidney, capsular tears, and renal pelvis or calyceal injuries. Critical injuries encompass kidney fragmentation and renal pedicle injuries (renal artery thrombosis, avulsion of renal vessels, and rupture of the pelviureteric junction). Minor and major renal trauma comprise 95% of cases of blunt renal trauma.

Ureteral injury. The overall incidence of traumatic ureteral injury is low and is usually associated with penetrating trauma or severe pelvic fractures. An expanding flank mass may be the only sign. Diagnosis is made by CT, IVP, or exploratory laparotomy. Late diagnosis occurs when urine extravasates into the abdomen.

Bladder injury. Frequently associated with pelvic fractures, especially in patients sustaining pubic rami, protruding acetabular, or Malgaigne fractures. Perforations may be intraperitoneal or extraperitoneal. Intraperitoneal lacerations are most common in patients who have been drinking, have a full bladder, and suffer blunt trauma from a steering wheel. Common presenting signs are gross hematuria and suprapubic tenderness. Diagnosis is made by retrograde cystography.

Urethral injury. Serious injury is rare, but if not properly managed, the outcome can be devastating (e.g., impotence, stricture). Urethral damage is subdivided into posterior urethral injury (superior to the urogenital diaphragm) and anterior urethral injury (distal to urogenital diaphragm). Posterior urethral injuries are most common in males (the urethra is only rarely injured in females) and accompanies pelvic fractures. Consider urethral injury in patients with perineal bruising, a boggy or high-riding prostate, blood at the meatus or the vagina, and inability to pass urine. Perform a urethrogram to visualize the extent and location of the injury. Posterior injury has a 20 to 30% association with bladder injury. Anterior urethral injury customarily occurs with straddle type trauma, manifesting as penile swelling or a large perineal or scrotal collection of fluid. *Do not pass a urethral catheter in any patient with suspected urethral injury, as the catheter may aggravate the injury.*

Treatment

Initial management is directed at restoring intravascular volume, careful monitoring of the patient, and ruling out serious extrapelvic injuries. Pelvic hemorrhage is most effectively controlled by stabilizing the pelvis, thereby permitting the closed retroperitoneal space to tamponade. Currently, *external pelvic fixation* is the preferred method for rapid control (can be applied in about 15 min), but the pneumatic antishock garment serves as a temporizing measure until more formal pelvic stabilization can be achieved. In cases where pelvic stabilization fails to control bleeding, prompt arteriography is indicated, with the expectation of stopping the bleeding by embolization of the involved vessel. Open pelvic fractures require thorough wound débridement (in the OR), appropriate pelvic stabilization, and a diverting colostomy (a multidisciplinary approach is necessary). Critical renal injuries (renal fragmentation, pedicle injuries) are the only true operative emergencies. Most renal injuries are managed expectantly (bed rest, analgesics, prophylactic antibiotics, serial ultrasonography) and have an excellent prognosis. Treatment of bladder and urethral injuries depends on the location and extent of injury, and definitive management is left to the urologic consultant.

Admission Criteria

Admission is mandatory in *all patients with an unstable pelvis, double breaks in the pelvic ring (type III), associated visceral injuries, and displaced fractures of the pelvis.* Isolated avulsion fractures of the pelvis that result from vigorous muscle contraction where the pelvis remains intact can be managed conservatively by providing adequate pain control and follow-up. Admission is generally recommended for *all patients with GU injury;* the final disposition of patients with blunt renal trauma and microscopic hematuria should be made in conjunction with a urologist after satisfactory assessment.

Suggested Readings

Schneider RE: Genitourinary trauma. Emerg Med Clin North Am 1993; 11:137–145.

Werkman HA, Jansen C, Klein JP, et al.: Urinary tract injuries in multiply injured patients: a rationale guideline for the initial assessment. Injury 1991;22:471–474.

4.7 BURNS

Description

More than 2 million Americans are burn victims each year. Isolated burns may be caused by the direct contact of the skin with a thermal source (a hot liquid or object, or fire) or may be a complication of a blunt or penetrating trauma (burning automobile, explosion, fall in attempt to flee fire). Inhalation injury and carbon monoxide poisoning (see section 7.8) frequently accompany burn trauma. Burns also take place when the skin comes in contact with an electrical current (household current, high-voltage current > 1000 volts, lightning), chemicals (acids, alkali, phenol, phosphorous), or radiation.

History

It is important to understand the circumstances surrounding the burn injury to properly assess and treat the patient. Specifically, the ED physician needs to know the etiology of the burn (brief scalding burn, flame contact, immersion of skin in hot liquid, electrical or chemical burn), the environment in which the burn happened (open or closed), the substances involved (plastic fire, chemicals, etc.), and other possible injuries sustained. Laryngeal burns have been reported following ingestion of microwave-heated foods and liquids. In addition, obtain an AMPLE history (see section 4.1).

Physical Examination

Note: *No matter how trivial a burn appears, assess the patient for possible significant complications.*

General. Verify the level of consciousness; confusion indicates either hypoxia or hypovolemia. Remove all clothing surrounding the burn area, taking care not to overlook the possibility of multiple trauma.

Vital signs. Be alert for signs of respiratory distress (tachypnea) and shock (tachycardia, hypotension).

HEENT. Look for evidence of thermal injury to the respiratory tract (singeing of eyebrows or nasal vibrissae, soot on face, carbonaceous sputum, hyperemic pharynx, hoarse voice, persistent cough). If there is any question, directly visualize the cords and epiglottis.

Lungs. Auscultate for stridor (signifying laryngeal edema). Hoarseness implies upper airway involvement. Rales, rhonchi, cough, and wheezing intimate lower airway damage.

Abdomen. Listen for bowel sounds (major burns are associated with a reactive ileus).

Extremities. Assess peripheral pulses, capillary refill, and sensation—especially in full-thickness and circumferential burns (progressive edema may lead to a compartment syndrome; see section 16.4).

Skin. Assess the depth, location (especially taking note of burns to the face, hands, feet, or genitalia) and percent of body surface area (BSA) affected. The "Rule of Nines" is a practical guide for determining the extent of burns. The adult BSA is divided into anatomic regions, each corresponding to a multiple of 9% of the total BSA: the head and neck make up 9%; the anterior trunk, 18%; the posterior trunk, 18%; each upper extremity, 9%; each lower extremity, 18%; and the perineum, 1%. Another useful reference is that the patient's palm (excluding fingers) represents approximately 1% of his or her total BSA.

Diagnostic Tests

Blood tests. Obtain blood samples for CBC, T&C, serum glucose, and electrolytes in seriously burned patients. Also obtain ABGs and carbon monoxide and methemoglobin levels in suspected inhalation injuries (burn in confined space, smoke exposure).

Urinalysis. Check for myoglobin, and consider pregnancy test in females of child-bearing age.

X-rays. A chest film is necessary in all possible inhalation victims. Additional x-rays are guided by the clinical findings.

Specific Conditions

Thermal Burns

Thermal burns are classified as follows:

- First-degree burns are limited to damage of the superficial epithelium. Clinically, they manifest as erythema of the skin (typified by a minor sunburn) with localized tenderness.
- Second-degree burns are partial-thickness injuries involving the epithelium and parts of the dermis. Typically, these burns display a red, moist, blistered appearance together with skin hypersensitivity and edema.
- Third-degree burns, also known as full-thickness burns, are characterized by total destruction of the skin and subdermal appendages (sweat and sebaceous glands, hair follicles). The skin appears charred or waxen with a whitish or gray color, and

unlike second-degree burns, third-degree burns appear dry. The burn surface is customarily pain free, being anesthetic to pinprick or touch.

- Fourth-degree burns involve complete damage to the skin and destruction of the underlying bone, fascia, and muscles.

Electrical burns

Electrical burns can be deceptive and are frequently more serious than they first appear. Besides causing localized thermal burns, electrical current can travel throughout the body; its path is influenced by various parameters, including voltage, amperage, and tissue resistance. Entrance and exit wounds frequently appear.

Possible complications following electrical injury include arrhythmias (especially if the current traverses across the thorax as in hand-to-hand electrical burns), fractures and dislocations (resulting from violent current-induced muscle contractions), myoglobinuria with renal failure (from extensive destruction of muscle), and neurologic damage (including spinal cord lesions). Lightning injuries are a type of high-voltage electrical injury, which may cause cardiac arrest, opisthotonic muscle contraction (resulting in fractures and dislocations), retinal detachment, rupture of the tympanic membrane, burns (uncommon, but may occur if clothing ignited), and skin patterning (tree- or fern-like patterns appear on skin).

Victims of conductive electrical injuries require comprehensive evaluation and management, which are best provided in a specialized burn center. Burn formulas for calculating fluid resuscitation do not apply to patients with conductive electrical injuries, because such patients require aggressive fluid resuscitation to mitigate the effects of rhabdomyolysis.

Chemical Burns

Chemical burns result from exposure of the skin to a variety of substances, including those commonly used as household cleaning agents. Alkali burns are able to penetrate the skin deeply (liquefaction necrosis), causing a more severe injury than acid burns (coagulation necrosis). Cutaneous injury from chemicals continues as long as the chemical remains in contact with the skin. Copious irrigation is essential in treating chemical burns, commencing at once (with tap water, if necessary) and continuing for at least 20 to 30 min. Do not attempt to neutralize the acid or alkali. Burns of the eye require special care (see section 14.4). All contaminated clothing should be removed, preferably in a designated "decontamination" area.

Hydrofluoric acid (employed in glass etching and used as a component of rust removers and semiconductors) is one the few chemicals with a specific antidote. If not properly treated, burns from this acid can cause extensive tissue destruction as well as systemic hypokalemia and hypomagnesemia. The patient who has exposure of the hands will complain of severe pain, usually in the nail bed area. After initial irrigation, cover the wounds with sterile gauze soaked with an iced solution of 25% magnesium sulfate. Remove the nail plates if hydrofluoric acid has penetrated beneath them. Definitive therapy of small burn areas consists of subcutaneous infiltration of a 10% solution of calcium gluconate or 10% magnesium sulfate, using a small-gauge needle, in amounts no greater than 0.5 mL/cm^2. In extreme cases, intraarterial calcium (10 mL of 10% calcium gluconate in 50 mL D_5W over 50 min) may be required.

Tar Burns

Tar burns are initially treated with immediate cooling and removal of the tar. Tar removal can be facilitated by use of various agents (Neosporin ointment, Tween 80, Medi-sol). Do not use a hydrocarbon solvent (gasoline, kerosene), as these are toxic themselves.

Treatment

The initial treatment of burns is based on the same principles and priorities outlined for other forms of trauma, namely securing the airway and supporting circulation. Patients with smoke inhalation should be provided 100% oxygen. A special priority when caring for the burn patient is to ensure arrest of the burning process by removing smoldering clothing or corrosive chemicals (brush powders from the skin; use copious irrigation). Further management is dictated by the severity of the burn, which in turn depends on the depth, extent, and location of the burn.

Few patients survive full-thickness burns that cover more than 70% of the body. The term *major burns* implies partial-thickness burns (first- or second-degree burns) that affect more than

20% of the BSA, or full-thickness burns (third-degree burns) that affect more than 10% of the BSA. Major burns require aggressive fluid replacement. Begin fluid resuscitation with lactated Ringer's (LR), calculating the total replacement dose in adults as follows:

$$\text{LR (mL)} = \text{Percent BSA burned} \times \text{Body weight (kg)} \times 2\text{–}4$$

One-half the calculated amount of fluid is given over the first 8 hr, and the other half is given over the subsequent 16 hr.

Supplemental measures include inserting an NG tube if patient experiences nausea, vomiting, or abdominal distention or if the patient has a major burn; providing adequate analgesia; removing all jewelry; performing an emergent escharotomy in circumferential extremity wounds that cause circulatory embarrassment or circumferential trunk or neck burns that impair respirations (limit the incision to insensate full-thickness burn and extend it the entire length of eschar), updating tetanus status, gently covering the burned skin with dry, clean linen if the burn is extensive, and providing local wound care.

Partial-thickness burns heal spontaneously, while scarring and contraction can occur with full-thickness burns. Most burns can be treated on an outpatient basis; however, specific therapy is controversial. Cold compresses can be applied to partial-thickness burns if they cover < 10% of the total BSA. Initial cleansing is with nonirritating solutions (saline or diluted chlorhexidine). Obviously, necrotic tissue is débrided, but blisters are often left intact. Prophylactic antibiotics are not indicated. Preferences for burn dressing vary widely among emergency medicine practitioners. Most use a topical antimicrobial agent (silver sulfadiazine or Bacitracin). Avoid use of silver sulfadiazine in patients with sulfa allergy and do not use on the face, as it may induce skin discoloration. Cover with a sterile occlusive dressing.

Patients with significant carbon monoxide levels (≥ 25%) following a fire and those with loss of consciousness, neurologic findings, seizures, or myocardial ischemia should be treated with hyperbaric oxygen.

Admission Criteria

Hospital admission is advised when *partial-thickness burns involve* > 15% of the total BSA or full-thickness burns affect > 3% of the total BSA. In addition, it is prudent to *lower the threshold for admis-*

sion in the elderly, patients with severe underling systemic disease, noncompliant patients, those with burns secondary to electricity or chemicals, those with suspected inhalation injury, and any patient with a burn involving the hands, face, perineum, or feet.

Transfer to a burn center is recommended when partial-thickness burns involve > 20% of the total BSA (or > 10% in patients older than 50 years) or full-thickness burns affecting > 10% total of the BSA. Transfer is also recommended for burns involving the face, eyes, ears, hands, feet, genitalia, perineum, or skin overlying major joints; significant electrical, lightning, and chemical burns; and inhalation injury. Arrangements for transfer should be made after the patient is stabilized. Contact must be physician to physician, and all pertinent documentation and information should accompany the patient.

Dispense adequate analgesics and burn supplies (topical antimicrobial, gauze dressings, sterile tongue depressors for application of ointments), along with written and oral instructions, and follow-up arrangements (patients should be seen 24 to 48 hr after initial treatment). Local wound cleansing followed by the application of a topical agent ought to be done once or twice daily. Full-thickness burns should be referred to a specialist.

Suggested Readings

Griglak MJ: Thermal injury. Emerg Med Clin North Am 1992; 10(2): 369–384.

Hobson MC, Burns BF, Smith DJ: Acute management of the burned patient. Plast Reconstr Surg 1992;89:1155.

Chapter 5

Gastroenterology

5.1 ACUTE ABDOMINAL PAIN

Description

There are essentially two types of abdominal pain: *visceral pain* and *parietal pain.* Visceral pain tends to be diffuse and poorly localized. It is often perceived in one of three general zones of the midline: *epigastrium* (associated with disorders of the stomach, duodenum, pancreas, liver, and biliary system), *periumbilical* (usually implies disease of the small intestine and cecum), and *hypogastrium* (commonly referred pain from the colon, rectum, and/or pelvis). Visceral pain also frequently evokes autonomic responses such as vomiting, tachycardia, bradycardia, and hypotension.

Parietal pain arises from irritation or inflammation of the abdominal skin, wall musculature, or parietal peritoneum. It is described as a sharp pain that lateralizes to one of four quadrants: right upper quadrant (RUQ), left upper quadrant (LUQ), right lower quadrant (RLQ), or left lower quadrant (LLQ). Voluntary muscular rigidity, known as *guarding,* can accompany parietal irritation (see Fig. 5.1.1).

History

Although up to one-half of cases of acute abdominal pain remain undiagnosed even after an ED evaluation, it is essential that the ED clinician obtain an accurate history to detect potentially life-threatening causes (perforated or ruptured viscus, GI hemorrhage, bowel necrosis or infarction, intraabdominal infection). Establish initial location of pain as well as radiation and current site of maximal intensity (localized pain that becomes generalized suggests a ruptured viscus with secondary peritonitis), onset

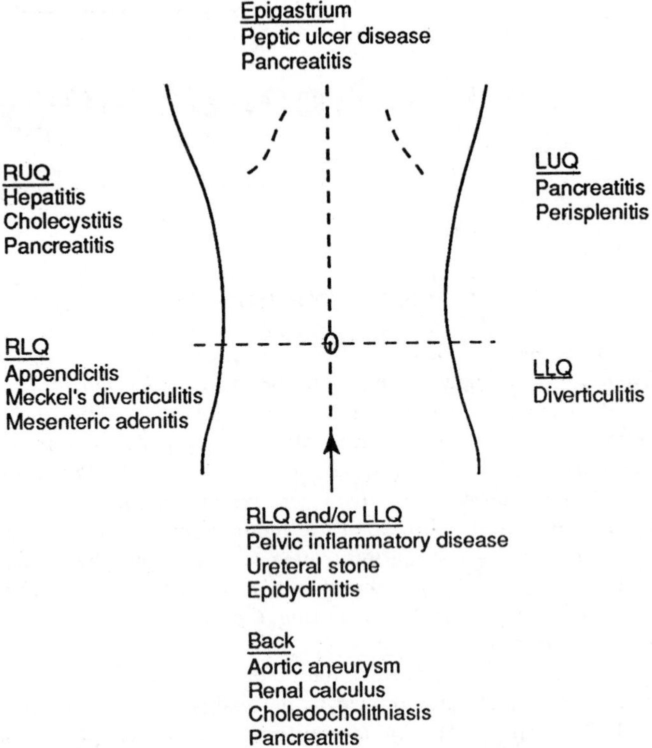

Figure 5.1.1. Abdominal pathology and site of maximum pain.

(abrupt, gradual), frequency (constant, intermittent), duration, quality (crampy, sharp), provocative or palliative maneuvers (food, bowel movements), and associated symptoms (fever, vomiting, diarrhea, constipation, dysuria, vaginal discharge, bleeding). In general, for the previously healthy individual, consider abrupt onset of abdominal pain lasts longer than 6 hr to be serious and of surgical significance. Moreover, the temporal relationship of pain and vomiting is important: Pain preceding vomiting implies a possible surgical abdomen, whereas vomiting before onset of pain is more characteristic of disorders not requiring surgery.

Inquire about previous episodes of abdominal pain (compare them with the character of the current pain) along with evaluation, diagnosis, and treatment. Obtain a complete OB-GYN history in all females of child-bearing age. In the general review of systems, cover potential sources of referred pain (myocardial, pulmonary) as well as potential metabolic and hematological causes (diabetic ketoacidosis, sickle cell disease, acute intermittent porphyria). Finally, ask about drug (antipyretics, antibiotics, and immunosuppressives may mask fever from intraabdominal infection) and/or alcohol use, prior abdominal surgery or trauma (consider possibility of spousal abuse), and any other underlying medical disorders (coronary or peripheral vascular disease).

Note: *The manifestations of acute abdominal disease may be blunted in the elderly.* Be particularly attentive for *mesenteric ischemia* when pain seems out of proportion to the clinical findings.

Physical Examination

It is important to repeat the physical examination to detect any subtle progression of the disease processes when the diagnosis is in doubt.

General. Note overall appearance (comfortable, ill, shocky) and color (pale, diaphoretic, cyanotic). Observe the patient's body position and movements. Patients with colic (renal or biliary) writhe in pain, while those suffering from peritonitis tend to lie still on their backs, often with their hips and knees flexed. Patients with pancreatitis or retroperitoneal disorders often favor a sitting position, leaning forward.

Vital signs. Verify blood pressure (hypotension accompanying abdominal pain is ominous) and pulse rate. Also test for orthostatic changes (volume depletion). Determine the rectal temperature.

HEENT. Inspect for icterus, pallor, and dryness of mucous membranes.

Chest. Regard abdominal wall motion with respirations. Listen for diminished or adventitious breath sounds (lower lobe pneumonia may present as abdominal pain).

Abdomen. It is advantageous to have the patient lie flat, with the hips and knees flexed (to relax abdominal wall musculature). Examine the abdomen for distention, appearance of scars (prior surgery), masses (check femoral and inguinal canals for hernias), dilated veins (portal hypertension), or skin lesions (bruises, striae) as well as visible peristalsis. Auscultate all four quadrants for quality and presence of bowel sounds, bruits, friction rubs, and succussion splash (ascites). Percuss and palpate gently and slowly at first, beginning at a site far from the area of complaint. Indicate areas of tenderness, guarding (voluntary, involuntary), and rebound (hallmark of peritonitis). Indirect tests for peritoneal irritation include having the patient cough and gently tapping the heels to elicit abdominal pain (also look at patient's face for grimacing).

Rectal. Examine for masses, fissures, tenderness, and prostate size. Check stool for blood.

Pelvic exam. Examine thoroughly, noting presence of discharge, bleeding, cervical motion tenderness, and uterine or adnexal enlargement or masses. A pelvic examination ought to be performed in all females with lower abdominal pain.

Male genitalia. Check for presence of hernia, scrotal masses, or tenderness.

Diagnostic Tests

CBC. The hemoglobin and hematocrit are altered with hemorrhage, dehydration, and anemias. Although an elevated WBC count implies possible infection or inflammation, a normal WBC count does not exclude infection (especially in elderly or immunosuppressed patients).

SMA. Obtain electrolytes (especially in patients with protracted vomiting or diarrhea and those on diuretics), serum glucose, BUN/creatinine, calcium, and liver function tests when indicated.

Amylase and lipase. Elevated in both pancreatic and nonpancreatic diseases (small bowel disorders, renal failure, facial trauma).

Pregnancy test. Order in all women of reproductive age with lower abdominal pain.

Type and screen. Order if GI bleeding is suspected (see section 13.1) or surgery is contemplated.

Urinalysis. A useful screening test for infection and diabetes (glucose and ketones) and to assess hydration (specific gravity).

ABG. Essential if respiratory distress is present or acid-base imbalance is suspected.

ECG. Mandatory for patients with a history of heart disease or cardiac risk factors (inferior wall myocardial infarction or angina may present as abdominal discomfort).

Nasogastric tube. Indicated for all patients with signs of intestinal obstruction or evidence of upper GI bleeding.

Routine X-rays. Order an upright CXR to exclude lower lobe pneumonia and to rule out the presence of free air under the diaphragm. If a gastric or duodenal perforation is suspected but free air is not apparent on x-ray, insufflate 200 mL of free air via a nasogastric tube and have the films retaken. Supine and upright films of the abdomen are also beneficial in patients with a possible obstruction or acute abdomen. Lateral decubitus films of the abdomen may substitute for an upright film when necessary.

Sonography. Abdominal and/or kidney sonograms may be helpful in detecting hepatobiliary or kidney disease and aortic aneurysm. Pelvic or transvaginal sonograms are both practical (can be done at bedside) and useful in the diagnosis of pelvic pain in females.

Miscellaneous studies. In selected cases, *GI endoscopy, radiographic contrast studies, CT,* and/or *abdominal angiography* may be advantageous.

Treatment

Provide basic supportive measures. Keep the patient NPO until a surgical cause can be excluded.

Traditional surgical dictum cautions against the use of analgesia in patients with undiagnosed abdominal pain because it may mask signs and symptoms. However, recent work questions this dictum and suggests small doses of an easily reversible analgesic (meperidine) may actually facilitate the exam. Nevertheless, it is best to discuss the use of analgesia with the surgical consultant before administrating the drug. Timely surgical consultation is essential in any patient suspected of harboring serious pathology.

Admission Criteria

Admit *all patients with severe pain, hypotension, sepsis, peritoneal signs, inability to take oral fluids,* and *patients at high risk for complications* (diabetics, patients taking steroids, elderly patients). The patient's functional status and home environment are also important considerations. Surgical consultation ought to be requested in *any patient for whom a serious disorder cannot be readily excluded,* and many patients require admission for further evaluation and observation even without a specific diagnosis. Appropriate instructions and follow-up should be arranged for any patient considered safe for discharge.

Suggested Readings

Aztard AR: Safety of early pain relief for acute abdominal pain. Br Med J 1992;305:554–556.

Silen W: Cope's early diagnosis of the acute abdomen, 18th ed. New York: Oxford University Press, 1991.

Vogt DP: The acute abdomen in the geriatric patient. Cleveland Clin J Med 1990;57(2):125–130.

5.2 APPENDICITIS

Description

Appendicitis is the most common cause of an *acute abdomen;* it occurs in all age groups, with the peak incidence being in the second and third decades of life. The condition usually arises from an obstruction of the lumen of the appendix (fecalith, tumor, foreign body, parasite), with subsequent inflammation. If left untreated, appendicitis progresses to gangrene, perforation, and abscess formation or peritonitis.

History

Appendicitis classically begins with diffuse periumbilical pain and subsequent anorexia, nausea, and vomiting (pain typically precedes vomiting). Characteristically, the pain shifts to the RLQ (2 to 12 hr after onset), becoming sharp and well localized. However, the pain may remain diffuse and never localize or begin in the RLQ. **Remember:** *45% of patients with appendicitis present atypically—because of the great variation in signs and symptoms, the diagnosis of appendicitis is frequently missed.* High-risk adult groups for perforation (due to delayed diagnosis of appendicitis) include the elderly, pregnant females, and patients on immunosuppressive therapy. Nonpregnant women of child-bearing age present the most difficult challenge in establishing the diagnosis.

Physical Examination

General. Note if patient appears toxic or in shock.

Vital signs. The rectal temperature rarely rises above 38.1°C (100.4°F) in the absence of perforation.

Abdomen. If symptoms have been present for several hours, percussion rebound *tenderness* of the RLQ can be elicited, with the maximum tenderness being at *McBurney's point. Rovsing's sign* is positive when there is referred tenderness to the RLQ upon palpation of the LLQ. *Muscle guarding* and resistance increase as inflammation progresses. Classic signs include the *psoas sign* (pain on passive hyperextension of the right hip) and the *obturator sign* (pain on passive internal rotation of the flexed right hip). Indirect tests for peritoneal inflammation include the *cough sign* (requesting the patient to cough while lying supine) and *heel jarring tests.*

Rectal. Right-sided rectal tenderness may be elicited. Test the stool for blood.

Pelvic exam. Must be done in all females to rule out disorders that can mimic appendicitis (ectopic pregnancy, acute salpingitis, pelvic inflammatory disease, ruptured corpus luteum cysts).

Diagnostic Tests

The diagnosis of appendicitis is a clinical one; while diagnostic studies may help confirm the diagnosis, appendicitis should never be excluded solely on the basis of ancillary tests.

CBC. Most patients (> 90%) will have either an elevated white count or a left shift. However, normal white blood cell counts can be seen with appendicitis (particularly in the elderly and immunocompromised patients). The hematocrit should be normal (think of cecal cancer in elderly patients with anemia and RLQ pain).

Urinalysis. Should be normal, although hematuria or pyuria may occur with ureteral irritation from a retrocecal appendix.

X-rays. Radiographs of the abdomen and chest are usually not helpful in proving the diagnosis (although the presence of a calcified appendolith favors a diagnosis of appendicitis), but they may aid in eliminating the presence of diseases that may imitate appendicitis.

Additional tests. Diagnostic ultrasound and barium enema may occasionally be helpful in difficult cases. A pregnancy test is mandatory in all females of child-bearing age with lower abdominal pain to rule out the possibility of ectopic pregnancy.

Admission Criteria

Any patient suspected of having acute appendicitis must be immediately hospitalized or taken to surgery. *In cases where the diagnosis is indefinite,* the patient ought to be observed in the hospital or an observation area.

Suggested Readings

Doherty GM, Lewis FR Jr: Appendicitis: continuing diagnostic challenge. Emerg Med Clin North Am 1989;7(3):537–553.

Graff L, Radford MJ, Werne C: Probability of appendicitis before and after observation. Ann Emerg Med 1991;20:503–507.

5.3 GALLBLADDER DISEASES

Description

Gallbladder disease typically arises from the presence of gallstones *(cholelithiasis)*. Cholelithiasis is detected in all age groups but is most prevalent in females between 30 and 80 years old. Pigmented stones occur in patients with sickle cell anemia and hemolytic anemia. Both *biliary colic* and *acute cholecystitis* arise from attempts to pass a stone through the cystic or common bile duct (Table 5.3.1). Biliary colic results from biliary spasm and is generally of short duration. In acute cholecystitis, there is a persistent obstruction, which causes ischemia, inflammation, edema, necrosis, and impaired venous drainage of the gallbladder. The

Table 5.3.1
Biliary Colic and Cholecystitis

Clinical Findings	Biliary Colic	Acute Cholecystitis	Complicated Cholecystitis
Pain	Crampy	Less steady	Steady > 4 hr
Nausea	Present	Present	Present
Vomiting	Variable	Mild	Mild
Onset	Related to meals (+)	Related to meals (±)	Related to meals (±)
Fever	Absent	Low grade	38.5°C (102°F)
WBC	Normal	Up to 15,000	> 15,000
Bilirubin	Normal	1.0–4.0 mg/dL	> 4.0 mg/dL
Course	Resolves in 1–4 hr	Resolves in 24–48 hr with treatment	Prolonged course despite treatment

pain of acute cholecystitis lasts longer and is often accompanied by fever, nausea, vomiting, and a leukocytosis.

History

Patients present with a variety of symptoms, ranging from mild, colicky RUQ pain following a meal (often a heavy meal of fatty or fried foods) to severe, crampy midepigastric pain. Pain may radiate to the right shoulder, back, or subscapular area. Vomiting is common and may provide variable relief. Frequently, patients will relate previous similar attacks.

Physical Examination

General. Patients with cholecystitis often appear sick and tend to avoid sudden motion, coughing, or deep inspiration. In contrast, patients with biliary colic are initially restless and uncomfortable but not toxic in appearance. Clinical jaundice implies a stone in the common bile duct *(choledocholithiasis)*.

Vital signs. Presence of fever generally signifies acute cholecystitis or cholangitis (fever typically absent in biliary colic).

Abdomen. Examination of the abdomen reveals tenderness or guarding in the RUQ (unilateral rectus guarding may be discovered). Tenderness becomes more localized with cholecystitis. A palpable, tender gallbladder is present in 15 to 30% of patients. *Murphy's sign* is RUQ tenderness along with a halting of inspiration during deep palpation. Bowel sounds are diminished. Generalized rebound tenderness may reflect a perforation.

Diagnostic Tests

CBC. WBC count may be mildly elevated (12,000 to 15,000/mm^3) in acute cholecystitis.

SMA. Elevations may be seen in liver enzymes, ALT and AST, alkaline phosphatase, and serum bilirubin (jaundice is usually clinically detectable when levels are greater than 2 to 3 mg/dL).

Amylase. Although nonspecific, serum amylase is elevated in 15% of patients and suggests choledocholithiasis and associated pancreatitis.

Urinalysis. Order to exclude urinary tract disease.

X-rays. The sensitivity of abdominal plain radiographs for gallstones is about 15%. If air is present in the biliary tree, suspect an emphysematous gallbladder or cholecystenteric fistula.

Diagnostic imaging. The choice of imaging study regularly depends on institutional preferences, with the two most commonly ordered tests being *ultrasonography* and *gallbladder nuclear scans.* Nuclear scanning affords the advantage of directly measuring cystic duct patency as well as providing an extremely high sensitivity and specificity (98% for both). Ultrasonography identifies most patients with symptomatic stones and is more accessible and more rapid than nuclear scanning. Furthermore, ultrasonography can identify other sources of RUQ pain.

Special Considerations

Emphysematous cholecystitis. Also known as *acute gaseous cholecystitis* or *gas gangrene* of the gallbladder. It primarily affects obese, elderly, immunosuppressed, or diabetic patients.

Perforation. Localized perforation may not be discovered until surgery.

Gallstone ileus. Results from the passage of a gallstone through a cholecystenteric fistula, possibly leading to mechanical obstruction of the bowel.

Acute cholangitis. A life-threatening situation caused by a bacterial infection in an obstructed biliary tree; often heralded by *Charcot's triad:* RUQ tenderness, jaundice, and spiking fevers. (The concomitant occurrence of shock and altered mental status is known as *Reynolds's triad.*)

Treatment

Emergency department management centers on ensuring adequate fluid status and control of pain and vomiting. Pain control can usually be achieved with meperidine (75 to 100 mg IV or IM q 2 to 4 hr). Ketorolac (30 mg IV or IM) is also effective in relieving pain. For patients with marked vomiting or ileus, an NG tube should be inserted. Employ parenteral antibiotics for suspected acute cholecystitis; patients who appear septic; and especially those with suspected ascending cholangitis, empyema of the gallbladder, or emphysematous cholecystitis (*gentamicin* 2.0 mg/kg IV loading dose plus *ampicillin* 2 g IV q 6 hr plus *metronidazole* 15 mg/kg IV loading dose) after blood cultures are obtained.

Surgical consultation is necessary for all patients with acute cholecystitis or complications associated with acute cholecystitis. The timing of cholecystectomy is controversial (some surgeons may operate in the first 24 hr before edema becomes pronounced, while others may elect to operate a couple of days following defervescence). Generally, early intervention is justified in toxic patients and those prone to complications.

Admission Criteria

Patients with a painful attack of cholelithiasis that is self-limited may be sent home after evaluation and treatment in the ED. *All patients with signs of acute cholecystitis* (toxic, febrile, leucocytosis) and *patients with biliary colic that does not resolve after ED therapy* require admission.

Suggested Readings

Diehl AK: Clinical evaluation for gallstone disease: usefulness of symptoms and signs in diagnosis. Am J Med 1990;89:29–33.

Marton KI, Doubilet P: How to image the gallbladder in suspected cholecystitis. Ann Intern Med 1988;109:722–729.

5.4 PEPTIC ULCER

Description

Peptic ulcer disease (PUD) characterizes a breakdown in the mucous membranes of the esophagus, stomach, or duodenum (most common location) caused by uncontrolled acid and pepsin in the gastric juice. Contributing factors to PUD include use of drugs such as aspirin and nonsteroidal antiinflammatory agents, infection with *Helicobacter pylori* (previously *Campylobacter pylori*), and stress.

History

Epigastric distress (described as a gnawing, dull, achy pain) that is occasionally relieved by antacids or milk and is frequently worse at night is the hallmark of PUD. However, this complaint is neither sensitive nor specific for PUD. In addition, the clinical history cannot differentiate duodenal from gastric ulcer disease. A sudden onset of severe, midepigastric pain that quickly generalizes over the entire abdomen with radiation to one or both shoulders implies an acute perforation; pain may become so severe that it provokes a syncopal event. Penetration of a peptic ulcer into another viscus (pancreas) causes a boring pain that radiates to the back. Significant vomiting is usually not a prominent feature with PUD, unless a gastric outlet obstruction or gastric malignancy is present. The course of luminal obstruction is generally insidious, with the patient noting early satiety and distention after ingestion of small quantities of food.

Physical Examination

Note: *The physical examination is typically unremarkable with uncomplicated PUD.*

Vital signs. Should remain normal in uncomplicated peptic ulcer disease but may become abnormal if complications arise (fever, tachycardia, hypotension).

Abdomen. Unremarkable except for slight epigastric tenderness in uncomplicated PUD. Diminished or absent bowel sounds, marked guarding or board-like rigidity indicates perforation. With escape of free air, there may be loss of liver dullness with tympany over the lower right rib cage. Signs and symptoms of acute pancreatitis (see section 5.7) may appear with posterior penetrating ulcers.

Rectal. Test the stool for blood. In perforation, large quantities of gastric fluid may escape, producing cul-de-sac tenderness.

Diagnostic Tests

CBC. The hematocrit may be increased secondary to volume depletion or it may be low if gastrointestinal bleeding has occurred; acute bleeds may not be reflected immediately in the hematocrit. The white cell count is normal in uncomplicated peptic ulcer but often elevated following perforation.

Amylase. Often elevated with a posterior penetrating ulcer.

X-rays. In perforation, an upright chest film is most sensitive for detecting free air under the diaphragm. If an upright chest is not possible, a lateral decubitus of the abdomen is satisfactory (position the patient for at least 5 min before taking the film).

Nasogastric tube. Aspiration of gastric contents can provide information about the presence of blood in the gastric fluid (bright red or "coffee grounds") as well as diagnose a gastric outlet obstruction (presence of > 300 mL of retained gastric contents 4 hr after a meal is significant).

Endoscopy. Consider in cases complicated by acute upper gastrointestinal bleeding (see section 5.6).

Treatment

Initial management will be guided by the degree of urgency of the situation. Volume resuscitation and rehydration are the first priorities if the patient appears hypotensive or dehydrated. Also supply supplemental oxygen. Type-specific or O negative blood should be provided as needed.

Nasogastric suction should be performed to treat luminal obstruction or ion preparation for surgical repair of a perforation.

Several pharmacologic agents are efficacious in outpatient treatment of PUD. The simplest therapy uses oral antacids (avoid sodium-containing products in patients with CHF or hypertension). Antisecretory drugs include H2 receptor antagonists *(cimetidine, ranitidine, famotidine,* and *nazatidine)* and proton pump inhibitors *(omeprazole).* Be aware of potential drug interactions (theophylline, warfarin, phenytoin) when prescribing these agents. Agents are also available to enhance mucosal defenses (sucralfate, bismuth, misoprostol). *Helicobacter pylori* is best treated with a regimen of bismuth and metronidazole plus tetracycline or amoxicillin. Other regimens include bismuth and clarithromycin plus tetracycline or amoxicillin. Encourage patients to avoid caffeinated beverages, smoking, and nonsteroidal antiinflammatory drugs. Intravenous H2 blockers may be used in severely ill patients.

Admission Criteria

All patients with significant complications (bleeding, perforation, penetration, gastric outlet obstruction, and refractory pain) require admission. Consult surgery or GI service when appropriate

Suggested Readings

Horowitz J, Kukora JS, Ritchie WP Jr: All perforated ulcers are not alike. Ann Surg 1989;209:693–696.

Sugawa C, Joseph AL: Endoscopic interventional management of bleeding duodenal and gastric ulcers. Surg Clin North Am 1992;72: 317–334.

5.5 INTESTINAL OBSTRUCTION

Description

Intestinal obstruction occurs when the normal flow of intestinal contents is blocked by either a mechanical or a functional obstruction, impairing intestinal motility. Obstruction may be complete or partial. If not treated expeditiously, mechanical obstruction can become lethal. The most common cause of *small bowel obstruction* (SBO) is postoperative adhesions, with hernias being the next most frequent source. Carcinoma is by far the most common etiology of *large bowel obstruction* (LBO) (Table 5.5.1).

Ileus is defined as a disruption of normal peristaltic motion of the gut, resulting in failure to propel intestinal contents. There are many etiologies for ileus (see Table 5.5.2). *Colonic pseudo-obstruction* (also called *Ogilvie's syndrome*) mimics the symptoms of mechanical obstruction, but there is an absence of obstructive lesions. Ogilvie's syndrome is most prevalent in elderly patients with chronic illnesses (CHF, myxedema, chronic renal failure).

History

Typically, acute intestinal obstruction is heralded by the gradual onset of crampy abdominal pain, followed by nausea, vomiting, and obstipation. In SBO the pain tends to localize more in the periumbilical region and occur paroxysmally at 5-min intervals. The pain from LBO tends to be less intense, localizing to the

Table 5.5.1
Intestinal Obstruction in Adults

Abnormalities within the lumen
- Gallstones
- Foreign bodies
- Polyps
- Fecal impaction

Intestinal wall abnormalities
- Tumor
- Ischemic strictures
- Intussusception
- Enteritis (regional, radiation)
- Diverticulitis

Extrinsic abnormalities
- Adhesions
- Hernia
- Tumor
- Volvulus
- Gynecologic disorders
- Intraabdominal mass (abscess, hematoma, foreign body, etc.)

Table 5.5.2
Causes of Ileus in Adults

Intraabdominal abnormalities
Peritoneal irritation (trauma, chemical, infection)
Vascular (mesenteric artery insufficiency, venous thrombosis, mesenteric vasculitis, bowel strangulation)
Extraperitoneal irritation (retroperitoneal hematoma, fracture, acute urologic disease)
Extraabdominal
Thoracic (pneumonia, inferior MI)
Systemic (electrolyte imbalance, sepsis, uremia, metabolic disorders)
Drug induced (anticholinergics, antihistamines, opiates)
Idiopathic

lower abdomen. Vomiting tends to occur later with LBO and is typically darker and more feculent. Continuous severe pain may suggest strangulation obstruction, a life-threatening condition. Inability to pass stool or flatus (obstipation) is seen with complete intestinal obstruction. However, the passage of flatus or feces for a brief period after onset of symptoms does not rule out the possibility of intestinal obstruction. Episodic explosive diarrhea in a patient with paroxysmal abdominal pain suggests partial intestinal obstruction.

Ileus is generally characterized by mild, constant abdominal pain. Colonic pseudo-obstruction often presents with massive abdominal distention, with or without vomiting or abdominal pain. Obtain a history that covers prior operative procedures, trauma, and known intraabdominal and pelvic pathology (tumor, gallstones, peptic ulcer disease, diverticulosis).

Physical Examination

General. Determine the overall appearance (restless, diaphoretic).

Vital signs. Tachycardia and hypotension may indicate severe volume depletion, sepsis, or peritonitis. Fever may be present.

Abdomen. Auscultate bowel sounds. In mechanical acute bowel obstruction, these are heard in rushes; are frequently high-pitched, tinkling, or musical; and are separated by quiet periods. Examine for distention (the higher the obstruction, the less the distention) and tympany. Palpate for abdominal tenderness (usually diffuse). Mild tenderness may accompany simple obstruction; however, localized tenderness, rebound, and guarding suggest peritonitis with possible strangulation. Inspect for surgical scars and external hernias. Ileus is generally associated with a silent abdomen (an absence of peristalsis) and variable abdominal distention. Colonic pseudo-obstruction typically presents with hypoactive to absent bowel sounds, a distended tympanic abdomen, and a palpable mass in the right side of the abdomen, indicating a dilated cecum.

Rectal. Examination may detect an obstructing mass. The presence of blood suggests a mucosal disruption (cancer, intussusception, strangulation, infarction).

Diagnostic Tests

SMA

A proximal SBO produces large amounts of vomitus, causing losses of water, sodium, chloride, hydrogen ions, and potassium. This leads to dehydration, azotemia, hypochloremia, hypokalemia, and metabolic alkalosis. A distal SBO may cause large fluid losses, but electrolyte abnormalities are less prominent. Ileus and colonic pseudo-obstruction may arise from electrolyte abnormalities.

CBC

Hemoconcentration may accompany dehydration. Leukocytosis may be present but is usually mild in SBO. Marked leukocytosis suggests strangulation and/or perforation.

X-Rays

Obtain an upright CXR (look for free air under the diaphragm) and upright and supine abdominal x-rays in all patients with possible intestinal obstruction. The hallmark of intestinal obstruction is the amassing of gas and fluid above the site of obstruction. A small bowel diameter > 3 cm or a large bowel diameter > 6 cm indicates intestinal distention.

With SBO the degree of small bowel dilation is disproportionate to the large bowel, with the obstructed small bowel revealing a stepladder pattern of air-fluid levels. The small bowel usually occupies the central abdomen, whereas the colon resides in the periphery and pelvis. When obstruction is complete, there will be little or no gas in the colon. LBO appears as a dilated large intestine on x-ray. If the ileocecal valve is competent, there is minimal small bowel gas; whereas an incompetent ileocecal valve allows accumulation of small bowel gas.

Sigmoid volvulus presents as a massively dilated colonic loop in the mid-abdomen; it looks like an inverted U, projecting upward from the pelvis to the abdomen. Ileus usually exhibits a uniform, diffuse gaseous distention throughout the GI tract, with nondifferential air-fluid levels seen on obstructive series. Colonic pseudo-obstruction is associated with a massive dilation of the ascending and transverse colon and a very dilated cecum; there is often no gas present in the left colon or air in the rectum.

Special Considerations

Strangulating obstruction. Results from impairment of the blood supply to the involved segment of the bowel. Strangulation frequently accompanies volvulus (the intestinal blood supply twists upon itself).

Sepsis. If the bowel obstruction remains unchecked, a gangrenous, infarcted bowel results. This allows bacteria to pass into the lymphatics and bloodstream, leading to septic shock.

Perforation. The part of the bowel proximal to the obstruction may overdistend and perforate. The cecum is the most common site for cecal rupture (a dilation > 11 cm in diameter is stated to be the danger point).

Closed-loop obstruction. Occurs when the colon becomes obstructed but the ileocecal valve remains intact, thereby permitting intestinal contents to enter the obstructed region and greatly overdistend the cecum. In closed-loop obstruction, a single loop of bowel is out of proportion to the remainder of the bowel.

Intussusception. Takes place when the bowel invaginates upon itself, resulting in a narrowing of the lumen and subsequent obstruction.

Treatment

Regardless of the cause or location of the obstruction, initial management includes replacement of fluids and electrolytes (LR), bowel decompression (NG tube), broad-spectrum antibiotics (gentamicin plus ampicillin plus clindamycin), and frequent monitoring of the patient's status. In cases of adynamic ileus secondary to an underlying medical disorder, employ the above measures in addition to managing the primary problem.

Surgical assessment should be prompt. The decision between operative and nonoperative management of intestinal obstruction depends on the patient's clinical status, response to fluid resuscitation, and response to decompressive maneuvers as well as the degree of suspicion for strangulation. The treatment of ileus is generally supportive and aimed at resolution of underlying causes. Treatment of colonic pseudo-obstruction is similar to that of ileus. Acute intervention is indicated if the cecal diameter is greater than 10 to 12 cm or there is evidence of progressive bowel ischemia or possible colonic or cecal perforation.

Admission Criteria

All patients with intestinal obstruction ought to be admitted to the surgical service.

Suggested Readings

Stack PS: Ogilvie's syndrome. Would you recognize it? Postgrad Med 1991;89:131–134.

Richards WO, Williams LJ: Obstruction of large and small intestine. Surg Clin North Am 1988;68:355–373.

Theuer C, Cheadle WG: Volvulus of the colon. Am Surg 1991;57:145–150.

5.6 GASTROINTESTINAL BLEEDING

Description

Bleeding can occur from any site along the gastrointestinal tract and is classified as either upper or lower tract bleeding, depending on whether the bleeding source is proximal or distal to the ligament of Treitz (second portion of duodenum) (Table 5.6.1).

History

A description of the bleeding can help distinguish upper from lower GI tract disease: *Hematemesis* (bright red blood implies a more active bleed than a coffee grounds appearance) almost always signifies upper gastrointestinal bleeding. *Melena* (passage of black tarry stools) implies a prolonged duration of blood in the

Table 5.6.1
Causes of Gastrointestinal Bleeding

Upper tract (proximal to ligament of Treitz)
- Peptic ulcer (duodenal, gastric, stomal, Zollinger-Ellison)
- Acute mucosal lesions (gastritis, Mallory-Weiss tears, stress ulcers in burn patients, ulcers associated with increased intracranial pressure)
- Varices (gastric, esophageal)
- Reflux esophagitis
- Vascular lesions (angiomata, Osler-Weber-Rendu, vasculitis)
- Neoplasms
- Hepatic trauma with hemobilia

Lower tract (distal to ligament of Treitz)
- Small intestine
  - Meckel's diverticulum
  - Intussusception
  - Regional enteritis
  - Neoplasm
  - Vascular malformations
  - Aortoenteric fistula (postsurgical repair of aorta)
- Colon
  - Diverticula
  - Neoplasm
  - Polyps
  - Colitis (ulcerative, Crohn's disease, ischemic, bacterial, protozoal)
  - Ectasias
- Rectal
  - Hemorrhoids
  - Proctitis
  - Fissures, fistulas

GI tract but does not differentiate upper from lower GI bleed. Bright red blood per rectum *(hematochezia)* suggests a lower tract source, although brisk upper tract bleeding can appear as red stool. Patients taking iron or bismuth preparations may have dark stools, but the consistency is not tarry as it is with blood and the heme test is negative. Try to exclude nongastrointestinal sources of bleeding (nosebleed, hemoptysis, vaginal bleeding) with the history and physical examination.

Presence and type of pain are clues: Crampy abdominal pain commonly accompanies the transit of large amounts of blood through the GI tract, while pain relieved by the onset of bleeding suggests peptic ulcer disease. Oppressive abdominal pain combined with a GI bleed is unusual and implies an underlying infection, ischemia, or inflammatory bowel disease. Inquire about the timing of vomiting. Vomiting, nausea or retching followed by pain and hematemesis is significant for a *Mallory-Weiss tear.* Carefully note drug use (especially aspirin, nonsteroidal antiinflammatory drugs, anticoagulants, corticosteroids). Past medical and surgical history should focus on prior bleeding episodes, ulcers, surgery (consider aortoenteric fistula in patients with a history of an aortic vascular graft), alcoholism, and liver disease. In rare cases, a family history may be helpful.

Physical Examination

General. Presence of pallor, diaphoresis, or restlessness implies massive bleeding. Also, if patient appears cachectic, look for signs of cancer (lymphadenopathy, mass) or other serious disease.

Vital signs. The pulse, blood pressure, and respirations assist in judging the degree of volume depletion. Unless the patient is clearly hypotensive, check for orthostatic changes.

Skin. Look for dermatologic stigmata of disease (purpura, telangiectasias, jaundice, spider angiomata, palmar erythema).

HEENT. Check the nose and throat for possible bleeding sources. The presence of hyperpigmentation spots on oral mucosa suggests *Peutz-Jeghers syndrome.*

Abdomen. Note bowel sounds, bruits, ascites, hepatosplenomegaly, tenderness, and rebound.

Rectal. Examine for hemorrhoids, masses, and fissures. Note the color of the stool and the reaction to hemoccult testing.

Diagnostic Tests

CBC. Hematocrit may acutely seem normal, frequently decreasing only after the patient receives fluid or hemoequilibrium occurs (6 to 24 hr). Repeat measurements are necessary. Type and cross-match for anticipated transfusion. Leukocytosis and thrombocytosis may be present with acute bleeding. Alcoholics in particular may present with thrombocytopenia.

PT/PTT. Check for coagulopathy.

SMA. A rise in BUN suggests an upper tract source of bleeding. Check liver function tests.

Nasogastric tube. Aids in locating the site of bleeding (upper versus lower), defining the activity of the bleed, and clearing the stomach of clots. Remember, a clear NG aspirate (without bile) is not a negative test, because bleeding may originate distal to the pylorus or the pylorus could be blocked by a tumor or stricture. Aspirate until you see a bilious return. Record whether coffee grounds or bright red blood is present.

Endoscopy and additional procedures. Fiberoptic endoscopy has become the optimal diagnostic procedure, allowing direct visualization of the lesion. The timing of emergency endoscopy is somewhat controversial. At present, it appears that the best indications for emergency esophagogastroduodenoscopy are (1) upper tract bleeding that does not cease with conservative management, (2) suspected variceal hemorrhage, and (3) suspected aortoenteric fistula. In acute lower gastrointestinal bleeding, perform sigmoidoscopy and consider colonoscopy. A radionuclide bleeding scan may be beneficial in deciding whether the bleeding source is located in the small or large intestine. Angiography is an additional diagnostic and therapeutic modality.

Treatment

Initiate resuscitation and stabilization as outlined in section 1.2. Blood product use is discussed in section 13.1. Saline nasogastric lavage is useful for gauging the activity of GI bleeding but has not been shown to promote hemostasis.

Bleeding varices can be treated with *sclerotherapy* and/or intravenous *vasopressin* (0.4 units/min IV). Vasopressin is contraindicated in patients with coronary artery disease or cerebral vascular disease. Supplemental intravenous nitroglycerin with the vasopressin regimen may increase efficacy. A Blakemore intraesophageal tube may be necessary when the above measures fail.

Admission Criteria

Acute gastrointestinal bleeding is associated with a 10% mortality rate. It is prudent to admit *all patients with gross gastrointestinal bleeding* (upper or lower), even if the patient is not severely ill, as the course may be unpredictable. *Patients who are still actively bleeding, are hemodynamically unstable, are > 55 years old, or have serious concomitant illness should be admitted to an intensive care setting.* Patients who bring up a few flecks of blood after repeatedly vomiting or who pass heme-positive stools without evidence of gross bleeding may be discharged after appropriate evaluation and observation. Early involvement of a gastroenterologist and/or surgeon is recommended for moderate to severe cases.

Suggested Readings

Marshall JB: Acute gastrointestinal bleeding. A logical approach to management. Postgrad Med 1990;87(4):63–70.

Papp JP: Management of upper gastrointestinal bleeding. Clin Geriatr Med 1991;7:255–264.

5.7 PANCREATITIS

Description

Acute pancreatitis results when pancreatic enzyme release produces inflammation and autodigestion of the pancreas.

History

Acute pancreatitis should be considered in patients presenting with upper abdominal pain, nausea, and vomiting. Pain is present in > 90% of cases of pancreatitis, ranging from mild to oppressive. Typically, pain localizes to the midepigastric region, but it may be diffuse or radiate to the back and is described as an incessant, boring pain. Onset is generally acute but may develop gradually (especially with underlying chronic pancreatitis). Some relief may be gained when the patient assumes a sitting posture and slumps forward. Anorexia, nausea, and vomiting are common accompanying symptoms.

The history focuses on questions pertinent to determining the etiology of the pancreatitis. *Cholelithiasis* (see section 5.3) and *alcoholism* (patients who present in alcohol withdrawal may have stopped drinking because of pancreatitis) are the most common causes. Inquire about previous similar episodes. Additional causes of pancreatitis include drugs (thiazide diuretics, sulfonamides, steroids, oral contraceptives, azathioprine, didanosine, stavudine), infections (viral, bacterial, parasitic), vasculitis, trauma, hypercalcemia, and hyperlipidemias (types I, IV, and V). It may also follow endoscopic retrograde choloagiopan-creatography (ERCP).

Physical Examination

The physical findings will vary with the severity and chronicity of the inflammatory process.

General. Look for sings of alcoholism; jaundice may be present in biliary pancreatitis as well. Tetany secondary to hypocalcemia and skin lesions secondary to fat necrosis are more unusual.

Vital signs. Check for low-grade fever, tachycardia, orthostasis, or frank hypotension (secondary to massive fluid sequestration or hemorrhage).

HEENT. Note presence of icterus.

Lungs. Listen for rales and percuss for pleural effusion (usually left sided).

Abdomen. The abdomen may be distended and tender, with decreased bowel sounds. Rebound may be present due to a severe chemical peritonitis. An abdominal mass *(pancreatic pseudocyst)* may be felt. While uncommon, look for ecchymosis in the periumbilical area (Cullen's sign) and flanks (Grey-Turner's sign) associated with hemorrhagic pancreatitis.

Rectal. A rectal exam must be performed in all patients with abdominal pain. Although pancreatitis does not cause heme-positive stool per se, there may be other disorders present that are causing the patient to bleed.

Diagnostic Tests

Amylase. Typically elevated in pancreatitis. However, increases in amylase levels are nonspecific and can occur naturally (macroamylassemia) or as a result of medications and other diseases that present with abdominal complaints (penetrated ulcer, small intestinal infarct, ruptured ectopic pregnancy, diabetic ketoacidosis, chronic renal insufficiency). More important, patients with pancreatitis may have normal amylase levels, either due to chronic calcific pancreatitis (the damaged pancreas cannot produce much amylase) or because of rapid clearance of amylase by the kidney. The level of amylase rise does not correlate with the severity of pancreatitis, although markedly elevated amylase levels are more common with biliary pancreatitis than alcoholic pancreatitis. Amylase elevations occur early in pancreatitis and can resolve within 2 to 3 days. Patients with pancreatitis who present late may have an elevated lipase and normal amylase.

Lipase. Possibly a more accurate indicator of pancreatic inflammation than serum amylase.

CBC. A leukocytosis is common, even in the absence of infection. The hematocrit may be elevated as result of hemoconcentration or decreased secondary to blood loss.

SMA. Glucose levels are elevated in roughly one-half the patients with pancreatitis. Calcium may be decreased (saponification). Bilirubin and alkaline phosphatase are more likely to be elevated with gallstone-induced pancreatitis than alcohol-associated pancreatitis.

ABG. Assess both acid-base status and oxygenation (adult respiratory distress syndrome).

X-rays. Check CXR for left pleural effusion or an adult respiratory distress syndrome (ARDS) pattern as well as for free air under the diaphragm. Review the KUB for gallstones, ascites, and pancreatic calcifications of chronic disease. The classical finding is a localized ileus, referred to as the "sentinel loop."

Additional imaging studies. Ultrasound and CT scan of the pancreas not only are helpful in confirming the diagnosis of pancreatitis but also assist in detecting complications such as pseudocysts, phlegmon, and biliary tract pathology. Order a CT and/or ultrasonography when confronted with biliary pancreatitis or a a complex case (persistent fever, pain, nausea, unclear etiology, palpable abdominal mass, worsening clinical condition).

Special Considerations

The presence of three or more of the following *(Ranson criteria)* has been shown to predict a more serious clinical course:

On Admission	Within First 48 hr
Age > 55	Hematocrit drop > 10%
WBC > 16,000/mm^3	BUN increase > 5 mg/dL
Glucose > 200 mg/dL	Calcium < 8.0 mg/dL
LDH > 350 IU/L	Po_2 < 60 mm Hg
AST > 250 IU/dL	Base deficit > 4 mEq/L
	Fluid sequestration > 6 L

Complications can be directly related to the pancreas *(pancreatic abscess, pancreatic pseudocyst, fistula, hemorrhagic necrosis, suppurative pancreatitis)* or to systemic manifestations (shock, respiratory distress syndrome, acute tubular necrosis). Patients with three or more Ranson criteria are at increased risk of systemic complications.

Treatment

Aggressive intravenous fluid replacement (isotonic crystalloids) is important. Correct any underlying electrolyte abnormalities (hypokalemia, hypocalcemia, hypomagnesemia). Continually monitor the patient's clinical and fluid status, using a Foley catheter, if necessary; and in unstable patients, conduct intravascular monitoring with a Swan-Ganz catheter.

Provide pain relief (*meperidine,* 1 to 2 mg/kg IV q 3 to 4 hr) in sufficient doses (adjust dosages when renal or liver dysfunction is present) once the diagnosis ensured. Continual NG suction is best reserved for patients with persistent vomiting. However, keep the patient NPO until he or she is largely pain free and bowel sounds are present. Do not give antibiotics routinely; use with documented infection (pancreatic diseases).

Admission Criteria

All patients with acute pancreatitis, regardless of severity, should be admitted. *Patients with greater than three risk factors* are best admitted to an ICU setting. Early surgical consultation is important in patients with suspected biliary pancreatitis, possible pancreatic abscess, and hemorrhagic or life-threatening pancreatitis as well as those for whom the diagnosis is uncertain.

Suggested Readings

Lankish PG, Schirren CA, Kunze E: Undetected fatal acute pancreatitis: why is the disease so frequently overlooked? Am J Gastroenterol 1991;86(3):322–326.

Lin XZ, Wang SS, Tsai YT, et al.: Serum amylase, isoamylase, and lipase in the acute abdomen. Their diagnostic value for acute pancreatitis. J Clin Gastroenterol 1989;11(1):47–52.

Ranson JHC: Risk factors in acute pancreatitis. Hosp Pract 1985;4:69–81.

5.8 DIARRHEA

Description

Diarrhea is an increase in the frequency, volume, and/or looseness of stools. There are many possible causes of diarrhea, but the majority of cases seen in the ED are of an acute-onset, infectious nature (labeled *gastroenteritis* when accompanied by nausea and vomiting). Infectious diarrhea can be divided into two types: *non-*

invasive and *invasive.* Noninvasive diarrhea is usually due to the presence of an *enterotoxin* in the intestinal lumen, with the typical patient being afebrile; there is also an absence of fecal leukocytes. Invasive diarrhea is characterized by direct infection of the intestine causing *mucosal ulceration,* causing a fever (systemic illness) and often generating fecal leukocytes.

History

Individuals vary greatly in their bowel habits, so the use of the term *diarrhea* is relative to a given individual's norm. Manifestations can range in severity from self-limited episodes to life-threatening illnesses. The medical history is geared toward eliciting a specific cause. A succinct description of the present illness is fundamental. It is particularly important to find out how long the diarrhea has been present (acute, chronic), and the quantity (volume, number of bowel movements in the past 24 hr), timing (especially nocturnal diarrhea), and quality (watery or bulky consistency, blood, mucous) of the stool. Ask about associated symptoms (nausea, vomiting, fever). Significant pain accompanying diarrhea is unusual and, if present (especially in the elderly), suggests ischemic bowel. Other important points to cover include exposure (similar symptoms in family members, friends, nursing home residents), recent dietary consumption (food poisoning), relation to food intake (abates with fasting, lactose intolerance), medication use (antibiotics, laxatives, magnesium-containing antacids), risk factors for HIV (see Table 5.8.1), history of inflammatory bowel disease (IBD) or other underlying systemic disorder (diabetes, scleroderma, hyperthyroidism, cystic fibrosis), prior surgery (postgastrectomy dumping syndrome), history of alcoholism, practice of anal intercourse (increases risk for *Campylobacter fetus,* gonorrhea, amebiasis, herpes simplex), pets (chickens, cats, and dogs are sources of *Campylobacter fetus*), and recent travel history (certain areas endemic for particular microbes).

Physical Examination

General. Note if the patient appears dehydrated, toxic or shocky. Assess for lymphadenopathy (AIDS, lymphoma).

Vital signs. Check a rectal temperature for fever (infection, inflammatory bowel disease) and note orthostatic changes in the blood pressure and/or pulse (dehydration). A relative bradycardia may accompany systemic *Salmonella* infection.

Table 5.8.1
Differential Diagnosis of AIDS-Related Diarrhea

Bacterial
- *Salmonella*
- *Shigella*
- *Campylobacter*
- *Neisseria gonorrhoeae*
- *Treponema pallidum*
- *Clostridium difficile*
- *Mycobacterium avium-intracellulare*

Protozoa
- *Giardia lamblia*
- *Cryptosporidium*
- *Entamoeba histolytica*
- *Isospora belli*

Viruses
- Cytomegalovirus (CMV)
- Herpes simplex

Noninfectious
- Kaposi's sarcoma
- AIDS-related enteropathy
- Lymphoma

Skin. Test skin turgor (dehydration), along with inspecting for skin lesions (rose spots, thrush, Kaposi's sarcoma), hyperpigmentation (Addison's disease), and purpura (vitamin K deficiency due to malabsorption).

Abdomen. Examine for masses, tenderness (localized, diffuse), peritoneal signs, bruits, hepatosplenomegaly, and distention.

Rectal. Assess rectal tone (patulous anus suggests frequent rectal intercourse), masses (impacted stool, villous adenoma), perianal abscesses, fistula (Crohn's disease), and examine the stool sample for gross or occult blood.

Diagnostic Tests

Note: *Systemically ill patients require standard laboratory tests, while minimally symptomatic patients with mild, acute symptoms may not require more than a stool sample.*

Stool. First, test for occult blood. Next, examine for PMNs (performed with either Gram's stain or methylene blue) (Table

5.8.2). Systemically ill patients (significant fever, blood or pus in stool) also require stool cultures *(Salmonella, Shigella, Yersinia, Campylobacter)*. In addition, a rectal swab—in an appropriate culture medium—is indicated when STD is considered (*Chlamydia,* gonorrhea, syphilis, herpes). If *Clostridium difficile* is suspected, send a blood or stool specimen to the lab for a toxin assay. Request ova and parasite analysis when the history is suggestive. A more reliable and less expensive assay, the ELISA test, has been developed to detect *Cryptosporidium* and *Giardia.*

Table 5.8.2
Fecal Leukocyte Testing

Positive PMNs
- Infectious agents
  - *Shigella*
  - *Campylobacter*
  - Enteroinvasive *E. coli*
- Inflammatory bowel disorders
  - Crohn's disease
  - Ulcerative colitis
  - Radiation colitis
  - Ischemic colitis

Negative PMNs
- Viral infections
  - Norwalk
  - Rotavirus
- Food poisoning
  - *Staphylococcus aureus*
  - *Bacillus cereus*
  - *Clostridium perfringens*
- Parasites
  - *Giardia lamblia*
  - *Entamoeba histolytica*
  - *Cryptosporidium*
- Miscellaneous
  - Irritable bowel syndrome
  - Enterotoxigenic *E. coli*

Variable
- *Salmonella*
- *Yersinia*
- *Vibrio parahaemolyticus*
- *Clostridium difficile*

CBC. Usually reserved for patients with concomitant fever and/or bloody stools. Serious bacterial infections and inflammatory bowel disease may generate a leukocytosis. Bleeding or chronic malabsorption may lead to anemia.

Blood cultures. Obtain if patient appears ill.

SMA. Obtain if diarrhea is severe or there are clinical signs of dehydration; hypokalemia and metabolic acidosis are most commonly detected.

Urinalysis. Reflects hydration status (specific gravity)

X-rays. Patients with significant abdominal pain, who appear ill, or have underlying inflammatory bowel disease require plain films of the abdomen. Review for toxic megacolon (abnormal distention) and thumbprinting (mesenteric ischemia).

Special Considerations

Food Poisoning

Staphylococcus aureus. Infection is transmitted by ingestion of contaminated food (especially dairy products, cream-filled pastries, custards, and mayonnaise) that contain a preformed toxin. After a short incubation period of 2 to 8 hr, an "explosive" onset of severe nausea, vomiting, abdominal cramping, and watery diarrhea occurs. Symptoms tend to resolve in 24 to 48 hr.

Clostridium perfringens. Diarrhea is caused by release of an enterotoxin following ingestion of anaerobic spore-forming rods found in improperly stored and cooked meat and poultry. The incubation period is 6 to 8 hr. Type A strains produce afebrile watery diarrhea, usually lasting 24 to 48 hr. Type C strains rarely produce fulminant and potentially fatal obstructive hemorrhagic jejunitis.

***Escherichia coli* (enterotoxigenic).** Heat-stable and -labile exotoxins (found in both water and food) that are responsible for more than half of cases of "traveler's diarrhea." Symptoms usually occur within 1st week of arriving to new region and are generally self-limited. Resultant watery diarrhea and abdominal cramps can be severe (lasting up to 1 week). Recently, a toxigenic, noninvasive *E. coli (0157:H7)* acquired from contaminated meat has been identified and gives rise to an acute, potentially lethal hemorrhagic colitis.

Vibrio cholera. Due to a heat-labile exotoxin (activates adenyl cyclase) and can lead to a severe life-threatening diarrhea (colorless, "rice water stool"; 20 to 25 L of fluid loss a day is possible). Diarrhea is sometimes combined with vomiting. Infection is transmitted via contaminated water or food with a 1- to 3-day incubation period. It is uncommon in the United States.

Vibrio parahaemolyticus. Toxin-mediated diarrhea transmitted via ingestion of raw or undercooked, contaminated saltwater seafood. The incubation period is 6 to 48 hr. Symptoms include abdominal cramps and diarrhea, which may be bloody. The infection is self-limited and symptoms last for less than 1 week.

Bacillus cereus. A Gram-positive rod that produces two discrete enterotoxins, one of which is heat-stable and often associated with fried rice. The incubation period is 2 to 4 hr. Symptoms include nausea and vomiting, which usually last less than 12 hr. The second is heat labile and is associated with underrefrigerated meats and vegetables. The incubation period is 6 to 14 hr. The primary symptom is diarrhea, which usually lasts 24 to 36 hr.

Infectious Bacterial

Clostridium difficile. Generally occurs subsequent to antibiotic therapy (especially clindamycin, ampicillin, or cephalosporins). A grayish yellow "pseudo-membrane" is found on sigmoidoscopy. Symptoms are variable and may include fever along with a watery diarrhea containing pus, mucus, and/or blood.

Campylobacter jejuni. A bacillus that causes diarrhea by invading and ulcerating mucosa in the terminal ileum. It is associated with ingestion of raw foods (poultry, clams), milk, and contaminated water. The incubation period is 2 to 4 days. Symptoms include fever, abdominal pain (may mimic appendicitis or pancreatitis), and a watery diarrhea that can progress to a bloody diarrhea. Diagnosis made by culture.

Campylobacter fetus. The organism directly invades the intestinal mucosa, with the highest concentration being in the ileum. It is transmitted by infected animals or animal products (meat cutters are at high risk). Onset is abrupt with high fevers (up to 40°C; 104°F), abdominal cramps, and frequent (6 to 10) daily bowel movements, which may contain gross blood or melena. Symptoms usually resolve in 2 to 4 days but may persist up to 3 weeks.

***Salmonella* species.** A tissue invasion of the mucosa occurs. Most cases are transmitted by contaminated foods (especially poultry), with symptoms (colicky abdominal pain, loose watery stools, chills and fever up to 40°C; 104°F) developing in 8 to 48 hr and subsiding in 2 to 5 days. *Enteric,* or *typhoid,* fever usually arises from *S. typhi* infection and is characterized by a sustained fever (often lasting 2 to 4 weeks), a quickly resolving diarrhea, headaches, abdominal pain, bacteremia, leukopenia, rose spots, and possible multiorgan failure. Intestinal hemorrhage or perforation may occur.

***Shigella* species.** Arises from infection with nonmotile Gram-negative bacillus and is transmitted via the fecal-oral route The incidence is higher in travelers and homosexual males. The incubation period is 36 to 72 hr. Symptoms range from a watery diarrhea along with a mild fever and malaise to severe manifestations (bacillary dysentery) characterized by high fevers, a bloody diarrhea mixed with mucus or pus, and tenesmus.

Yersinia enterocolitica. Diarrhea arises from direct tissue invasion, with transmission via contaminated food. Fever, abdominal pain, and diarrhea (may be bloody) commonly occur together. In addition, infection of the terminal ileum accompanied by mesenteric lymphadenopathy may take place and mimic appendicitis.

Viral

Parvovirus (Norwalk agent, Hawaii agent). Infects all age groups and has been implicated in several diarrhea epidemics. Viral-related gastroenteritis is typically a diagnosis of exclusion, distinguished by an absence of fecal leukocytes in the stool and no extenuating circumstances (no history of ingestion of contaminated food). Symptoms are self-limited.

Rotavirus. Primarily affects infants but may occur in adults.

Parasitic

Giardia lamblia. One of the most common parasitic infections in the United States, with the organism residing in the duodenum and jejunum. Infection is most prevalent in travelers to endemic regions, homosexual males, and immunodeficient persons. Transmission may be person-to-person or waterborne (mountainous regions). The clinical picture varies from asymptomatic to intermittent watery diarrhea to acute-onset watery diarrhea with abdominal cramps and flatulence. Definitive diagnosis requires identification of the cyst or trophozoite forms of the parasite in duodenal aspirates or stool samples.

Entamoeba histolytica. Causes *amebiasis,* especially in travelers, institutionalized patients, and homosexual males. The primary site of invasion is the cecum; but the rectum may become infected, developing ulceration, which leads to rectal pain, tenesmus, and urgency. Symptoms are highly variable, ranging from an asymptomatic carrier state to abdominal pain along with numerous loose stools to a full-blown bacillary dysentery (high fever, bloody diarrhea, prostration). Complications include ameboma of the cecum or terminal ileum, intestinal stricture, and hepatic abscess.

Isosporiasis belli. A coccidial parasite and the most widespread cause of diarrhea in AIDS patients. The clinical picture is chronic watery diarrhea and weight loss. Blood eosinophilia may occur. The diagnosis is established by identifying oocytes in the stool, demonstrated with acid-fast staining.

Cryptosporidium. Causes enterocolitis in both normal and immunocompromised hosts. Waterborne transmission and acquisition by international travelers have been documented. In immunocompetent hosts, the incubation period is roughly 1 week and symptoms include watery nonbloody diarrhea, sometimes accompanied by abdominal pain, nausea, fever, anorexia, and weight loss. In immunocompromised hosts and particularly AIDS patients, the secretory diarrhea is chronic, profuse, and unremitting and respiratory tract involvement may occur.

Fungal

Candida albicans. May be pathogenic in immunosuppressed patients. The gastrointestinal tract may be involved anywhere from the mouth to the anus, and severe diarrhea may be a symptom.

Treatment

The major cause of morbidity and mortality related to diarrhea is *intravascular volume depletion* and associated *electrolyte imbalances.* If possible, encourage oral repletion with balanced rehydration solutions (a simple home-made oral rehydration solution is created by mixing 1 teaspoon of table salt, 4 heaping tablespoons of sugar, 1 teaspoon of sodium bicarbonate, and 1 L of water). With serious volume depletion, administer intravenous boluses (250 to 500 mL over 1 hr) of crystalloids (NS or lactated Ringer's); frequently reassess the patient, titrating further infusions based on the patient's clinical status. Recheck electrolyte values when imbalances are present.

Patients with acute diarrhea of < 24 hr duration that is accompanied by fever, tenesmus, heme-positive stools, or dehydration and who have fecal leukocytes may be treated empirically with *ciprofloxacin* (500 mg PO BID for 3 to 5 days) or *norfloxacin* (400 mg PO BID for 3 to 5 days) pending toxin and culture data. If contraindications to fluoroquinolones exist, *trimethoprim/sulfamethoxazole* (1 DS tablet PO BID for 5 days) may be substituted.

Use *metronidazole* (250 mg PO QID for 7 to 10 days) or *vancomycin* (125 mg PO QID for 7 days) for suspected antibiotic-related *C. difficile* infection. Suspected *Giardia* infections are treated with *metronidazole* (250 mg PO TID for 5 days), while amebiasis is treated with *metronidazole* (750 mg TID for 10 days); alcohol ingestion needs to be avoided for 48 hr following metronidazole ingestion because of a disulfiram-type reaction. Mild to moderate exacerbations of ulcerative colitis may be treated with *sulfasalazine* (1.0 g PO q 6 h) or *mesalamine* (1.0 g PO q 6 h) supplemented with corticosteroid enemas.

In up to 50% of patients with AIDS-related diarrhea, no organism can be identified. Recent studies have suggested that the *macrolides* (azithromycin) may be beneficial for empirical treatment of nonbacterial infections, while paromomycin (500 mg PO QID for 14 days) may be effective therapy for *Cryptosporidium* or *Isospora belli.*

Until recently, the use of antimotility agents was considered taboo. Recent studies have modified this position, and the judicious use of *loperamide* (4 mg initially, followed by one 2-mg capsule after each stool, up to 16 mg total a day) for nontoxic adults is considered acceptable. Bismuth subsalicylate (2 tablets or 30 mL QID) reduces symptoms of traveler's diarrhea.

Admission Criteria

Factors guiding the need for admission include *clinical status* (toxic appearance, significant volume depletion with ongoing diarrhea loss), *underlying medical conditions* (immunosuppressed, inflammatory bowel disease), *age* (elderly more susceptible to complications arising from fluid loss), and *social situation.*

Suggested Readings

Goodman LJ, Trenholme GM, Kaplan RL, et al.: Empiric antimicrobial therapy of domestically acquired acute diarrhea in urban adults. Arch Int Med 1990;150:541–546.

Guerrant RL, Bobak DA: Bacterial and protozoal gastroenteritis. N Engl J Med 1991;325:327–333.

Murphy GS, et al.: Ciprofloxin and loperamide in the treatment of bacillary dysentery. Ann Intern Med 1993;118:582–586.

5.9 ACUTE HEPATITIS

Description

Hepatitis, an acute ailment of the liver, is most commonly caused by one of several viruses that gives rise to hepatocellular inflammation, damage, and dysfunction. The diagnosis of acute viral hepatitis depends on a combination of clinical and biochemical findings.

History

Prodromal symptoms of viral hepatitis are nonspecific and include anorexia, nausea and vomiting, arthralgias, arthritis, urticaria, myalgias, low-grade fever, rash, dark urine, and clay-colored stools. The rapidity of onset depends on the etiology of hepatitis (fairly abrupt onset with hepatitis A; more indolent with hepatitis C). The severity of the illness is contingent on the etiology, extent of underlying liver pathology, and the interaction between host factors and the offending agent (in immunocompromised patients strongly consider the possibility of cytomegalovirus or toxoplasmosis). In jaundiced patients, ask about RUQ pain. Establish the following data: past history of hepatitis, contact with hepatitis infected individuals, prescribed medications, use or exposure to alcohol or other hepatotoxins (mushrooms), blood transfusions, intravenous drug abuse, travel history, sexual preference, heavy tattooing, and underlying disorders (hemodialysis, recent surgery, organ transplantation). In pregnant females who are near term consider *cholestatic jaundice of pregnancy* or *acute fatty liver of pregnancy*.

Physical Examination

General. Physical findings are variable, and patients may range from being comfortable and non–ill appearing to toxic or shocky.

Vital signs. Always check a rectal temperature. Do orthostatic pulse and pressure readings.

HEENT. Look for icterus.

Neck. Check for adenopathy.

Abdomen. Evaluate for RUQ tenderness as well as hepatomegaly (70% of cases) and splenomegaly (20% of cases). Check for ascites.

Rectal. Test the stool for blood.

Extremities. Look for edema or track marks. Arthralgias or frank arthritis may be present.

Skin. Note jaundice. Look for spider angiomata, palmar erythema (chronic alcohol abuse) and urticaria.

Neurologic. Note lethargy, confusion, stupor, or level of coma. Check for asterixis.

Diagnostic Tests

General Tests

CBC. Typically a mild anemia; a low, normal, or mildly elevated WBC count and a lymphocytosis > 35% are present. If the clinical picture and CBC suggest infectious mononucleosis, order a monospot or heterophile antibody test.

SMA. The liver function tests (LFTs) serve as a useful screening test for hepatocellular injury. While nonspecific, LFTs (AST, ALT, alkaline phosphatase, total bilirubin, GGTP) are sensitive for liver pathology. Serum bilirubin levels > 20 mg/dL indicate severe disease; but the degree of transaminase elevation is not predictive. With alcoholic-related liver disease, the increase in AST is disproportionate when compared to the ALT (AST:ALT ratio > 2 is characteristic of acute alcoholic hepatitis). Assess additional biochemical markers of liver function (serum protein, albumin, glucose).

PT. Depends on liver-synthesized clotting factors; mild elevations are not abnormal with hepatitis. Significant prolongation of PT (> 3 sec) conveys a poor prognosis.

PTT. May be elevated in severe disease.

Antibodies

Order the full-battery of hepatitis serologic studies when viral hepatitis is considered. This includes anti-HAV, HBsAg, anti-HBs, anti-HBc, and hepatitis C testing (Table 5.9.1). Antibody to *hepatitis A* appears early in the course of the illness; with IgM antibodies initially appearing, peaking within the 1st week of clinical disease, and disappearing in following 3 to 6 months. IgG antibody to HAV emerges after 1 month and persists for years.

The earliest serologic marker for *hepatitis B* (HBV) is *hepatitis B surface antigen* (HBsAg), which can be detected in the serum before clinical symptoms become apparent (as early as 1 week postinoculation). HBsAg normally disappears with resolution of infection; persistence beyond 6 months indicates a chronic carrier state. Antibodies to the *hepatitis B core Ag* (anti-HBc) also surface promptly (appearing 3 to 4 weeks after HBsAg arises), and may be the only marker present following disappearance of HBsAg (core window) in patients with *active* hepatitis B. Generally anti-HBc levels decline, but levels may remain high in chronic carriers.

Hepatitis B e antigen (HBeAg) appears shortly after HBsAg develops, and its presence indicates a high state of infectivity. Continuance of HBeAg levels beyond 3 months increases the likelihood of chronic hepatitis B infection, while the appearance of antibody to HBeAg (anti-HBe) usually coincides with disappearance of HBeAg, indicating probable resolution of infection. A

Table 5.9.1
Serologic Marker Patterns for Hepatitis A and B

Anti-HAV (IgM)	HBsAg	Anti-HBc (IgM)	Anti-HBs	Interpretation
+	−	−	−	Acute hepatitis A infection
−	+	−	−	Early acute hepatitis B infection (preclinical)
−	−	+	−	Acute hepatitis B infection (core window period)
−	+	±	−	Chronic hepatitis (anti-HBc may be positive for IgG); consider testing for HDV
−	−	−	+	Vaccination or recovery (with recovery, anti-HBc may be positive for anti-HBc IgG)
+	+	−	−	Acute hepatitis A superimposed on chronic hepatitis B
−	−	−	−	Look for cause other than hepatitis A or B

specific antibody to HBsAg (anti-HBs) appears in individuals successfully vaccinated against hepatitis B as well as those people with successful recovery. A recently developed DNA assay for HBV infected serum is now available.

Hepatitis D infection may also be tested for (assay based on antibody detection). Diagnosis of hepatitis C is predicated on an enzyme immunoassay, which exhibits only a moderate sensitivity and specificity. Other viral causes (Epstein-Barr virus, cytomegalovirus) can be diagnosed by specially requested tests.

Special Considerations

Hepatitis A (HBA). Usually transmitted via the fecal-oral route and has been associated with sewage-contaminated shellfish. The incubation period is short (roughly 15 to 50 days). Close to 50% of the American population has undergone subclinical infection with hepatitis A and displays hepatitis A antibodies (positive IgG). Patients with HAV are most infectious for 2 weeks before icterus and 1 week after the onset of jaundice.

Hepatitis B (HBV). Transmitted by percutaneous, oral-fecal, oral-oral, and venereal routes. High-risk groups include intravenous drug abusers, homosexuals, medical personnel, and blood transfusion recipients. The incubation period is long (roughly 50 to 150 days). Patients are a communicable risk for infection for up to 6 weeks before the onset of symptoms and remain infectious as long as HBsAg can be detected in the serum.

Hepatitis C (HBC). Spread by percutaneous route and currently the most common cause of posttransfusion hepatitis. The incubation period is roughly 25 to 75 days. Antibody to hepatitis C virus is present in 0.5% of blood donors with normal ALT levels.

Hepatitis D (HBD). Known as the delta agent; causes infection only in individuals already infected by hepatitis B. Route of transmission is similar to that of HBV.

Hepatitis E (HBE). Spread by fecal-oral route and commonly implicated in hepatitis epidemics in developing countries. It usually affects adults and has a high mortality in pregnant women. Although rare in the United States, it has been reported in immigrants. No serologic markers are currently available.

Fulminant hepatitis. Rare with hepatitis A, but occurs in up to 2% of cases of hepatitis B and C infections. Fulminant hepatitis is more prevalent when HDV is combined with HBV infection. Extensive necrosis of the liver takes place, leading to a progressive jaundice, toxemia, GI symptoms, hemorrhagic abnormalities, and hepatic encephalopathy. Ascites appears within 8 weeks of onset of symptoms. The earliest laboratory finding is a prolongation of the PT. Treatment is mainly supportive, with the only effective therapy being liver transplantation.

Chronic persistent hepatitis. Associated with hepatitis B or hepatitis C; characterized by persistent elevation of serum transaminases for > 6 months. Despite complaints of continual fatigue, anorexia, and/or malaise, the prognosis for recovery is generally good.

Chronic active hepatitis. Complication of hepatitis B and C infection, frequently leading to irreversible liver disease (cirrhosis).

Epstein-Barr virus. A herpes virus that is transmitted during oral-oral contact or parenterally. May lead to a mild hepatitis accompanied by nausea, vomiting, and jaundice (10 to 20% of infected individuals). Serum aminotransferases are moderately elevated (300 to 500 IU/L). The hepatitis is usually part of the clinical syndrome of infectious mononucleosis.

Cytomegalovirus. A herpes virus that can produce a syndrome like infectious mononucleosis but without adenopathy or tonsillopharyngeal involvement. Liver involvement mimics the more common forms of viral hepatitis, but it is usually milder than other manifestations.

Drug-induced liver disease. May result from immunologic-mediated mechanisms (isoniazid, phenytoin, methyldopa, sulfonamides, oral contraceptives) or from direct toxicity (acetaminophen overdose, alcohol, Amanita mushroom poisoning).

Vascular occlusion. Also referred to as Budd-Chiari syndrome (an occlusion of the hepatic veins); can produce clinical findings resembling acute hepatitis. It occurs with myeloproliferative disorders, bone marrow transplants, and oral contraceptive use.

Treatment

Most patients who are able to eat and drink do not require admission. It should be explained to these patients that there is no specific therapy for hepatitis. They should be counseled to avoid alcohol and other toxins and to discontinue all potentially hepatotoxic drugs. Isolation is not necessary. Stool precautions and careful hygiene are reasonable. It may be appropriate for the patient to avoid contact with children and chronically ill or elderly adults until the diagnosis is clear. Patients should have weekly follow up arranged as outpatients for blood testing until recovery demonstrated. See section 9.8 for issues relating to postexposure prophylaxis to infected blood and body fluid.

Admission Criteria

Admit *patients who display the following:*

- Inability to keep fluids down with consequent dehydration;
- Gl bleeding or other signs of coagulopathy;
- PT prolonged by > 3 sec over control;
- Hypoglycemia (< 45 mg/dL);
- Bilirubin > 20 mg/dL;
- Signs of fulminant hepatic failure (encephalopathy, ascites, pedal edema, shock); and
- Concurrent complicating illnesses.

Suggested Readings

Ergun GA, Miskovitz PF: Viral hepatitis. The new ABC's. Postgrad Med 1990;88:69–76.

Lee WM: Acute liver failure. N Engl J Med 1993;329:1862–1867.

5.10 CIRRHOSIS

Description

Cirrhosis of the liver is an irreversible pathologic process where hepatocellular injury results in diffuse hepatic fibrosis and distortion of the normal lobular and vasculature architecture of the liver into structurally abnormal nodules. The liver has a limited range of response to injury, so the ultimate histology pattern observed in cirrhosis is similar regardless of the underlying etiology. *Alcohol (Laennec's cirrhosis)* is the most common cause in the United States and Europe, followed by *chronic viral hepatitis,* caused by either *hepatitis B* or *hepatitis C virus.* Other less common etiologies include drugs and toxins, cholestatic liver disease (primary biliary cirrhosis, sclerosing cholangitis), metabolic disorders (hemochromatosis, Wilson's disease, α-1-antitrypsin deficiency), venous outflow obstruction (Budd-Chiari syndrome, chronic right heart failure), and miscellaneous causes (cystic fibrosis, sarcoidosis).

History

The onset of symptoms is ordinarily insidious. Symptomatic cirrhosis is characterized by a general deterioration in health, including chronic fatigue, poor appetite, weakness, and wasting (weight loss may be masked by ascites and edema). Nausea, vomiting, and diarrhea are common complaints. Females of childbearing age suffer menstrual abnormalities (usually amenorrhea), whereas in males there is a loss of libido. Severe pruritus is associated with biliary cirrhosis. Important historical information is similar to that needed for hepatitis (see section 5.9).

Physical Examination

General. Patients appear chronically ill.

Vital signs. Patients are prone to hypothermia.

Skin. Check for spider nevi (usually on upper half of body) and telangiectasias of exposed areas. Slate gray coloring of the skin is seen with hemochromatosis (known as bronze diabetes); alopecia is also a prominent feature.

HEENT. Inspect for glossitis, cheilosis, parotid enlargement, and Kayser-Fleischer rings in the cornea (Wilson's disease). Scleral icterus appears when bilirubin values are > 3 mg/dL.

Chest. Observe for gynecomastia and dilation of superficial veins.

Heart. Note if size is increased (CHF).

Abdomen. Palpate for hepatomegaly and splenomegaly. Look for dilation of superficial veins of the abdomen (caput medusae). Percuss for ascites (late finding).

Genitalia. Assess for testicular atrophy.

Rectal. Check stool for occult blood. Hemorrhoids are frequently present (portal hypertension). **Note:** *Do not incise or excise the hemorrhoids of a cirrhotic in the ED.*

Extremities. Note palmar erythema (especially of thenar and hypothenar eminence), peripheral edema, and Duputyren's contracture (contracture of palmar fascial bands).

Neurologic. Examine for asterixis (flapping tremor is best seen with arms outstretched and wrists in hyperextension) and altered mental status (hepatic encephalopathy).

Diagnostic Tests

CBC. Anemia is a frequent finding (chronic disease, nutritional factors, GI bleed). The WBC count may be low, normal, or elevated. Thrombocytopenia may occur (splenic sequestration, bone marrow toxicity from ethanol).

Serum glucose. Profound hypoglycemia may appear in patients with alcohol-related cirrhosis or fulminant hepatic failure.

SMA. Check for hyponatremia (dilutional, SIADH, inappropriate diuretic use); hypokalemia (gastrointestinal losses, secondary hyperaldosteronism, diuretic use); elevated BUN:creatinine ration (dehydration, hepatorenal syndrome); decreased serum albumin; and elevations of AST, ALT, alkaline phosphatase (elevation of alkaline phosphatase out of proportion to other enzymes suggests biliary cirrhosis), and bilirubin. Marked elevation of blood ammonia levels (> 200 mg/dL) may be seen in patients with hepatic encephalopathy.

PT/PTT. Coagulation abnormalities result from failure of synthesis of clotting factors in the liver.

ABG. Arterial hypoxemia is common in decompensated patients. Various acid-base disturbances can occur, with respiratory alkalosis (pH around 7.5) being the most common.

Endoscopy. May be necessary emergently in suspected bleeding varices.

Special Considerations

For varices, see section 5.6.

Ascites

Ascites results from increased sinusoidal pressure, hypoalbuminemia, abnormal hepatic and abdominal lymph production, and abnormal salt and water retention by the kidneys. Generally, ascites causes little more than unsightly abdominal distention and discomfort. However, if it becomes massive, ascites can lead to respiratory embarrassment. Initial management should be conservative, emphasizing sodium restriction and bed rest. In patients not responding to conservative measures, give *spironolactone* starting at 50 mg BID. Abdominal paracentesis should be reserved for patients in respiratory distress, extreme discomfort, or suspected spontaneous bacterial peritonitis. If large volumes of ascitic fluid are to be removed (4 to 6 L), concomitantly administer intravenous *albumin* (8 to 10 g/L of ascitic fluid removed).

Spontaneous Bacterial Peritonitis

Spontaneous bacterial peritonitis (SBP) arises from an infection of ascitic fluid and is a serious complication in cirrhotics. The designation "spontaneous" implies that there is no evidence of perforation of the gut and infection of the ascitic fluid is thought to result from transient bacteremia. Differentiation of SBP from primary peritonitis is important since the management differs. Infection usually results from a single organism with SBP (usually *E. coli* or *Klebsiella*); a multiorganism infection occurs with peritonitis secondary to a perforated viscus. SBP is tentatively diagnosed by paracentesis—review a Gram stain (positive in only half of infections) and a WBC count (PMNs > 250 to 300 cells/mm^3 suggests SBP) and order a culture and sensitivity. Begin antibiotic therapy (cefotaxime, 1.5 to 2.0 g IV q 6 hr) before culture results.

Hepatorenal Syndrome

Patients with cirrhosis can develop renal failure from a variety of mechanisms, ranging from urinary tract infection and prerenal azotemia to intrarenal causes such as acute tubular necrosis. Hepatorenal syndrome is an entity unique to decompensated cirrhotics wherein patients develop functional renal failure in the absence of other known causes of renal failure. It is almost universally fatal and probably represents a disturbance in the normal homeostatic mechanisms of renal perfusion. The only effective current therapy is liver transplantation.

Hepatic Encephalopathy

Hepatic encephalopathy is a complex neuropsychiatric syndrome characterized by mood changes, confusion, drowsiness, disorientation, and even coma. The exact primary cause of hepatic encephalopathy is unclear, but recent evidence implicates the accumulation of toxins that the liver can no longer metabolize. Factors that can precipitate hepatic encephalopathy include gastrointestinal bleeding, azotemia, a high protein diet, drugs (sedatives, tranquilizers, excessive diuretic use), metabolic imbalances (hypokalemia), and infection (urinary tract infection, aspiration pneumonia, spontaneous bacterial peritonitis). In addition to the typical stigmata of cirrhosis, patients with hepatic encephalopathy may demonstrate fetor hepaticus (musty odor of the breath) and asterixis. Once the ABCs are secured, attempt to improve mental status by correcting fluid-electrolyte imbalances, providing adequate nutrition (withhold dietary protein), treating infection, and cleansing the gut (eliminate any endogenous toxins, reduce absorption of gut-derived bacterial protein). The most popular agent is *lactulose,* which can be given orally or via nasogastric tube in 15- to 30-mL doses 3 to 4 times daily (the goal is two to three loose stools per day). A lactulose-retention enema (leave in place 30 to 60 min) can also be used—mix 300 mL of lactulose syrup with 700 mL of tap water. Additional measures include *neomycin* (1 g PO or via NG q 6 to 12 hr), metronidazole (250 mg PO TID), and *flumazenil* (a benzodiazepine receptor antagonist that may reverse the effects of the inhibitory neurotransmitter GABA).

Treatment

Short of liver transplantation, there is no specific therapy for cirrhosis (an exception is patients with cirrhosis secondary to hemochromatosis or Wilson's disease) (Table 5.10.1). Treatment is geared toward elimination of the potential hepatotoxic agent and aggressive management of complications. Avoid the use of narcotics, tranquilizers, and sedatives, especially those excreted by the liver (if the patient is severely agitated, employ *oxazepam,* 10 to 30 mg PO TID, which is not metabolized by the liver). Abstinence from alcohol is the single most effective therapy in improving survival in patients who have cirrhosis secondary to alcohol abuse. Pa-

Table 5.10.1
Pugh Staging of Cirrhosis

Parameter	Points[a]		
	1	2	3
Encephalopathy	None	Mild	Advanced, coma
Ascites	Absent	Slight	Moderate
Bilirubin (mg/dL)	< 2.0	2.0–3.0	> 3.0
Albumin (g/dL)	> 3.5	2.8–3.5	< 2.8
Prothrombin time (sec prolonged)	1.0–4.0	4.0–6.0	> 6.0

[a]Class A, 5–6 points (6.4 years average survival); class B, 7–9 points (1–5 years average survival); class C, 10–15 points (2 months average survival).

tients suffering from intense pruritus secondary to accumulation of bilirubin (biliary cirrhosis) may benefit from the use of an anion exchange residue such as *cholestyramine* (4 g PO TID).

Admission Criteria

Admit *patients with new-onset ascites or hepatic encephalopathy* or who *may be septic* (including spontaneous bacterial peritonitis). Also *patients who have intractable nausea and vomiting with moderate to severe dehydration; gastrointestinal bleeding* (if the patient is hemodynamically unstable or experiencing active bleeding, admit to the ICU); and *hypoglycemia* (< 60 mg/dL).

Patients with chronic ascites or patients with a history of hepatic encephalopathy who are mildly encephalopathic (stage I) can often be managed as outpatients

Suggested Readings

Pomier-Layrargues G: Flumazenil in cirrhotic patients in hepatic coma. Hepatology 1994;19:32–35.

Runyon BA: Care of the patient with ascites. N Engl J Med 1994;330: 337–342.

Chapter 6

Metabolism

6.1 DIABETIC COMA AND HYPERGLYCEMIA

Diabetic Ketoacidosis

Description

Diabetic ketoacidosis (DKA) is the most frequently encountered endocrine emergency. It is characterized by hyperglycemia, ketoacidosis, dehydration, and electrolyte imbalances. Shock occurs when volume depletion is profound, whereas a metabolic acidosis accompanies accelerated ketogenesis.

History

Although DKA generally occurs in known or newly diagnosed type I (insulin- dependent) diabetics (IDDM), it may also appear in elderly type II diabetics. Establish the patient's prior diabetic history—years since diagnosis, level of control, previous hospitalizations, diabetic complications, and current insulin or drug regimen. Always look for the event precipitating DKA. Frequently, patients report a minor illness with poor oral intake and decreased or discontinued insulin use. Other possible causes include myocardial infarction, stroke, pancreatitis, pregnancy, infection, or stress of any nature. The presenting symptoms are variable. Anorexia, abdominal pain, nausea, vomiting, lethargy, tachypnea, change in mental status, or coma should alert one to the diagnosis. Complications of DKA include hypothermia, hypotension, shock, gastric atony, gastrointestinal bleeding, pulmonary aspiration, respiratory distress syndrome, thrombosis, and hemorrhagic diathesis.

Physical Examination

Vital signs. Check for orthostatic changes. Note the respiratory rate and pattern (Kussmaul breathing). Obtain a rectal temperature to ensure accuracy of the recording (hypothermia, as well as hyperthermia, may accompany infection).

HEENT. Examine for infection of the sinuses, pharynx, gums, or tympanic membranes. A musty or fruity odor (ketones) may be detected on the breath.

Neck. Check jugular veins. Test for meningismus.

Lungs. Listen for rales or wheezes.

Abdomen. Auscultate for bowel sounds. Observe for abdominal distention (gastric atony, gastrointestinal bleeding). Severe ketonemia can provoke severe abdominal complaints.

Extremities. Inspect carefully for skin ulcers, cellulitis, or abscesses (especially the lower extremities).

Neurologic. Note level of consciousness. Examine for focal deficits. The level of consciousness generally correlates with serum osmolarity, not pH.

Diagnostic Tests

SMA. Do a fingerstick glucose. Serum glucose is usually > 300 mg/dL, although the range is highly variable. Two classes of DKA patients with unimpressive glucose elevations are pregnant females and alcoholics. Serum potassium (K^+) levels may be low, normal, or high; while higher serum potassium levels tend to be the rule, there is almost always a total body deficit of potassium in DKA. An initially low serum potassium level attests to severe depletion and mandates a need for aggressive replacement. Serum sodium will be artificially lowered by 1.6 mEq/L for each 100 mg/dL increase in glucose. DKA may also elevate amylase levels.

ABG. Check the pH at regular intervals (can use venous sample).

Urinalysis. Employ a test strip for ketones, nitrites, and leukocyte esterase. Obtain a microscopic analysis to screen for infection.

Serum ketones. Beta-hydroxybutyrate (BHOB) may be the predominant ketone found in the blood during DKA, especially in the face of hypoxia and decreased perfusion, conditions that lower the redox potential. The nitroprusside reaction tests for acetone and acetoacetate but not BHOB. Results may be misleading, with reported ketone concentrations being low at presentation because of the preponderance of BHOB.

CBC. Order a WBC count with differential (may be elevated even in the absence of infection).

PT/PTT. Note any coagulopathy.

ECG. Indicated in the majority of adults with DKA. Besides detecting myocardial ischemia, the ECG provides rapid information regarding the potassium level (high potassium levels are associated with peaked T waves and widened QRS complexes).

X-rays. A chest film is often useful in seeking underlying complications (pneumonia, CHF).

Treatment

The key to successful management is adequate fluid restoration and supplemental insulin therapy, along with compulsive monitoring of vital signs, intake and output (I&O), serum glucose, pH, and potassium. Start a flow sheet in the emergency department.

The fluid deficit in the typical adult with DKA ranges from 3 to 5 L. In patients with normal cardiac function, give normal saline as a bolus, 1 L over 30 to 60 min, followed by a 2nd L infused over 1 to 2 hr. Further fluid therapy should be guided by the patient's clinical status. Shock may warrant more rapid infusion. Avoid overzealous replacement, which can induce cerebral and/or pulmonary edema. Hyperglycemia tends to correct more rapidly than acidosis, requiring the addition of glucose to the intravenous fluids during the course of therapy; when a patient's blood sugar reaches 250 mg/dL, switch to D_5half-NS or D_5NS.

The administration of normal saline alone can lower blood glucose by 15 to 20% in the 1st hour. The goal of therapy is to lower serum glucose by approximately 100 mg/dL/hr. Most often, insulin is given via the intravenous route in DKA (especially in the shocky patient, to avoid erratic absorption); an intravenous bolus of 0.1 to 0.2 units/kg is followed by an infusion of 0.1/unit/kg/hr. Predicate subsequent dosing on the patient's clinical status, along with glucose (check every 30 min), electrolyte, osmolality, and pH levels.

Correct electrolyte abnormalities. Once normal renal function has been restored, add 20 mEq of potassium to the 1st L of fluid if the patient is *hypo*kalemic; for *normal* potassium values (3.5 to 5.5 mEq/L), add 20 to 40 mEq to the 2nd L of fluid; and withhold potassium supplementation from patients who are *hyperkalemic* (serum potassium > 5.5 mEq/L). *Except in extreme hypokalemia, do* not *give potassium at a rate exceeding 10 mEq/hr through a peripheral vein or 20 mEq/hr through a central vein (this should be done under cardiac monitoring)*. Both the serum potassium and serum phosphorus levels fall following fluid and insulin therapy. While a portion of the potassium replacement can be given as potassium phosphate, aggressive phosphate repletion is not necessary (too quick a correction of phosphate may cause hypocalcemia and tetany).

Restrict the use of sodium bicarbonate to patients with hyperkalemia and/or severe acidosis. A number of deleterious effects are associated with imprudent use of bicarb (hyperosmolarity, alkalosis, paradoxical CSF acidosis).

Hyperosmolar Nonketotic Coma

Description

Patients with hyperosmolar nonketotic coma (HNKC) customarily demonstrate a serum glucose > 600 mg/dL and a serum osmolarity > 350 mOms/L. Typically, there is an absence of ketoacidosis, although mixed cases can occur. The diagnosis of HNKC needs to be considered in any elderly patient with an altered mental status.

History

Inquire about preceding history of diabetes (solicit additional sources such as family, friends, old medical records, private physician). HNKC is most prevalent in older type II (non-insulin-dependent) diabetics (NIDDM) with mild renal dysfunction (although one-half of cases lack prior history of diabetes). The presentation is frequently subacute and may be a consequence of stroke, MI, GI hemorrhage, or infection. The use of certain medications (corticosteroids, diuretics, phenytoin) is also associated with exacerbating HNKC. Accompanying glycosuria induces a profound osmotic diuresis, leading to complications such as dehydration, electrolyte imbalance, and shock. In addition, patients with HNKC are often lethargic and unable to take fluids by mouth, further exacerbating volume depletion. Mental status changes are common with HNKC (severity of mental status changes corresponds to osmolarity). Coma, seizures, and even focal deficits may result from hyperosmolar state.

Physical Examination

The physical exam is essentially the same as for the patient with DKA, although signs of dehydration (decreased skin turgor, dry mucous membranes) are frequently unreliable in the elderly. In addition, urine output may be deceptively normal secondary to the osmotic diuresis.

Diagnostic Tests

The same laboratory studies (glucose, electrolytes, BUN, creatinine, CBC, ABG, etc.) ordered for DKA are obtained in patients with suspected HNKC. Blood glucose levels regularly are > 600 mg/dL and may be > 2000 mg/dL. *Osmolarity* is calculated using the following formula:

$$\text{Osmolarity} = 2 \times \text{Serum sodium} + \text{Blood glucose}/18 + \text{BUN}/2.8$$

Most patients are azotemic, due to a combination of prerenal and renal etiologies. Hematocrit and hemoglobin are often elevated subsequent to hemoconcentration. A conscientious investigation for underlying illness (CXR, ECG, blood and urine cultures, CT of head) is essential.

Treatment

The paramount goals of ED management are to restore the intravascular volume (the average patient with HNKC has an 8- to 12-L fluid deficit) and correct hyperosmolality. Initiate fluid therapy with normal saline until blood pressure, pulse, and urine output are normalized; once these parameters are secured, change the intravenous fluid to 0.5 normal saline at a rate of 250 to 500 mL/hr, adjusting the rate as needed. If the patient is in shock or hypotensive, administer *isotonic saline;* if the patient is hypertensive or severely hypernatremic (> 160 mEq/L), give *half-normal saline.* Patients with large fluid losses or those with underlying cardiac or renal disease may require invasive monitoring to guide fluid replacement.

Administer insulin cautiously (too rapid a drop in blood glucose can induce cerebral edema). Low doses of insulin (10- to 20-unit IV bolus) are generally adequate.

Correct electrolyte imbalances. Total potassium depletion is usually greater in HNKC than in DKA. Once adequate renal function is established, give potassium (10 to 15 mEq/hr) to the normokalemic or hypokalemic patient. This is best done under cardiac monitoring.

Avoid phenytoin if seizures occur in the patient with HNKC. It is generally ineffective and inhibits the release of endogenous insulin.

Hyperglycemia

Description

If a diabetic patient with an elevated serum glucose is well perfused, nonacidotic, and displays a normal serum osmolarity, that patient is simply hyperglycemic.

History

Hyperglycemia is suggested by polyuria, polydipsia, and nocturia as well as increasing fatigue, lethargy, weight loss, visual disturbances, and headache. Other complaints may include pain or numbness in the feet and/or hands secondary to diabetic neuropathy. The most important task is finding out why the patient's diabetes is uncontrolled. Investigate thoroughly for noncompliance with diet or medication and seek possible sources of infection. Other conditions that may promote hyperglycemia in the diabetic include drugs (glucocorticoids, estrogens, propanolol), pregnancy, emotional stress, or a change in physical activity level.

Physical Examination

Address any abnormal vital signs; orthostatic pulse and blood pressure measurements assist in evaluating the volume status. Diabetics are particularly prone to complications involving the eyes, kidneys, and feet (due to microvascular disease).

Diagnostic Tests

Basic laboratory studies besides glucose determinations include plasma electrolytes, BUN, creatinine, ketones, and a urinalysis to exclude the possibility of DKA or HNKC.

Treatment

Hyperglycemic patients can be effectively managed by oral hydration and subcutaneous insulin. These patients do not universally need intravenous fluids or intravenous insulin; in fact, an aggressive approach may be dangerous. If subcutaneous insulin is used, observe the patient for 2 to 4 hr in the ED; a repeat fingerstick or serum glucose should be performed before discharge.

Admission Criteria

Although all patients with DKA and HNKC require admission, most patients with simple hyperglycemia can be treated in the ED and discharged with outpatient follow-up. Exceptions include *hyperglycemic patients who are vomiting, are unable to take fluids or medications, or are becoming significantly dehydrated* (especially type I diabetics who are prone to develop DKA).

Suggested Readings

Israel RS: Diabetic ketoacidosis. Emerg Med Clin North Am 1989;7(4): 859–871.

Pope DW, Dansky D: Hyperosmolar hyperglycemic nonketotic coma. Emerg Med Clin North Am 1989;7(4):849–857.

Siperstein MD: Diabetic ketoacidosis and hyperosmolar coma. Endocrinol Metab Clin North Am 1992;21(2):415–432.

6.2 HYPOGLYCEMIA

Description

The central nervous system depends on glucose as its sole fuel source. Normally (although variable), signs and symptoms of hypoglycemia do not manifest until the plasma glucose is < 55 mg/dL.

Hypoglycemia occurs most commonly in diabetic patients who take an inappropriate dose of either insulin or oral hypoglycemic agent. Other causes of hypoglycemia include *fasting hypoglycemia* (underproduction of glucose caused by acquired liver disease, drugs such as ethanol or salicylates, or overuse of glucose as occurs with insulinomas) or *postprandial hypoglycemia* (rapid gastric emptying, idiopathic).

History

Obtain a clear history of the episode that prompted the emergency department visit. Inquire about underlying diabetes, alcoholism, or major systemic disease and the most recent dose of insulin or oral hypoglycemic, if taken. Ask about occurrence of previous hypoglycemic episodes and the symptoms of all episodes as well as their relation to eating or fasting.

Symptoms of hypoglycemia can be divided into *adrenergic* and central nervous system *(neuroglycopenic)* symptoms. Adrenergic manifestations tend to have a more sudden onset and are typically postprandial complaints. These include anxiety, irritability, palpitations, sweating, tachycardia, and tremor. Neuroglycopenic symptoms typically demonstrate a more gradual onset and are usually fasting complaints. These include headache, fatigue, confusion, amnesia, seizures, loss of consciousness, irrational behavior, a glassy-eyed stare, diplopia, and dysarthria. There can be a wide gamut of additional presenting complaints in hypoglycemia, including focal neurologic deficits, focal seizures, isolated aglossia, and acute violent behavior. Hypoglycemia should be suspected with any case of altered mental status, neurologic abnormality, or bizarre behavior.

Physical Examination

General. Note if the patient is obese (insulinoma, diabetes) or cachectic (malnutrition).

Vital signs. Check for tachycardia. Note if the patient is hyperthermic or hypothermic.

Skin. Inspect for diaphoresis. Look for stigmata of alcohol abuse.

Abdomen. Examine for hepatomegaly, splenomegaly, or ascites.

Neurologic. Determine the level of consciousness and mentation. Do a thorough neurologic examination, and look for focal deficits. Examine for tremor.

Diagnostic Tests

SMA. Do an immediate fingerstick glucose to estimate serum glucose; confirm with a formal plasma glucose. Spuriously low glucose values can accompany leukocytosis.

Specific assays. Order serum insulin and C peptide assays when insulinoma or surreptitious insulin use is suspected.

Treatment

Do not wait for the formal glucose determinations to return before treating hypoglycemia suggested by a lab stick. Patients with mild symptoms and hypoglycemia may be treated initially with oral solutions (fruit juice, oral D_{50}). Offer more complex carbohydrates as symptoms resolve. Alcoholics at risk for malnutrition require thiamine (100 mg IV or IM) administration as well. Patients with more pronouned symptoms (altered mental status) need intravenous glucose (1 amp of D_{50} raises serum glucose approximately 180 mg/dL). Some patients may require a second or third ampule. Detrimental side effects of D_{50} include volume overload, CHF, and hypokalemia. For patients at risk of recurrent hypoglycemia (large insulin overdose or oral hypoglycemia OD), initiate intravenous D_5 or D_{10}. If there is a problem obtaining intravenous access, glucagon (1 to 2 mg IV) may serve as a temporizing measure. Side effects of glucagon include nausea and vomiting. Hepatic glycogen stores cannot be restored with intravenous glucose; instead, enteral intake is required to rebuild glycogen stores.

Admission Criteria

Patients with serious or life-threatening symptoms of hypoglycemia (seizures, coma), *who have ingested long-acting sulfonylureas or self-administered insulin and exhibit persistent hypoglycemia, or who have hypoglycemia due to alcoholism or hepatic disease* require admission. *Alcoholics who have taken insulin and become hypoglycemic* should also be admitted. *Patients with hypoglycemia and no obvious cause* need to be admitted for further evaluation.

Diabetics with hypoglycemia that resolves quickly and who have a reason for the episode (took insulin but did not eat usual meals due to unusual circumstances) do not require admission. However, diabetics who have a concomitant acute illness that prevented eating or who cannot eat properly or take medications without better social supports may need to be admitted for further observation and adjustment of medications.

Suggested Readings

Browning RG. Dextrose: antidote or toxin. Ann Emerg Med 1990;19: 683–685.

Blackman JD, Towle VL, Lewis GF, et al.: Hypoglycemic thresholds for cognitive dysfunction in humans. Diabetes 1990;39(7):828–835.

Slama G, Traynard PY, Desplanque N, et al.: The search for an optimized treatment of hypoglycemia. Arch Intern Med 1990;150(3):589–593.

6.3 THYROID STORM

Description

Thyroid storm is a severe and life-threatening form of thyrotoxicosis. It is manifested by exaggerated symptoms of thyrotoxicosis, including fever and neurologic, cardiovascular, gastrointestinal, and hepatic dysfunction. The following conditions may provoke thyroid storm in an untreated or inadequately treated patient with hyperthyroidism: surgery in a poorly prepared hyperthyroid patient; vigorous palpation of an enlarged, toxic thyroid gland; trauma; underlying illness (pneumonia, influenza, DKA); radioactive iodine therapy; exposure to inorganic iodine (cough syrups, vitamins) or organic iodine compounds (angiography, cardiac catheterization, intravenous pyelogram); and abrupt withdrawal of propanolol or antithyroid medication.

History

Common symptoms include weakness, weight loss, heat intolerance, diplopia, fever, palpitations, chest pains, anxiety, tremor, agitation, confusion, psychosis, diarrhea, nausea, and vomiting. Recent infections, trauma, or medical procedures should be noted. Past medical history should include any chronic medical problems, previous thyroid disease, and all medications along with dosages. The elderly may display apathetic hyperthyroidism, presenting a subtle clinical picture of weight loss, weakness, apathy, and worsening of underlying cardiac disease.

Physical Examination

General. Observe for restlessness, agitation, confusion, tremulousness, and jaundice. Note the level of consciousness.

Vital signs. Check for fever, tachycardia (often out of proportion to fever), and tachypnea.

HEENT. Check for lid lag, extraocular muscle weakness, and exophthalmos.

Neck. Palpate the thyroid gland; if the gland is enlarged, note consistency, size, and nodularity. Bruits may be heard over the thyroid gland.

Lung. Listen for rhonchi and rales (CHF, pneumonia).

Heart. Auscultate rate, rhythm (frequently irregular due to atrial fibrillation), murmurs, and gallops.

Abdomen. Check for liver enlargement and splenomegaly.

Neurologic. Examine for peripheral muscle weakness and presence of tremor. Check for brisk deep tendon reflexes.

Skin. Usually warm, moist, and smooth. Look for pedal edema.

Diagnostic Tests

The diagnosis is based on clinical evaluation. Laboratory data will confirm the diagnosis, but therapy cannot wait.

CBC. Check hematocrit and WBC count with differential.

SMA. Note electrolytes, glucose, and liver function tests.

Thyroid function tests. Obtain TSH, free T_4, and T_3 RIA. However, results will not usually be available to the ED physician.

Urinalysis. Screen for infection.

X-rays. Review CXR for cardiomegaly as well as pulmonary infiltrates.

ECG. Inspect for aberrant rhythms, tachycardia, or signs of ischemia.

Treatment

Management of thyroid storm requires a four-pronged approach: general supportive measures, therapy against the thyroid gland, mediation of peripheral thyroid hormone effects, and correction of underlying illness or precipitating event.

Administer *propylthiouracil* (200 to 250 mg q 4 hr PO) or *methimazole* (20 to 25 mg q 4 hr PO) to inhibit thyroid hormone synthesis. Use *sodium iodide* (1 to 2 g/day IV) or *Lugol's iodide* (5 drops q 4 hr PO) to block thyroid hormone release. Give iodide preparations 30 to 60 min after antithyroid drugs to prevent iodide-induced thyrotoxicosis. If necessary, administer these medications through an NG tube.

Beta-blockers—*propanolol* (1 to 5 mg q 4 hr IV) or *metoprolol* (5 mg IV q 5 min for three doses)—limit overstimulation by the sympathetic nervous system. Use β-blockers with caution in asthmatics. *Dexamethasone* (2 mg q 6 hr IV or IM) helps to further limit the conversion of T_4 to T_3. *Digoxin* may be employed for treating atrial fibrillation (see section 1.6).

Supportive measures include reduction of fever with antipyretics (use acetaminophen, cooling blankets, or sponge baths—*avoid aspirin,* since it may provoke thyroid hormone release), correction of fluid and electrolyte imbalances, and treatment of any coexisting infections or medical problems.

Admission Criteria

All patients in thyroid storm require admission, preferably to an ICU-type setting. *Patients with lesser degrees of uncontrolled hyperthyroidism* should be admitted *if they demonstrate significant cardiac abnormalities, are acutely infected, or do not have ready access to close outpatient follow-up.*

Suggested Readings

Gavin LA: Thyroid crises. Med Clin North Am 1991;75(1):179–193.
Roth RN, McAuliffe MJ: Hyperthyroidism and thyroid storm. Emerg Med Clin North Am 1989;7(4):873–883.

6.4 MYXEDEMA COMA

Description

Inadequate production of thyroid hormone can result from a variety of causes, but the most common etiologies are chronic Hashimoto's thyroiditis and prior ablative or surgical therapy for hyperthyroidism. Hypothyroidism initially manifests as cold intolerance; thick, dry skin; hoarse voice; constipation; retarded speech and reactions; and apathy. Progression to obtundation and coma accompanied by hypothermia (< 35.0°C, 95.0°F) implies myxedema coma, a condition primarily affecting patients over age 75 with underlying sepsis, hypothermic exposure, or drug or alcohol ingestion.

History

The clinical picture depends on the age and sex of the patient, the site of the defect in thyroid hormone production (thyroid or pituitary), and the rate of development of deficiency. The slow progression of symptoms and their nonspecific nature as well as the patient's apathy in regard to complaints often delay or obscure the diagnosis. Early symptoms include constipation, skin changes, edema, anovulation, headache, arthralgias, hoarseness, cold intolerance, and fatigue. Patients who quickly develop hypothyroidism may complain of myalgias, arthralgias, and paresthesias.

Physical Examination

Vital signs. Hypertension (diastolic) and bradycardia may appear. Severely myxedemic patients may be hypothermic (remarkable for absence of shivering).

Skin. Note coarse, dry, or myxedematous quality.

HEENT. Myxedema facie's is characterized by facial puffiness, periorbital edema, ptosis, coarse skin, thinning eyebrows, and macroglossia.

Neck. Look at the neck for scar suggestive of thyroid surgery. Check thyroid size for presence of goiter or nodules.

Heart. Heart sounds may be distant due to chronic pericardial effusion.

Abdomen. Megacolon is a common finding; check for abdominal distention, diminished bowel sounds (paralytic ileus), distended bladder (urinary retention), and fecal impaction.

Extremities. Note the presence of nonpitting edema.

Neurologic. Motor strength may be diffusely decreased. Peripheral sensory neuropathy may be present. Deep tendon reflexes are likely to be diminished or delayed (especially in the relaxation phase, "hung-up" relaxation). Patients may be dull in affect, apathetic, obtunded, or even comatose.

Diagnostic Tests

SMA. Hyponatremia and hypoglycemia may occur.

CBC. A macrocytic anemia may be present.

ABG. Often reveals hypercapnia and hypoxia; respiratory failure is the major cause of death in myxedema coma.

Thyroid function tests. Useful in guiding future therapy but does not assist in the ED management. *Do not delay treatment* while waiting for laboratory results to return.

Serum cortisol. Draw a level early (before administration of corticosteroids).

ECG. Often reveals sinus bradycardia, low voltage, flattening or inversion of T waves, and prolongation of the PR interval.

Echocardiogram. Order if you suspect pericardial effusion.

Treatment

Prompt recognition and management are mandatory to prevent the high morbidity and mortality seen with myxedema coma.

There are two phases to treatment: (1) supporting the vital signs and (2) hormonal or drug therapy. Supportive care focuses on the "hypos": hypoadrenalism, hypocontractility, hypometabolism, hypoosmolality, hypothermia, and hypoventilation. While hypoventilation usually responds to hormonal therapy, the complications of hypothyroidism (macroglossia, goiter, edema) may provoke airway obstruction. If endotracheal intubation is required, try to avoid the use of paralytic agents and CNS depressants. Replace volume with extreme caution; even though these patients may be fluid depleted, they are prone to heart failure. Accompanying hyponatremia may be severe. Since these patients have a fragile cardiovascular system, continuous ECG monitoring is mandatory. Consider invasive monitoring. Hypothermia can generally be treated with a heating blanket. If an acute myocardial infarction is ruled out, thyroid-hormone replacement can be started with *levothyroxine sodium* (Levothroid, Synthroid). Administer a dose of 50 to 100 μg IV Q 6 to 8 hr for 24 hr and then 75 to 100 μg IV every day until oral intake is possible. In addition, give *hydrocortisone* (100 mg IV q 8 hr). Clinical improvement from myxedema coma usually occurs within 24 to 36 hr, although the need for mechanical ventilation may persist beyond this time.

Admission Criteria

Patients with simple hypothyroidism can be started on therapy in the ED and followed up as outpatients. *Patients with frank myxedema coma* require admission to an intensive care bed.

Suggested Readings

Mitchell JM: Thyroid disease in the emergency department. Thyroid function tests and hypothyroidism and myxedema coma. Emerg Med Clin North Am 1989;7(4):885–902.

Myers L, Hays J: Myxedema coma. Crit Care Clin 1991;7(1):43–56.

6.5 ADRENAL CRISIS

Description

Adrenal insufficiency occurs in a variety of ED settings. An acute adrenal crisis may appear in patients receiving anticoagulant therapy who bleed into their adrenal glands or in patients with overwhelming sepsis who develop adrenal hemorrhage—a condition referred to as *Waterhouse-Friderichsen syndrome.* Sepsis-related adrenal hemorrhage most frequently arises from meningococcemia but also complicates infectious pneumococcus with *Staphylococcus* or *Hemophilus influenzae.*

Chronic adrenal insufficiency may be the result of granulomatous infection of the glands, autoimmune disease, or invasion by metastatic tumor. Patients with preexisting adrenal insufficiency may proceed to an acute adrenal crisis when illness or stress (surgery, trauma) increases metabolic demands. However, *the most common cause of adrenal insufficiency seen in the ED is abrupt withdrawal of glucocorticoids in a patient who is steroid dependent.* Assume all patients taking > 5 mg/d of prednisone (or its equivalent) for 2 weeks or more to be steroid dependent (Table 6.5.1).

History

The majority of patients with adrenal insufficiency complain of nonspecific symptoms such as weakness, anorexia, nausea, vomiting, and weight loss. Accompanying hyperpigmentation is typically a diffuse darkening of both exposed and unexposed areas of skin, including elbows or creases of the hand, as well as a heightened pigmentation of such areas as the nipples. Gastrointestinal complaints range from mild anorexia to severe vomiting, diarrhea, and abdominal pain (may mimic an acute abdomen).

Table 6.5.1
Equivalent Doses of Corticosteroids

Drug	Equivalent Dose (mg)
Short acting	
Cortisone	25
Hydrocortisone	20
Prednisone	5
Prednisolone	5
Methylprednisolone	4
Intermediate acting	
Triamcinolone	4
Long acting	
Dexamethasone	0.5–0.75
Betamethasone	0.6

Personality changes, including irritability and restlessness, may be related by the patient or family members. Determine onset and duration of symptoms, any recent stress or intercurrent illness, associated complaints (fever, chills, back pain), underlying disorders (tuberculosis, tumor, autoimmune disease, asthma), medications (especially anticoagulants) and compliance with or recent discontinuation of corticosteroid therapy.

Physical Examination

General. Inspect for hyperpigmentation or vitiligo.

Vital signs. Check for hypotension, including orthostatic changes. Note fever.

HEENT. Look for bluish black hyperpigmented patches on the mucous membranes.

Neck. Palpate the thyroid for enlargement.

Abdomen. Examine the abdomen carefully if the patient has gastrointestinal complaints to rule out the possibility of unrelated abdominal disease.

Neurologic. Examine for mental status changes and focal deficits.

Diagnostic Tests

SMA. Analyze for characteristic hyponatremia, hyperkalemia, hypoglycemia, and anion gap acidosis.

CBC. An elevated hematocrit may be due to fluid depletion and hemoconcentration. An eosinophilia often accompanies adrenal insufficiency. The WBC count may be depressed, or a relative lymphocytosis can occur with adrenal insufficiency.

Endocrinology studies. Order serum cortisol levels and ACTH to guide future management.

CXR. A small, slender cardiac silhouette may be present in chronic adrenal insufficiency. Also look for evidence of a concomitant illness such as TB.

Treatment

Give immediate intravenous steroid replacement in patients with suspected adrenal crisis: *hydrocortisone* (Solu-Cortef; 100 mg IV bolus, followed by 50 mg IV q 4 to 6 hr for 48 hr). If panhypopituitarism is considered, administer dexamethasone (Decadron; 5 to 10 mg IV) instead of hydrocortisone (dexamethasone, unlike hydrocortisone, does not interfere with the ACTH-stimulation test or plasma-cortisol assay). However, dexamethasone lacks the mineralocorticoid activity of hydrocortisone and must be supplemented with mineralocorticoid therapy: *fludrocortisone acetate* (Florinef; 0.1 to 0.2 mg IM).

Treat hypotension aggressively. Treat underlying causes (sepsis, coagulopathy).

Admission Criteria

All patients in adrenal crisis should be admitted for continued therapy and observation.

Suggested Readings

Chin R: Adrenal crisis. Crit Care Clin 1991;7(1):23–42.

Waise A, Young RJ: Pitfalls in the management of acute adrenocortical insufficiency. J R Soc Med 1989; 82:741–742.

Hypercalcemia

Etiology

The three main causes of hypercalcemia seen in the ED are *malignancy* (breast, lung, prostate, multiple myeloma), *hyperparathyroidism* (triad of nephrolithiasis, metabolic bone disease, hypercalcemia), and *granulomatous disease* (sarcoidosis, TB).

History

Symptoms of hypercalcemia include lethargy, stupor, increased thirst, malaise, fatigue, weakness, anorexia, constipation, and polyuria. Mentation may be depressed or abnormal; frank psychosis and even coma may occur. The patient should be questioned closely about diet (milk, alkali), medications (especially thiazide diuretics, lithium, estrogens), and underlying diseases (especially tumor) as well as symptoms unique to the many syndromes listed above. Pancreatitis and peptic ulcer are also associated with hyperparathyroidism. A history of renal stones can be relevant.

Physical Examination

General. Note level of alertness. Look for evidence of malignancy (wasting, cachectic appearance).

Vital signs. Hypertension is a common finding.

HEENT. Note conjunctivitis or band keratopathy on eye exam.

Neck. Palpate the thyroid for size and consistency. Palpate for adenopathy.

Lungs. Listen for rales, dullness, or a rub (tumor).

Breasts. Palpate for masses and axillary nodes.

Abdomen. Bowel sounds may be decreased. Palpate for hepatosplenomegaly or presence of masses. Palpate groin for adenopathy.

Neurologic. Reflexes may be depressed and motor strength decreased.

Diagnostic Tests

SMA. Check a stat serum calcium as well as electrolytes. Normally, serum calcium is between 8.9 and 11 mg/dL (4.4 and 5.5 mEq/L). Approximately 40% of the total serum calcium is bound to serum proteins, with the unbound ionized fraction (normal values of 4.4 to 5.1 mg/dL; 2.2 to 2.6 mEq/L) being the biologically active form. For each decrease of 1 g/dL of serum albumin, the serum calcium level will drop 0.8 mg/dL. A corrected serum calcium level > 11 mg/dL (ionized calcium level > 5.2 mg/dL) is diagnostic of *hypercalcemia*. Hypercalcemic patients may be hypokalemic. Also, hypopsophatemia may occur. Assess renal function (creatinine, BUN). An elevated alkaline phosphatase suggests bony involvement.

CBC. Confirm the hematocrit and WBC count.

Urinalysis. Check for proteinuria. Bence-Jones proteinuria is not routinely detected by the urine test strip; you must order a specific test that employs heating or the addition of sulfosalicylic acid.

ECG. Manifestations of hypercalcemia include shortening of the QT interval, widening of T waves, and ST-T wave coving.

X-rays. A CRX is necessary for screening purposes; other x-rays should be ordered selectively (bony films may reveal metastasis or Paget's disease).

Treatment

Aggressively hydrate the patient; urinary calcium excretion is enhanced by intravenous saline. If the patient is young and has no history of cardiac disease, give an intravenous bolus of normal saline (500 mL) followed by 250 to 500 mL/hr. For elderly patients or those with underlying cardiac disease, consider invasive monitoring.

Once adequate hydration is obtained, give *furosemide* (20 to 60 mg IV q 2 to 6 hr) to enhance diuresis. Aim for a urine output of 200 to 500 mL/hr. Carefully monitor the patient's hemodynamic status as well as electrolyte values.

Use steroids if the hypercalcemia is due to adrenal insufficiency, hypervitaminosis A or D, sarcoidosis, breast cancer, or a myeloproliferative disorder. The dose of *hydrocortisone* is 100 to 200 mg IV q 6 hr.

Alternative therapies include *etidronate disodium* (7.5 mg/kg/d IV), *calcitonin* (4 U/kg IV, IM, or SQ), and *plicamycin* (25 μg/kg in 500 mL D5W IV over 4 to 6 hr). In extremely severe cases, consider *dialysis* (particularly for patients with compromised renal function).

Admission Criteria

Patients with hypercalcemia (levels > 12 mg/dL) require admission for further evaluation and therapy. Patients with hypercalcemia in the range of 10.5 to 12 mg/dL may be investigated as outpatients after discussion with the consultant.

Suggested Readings

Attie MF: Treatment of hypercalcemia. Endo Metabol Clin North Am 1989;18(3):807–828.

Olinger ML: Disorders of calcium and magnesium metabolism. Emerg Med Clin North Am 1989;7(4):795–822.

Hypocalcemia

Description

Hypocalcemia occurs in a variety of clinical settings: hypoparathyroidism, malabsorption, renal disease, and secondary to medications (anticonvulsants, hydrofluoric acid exposure, chemotherapeutic agents). In critically ill patients, hypocalcemia may accompany acute pancreatitis and rhabdomyolysis. The potential for hypocalcemia also exists when massive blood transfusions are used.

History

Hypocalcemia principally affects the nervous system, both *centrally* and *peripherally*. Classically, patients exhibit an *altered mental status,* ranging from confusion, psychosis, and lethargy to coma and seizures. The cardinal peripheral nervous system manifestation is *tetany.* Patients may also complain of paresthesias (particularly involving the perioral area and hands and feet). When severe, hypocalcemia can cause muscle weakness or laryngospasm. GI complaints (vague crampy abdominal pain, nausea, vomiting) are also common. Establish the onset and duration of symptoms. Ask about possible precipitating factors such as medications, surgery, trauma, radiation therapy (particularly of neck region), use of alcohol or drugs, and dietary history.

Physical Examination

General. Determine the mental status as well as overall appearance (chronically ill, malnourished). Pseudohypoparathyroidism is characterized by a round face, chondrodystrophy, short stature, and mental retardation.

Vital signs. Check the pulse (tachycardia is common). Check respiration (the presence of tachypnea in an otherwise healthy patient complaining of tetany symptoms suggests the possibility of hyperventilation syndrome) and temperature (fever).

Skin. Inspect for dryness of skin and hair as well as alopecia. Vitiligo and mucocutaneous candidiasis suggest *idiopathic hypoparathyroidism.*

HEENT. Examine the eyes for subcapsular cataracts and papilledema; both can be seen with hypocalcemia.

Neck. Auscultate for stridor (laryngospasm). Inspect for surgical scars as well as radiation ports.

Cardiovascular. Examine for evidence of CHF (rales, S_3, distended neck veins).

Neurologic. Test for *Chvostek's sign* (twitching of the facial muscles elicited by a sharp tap of the facial nerve in front of the ear), *Trousseau's sign* (inflate a blood pressure cuff on the arm or leg; a carpopedal spasm will occur within 3 min if hypocalcemia is present), and hyperreflexia.

Diagnostic Tests

SMA. Hypocalcemia is diagnosed when the "corrected" serum calcium is < 8.5 mg/dL. If available, order *serum ionized calcium* levels. Also check serum magnesium (hypomagnesemia can mimic findings of hypocalcemia), potassium (hypokalemia may mask tetany from hypocalcemia), chloride, phosphorus, serum creatinine (a low serum phosphate combined with an elevated serum creatinine implies renal insufficiency), amylase (pancreatitis) and creatinine phosphokinase (rhabdomyolysis) levels.

ABG. Ensure adequate ventilation.

Parathyroid hormone levels. Does not assist in the immediate ED management but aids future therapy.

ECG. Review for prolongation of the QT interval.

Treatment

Airway control is the foremost concern. If laryngospasm and tetany preclude nasotracheal or orotracheal intubation, a surgical airway (cricothyrotomy) is mandated. Definitive treatment of *hypocalcemia* is attained with *calcium gluconate* (10 to 20 mL of a 10% solution given IV over 10 min; mix the calcium gluconate solution with 100 mL NS or D_5W to avoid irritation to veins). Except in extreme emergencies, it is best to not use *calcium chloride,* as this agent is very sclerosing to the vein. *Use calcium with extreme caution in patients on digitalis therapy, and avoid calcium use if digitalis toxicity is suspected.* If symptoms of hypocalcemia persist, a continuous infusion of calcium gluconate (1 to 2 mg/kg/hr) can be given. In addition, in patients with suspected hypomagnesemia, deliver parenteral magnesium: *magnesium sulfate* (1 to 2 g IV over 30 to 60 min). Recheck serum calcium levels every 1 to 4 hr, until the patient stabilizes. Place the patient on a cardiac monitor during restoration therapy; normalization of the QT interval serves as a rough guide to adequate calcium replacement.

Admission Criteria

All patients with symptomatic hypocalcemia require admission to a monitored bed until the hypocalcemia is corrected and the underlying etiology determined.

Suggested Readings

Olinger ML: Disorders of calcium and magnesium metabolism. Emerg Med Clin North Am 1989;7:795–822.

Zaloga GP, Chernow B: Hypocalcemia in critical illness. JAMA 1986;256: 1924–1927.

6.6 HYPONATREMIA

Description

Hyponatremia is defined as a serum sodium (Na^+) < 135 mEq/L and implies an excess of plasma water in relation to sodium. Total body sodium or total body water may be low, normal, or elevated in hyponatremia. The symptoms and signs associated with hyponatremia include hypotension, anorexia, nausea, vomiting, confusion, seizures, and coma. Symptoms depend on the rate of the fall of serum sodium as well as the absolute level.

History

Ask about underlying systemic disease (cirrhosis, renal disease, CHF, hypothyroidism, Addison's disease). Establish medication history, including diuretics and drugs (chlorpropamide, carbamazepine, clofibrate, cyclophosphamide, narcotics, tricyclic antidepressants) known to provoke syndrome of inappropriate antidiuretic hormone (SIADH). Also, consider the possibility that the patient is drinking excessive quantities of free water (frequently, there is an underlying psychiatric history). A recent history of nausea, vomiting, or diarrhea may suggest gastrointestinal loss of sodium. Acute, severe (< 115 mEq/L) hyponatremia often manifests as an altered mental status (lethargy, confusion, irritation, seizures).

Physical Examination

Vital signs. Check for hypertension (volume overload) or hypotension (volume depletion).
HEENT. Look for signs of dehydration.
Neck. Check for jugular venous distention.
Lungs. Listen for rales (CHF, pneumonia).
Heart. Note the presence of gallops or rubs.
Abdomen. Palpate and percuss for ascites (cirrhosis).
Back. Check for presacral edema.
Extremities. Note peripheral edema.
Neurologic. Check relaxation time of deep tendon reflexes.

Diagnostic Tests

SMA. Check all electrolytes, BUN, and creatinine. It is important to remember that osmotically active substances (glucose, mannitol, lipids, and proteins) draw water from the extravascular space and cause a spurious lowering of serum sodium. This factitious hyponatremia is most commonly seen with elevated serum glucose. For every 100 mg/dL elevation in glucose, the sodium value decreases by 1.6 mEq/L. Symptomatic hyponatremia does not usually occur until the plasma sodium falls below 120 mEq/L.

Urine electrolytes. Urine sodium may be helpful (Table 6.6.1).

Osmolarity. Check both urine and serum osmolarity.

Special Considerations

SIADH is a diagnosis of exclusion, requiring the following criteria: (1) hyponatremia and serum hypoosmolality, (2) urine osmolality greater than serum osmolality, (3) urinary sodium > 20 mmol/L, (4) normal renal and endocrine function, and (5) no history of diuretic use.

Table 6.6.1
Differential Diagnosis of Hyponatremia

Plasma Volume	Edema	Urine Sodium	Treatment
Increased			
Cirrhosis, neprosis, CHF	Present	Low (< 30 mEq/L)	Restrict water and salt; use diuretics
Decreased			
GI losses	Absent	Low	Normal saline (IV)
Addison's	Absent	Elevated (> 30 mEq/L)	Normal saline (IV)
Salt-wasting nephropathy	Absent	Elevated	Normal saline (IV)
Diuretics	Absent	Elevated early; usually low	Normal saline (IV)
Normal			
Factitious	Absent	Normal	Treat underlying condition
Hypothyroidism	Absent	Normal or elevated	Treat underlying condition
SIADH	Absent	Very high (> 50 mEq/L)	Restrict water
Water intoxication	Absent	Normal or low	Restrict water

Treatment

Definitive treatment depends on the *specific etiology of hyponatremia, acuity of onset, severity of clinical findings,* and *the patient's volume status* (see Table 6.6.1 for details). **Note:** *Caution is essential when treating hyponatremia—too rapid a correction* (> 20 to 25 mEq/L in 24 hr) *may lead to permanent neurologic damage and central pontine myelinolysis.*

When hyponatremia is severe and leads to seizures or coma, consider hypertonic saline therapy (1 L of 3% NS contains 500 mEq of sodium). If the patient is volume depleted, restore with normal saline or hypertonic saline. The amount of sodium required to correct the deficit can be calculated by the following formula:

$$\text{Sodium deficit} = (\text{Desired sodium} - \text{Observed sodium}) \times 0.6 \times \text{Weight (kg)}$$

where *desired serum sodium* is usually taken as 140 mEq/L. An infusion of 1 mL/kg/hr of 3% saline solution raises the serum sodium concentration approximately 1 mEq/hr. For patients with a normal or expanded extracellular fluid volume, concomitantly restrict water intake and carefully create a diuresis: furosemide (40 mg IV) or bumetanide (1 mg IV).

As a general rule, correct the sodium at the same rate it was lowered; *do not* increase serum values more than 12 mEq in 24 hr, and stop aggressive therapy once sodium values reach 125 mEq/L.

Suggested Readings

Cheng JC, Zikos D, Peterson DR et al.: Symptomatic hyponatremia: pathophysiology and management. Acute Care 1989;15:270–292.

Sterns RH: The management of hyponatremic emergencies. Crit Care Clin 1991;7(1):127–142.

6.7 HYPERNATREMIA

Description

Hypernatremia is defined as a serum sodium > 145 mEq/L. Hypernatremia indicates a deficit of total body water relative to total body sodium. This most commonly arises from excessive loss of hypotonic fluids (vomiting, NG suction, diarrhea, sweating, osmotic diuresis) or inadequate intake of water (debilitated or comatose patient). Additional causes include diabetes insipidus (nephrogenic or pituitary) or excessive sodium accumulation (administration of hypertonic saline or sodium bicarbonate).

History

Suspect the diagnosis of hypernatremia in all patients with an altered mental status, and decreased access to free water (nursing home patients, history of paraplegia or CVA). Like hyponatremia, the severity of manifestations adheres to both the absolute increase in serum sodium and the rate of accumulation. The central nervous system is most vulnerable to hypernatremia (causes dehydration of brain cells). Subsequent symptoms include thirst, polyuria, nocturia, anorexia, lethargy, nausea, vomiting, agitation, and muscular irritability, with possible seizures, respiratory paralysis, and death. Ask about underlying disorders (tumor, CVA, CNS infection, recent brain surgery or trauma) that could cause central diabetes insipidus (DI) as well as drugs (lithium, demeclocycline, loop diuretics) that could provoke DI.

Physical Examination

General. Observe body habitus (cachexia) along with mental status (lethargy, comatose).

Vital signs. Check for signs of volume depletion (hypotension, tachycardia, orthostatic changes).

HEENT. Check for dry mucous membranes.

Skin. Note decreased turgor.

Diagnostic Tests

SMA. Assess electrolytes, glucose, BUN, and creatinine along with serum osmolality.

CBC. Check WBC count for infection; check hematocrit (may be elevated with dehydration).

Urinalysis. Order urine osmolality, sodium, and creatinine. Check for signs of infection. Consider monitoring urine output (oliguria).

Treatment

The first priority is ensuring adequate circulation; correct any volume deficits with normal saline. The total body water (TBW) deficit can be estimated from the following formula:

$$\text{TBW deficit} = 1 - (\text{Measured sodium}/\text{Desired sodium}) \times 0.6 \times \text{Weight (kg)}$$

where *desired serum sodium* is usually taken as 140 mEq/L.

Once the hemodynamic status is stabilized, correct hypernatremia with D_5W or half-normal saline. *Do not* decrease serum sodium by more than 2 mEq/L/hr (it is possible to induce cerebral edema with overzealous correction). As a general rule, the sodium should be deceased at the same rate it was elevated.

Suggested Readings

Oh MS, Carroll HJ: Disorders of sodium metabolism: hypernatremia and hyponatremia. Crit Care Med 1992;20(1):94–103.

Votey SR, Peters AL, Hoffman JR: Disorders of water metabolism: hyponatremia and hypernatremia. Emerg Med Clin North Am 1989; 7(4):749–769.

6.8 HYPOKALEMIA

Description

Hypokalemia is defined as a serum potassium (K^+) < 3.5 mEq/L, although the serum potassium is only a rough reflection of total body potassium stores, since potassium is predominantly an intracellular cation. Causes of potassium deficiency include *renal-related* etiologies (diuretics, renal tubular disease, hyperaldosteronism), *GI losses* (vomiting, NG suction, diarrhea, fistula), *intracellular shifts* (alkalosis, insulin, β-2-agonists, hypokalemic periodic paralysis), and *poor intake* (elderly, alcoholic, anorexic patients).

History

Manifestations of mild to moderate hypokalemia include weakness, muscle cramps, constipation, ileus, and hyporeflexia; whereas *severe hypokalemia* (< 2.5 mEq/L) can lead to a flaccid paralysis, tetany, rhabdomyolysis, respiratory arrest, and cardiac disturbances.

Physical Examination

Vital signs. Assess pulse, blood pressure (hypokalemia combined with hypertension suggests renovascular disease, primary aldosteronism, Cushing's syndrome) and respiratory rate.

Skin. Inspect for bruising and/or tissue destruction.

Abdomen. Check for presence of ileus.

Neurologic. Check for muscle strength and hyperreflexia. Assess mental status.

Diagnostic Tests

SMA. Send stat potassium specimen. Check renal function and calcium (Ca^{++}) and magnesium (Mg^{++}) levels.

ABG. As a general rule, for every increase of 0.1 pH unit secondary to metabolic alkalosis, the potassium decreases by 0.3 mEq/L.

Digitalis. Hypokalemia increases susceptibility to digitalis toxicity.

ECG. Abnormalities include flattening or inversion of T waves, appearance of U waves, ST-T wave depressions, and when severe, atrioventricular blocks and cardiac arrest.

Treatment

The safest method of correcting mild to moderate hypokalemia is orally (KCl tabs or elixir). Patients with severe hypokalemia (especially if accompanied by ECG changes or neuromuscular problems) and patients who cannot take oral supplements require intravenous potassium replacement. Add 10 to 20 mEq to each liter of NS or dilute 10 mEq KCl in 100 mL NS; do not exceed 20 mEq/hr of potassium. Higher concentrations are best given through a central line, if available, since potassium is an irritant to the veins. Intravenous replacement is best performed with continuous cardiac monitoring. As a general rule, it takes 40 to 50 mEq of potassium to raise serum potassium by 1 mEq/L. Calcium and magnesium deficiencies may cause hypokalemia to be refractory to replacement and call for concurrent correction.

Suggested Readings

Freedman BI, Burkart JM: Endocrine crises. Hypokalemia. Crit Care Clin 1991;7(1):143–153.

Whang R, Whang DD, Ryan MP: Refractory potassium repletion. A consequence of magnesium deficiency. Arch Intern Med 1992;152:40–43.

6.9 HYPERKALEMIA

Description

Hyperkalemia implies a serum potassium > 5.5 mEq/L. A rapidly rising potassium level is especially dangerous and life-threatening.

Causes include *spurious* or *pseudohyperkalemia* (prolonged or tight tourniquet, repetitive fist clenching during phlebotomy, use of a narrow catheter or needle, blood drawn from an arm with a potassium infusion, marked leukocytosis > 50,000/mm^3, thrombocytosis), *decreased potassium excretion* (acute or chronic renal failure, adrenal insufficiency, potassium sparing diuretics, ACE inhibitors), *intracellular to extracellular shifts* (acidosis, burns, crush injuries, tumor lysis syndrome, rhabdomyolysis, hyperkalemic periodic paralysis, acute digitalis overdose, succinylcholine, nonsteroidal antiinflammatories, nonselective β-blockers, insulin deficiency), and *excessive potassium intake* (iatrogenic oral or intravenous potassium supplementation, high-dose potassium salts of penicillin, blood transfusions). In addition, hyperkalemia has been reported in AIDS patients who use pentamidine or high-dose trimethoprim.

History

Complications resulting from hyperkalemia include impaired neuromuscular conduction, which leads to weakness (initially more conspicuous in lower extremities), paresthesias, hyporeflexia, and if severe, a flaccid quadriplegia and/or respiratory paralysis; GI disturbances (anorexia, nausea, vomiting, abdominal cramping, diarrhea); and cardiovascular disorders (bradycardia, palpitations, syncope, cardiac arrest).

Physical Examination

Vital signs. Check the pulse (heart rate may be slow or rapid), blood pressure (consider adrenal insufficiency when hypotension is combined with hyperkalemia), temperature, and respiratory rate (respiratory arrest possible).

Heart. Auscultate for rate and rhythm disturbances.

Abdomen. Evaluate for abdominal aneurysm (can impair renal blood flow).

Pelvic and rectal. Perform to rule out obstructive uropathy.

Extremities. Inspect for arteriovenous fistula (chronic renal failure), evidence of tissue trauma or destruction (rhabdomyolysis), rash (malar rash of systemic lupus erythematosus), and pigmentation changes (bronze discoloration associated with Addison's disease).

Neurologic. Examine for weakness (symmetrical), paresthesias, and areflexia.

Diagnostic Tests

SMA. Send stat potassium level (plasma potassium concentration is more accurate than serum levels). Electrolytes, BUN, creatinine, glucose, and CPK may help determine the etiology of hyperkalemia.

CBC. Spurious hyperkalemia occurs when pronounced leukocytosis (> 50,000/mm^3) or thrombocytosis (platelet counts > 750,000/mm^3) is present.

Urinalysis. Assess urine sediment (crystals, casts, RBCs, WBCs) for clues to renal insufficiency.

ABG. Serum potassium levels rise approximately 0.7 mEq/L for each 0.1 pH unit decline in acidosis.

ECG. Readily accessible and can identify patients at risk for conduction disturbances. Inspect for tall or peaked T waves, depressed ST segments, prolongation of the PR and QRS intervals, diminished P waves or atrial arrest, and widening of the QRS complex. A sine-wave pattern in a patient at risk for hyperkalemia necessitates emergent treatment. Terminal events (V-fib) appear when potassium concentrations are greater than 10 mEq/L.

Treatment

Foremost, confirm that the potassium level is elevated, and place the patient on a cardiac monitor. If levels exceed 6.5 mEq/L (especially if ECG changes, muscular paralysis, or respiratory compromise is present), begin emergent therapy.

Calcium provides the most immediate (although transient) reversal of hyperkalemic-related cardiac toxicity. Give 5 to 10 mL of *calcium gluconate* (10% solution) by slow IVp over 2 to 5 min. Calcium chloride provides a higher concentration of elemental calcium but is more sclerotic to the veins. **Note:** *Avoid the use of calcium products if digitalis toxicity is considered.*

Supplemental therapy also incorporates medications inducing a redistribution of potassium. *Insulin* (5 to 10 units of regular insulin IV) given together with glucose (50 mL IV bolus of $D_{50}W$) lowers serum potassium within 30 min; the effect lasts for several hours. Follow glucose levels carefully to avoid iatrogenic hypoglycemia. Administer *sodium bicarbonate* 1 to 2 amps (44 to 88 mEq) IVp over 5 min, which also causes an intracellular shift of potassium (especially helpful if acidosis present). Bicarb achieves an effect in about 15 min but is not without hazard (volume overload, hypernatremia, hyperosmolarity). *Albuterol,* given as a nebulized β-agonist, is also effective in temporarily lowering serum potassium levels, particularly in uremic patients.

Methods to reduce total body potassium load include *ion-exchange resins* (Kayexalate; supplied as a 20 to 50 g PO dose dissolved in 100 mL 20% sorbitol solution or, for patients unable to take it orally, 50 g PR in 200 mL 20% sorbitol as an enema)—use with caution in patients with history of CHF because of sodium load. Other treatment includes (40 to 80 mg IVp) in patients with adequate renal function (pay strict attention to fluid balance) and hemodialysis or peritoneal dialysis, if the underlying renal insufficiency or potassium elevation persists despite the aforementioned measures.

Suggested Readings

Allon M, Copkney C: Albuterol and insulin for treatment of hyperkalemia in hemodialysis patients. Kidney Int 1990;38:869–871.

Zull DN: Disorders of potassium metabolism. Emerg Med Clin North Am 1989;7(4):771–794.

Chapter 7

Toxicology

7.1 DRUG EXPOSURE: INITIAL APPROACH AND SUPPORTIVE CARE

History

Appropriate care of a drug exposure depends on identification of the exposure as toxic and knowledge of the toxin involved, its pharmacokinetics, and the target organs. Determine the route of exposure: inhalation, dermal, ocular, oral, or intravenous. If the patient is unable or unwilling to give a history, questions should be directed to family, friends, or prehospital personnel. Pertinent bottles or containers should be obtained. Important historical points include (1) name, quantity, time, and route of exposure; (2) signs and symptoms since exposure; (3) chronic illnesses and medications and their doses; (4) prior drug use; (5) history of concomitant trauma; and (6) possibility of pregnancy.

Physical Examination

General. Observe agitation, stupor, and level of alertness.

Vital signs. A rectal temperature (to ensure an accurate core temperature) must be checked in addition to pulse, blood pressure, and respiratory rate.

Skin. Note whether the patient is flushed, pale, or cyanotic. Look for track marks as evidence of intravenous drug use.

HEENT. Evaluate for signs of head trauma (hemotympanum, CSF rhinorrhea, Battle's sign). Check pupils for miosis, mydriasis, or anisocoria. Note evidence of airway obstruction or pharyngeal irritation. Establish that the gag reflex is intact (patient can protect his or her airway).

Neck. Check for meningeal signs, thyromegaly, or crepitus.

Lungs. Note asymmetric breath sounds (pneumothorax), rales, rhonchi, or wheezes.

Abdomen. Listen for bowel sounds and check organ size.

Neurologic. Observe and describe the level of lethargy or agitation. Note any cranial nerve, motor, or sensory deficits.

Specific Toxicological Syndromes

Hypertension with tachycardia. Amphetamines, bretylium, cocaine, ephedrine, epinephrine, pseudoephedrine, hypnosedative or alcohol withdrawal, levodopa, MAO inhibitors, marijuana, phencyclidine, antihistamines, LSD, polycyclic antidepressants, antipsychotics, nicotine, or organophosphate insecticides.

Hypertension with normal or slowed pulse. Clonidine, epinephrine, ergot, or phenylpropanolamine.

Hypotension with bradycardia. Barbiturates, benzodiazepines, clonidine, tetrahydrozoline, β-blockers, calcium channel blockers, cyanide, cyclic antidepressants, digoxin, fluoride, nicotine, opioids, organophosphate insecticides, propoxyphene, and sympatholytic antihypertensives.

Hypotension with tachycardia. Carbon monoxide, cyanide, cyclic antidepressants, theophylline, iron, nitroprusside, nitrites, phenothiazines, hydralazine, disulfiram-ethanol interaction, caffeine, terbutaline, metaproterenol, antipsychotic agents, colchicine, arsenic, amatoxin-containing mushrooms, or one of many plant toxins.

Tachypnea. Salicylates, pentachlorophenol, metabolic acidosis with respiratory compensation, carbon monoxide, cyanide, hydrogen sulfide, amphetamines, cocaine, or theophylline.

Respiratory depression. Antipsychotics, chlorinated hydrocarbon solvents, clonidine, cyclic antidepressants, ethanol, barbiturates, benzodiazepines, opioids, botulism toxin, cobra envenomation, neuromuscular-blocking agents, nicotine, organophosphate insecticides, strychnine, or tetrodotoxin.

Hyperthermia. Amoxapine; amphetamines; LSD; anticholinergics; antihistamines; polycyclic antidepressants; cocaine; MAO inhibitors; phencyclidine; pentachlorophenol; thyroid hormone; ethanol, barbiturate, or benzodiazepine withdrawal; salicylates; or metal or polymer fume fever.

Hypothermia. Ethanol, barbiturates, benzodiazepines, isopropyl alcohol, opioids, phenothiazines, or cyclic antidepressants.

Seizures. Amphetamines; amoxapine; antipsychotics; antihistamines; β-blockers; boric acid; camphor; cocaine; chlorinated hydrocarbon solvents and insecticides; cicutoxin; citrate; carbon monoxide; cyanide; carbamazepine; polycyclic antidepressants; ethanol, barbiturate, or benzodiazepine withdrawal; phencyclidine; phenylpropanolamine; phenothiazines; theophylline; DET; ethylene glycol; fluoride; isoniazid; lead; lithium; lidocaine; mercury; meperidine; phenol; phenylbutazone; nicotine; NSAID; propoxyphene; salicylates; strychnine; or organophosphate insecticides.

Muscle weakness. Barium, botulism toxin, cobra toxin, gasoline sniffing, magnesium, mercury, nicotine, organophosphate insecticides, paralytic shellfish, hydrocarbon solvents, thallium, or toluene.

Mydriasis. Amphetamines, atropine, antihistamines, caffeine, cocaine, dopamine, LSD, MAO inhibitors, methanol, nicotine, glutethimide, or cyclic antidepressants.

Miosis. Barbiturates, clonidine, ethanol, isopropyl alcohol, nicotine, opioids, organophosphates, phencyclidine, phenothiazines, tetrahydrozoline, or triazolam.

Nystagmus. Barbiturates, carbamazepine, ethanol, ethylene glycol, lithium, organophosphates, phenytoin, or phencyclidine.

Odors. Acetone or ketone odor from chloroform or isopropyl alcohol; acidic or pear-like odor from paraldehyde or chloral hydrate; bitter almonds odor from cyanide; smell of carrots from cicutoxin; garlic odor from arsenic, dimethyl sulfoxide, organophosphates, phosphorus, selenium, or thallium; odor of mothballs from naphthalene or paradichlorobenzene; or odor of wintergreen from methyl salicylate.

Hypokalemia. Barium, β-adrenergics, caffeine, epinephrine, theophylline, or toluene.

Hyperkalemia. Alpha-adrenergics, β-blockers, digitalis glycosides, oleander, fluoride, or lithium.

Anion gap metabolic acidosis. Acetylene, benzyl alcohol, β-adrenergics, boric acid, caffeine, carbon monoxide, epinephrine, ethanol, ethylene glycol, formaldehyde, hydrogen sulfide, ibuprofen, iron, isoniazid, methanol, methylphenidate, salicylates, or theophylline.

Osmolal gap. Acetone, ethanol, ethyl ether, ethylene glycol, isopropyl alcohol, mannitol, methanol, propylene glycol, or trichloroethane.

Diagnostic Tests

Routine chemistries. Glucose, electrolytes, BUN, and creatinine may provide beneficial information and assist in the calculation of the *anion gap* and *serum osmolality*.

Arterial blood gas. Helpful for determination of acid-base status, oxygenation carboxyhemoglobin (CoHb), and methemoglobin. Remember that carboxyhemoglobin and methemoglobin levels are equivalent on arterial and venous specimens and that the decision to intubate the trachea is a clinical decision that is not based on ABG results. Also, currently available pulse oximeters will give no indication of carboxyhemoglobin or methemoglobin levels.

Radiographs. X-rays may be beneficial to help localize orally ingested button batteries or the illicit drugs of "body packers." Other agents (chloral hydrate, calcium, heavy metals, iodides, iron, psychotropics, enteric coated drugs, and solvents) may be identified on a KUB. Remember the mnemonic CHIPES. However, their absence does not preclude a lethal ingestion.

Drug levels. Specific drug assays should be ordered selectively based on the clinical assessment. Common exposures in which the levels will actually alter therapy include acetaminophen, aspirin, carboxyhemoglobin, digoxin, ethylene glycol, iron, lithium, methanol, methemoglobin, red blood cell cholinesterase (for organophosphate insecticides), theophylline, lead, cadmium, mercury, and arsenic. *Aspirin and acetaminophen levels should be obtained routinely in all intentional overdoses because the preliminary signs and symptoms of these ingestants may be elusive.* In the majority of cases, drug levels and toxicological screens are not beneficial and treatment is based on clinical parameters.

Treatment

Protect and maintain the airway. Provide appropriate ventilation and oxygenation. Maintain circulatory status appropriate for age and prevent tissue hypoperfusion.

Prevent further exposure or absorption via decontamination. Dermal, ocular, and buccal exposures can be safely decontaminated with copious local irrigation (normal saline or water). Water is contraindicated for elemental sodium or lithium. Inhalational exposures require removal from the source and administration of supplemental oxygen.

Oral ingestions should be treated with *activated charcoal* (1 g charcoal/kg body weight) and 70% sorbitol (2 mL/kg body weight). Activated charcoal should not be used in isolated caustic ingestions (it is minimally effective and makes subsequent endoscopy difficult). Repeated doses are dictated by the severity and type (particularly sustained-release preparations) of the overdose. *Do not employ multiple doses of cathartics when using a multiple dose–activated charcoal regimen.* Contraindications to the use of sorbitol include abdominal trauma, intestinal obstruction, or adynamic ileus. Anyone given sorbitol should be monitored for hypokalemia and hypomagnesemia. *Gastric lavage* may be considered before activated charcoal use if the ingestion occurred less than 60 min earlier and if the airway is protected. The use of ipecac is not recommended in the hospital setting.

The rules of gastric lavage for an adult are as follows:

- Always protect the airway;
- Place the patient in the left lateral decubitus position with the head tilted down;
- Use a 36 to 40 French Lavacuator hose or Ewald tube and confirm tube placement; and
- Use the barrel of a 60-mL syringe as a funnel and lavage aliquots of 200 mL (equal portions of activated charcoal and water).

Another modality for gastrointestinal decontamination is whole-bowel irrigation (WBI). WBI involves the administration of 2 L/hr of a balanced electrolyte solution of polyethylene glycol (GoLYTELY or Colyte) by mouth or NG tube until the rectal effluent is clear. WBI is particularly indicated for the following situations: late presentation (> 1 to 2 hr) of a potentially severe overdose, ingestion of delayed release preparations (e.g., theophylline, lithium, and potassium chloride), iron ingestions, and body packers or stuffers.

Increase elimination. Activated charcoal will enhance the elimination of virtually every oral ingestant—*except* ethanol, ethylene glycol, methanol, lithium, corrosives, and iron. Forced diuresis is not recommended, because drug elimination via renal excretion is usually independent of urine flow rates. It is important to ensure that every patient is euvolemic. Remember that the osmotic load of orally administered sorbitol may cause 3 to 4 L of fluid to be sequestered in the gut and cause a relative intravascular hypovolemia. Ion trapping is based on the principle that dissociable substances cross cell membranes more easily in the un-ionized state. Urinary acidification is not recommended; however, urinary alkalinization with 1 to 1.5 mEq/kg sodium bicarbonate IVp along with 2 amps (50 mEq/amp) sodium bicarbonate in 1 L D_5W with 20 mEq potassium chloride will increase the excretion of salicylates, phenylbutazone, phenobarbital, and isoniazid. It is important to supplement the potassium, to facilitate urinary alkalinization, and to measure urine pH to ensure that it remains > 7.5.

Achieve extra-corporeal elimination. *Drugs amenable to hemodialysis* include bromide, boric acid, chloral hydrate, ethanol, ethylene glycol, isopropyl alcohol, lithium, methanol, and salicylic acid. *Drugs amenable to hemoperfusion* include carbamazepine, chloramphenicol, phenytoin, ethchlorvynol, glutethimide, methaqualone, methotrexate, methylphenobarbital, diquat, paraquat, pentobarbital, phenobarbital, podophyllum, theophylline, and the digoxin-Fab fragment complex.

Provide antidotes as indicated in Table 7.1.1.

Admission Criteria

All patients who do not respond immediately to therapy or who have ingestions with possible late-onset effects should be admitted. If available, they should be admitted to the service of a medical toxicologist.

Suggested Readings

Kulig K: Initial management of ingestions of toxic substances. N Engl J Med 1992;326:1677–1681.

Olson KR, Pentel PR, Kelley MT: Physical assessment and differential diagnosis of the poisoned patient. Med Toxicol 1987;2:52–81.

Perrone J, Hoffman RS, Goldfrank LR: Special considerations in gastrointestinal decontamination. Emerg Med Clin North Am 1994; 12(2):285–299.

7.2 OPIOID POISONING

Description

Mild opioid intoxication gives rise to marked euphoria, often accompanied by anorexia, nausea, vomiting, constipation, and decrease in libido. A decline in mentation and depression of consciousness with eventual coma results from significant opioid

Table 7.1.1
Commonly Used Antidotes

Antidote	Description of Antidote/Toxin	Adult Dose and Comments
Activated charcoal	An adsorbent that adheres to many toxic drugs and chemicals; used for gastrointestinal dialysis	Give 6 g PO q 24 hr.
Antivenin (crotalidae); polyvalent (Wyeth)	Crotalid snakebites	Give 5–8 vials for minimally severe bites, 8–12 vials for moderately severe bites, and 12–30 vials for very severe bites: 1 vial q 15–20 min. Always call the regional Poison Control Center.
Antivenin (latrodectus mactans; MSD)	Black widow spider bites (bradydysrhythmias)	
Atropine	Cholinesterase inhibitors, organophosphate insecticides (malathion, parathion), cholinergic agents (neostigmine, pilocarpine, methacholine), and certain mushrooms	Give 1–2 mg by slow IVp until desired effect is achieved (normal heart rate, dilated pupils, dry mouth).
Botulinal antitoxin (ABE, trivalent)	Botulism (available from local health department or the Centers for Disease Control and Prevention)	Contact the CDC for specific dosage instructions (404-329-3753).
Calcium chloride	Calcium-channel blockers, hydrofluoric acid, fluorides, ethylene glycol	Give 1 g over 5 min by IV infusion with continuous cardiac monitoring; may be repeated often in life-threatening situations, but the serum calcium level should be monitored after the third dose. Concomitant magnesium administration may be needed.

Table 7.1.1—*Continued*

Antidote	Description of Antidote/Toxin	Adult Dose and Comments
Calcium disodium ethylene amine-tetraacetic acid (CaEDTA)	Copper, zinc, lead, cadmium	Give 25 mg/kg q 8 hr IV.
Calcium gluconate	Hydrofluoric acid burns, black widow spider bites	Infiltrate each square centimeter of burn with 0.5 mL of 10% solution SQ, using a 25-gauge needle; may be given intraarterially as 10 mL of 10% solution in 50 mL of D_5W via infusion pump over 4 hr.
Cyanide kit (amyl nitrite, sodium nitrite, sodium thiosulfate)	Cyanide (potassium cyanide, hydrocyanic acid, laetrile, nitro-prusside sodium)	Break pearl and hold it under patient's nose; give 10 mL of 3% sodium nitrite solution IV at 2.5–5.0 mL/min, then give 12.5 g of sodium thiosulfate by slow IV infusion.
Deferoxamine (Desferal)	Iron (acute and chronic)	DFO challenge test: give 50 mg/kg IM up to a maximum of 2 g every 6–8 hr until urine is no longer red; if hypotensive, give 15 mg/kg/hr by slow IV infusion. Watch for drug-induced hypo-tension or rash.
Dextrose in water (50%)	Hypoglycemic agents (patients with altered mental status)	Give 25 g IVp; if the patient responds or the blood glucose is < 60 mg/100 mL, give a repeat dose and begin an IV infu-sion of $D_{10}W$.

Table 7.1.1—*Continued*

Antidote	Description of Antidote/Toxin	Adult Dose and Comments
Digoxin-specific antibody fragments	Digitalis glycosides	Equimolar to ingestions; the number of vials required is equal to the number of milligrams of digoxin ingested divided by 0.6. If the amount of drug ingested is unknown and the patient has life-threatening dysrhythmias, give 10–20 vials IV. If the serum digoxin concentration is known, the number of vials to administer is equal to [the concentration (ng/mL) × 5.6 × weight (kg)]/600.
Dimercaprol (BAL; British antilewisite)	Arsenic, gold, mercury, lead poisoning	Arsenic poisoning: give 3–5 mg/kg by deep IM injection q 4 hr until GI symptoms resolve. Lead poisoning: give 3–5 mng/kg IM q 4 hr for 2 days, then q 4 1–2 hr for up to 7 more days. Mercury poisoning: give 3–5 mg/kg IM q 4 hr for 2 days, then 3 mg/kg q hr for 2 days, then 3 mg/kg q 12 hr for 7 more days.
2,3-dimercaptosuccinic acid (DMSA)	Chelator for lead, arsenic mercury	Give 10 mg/kg q 8 hr for 5 days.
Diphenhydramine	Phenothiazines, haloperidol, thioxanthines	Give 50 mg IM or IV to relieve drug-related dystonias.

Table 7.1.1—*Continued*

Antidote	Description of Antidote/Toxin	Adult Dose and Comments
Ethanol	Methanol, ethylene glycol	Give a loading dose of 1 g/kg of a 10% solution by slow IVp, followed by an infusion of 130 mg/kg/hr. If the patient is being dialyzed, give 250–300 mg/kg/hr to maintain levels. Chronic alcoholics may require higher doses.
Flumazenil (Romazicon)	Benzodiazepines	Give 0.2 mg IVp; can be repeated q 5–10 min as needed up to a total of 1 mg.
Folinic acid, folic acid	Methyl alcohol, methotrexate	Give 1 mg/kg up to 50 mg by slow IV infusion of folinic acid, followed by 1 mg/kg up to 50 mg IV q 4 hr for 6 doses of folic acid.
Glucagon	Insulin, oral hypoglycemics, β-blockers, calcium antagonist OD	Give 1–4 mg by slow IVp; may be repeated.
Glucose	Insulin, oral hypoglycemics	Give 25 g (1 amp) D_{50} IV; repeat, depending on glucose level.
Ipecac syrup	Emetic	Give 30 mL PO or via NG tube, followed by 300 mL of fluid; may be repeated in 30 min, if emesis does not occur.
Methylene blue	Methemoglobin (levels > 20%)	Give 1–2 mg/kg IV (0.2 mL/kg of a 1% solution).
4-methylpyrazole	An investigational drug used for methanol and ethylene glycol ingestions	Give 15 mg/kg PO, followed by 10 mg/kg q 12 hr until levels of toxin are undetectable.

Table 7.1.1—*Continued*

Antidote	Description of Antidote/Toxin	Adult Dose and Comments
N-acetyl cysteine	Acetaminophen	Give initial dose of 140 mg/kg PO, then 70 mg/kg q 4 hr up to 17 doses PO.
Nalmefene (Revex)	Opiates	Give 0.5 mg IVp; can be repeated q 2–5 min to a total of 1.5 mg.
Naloxone (Narcan)	Opiates, clonidine OD	Give 2 mg IM or IVp; can be repeated up to a total dose of 10–20 mg. Some opiates (propoxyphene, meperidine, codeine) may require high doses. If patient responds, give the total dose necessary to reverse the opiate effects q 1 hr by IV infusion.
Nicotinamide	Vacor rodenticide	Give 500 mg IM or slow IVp, then give 100–200 mg IM or IV q 4 hr for up to 48 hr.
Oxygen (hyperbaric)	Carbon monoxide, cyanide, hydrogen sulfide	Use the highest concentration possible. If the patient is breathing independently, use a nonrebreathing mask with 100% oxygen. If the patient is being mechanically ventilated, use 100% oxygen.
D-penicillamine	Copper, lead, mercury, arsenic	Give 0.75–1.50 g daily; do not exceed a daily dose of 2 g. High incidence of side effects (fever, rash, bone marrow depression, proteinuria).

Table 7.1.1—*Continued*

Antidote	Description of Antidote/Toxin	Adult Dose and Comments
Physostigmine (Antilirium)	Anticholinergic agents and tricyclic antidepressant poisoning	Give 0.5 mg by slow IVp as a test dose, followed by up to 1.5 mg IV over 5 min to a total of 2 mg. Can cause seizures and should not be used routinely. Indications in anticholinergic poisoning include SVT with hypotension, seizures and arrhythmias unresponsive to conventional agents, and extreme agitation or delirium.
Polyethylene glycol (GoLYTELY)	Use as a general GI decontaminant to produce whole-bowel irrigation	Give 2 L/hr PO or via NG tube; continue administration until the watery stool is clear and free of solid matter. Indicated for serious ingestions presenting late (after 2 hr), ingestions of sustained-release medications, and iron ingestions.
Pralidoxime	Organophosphates	Give 25–50 mg/kg, not to exceed 2 g IM. Most effective within 24 hr postexposure. Used concomitantly with atropine.
Protamine sulfate	Heparin	Use 1 mg to neutralize 100 units of heparin; do not exceed 50 mg. Give as IV infusion over 5 min.

Table 7.1.1—*Continued*

Antidote	Description of Antidote/Toxin	Adult Dose and Comments
Pyridoxine hydrochloride	Ethylene glycol, isoniazid, mushrooms containing monomethylhydrazine	Glycol poisoning: give 100 mg IV daily for ethylene. Isoniazid poisoning: give 1 g/g ingested up to a maximum of 5 g IV.
Sodium bicarbonate (5% solution)	Salicylates, tricyclic antidepressants, phenobarbital	Give 2 mEq/kg by slow IVp, thereafter give a constant infusion in 500 mL D_5W. Attempt to maintain atrial pH of 7.50–7.55 and urine pH of 8.0–9.0.
Sorbitol	General (cathartic, sweetener for activated charcoal)	Give 1 g/kg PO or via NG tube. Excessive use can lead to diarrhea.
Thiamine hydrochloride	Thiamine deficiency, ethylene glycol	Give 100 mg IM or by slow IVp. Indicated for all alcoholics and malnourished patients.
Vitamin K	Coumarin, indanedione anticoagulants	Give 10 mg SQ, based on prothrombin time.

overdoses. Respiratory depression can ultimately ensue, followed by hypoxia or apnea, with sequelae of anoxic encephalopathy or death from asphyxiation, when opioid toxicity is extreme. Noncardiogenic pulmonary edema may result from a variety of mechanisms. Hypotension and bradycardia can lead to circulatory collapse and cardiopulmonary arrest. Miosis is characteristic of opioid overdose. However, meperidine (Demerol) may dilate the pupils, and severe hypoxia can cause normal, dilated, or fixed and constricted pupils. In addition, patients with mixed drug overdoses may have variable pupillary light reactions. Heroin mixed with scopolamine, an anticholinergic agent that causes dilated pupils, has become popular of late. Hence, the absence of miotic pupils does not rule out opioid overdose. Table 7.2.1 presents a classification of opioids, and Table 7.2.2 lists clinical features.

History

If the patient is able to give a history, the quantity, type, and time of opioid administration should be determined. Use of other drugs should be elicited. Chronic abusers should be asked how many years they have been using opioids, their usual mode of ad-

Table 7.2.1
Classification of Opioids

Classification of Opioids
Natural opium
Opium
Paregoric (camphorated tincture of opium)
Morphine
Codeine
Synthetic derivatives
Morphine and codeine congeners
Heroin
Hydromorphone (Dilaudid)
Oxymorphone (Numorphan)
Hydrocodone (Hycodan)
Oxycodone (Percodan)
Methadone and congeners
Meperidine (Demerol)
Anileridine (Leritine)
Diphenoxylate (Lomotil)
Methadone (Dolophine)
L-α-acetylmethadol (LAAM)
Propoxyphene (Darvon)
Others
Pentazocine (Talwin)
Butorphanol (Stadol)
Nalbuphine (Nubain)
Buprenorphine (Buprenex)
Fentanyls and designer opioids
Fentanyl (Innovar, Sublimaze)
Sufentanil
3-methyl fentanyl (China white)
Lofentanil
Carfentanil

Table 7.2.2
Clinical Features of Opioid Intoxication

Clinical Presentation	Cause
Pinpoint pupils	Stimulation of cranial nerve III nucleus
Coma	Agonist at opioid receptors
Respiratory depression	Depression of medullary respiratory center
Bradycardia	↓↓ sympathetic tone, ↑↑ parasympathetic tone
Hypotension	Peripheral arteriolar and venous dilation
Hypothermia	Peripheral vasodilation; CNS depression
Pulmonary edema	↑↑ pulmonary vascular permeability
Seizures (morphine, fentanyl, meperidine, propoxyphene)	Epileptogenic effects of compound and the metabolites

ministration, and their enrollment in any detoxification or methadone programs. Past medical history should include common complications of abuse: hepatitis, endocarditis, pneumonia, and AIDS as well as previous episodes of overdose. Alcohol consumption should be noted and quantified. Be aware that life-threatening complications can arise in patients taking opioid derivatives (i.e., dextromethorphan or meperidine) with monoamine oxidase inhibitors. Furthermore, certain designer drugs, like 3-methyl fentanyl are up to 6000 times more potent than morphine. On the street, these drugs may be referred to as *China white* or *Persian white.*

Physical Examination

General. Note the level of consciousness and affect.

Vital signs. Monitor for hypotension, hypothermia, bradycardia, and decreased rate or depth of respiration.

HEENT. Examine for signs of cerebral trauma. Always check pupillary light responses and fundi.

Neck. Note if supple.

Lungs. Listen for rales.

Skin. Note track marks around extremities, neck, or clavicle or evidence of peripheral cyanosis.

Heart. Listen for new murmurs, consistent with endocarditis.

Neurologic. Do as thorough an examination as possible and repeat it intermittently to monitor alterations of coma.

Diagnostic Tests

SMA. Check glucose by fingerstick. Note electrolyte imbalances if indicated.

Toxicology. Opioids can be qualitatively identified in urine or quantified in serum for medicolegal purposes. However, these results are irrelevant when dealing with an acute overdose. The fentanyls and designer opioids will not be identified on routine tox screens and require special RIA techniques for detection. A positive response to naloxone in the face of a drug screen negative for opioids should lead one to consider a fentanyl or designer-like drug OD. Serum alcohol, acetaminophen, and salicylate levels should be drawn on comatose patients who do not respond or respond incompletely to treatment for opioid overdose.

Treatment

Ensure airway, breathing, circulation, and decontamination. Give naloxone (Narcan; 2 mg IV, IM, SC, or via endotracheal tube). An alternative narcotic antagonist is nalmefene (Revex; 0.5 mg IV, with repeat doses Q 2 to 5 min for a total of 1.5 mg). Intravenous naloxone should result in an increased respiratory rate and improved mental status within 1 to 2 min. If no change occurs, a 4-mg dose should be administered. Remember that a propoxyphene, methadone, or pentazocine overdose may require 10 to 20 mg naloxone for reversal of the CNS depressant effects. If opiate dependence is strongly considered, you may elect to titrate the dose of naloxone (starting with a 0.4-mg dose) to avoid abrupt withdrawal. When intravenous access cannot be obtained rapidly, patients with stable vital signs and an adequate airway may receive the same dose intramuscularly; a response should be seen within 5 min. If intravenous access cannot be obtained and the vital signs remain unstable, the patient should be intubated and administered the same dose via the endotracheal tube; anticipating a response within 2 min.

If naloxone fails to fully resolve the patient's status (i.e., the patient is not breathing and/or talking normally), consider a concomitant problem such as a mixed overdose, head injury, hypoxic brain injury, or CNS infection. The standard 6-hr observation period is generally adequate to exclude toxicity from opioid ingestion, with the possible exception of diphenoxylate (Lomotil) ingestions. Naloxone lasts for 20 to 60 min, while nalmefene lasts 2.5 hr. The half-life of the ingestant is usually longer than that of naloxone and the type and quality of the ingestant are often unknown. Problems arise when the patient wishes to leave while he or she is lucid, but the half-life of the ingestant will outlast the naloxone. In this case, every effort must be made to persuade the patient to stay, including if necessary, physical or chemical restraints of the irrational patient (see section 19.2).

Further treatment via the general approach to drug ingestion outlined in section 7.1 should be given to those patients who do not respond or respond incompletely to naloxone therapy. Patients who remain comatose should be evaluated as detailed in section 3.1. **Always remember:** *Half of drug deaths result from underlying infection or injury!*

Admission Criteria

Patients with continued unexplained altered mental status or abnormal vital signs will require admission. Some clinicians believe that patients who respond to naloxone and show no return of respiratory depression, sedation, or miosis 4 hr after their last naloxone dose may be safely discharged.

Suggested Reading

Ellenhorn JM, Barceloux DG: Medical toxicology: diagnosis and treatment of human poisoning. New York: Elsevier, 1988.

Ford M, Hoffman RS, Goldfrank LR: Opioids and designer drugs. Emerg Med Clin North Am 1990;8:495–511.

7.3 SEDATIVE HYPNOTICS POISONING

Description

Sedative hypnotics available in this country include barbiturates, benzodiazepines, meprobamate, ethchlorvynol, glutethimide, and methaqualone. The use of these products is associated with a high incidence of addiction, suicide, and accidental death. Although benzodiazepines are one of the most commonly prescribed medications in the world and are associated with widespread abuse and addiction, death secondary to a pure benzodiazepine overdose is rare.

Both barbiturates and benzodiazepines are central nervous system depressants. Although all systems in the body are affected by this central inhibition, the respiratory drive is much more depressed in poisonings with barbiturates than with benzodiazepines. The addition of other respiratory depressants, such as ethanol, can cause apnea at much lower levels of either substance. Both are metabolized by hepatic mixed-function oxidases and thus demonstrate prolonged half-lives in hepatic failure.

Clinical Presentation

Determining the exact agent ingested is consequential; the onset and duration of the action of barbiturates and benzodiazepines vary between particular agents in each class. Shorter-acting products may take 10 to 30 min to show effects and are more likely to cause respiratory depression, whereas symptoms from longer-acting substances may require more than 1 hr to develop (see Table 7.3.1). Both barbiturates and benzodiazepines can cause coma.

Cardiovascular collapse is extremely rare with benzodiazepines but not uncommon with large ingestions of barbiturates. Hypotension, bradycardia, diaphoresis, and decreased urinary output can all be manifestations of shock secondary to a depression in myocardial contractility associated with severe barbiturate poisoning. The most common cause of morbidity and mortality from barbiturate or benzodiazepine poisoning is respiratory depression.

Table 7.3.1
Duration of Action of Sedative Hypnotics

Duration of Action	Barbiturates	Benzodiazepines
Ultrashort	Thiopental (Pentothal) Methohexital (Brevital)	Midazolam (Versed) Temazepam (Restoril) Triazolam (Halcion)
Short	Pentobarbital (Nembutal) Secobarbital (Seconal)	Alprazolam (Xanax) Oxazepam (Serax) Diazepam (Valium)
Intermediate	Amobarbital (Amytal) Butalbital (Fiorinal)	
Long	Phenobarbital (Luminal) Barbital Primidone (Mysoline)	Lorazepam (Ativan) Flurazepam (Dalmane) Clonazepam (Klonopin) Chlordiazepoxide (Librium)

Physical Examination

General. Note the level of consciousness, especially the respiratory status.

Vital signs. Observe for hypothermia, respiratory depression, and hypotension.

HEENT. Check for the gag reflex in patients with an altered mental status. Check pupillary reaction and eye movements for nystagmus. Note that patients with severe barbiturate poisoning may eventually recover full neurologic function, even after presenting with fixed and dilated pupils (as long as the patient has not suffered an hypoxic brain injury).

Lungs. Pulmonary edema has been reported.

Neurologic. Severely poisoned patients may be hyporeflexic or areflexic and comatose.

Diagnostic Tests

Chemistries. Check glucose (bedside Dextrostix) and other chemistries as indicated.

ABG. Respiratory depression will often first manifest as an elevated PCO_2. Pulmonary edema (barbiturate poisoning) would be suggested by hypoxia and a low PO_2 or oxygen saturation.

Toxicology screens. Serum barbiturate levels are available to confirm the diagnosis, but clinical correlation is extremely important since blood levels are notoriously inaccurate in predicting the level of intoxication. Benzodiazepine levels are usually not available and are never clinically useful. The use of ethanol will cause a synergistic clinical sedation out of proportion to the ingested dose, so alcohol levels should also be obtained.

Treatment

Always protect the patient's airway and assist ventilation as needed *(the major hazard of sedative or barbiturate OD is respiratory depression)*. Monitor both pulse oximeter and ABGs for evidence of respiratory insufficiency.

Warm hypothermic patients (see section 18.2). Resuscitate hypotensive patients with intravenous fluids first. If there is no response in blood pressure to the administration of 2 to 3 L of normal saline or lactated Ringer's, vasopressors such as dopamine or norepinephrine should be employed. Follow the general approach for decontamination and use of activated charcoal.

Alkalinizing the urine may increase excretion of long-acting barbiturates such as phenobarbital. Hemodialysis and hemoperfusion are effective in removing long-acting barbiturates but are rarely necessary. Severely poisoned patients with unstable vital signs such as refractory hypotension despite aggressive therapy are candidates for hemodialysis or hemoperfusion. Patients with extremely high levels and renal failure may also be candidates for hemodialysis.

Flumazenil (Romazicon) is a competitive antagonist of benzodiazepines in the CNS (it does not alter the metabolism of benzodiazepines but only displaces them from receptor sites). Flumazenil effectively reverses respiratory and mental status depression caused by benzodiazepine overdoses. The usual starting dose is 0.2 mg, IV, which can be repeated several times to total of 1 mg if there is no response. The half-life of flumazenil is 45 to 60 min; patients must, therefore, be observed for the return of respiratory depression as the flumazenil is metabolized. Patients on chronic doses of benzodiazepines may suffer withdrawal if administered flumazenil. Seizures and dysrhythmias have been reported in patients given flumazenil after ingestions of polycyclic antidepressants and chloral hydrate. For this reason it should not be administered routinely to all overdosed patients with altered mental status.

Admission Criteria

The most important point is to *rely on physical examination* rather than blood levels to determine the need for admission.

Suggested Readings

Baltarowich L: Barbiturates. Top Emerg Med 1985;7:46–54.

Osborn H, Goldfrank LR: Sedative-hypnotic agents. In Goldfrank LR, Flomenbaum NR, Lewin NA, et al.: Goldfrank's toxicologic emergencies. Norwalk, CT: Appleton & Lange, 1994.

7.4 ANTICHOLINERGIC AND POLYCYCLIC ANTIDEPRESSANT POISONING

Anticholinergic medications are available in a variety of prescription and over-the-counter medications. Common preparations are listed in Table 7.4.1.

Table 7.4.1
Anticholinergics

Antidepressants
- Amitriptyline (Elavil)
- Imipramine (Tofranil)
- Doxepin (Sinequan)
- Maprotiline (Ludiomil)
- Amoxapine (Asendin)
- Nortriptyline (Pamelor)
- Desipramine (Norpramin)
- Protriptyline (Vivactil)
- Trazodone (Desyrel)

Antiemetics
- Prochlorperazine (Compazine)
- Droperidol (Anapsine)
- Atropine

Antihistamines
- Diphenhydramine (Benadryl)
- Hydroxyzine (Vistaril)
- Chlorpheniramine (Chlor-Trimeton)

Anti-Parkinson drugs
- Benztropine (Cogentin)
- Trihexyphenidyl (Artane)

Antispasmodics
- Dicyclomine (Bentyl)
- Propantheline (Pro-Banthine)

Antipsychotics
- Haloperidol (Haldol)
- Chlorpromazine (Thorazine)
- Thioridazine (Mellaril)
- Trifluoperazine (Stelazine)
- Thiothixene (Navane)

Muscle relaxers
- Cyclobenzaprine (Flexeril)

Anticonvulsants
- Carbamazepine (Tegretol)

Ophthalmoplegics
- Tropicamide (Mydriacyl)
- Scopolamine (Dramamine)

Sleeping pills
- Pyrilamine maleate (Compoz)

Clinical Presentation

The clinical effects can be remembered as:

Hot as a hare;
Blind as a bat;
Dry as a bone;
Red as a beet; and
Mad as a hatter.

Peripheral effects of anticholinergic medications include dry skin and mucous membranes. Suppression of cholinergic sweat glands and agitation can result in hyperthermia. Blockade of cholinergic receptors on urinary bladder and intestinal smooth muscle leads to urinary retention and ileus. Pupils are often dilated, and vision is blurred. Although rare, blockade of smooth muscle receptors on large vessels combined with tachycardia can raise blood pressure. Cutaneous blood vessels may be dilated with flushing noted on physical examination. Decreased vagal tone results in tachycardia.

In addition to these anticholinergic effects, cyclic antidepressants also display cardiovascular toxicity, including mimicking the actions of class 1A antiarrhythmics (myocardial depression and cardiac conduction disturbances), blocking the fast sodium channels in cardiac conduction tissue, blocking the reuptake of norepinephrine (precipitating tachycardia), and demonstrating an α-blocking action (leading to vasodilation). Central effects of anticholinergic medications include agitation, hallucinations, and confusion, and can progress rapidly to coma and convulsions. Amoxapine toxicity has been associated with intractable seizures.

Physical Examination

General. Note the level of consciousness, the presence of a gag reflex, and the patency of the airway.

Vital signs. Note hyperthermia, hypotension (check for orthostatic changes), and tachycardia or bradycardia.

HEENT. Pupils are classically dilated. Mucous membranes are often dry, and vision may be blurred.

Abdomen. Bowel sounds may be decreased or absent. Urinary retention may present as a distended bladder.

Skin. Note lack of perspiration, especially in the axilla, since this lack of axillary perspiration may be the only clinical difference between anticholinergic and sympathomimetic poisoning.

Neurologic. Look for myoclonus, hyperactive DTRs, and the Babinski sign.

Diagnostic Tests

Chemistries. Check electrolytes, especially potassium, and note renal function.

Blood toxicology testing. Drug levels are poor predictors of toxicity and should not be used as guides to therapy.

ABG. Acidosis tends to precipitate dysrhythmias, and efforts should be aimed at maintaining serum pH above 7.40.

ECG. Conduction abnormalities are the hallmark of cyclic antidepressant and antihistamine cardiac toxicity. While sinus tachycardia is the earliest and most common cardiac manifestation, QRS widening >120 msec is the hallmark of severe toxicity and heralds a higher incidence of serious side effects (i.e., seizures or ventricular dysrhythmias). QT prolongation can also occur.

Treatment

Maintain airway patency and assist ventilation as necessary. Patients can deteriorate from normal mentation and cardiac rhythm to seizures and cardiac dysrhythmias very quickly. All patients with consistent histories or signs and symptoms of severe poisoning with these medications should be closely monitored. Provide gut decontamination with lavage and activated charcoal.

Sodium bicarbonate is the treatment of choice for conduction abnormalities, ventricular dysrhythmias, and hypotension unresponsive to intravenous fluids. Alkalization is achieved by infusing 1 to 2 amps (1 to 2 mEq/kg) of sodium bicarbonate; followed by an infusion of 2 amps of sodium bicarbonate in 1 L of D_5W at 50 to 100 mL/hr. The goal of alkalization is an arterial pH of 7.5 to 7.55. In unstable patients, alkalization can be supplemented by intubation with hyperventilation. The following are indications for alkalization:

- QRS duration > 100 msec;
- Ventricular dysrhythmias, including frequent PVCs;
- Hypotension;

- Cardiac arrest; and
- Altered mental status, including seizures (controversial).

Resuscitate hypotensive patients with intravenous fluids (e.g., isotonic crystalloids) first (2 to 3 L), followed by sodium bicarbonate and then a vasopressor. Remember that cyclic antidepressants block α-receptors in peripheral blood vessels and deplete catecholamines. It is best to begin pressor therapy with a direct pressor, α-agonist such as levoephedrine or phenylephrine.

Dysrhythmias refractory to sodium bicarbonate can be difficult to manage. Either phenytoin or lidocaine can be used as a second-line antidysrhythmic therapy. Class 1A antidysrhythmics are contraindicated. Seizures may also be refractory to conventional management. Benzodiazepines (such as lorazepam, 2 mg IV) are first-line agents. Phenobarbital (up to 30 mg/kg IV) may have greater efficacy than phenytoin in controlling refractory or persistent seizures.

Physostigmine is an anticholinesterase that has been used to reverse anticholinergic poisoning. However, physostigmine can lower the seizure and possibly can result in severe bradycardia and asystole. Its use is, therefore, not recommended routinely in these patients. It may be helpful in diagnosing patients with an unknown overdose (a clear-cut response implies poisoning with an anticholinergic agent). However, the QRS interval on the ECG must be < 100 msec, and physostigmine must be given slowly (1 to 2 mg IV over 5 min).

Admission Criteria

In patients ingesting only polycyclic antidepressant medications, data support medical clearance if no symptoms are noted after 6 hr of observation. *Symptomatic patients, including those with altered mental status, bradycardia or tachycardia, and a widened QRS interval* require admission and careful observation in a monitored setting such as an ICU.

Suggested Readings

Pentel PR, Benowitz NL: Tricyclic antidepressant poisoning: management of arrhythmias. Med Toxicol 1986;1:101–121.

Pimentel L, Trommer L: Cyclic antidepressants: a review. Emerg Med Clin North Am 1994;12:533–547.

7.5 SYMPATHOMIMETICS: COCAINE AND AMPHETAMINES

Description

Amphetamines may be abused via oral, inhalational, or intravenous routes (Table 7.5.1). Orally, absorption is complete within 6 hr. Amphetamine and its analogues have variable peripheral and central α- and β-adrenergic effects; these agents cause increased systolic and diastolic blood pressure, initially with bradycardia. Higher doses lead to tachycardia and dysrhythmias. The CNS properties include increased alertness, euphoria, anorexia, anxiety, confusion, seizures, and hyperpyrexia. Amphetamine psychosis involves paranoid delusions, hallucinations, and bizarre behavior in the setting of chronic abuse. Tactile hallucinations (bugs on the skin) are distinctive features of amphetamine and cocaine abuse.

Cocaine is a local anesthetic that causes CNS stimulation and blocks the reuptake of neurotransmitters. As the lower brain centers are stimulated, seizures result. Nasal insufflation causes peak cocaine plasma levels within 30 min, while smoking (crack or free-basing) leads to peak elevations within 2 to 5 min. Cocaine is rapidly hydrolyzed by plasma and liver cholinesterase. Metabolites are detectable in the urine up to 140 hr postuse, depending on the assay used. Furthermore, the presence of ethanol may prolong the half-life of cocaine (forming the metabolite cocaethylene). In addition, cocaine is commonly taken in combination with heroin (speedball). As with amphetamines, elevations of blood pressure and pulse are common; although late in intoxication, hypotension and cardiovascular collapse may transpire.

Table 7.5.1
Sympathomimetic Terminology

Common Name	Street Terminology
Amphetamines	Bennies, speed
DOM, STP	Serenity, peace pill
DOB	Golden eagle, tile
Methamphetamine	Crank, speed
MDA	Love pill
MDMA	Adam, ecstasy
MDEA	Eve
Cocaine	Crack, coke, toot, snow

Hyperthermia is a common complicating factor. Rhabdomyolysis is common in both cocaine and amphetamine overdoses and may result in significant morbidity.

History

Acutely intoxicated patients may present with a variety of complaints, including palpitations, chest pain, headache, or feeling tense and out of control. More serious presentations include seizures, stroke, tachyarrhythmias, and hyperthermia. Patients must be questioned as to the kind and quantities of drugs taken as well as the route of administration. Remember that some of the designer amphetamines have half-lives greater than 24 hr. Patients who inject should be questioned concerning other complications of intravenous drug use. Adverse effects from the use of amphetamines and cocaine, such as stroke and acute myocardial infarction, may occur several weeks after the last exposure.

Physical Examination

General. Note agitation, altered state of consciousness, and diaphoresis.

Vital signs. Check for tachycardia, increased blood pressure (in severe intoxication, hypotension may occur), hyperthermia, and rapid respiratory rate.

HEENT. Pupils will be dilated. Check the nasal septum for perforation.

Lungs. Listen for rales (failure, infection), decreased breath sounds (pneumothorax), and palpable subcutaneous emphysema (pneumomediastinum, pneumothorax).

Heart. Check for murmurs (endocarditis), S_3, S_4 (cardiomyopathy, acute ischemia, CHF), and Hamman's sign (crunching or crackling sound when pneumomediastinum is present).

Abdomen. Bowel sounds should be increased.

Back. Pain may indicate renal infarction or significant rhabdomyolysis.

Rectal. Do not fail to consider body packing, particularly in those patients with prolonged toxicity or those who may be in incarceration.

Extremities. Note any fresh track marks, cellulitis, ulcers, or muscle tenderness.

Neurologic. Do as complete an examination as possible.

Note: *The presence of diaphoresis and increased bowel sounds helps to differentiate sympathomimetic toxicity from anticholinergic overdose.*

Diagnostic Tests

CBC. Check hematocrit and WBC count.

SMA. Note any electrolyte imbalances and increased CPK (evidence of rhabdomyolysis).

Urinalysis. Note evidence of heme on dipstick without red blood cells on microscopic exam (as evidence of rhabdomyolysis).

ABG. Useful in patients with respiratory abnormalities.

ECG. Note any arrhythmias. Rule out acute infarction. Patients with prolonged chest pain should have serial ECGs.

Drug levels. Cocaine metabolites and amphetamines may be detected in the urine for legal purposes. Treatment depends on clinical signs and symptoms.

CXR. Patients who smoke cocaine are susceptible to atelectasis, pneumonia, pulmonary infarct, pneumothorax, pneumomediastinum, hemothorax, and pulmonary edema.

Abdominal plain films. Order if you suspect the patient of being a body packer or stuffer or if patient has acute abdominal complaints.

CT scan of head. Indicated in patients with persistent altered mental status, first-time seizures, or focal neurologic findings after ingesting sympathomimetics.

Treatment

Provide any necessary life support: airway, breathing, circulation, control of hyperthermia. With oral ingestions, provide gut decontamination (e.g., lavage, WBI) as indicated. If vital signs are stable and the patient is agitated, maintain verbal contact and decrease environmental stimulation.

Intravenous access and ECG monitoring are essential. Sedation with benzodiazepines (lorazepam or diazepam) is suggested if agitation, seizures, hypertension, or tachycardia are present. Ensure euvolemia, as many of these patients are relatively dehydrated and are at increased risk of rhabdomyolysis. Avoid acidosis.

Monitor blood pressure closely. Usually, the hypertension and tachycardia associated with cocaine use are transient. If hypertensive crisis occurs, β-blockers are contraindicated (because of the unopposed α-stimulation). The best treatment may be with an easily titratable vasodilator (nitroprusside or nitroglycerin) or an α-blocker (phentolamine). However, beware of tachycardia. Treat hyperthermic crisis aggressively (see section 18.1).

Controversy exists regarding the use of lidocaine for ventricular dysrhythmias that develop early in course of cocaine toxicity (e.g., lidocaine may potentiate the effects of cocaine on the myocardium). Titratable, rapid-acting β1-selective blockers (Esmolol) may be used for the treatment of supraventricular tachycardias if sedation fails.

Body stuffers or packers should be treated in an ICU until all packets have passed through the GI tract. Use activated charcoal with sorbitol, followed by whole-bowel irrigation if the packets are not immediately passed. Surgical consultation for removal is indicated with intestinal obstruction, when signs indicate leakage or rupture, or if the packets remain immobile for > 48 hr.

Admission Criteria

Patients with mild intoxication can be treated in the ED. *All patients who are body stuffers or packers and patients with serious complications* should be admitted, *including those with the following:*

- Cardiac arrhythmias or acute myocardial infarction;
- Seizures;
- Hyperthermia;
- Rhabdomyolysis;
- Hypertensive crisis;
- Cerebrovascular accident; and
- Severe psychotic problems.

Suggested Readings

Derlet RW, Albertson TE: Emergency department presentation of cocaine intoxication. Ann Emerg Med 1989;18:182–186.

Ettinger NA, Albin RJ: A review of the respiratory effects of smoking cocaine. Am J Med 1989;87:664–668.

Spivey WH, Euerle B: Neurologic complications of cocaine abuse. Ann Emerg Med 1990;19:1422–1428.

7.6 SALICYLATE POISONING

Description

Salicylates are used as both analgesics and antiinflammatories and are found in a variety of prescription and over-the-counter medications (e.g., Pepto-Bismol). An exceptionally high concentration of salicylate compound occurs in the topical preparation methyl salicylate, also known as oil of wintergreen (1 teaspoon contains the equivalent of 7.5 g of aspirin). Presentations can be acute or chronic and may result from either ingestion (intentional or accidental) or dermal absorption. Toxic doses of salicylates initially stimulate central respiratory centers, leading to hyperventilation and a respiratory alkalosis. Renal excretion of bicarbonate returns the serum pH toward normal, but usually cannot completely compensate. Sodium and potassium accompany the excretion of bicarbonate in the urine, often leading to electrolyte imbalances. In a large acute or chronic ingestion, a metabolic acidosis develops. Salicylate toxicity also interferes with cellular metabolism (uncoupling oxidative phosphorylation and interrupting glucose and fatty acid metabolism). In addition, severe acute or chronic overdoses of salicylates can cause cerebral and/or pulmonary edema. Acute ingestions of < 150 mg/kg of salicylate generally do not create significant problems, while doses of 150 to 300 mg/kg are capable of generating mild to moderate symptoms. Severe intoxication takes place with ingestions > 300 mg/kg. Chronic intoxication is generally associated with doses of 100 mg/kg/day or greater for more than 2 days.

Salicylates are weak acids. Ordinarily, they are rapidly absorbed and are converted to an ionized particle that binds with serum proteins. Serum levels typically are detectable 15 to 30 min after ingestion. However, absorption of enteric-coated preparations can be delayed or erratic. Aspirin, when ingested in large amounts, can form concretions or bezoars in the stomach, resulting in unpredictable and prolonged serum levels. Absorption of aspirin and related compounds can also be hampered by salicylate-induced pylorospasm as well as coingestions. Normal metabolism principally occurs in the liver. However, when hepatic enzyme systems become saturated, salicylate excretion shifts to the renal pathways. Moreover, when salicylate concentrations approach toxic levels, protein binding is exceeded and a greater percentage of salicylate molecules transform to a free, nonionized form. It is the nonionized configuration of salicylate that is capable of crossing cellular membranes (e.g., proximal tubules of the kidney, the blood-brain barrier) and producing toxic effects in the body's tissues. Metabolic acidosis also favors a shift in the equilibrium to the nonionized molecule.

All the above factors contribute to difficulty in interpreting serum salicylate levels and the nomogram is often not applicable. However, levels of 80 mg/dL and above are very serious, especially if a concomitant acidosis is present. Symptomatic patients should be treated regardless of the nomogram plot. The nomogram is not useful for sustained-release products or multiple or chronic ingestions. A repeat salicylate level should be obtained in all patients with suspected ingestions several hours after the initial level to (1) document a falling serum salicylate concentration before medical clearance in asymptomatic individuals and (2) follow the clinical course of symptomatic patients.

History

The history should include not only the quantity of salicylate ingested but whether the ingestion or exposure occurred as a single, acute event or was the result of multiple chronic ingestions. Gastrointestinal symptoms often initially predominate in acute ingestions. Nausea, vomiting, and abdominal pain are the most common complaints, but hematemesis is also reported. Hyperventilation, dehydration, diaphoresis, headache, ataxia, and tinnitus are also related. More severe overdoses (> 300 mg/kg) can present as lethargy, cardiovascular abnormalities, coagulation disorders, hyperthermia, pulmonary edema, and coma. In acute poisoning, levels usually correlate well with severity of symptoms.

The paramount feature of chronic poisoning with salicylates is mental status changes (e.g., confusion, drowsiness, slurred speech, agitation, seizures) with or without dehydration. The diagnosis is frequently overlooked because of the nonspecific nature of symptoms and because a majority of the victims of chronic toxicity are elderly. These patients are easily mistaken for being septic; therefore, salicylate toxicity should be part of the differential in all elderly patients with an altered mental status or unexplained acid-base disturbances. Serum salicylate levels are notoriously inaccurate in predicting toxicity secondary to chronic poisonings. Cerebral and pulmonary edema are more common in chronic salicylate poisoning than in an acute overdose. Morbidity and mortality rates also tend to be higher in chronic intoxications. The distinction between acute and chronic poisoning becomes less clear as time progresses following the ingestion.

Physical Examination

Vital signs. Hyperventilation and hyperthermia are often noted. Blood pressure is usually initially stable.

HEENT. Tinnitus or deafness may be found. Examine fundi for papilledema.

Lungs. Listen for rales as an early indication of pulmonary edema.

Abdomen. Check for tenderness, guarding, and peritoneal signs (consider possibility of perforation).

Rectal. Check the stool for blood.

Skin. Diaphoresis may be profuse.

Neurologic. Altered mental status, convulsions, or coma are poor prognostic findings. Paratonia (muscle rigidity) is seen with serious salicylate overdose.

Diagnostic Tests

Serum Salicylate Levels

Blood should be immediately sent for testing of salicylate levels in suspected patients or those with compatible histories or symptoms consistent with salicylate ingestions. Repeat levels 2 to 4 hr after the first level can help determine the course of the ingestion (to identify the peak level and prolonged absorption and sustained plasma levels, which appear with sustained-release compounds, tablet masses, or bezoar). Patients with chronic ingestions of salicylates can have serum levels within therapeutic ranges and still be severely toxic.

Bedside "Qualitative" Salicylate Testing

The presence of salicylates can be quickly confirmed by adding several drops of 10% ferric chloride to 1 mL of the patient's urine (a purple color indicates presence of salicylates). This is a qualitative not a quantitative test. Another quick bedside test for salicylates utilizes the Ames Phenistix (normally used to diagnose PKU in infants); it turns brown when either salicylates or phenothiazines are present in urine or blood.

Electrolytes

Serum glucose (hypoglycemia may be present) and electrolytes (calculate anion gap) should be frequently monitored. Pay careful attention to potassium levels (although serum potassium levels may appear normal initially, potassium depletion occurs through increased renal excretion caused by salicylate toxicity as well as intracellular shifting with the correction of acidosis).

Other Tests

ABG. Should be drawn periodically to aid in guiding therapy.

PT/PTT. Coagulation parameters should be monitored (clotting problems are more likely in chronic ingestions).

Urinalysis. Check for ketones.

CXR. Order if you suspect pulmonary edema (pulmonary edema occurs with a normal size heart).

CT head. If there is no improvement in mental status, look for hemorrhage and cerebral edema.

Treatment

Provide basic life support with special attention to the airway. Provide gut decontamination as indicated.

Virtually every patient with salicylate toxicity will be dehydrated (fluid is lost through vomiting, sweating, hyperventilation, and increased renal excretion). Hydration can be initiated concomitantly with alkalization by administering 1 to 2 mEq/kg of sodium bicarbonate IVp followed by an infusion of 88 mEq/L (2 amps) of sodium bicarbonate in D_5W at a rate of 10 to 15 mL/kg/hr over the first 1 to 2 hr until adequate urine flow is established. You must monitor the patient conscientiously, especially safeguarding against the development of pulmonary edema. A Foley catheter should be placed to monitor urine output as well as urinary pH. Alkalinizing the urine (pH $>$ 8) will increase salicylate excretion. Additional bicarbonate boluses may be needed (keep the serum pH around 7.5). Patients in shock may require more aggressive fluid administration (if there is evidence of a GI bleed, blood products may be required; see section 13.1).

Although initial serum potassium (K^+) levels may be reported as normal, hypokalemia generally occurs with salicylate poisoning. Total body potassium is lost via increased renal excretion and vomiting, with further decreases resulting from intracellular shifts. Unless renal failure is present, early use of potassium supplements is essential once urine flow is established (add 20 mEq to each liter of intravenous fluid). It will also be difficult to alkalinize the urine unless potassium depletion is corrected. Potassium levels need to be followed serially, and the patient should be on a cardiac monitor while potassium is given.

Hemodialysis is indicated for the patient:

- Who is deteriorating in spite of supportive care and alkaline diuresis;
- With renal failure;
- With persistent CNS disturbance (e.g., coma, seizures);
- With ARDS in whom salicylate levels are not rapidly falling;
- With congestive heart failure or noncardiogenic pulmonary edema; and
- Whose salicylate levels are > 100 mg/dL.

Activated charcoal absorbs salicylates well, and multiple doses may be effective in more rapidly eliminating serum salicylates. Surgical or endoscopic removal or concretions may be necessary (can attempt to dislodge with lavage).

Admission Criteria

Symptomatic patients, patients with renal failure, and patients with suspected toxic ingestions in whom serum salicylate levels are rising should be admitted. *Patients who have ingested enteric-coated tablets* may have prolonged absorption and should be monitored for extended periods until falling levels are documented and the patient is asymptomatic.

Suggested Readings

Dugandzic RM, Therny MG, Dickinson MG, et al.: Evaluation of the validity of the Dome nomogram in the management of acute salicylate intoxication. Ann Emerg Med 1989;18:1186–1190.

Yip L, Dart RC, Gabow PA: Concepts and controversies in salicylate toxicity. Emerg Med Clin North Am 1994;12:351–364.

7.7 ACETAMINOPHEN POISONING

Acetaminophen (*N*-acetyl-*p*-aminophenol; APAP) is one of the most common poisoning agents reported to the American Association of Poison Control Centers. Many APAP products contain other substances such as opiates, salicylates, or antihistamines. APAP intoxication may result in centrilobular hepatic necrosis. The potentially hepatotoxic dose of APAP in adults is considered to be an ingestion of greater than 140 mg/kg (or >7.5 g in the average adult). Chronic alcoholism increases the susceptibility of the liver to hepatotoxicity. Additional predisposing factors to acetaminophen toxicity are poor nutrition, renal insufficiency, and chronic cardiopulmonary insufficiency.

The peak serum levels of APAP occur at 30 to 120 min after therapeutic dosing. The serum concentration measured 4 to 24 hr after a single large overdose seems to be the best predictor of hepatotoxicity. For this reason, a nomogram has been devised to predict the occurrence of toxicity and guide management. Levels drawn before 4 hr after ingestion are not useful. Patients falling within the "possible hepatic toxicity" zone require treatment with *N*-acetylcysteine (NAC) (Fig. 7.7.1).

History

Most patients are initially asymptomatic even after toxic ingestions of APAP. If a combination of products is ingested, symptoms may be consistent with intoxication of these compounds. Massive ingestions of APAP often lead to nausea and vomiting, and patients presenting several hours or days following a toxic ingestion may show signs of hepatic or renal failure. Hepatotoxicity is usually not evident for 24 to 36 hr after toxic ingestions.

Physical Examination

Note: *The physical examination of patients who have ingested toxic amounts of APAP is often entirely normal.*

HEENT. Icterus may be present in late presentations.
Abdomen. Check for hepatomegaly or hepatic tenderness.
Skin. Observe for jaundice.

Diagnostic Tests

Serum APAP levels. Should be routinely ordered in all overdose patients, because of the tendency for overdose victims to conceal information about an ingestion. Levels of APAP are most accurate if drawn at 4 hr, but levels drawn after 4 hr may be plotted on the nomogram to assess the likelihood of toxicity. If the time of ingestion is unknown, find out when the patient was last seen and develop a worst-case scenario. New "extended

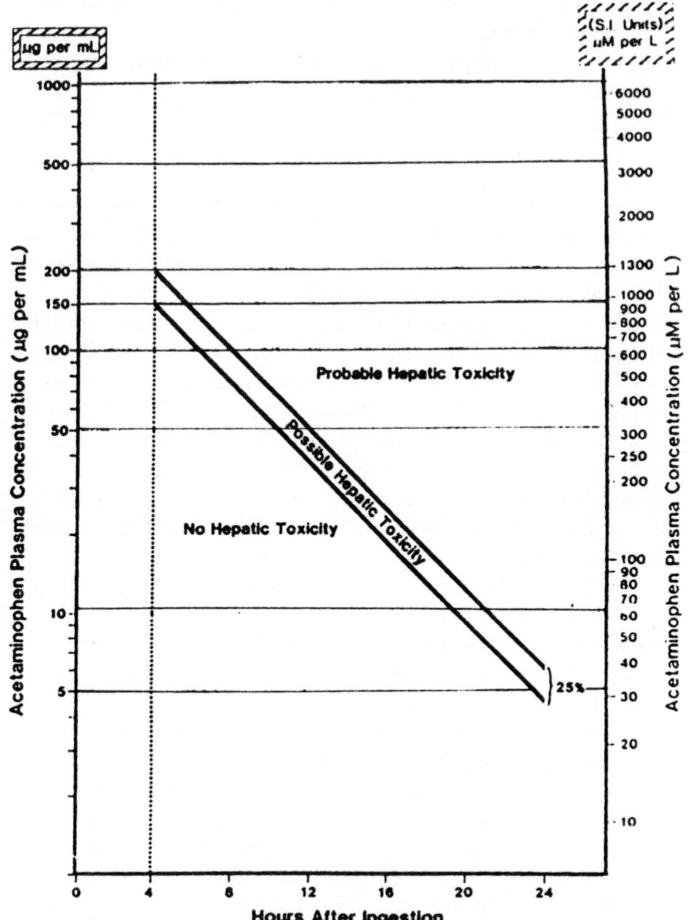

Figure 7.7.1 Rumack-Matthew nomogram for acetaminophen poisoning.

relief" preparations of APAP require a repeat level 4 hr after the initial one. Both results should be plotted on the nomogram.

SMA. Electrolytes and renal function should be monitored. Hepatic enzymes should be evaluated and followed in all patients throughout their course.

PT. May be the most sensitive indicator of hepatotoxicity and should be followed serially.

Treatment

Supportive care should be initiated as for all overdose victims. Gastric-emptying procedures can be performed if these patients present less than 1 hr after ingestion. One oral dose of activated charcoal should be administered (1 g/kg).

A 4-hr postingestion APAP level should be drawn and checked. If the serum level falls within or above the possible toxicity zone on the nomogram, NAC should be administered as an antidote. NAC acts like glutathione and detoxifies the hepatotoxic intermediary metabolite. Studies have shown that NAC is effective in preventing hepatotoxicity if therapy is begun within 24 hr after the ingestion, and more recent evidence suggests that late administration of NAC may also help to treat fulminant hepatic necrosis.

NAC is administered as an oral loading dose of 140 mg/kg, and then every 4 hr at 70 mg/kg for a total of 17 doses. If APAP levels are delayed or not available, or the patient presents late after the ingestion, empiric treatment is recommended, particularly if there is a history of ingestion over 140 mg/kg. If the patient vomits the loading dose, an antiemetic like metoclopramide (up to 2 mg/kg IV in 50 mL normal saline over 15 min) or ondansetron (up to a total of 32 mg in 50 mL D_5W over 15 min) in sufficiently high doses should be given and the NAC dose should be repeated. The administration of oral-activated charcoal before NAC will not adversely affect the outcome since the loading dose of NAC is so large. Patients refusing NAC or unable to tolerate it because of its smell may receive doses by nasogastric tube. An intravenous preparation of NAC may soon be available. In an emergency, the oral preparation may be given intravenously provided it is diluted to a 3% solution in D_5W and infused over 1 hr.

Admission Criteria

All patients requiring NAC therapy should be admitted.

Suggested Readings

Anker AL, Smilkstein MJ: Acetaminophen: concepts and controversies. Emerg Med Clin North Am 1994;12:335–349.

Borkovsky HL: Acute hepatic and renal toxicity from low doses of acetaminophen. Hepatology 1994;19:1141–1143.

7.8 CARBON MONOXIDE POISONING

Description

Carbon monoxide (CO) intoxication is the leading cause of poisoning deaths each year in the United States. Occupational groups at risk include toll and turnstile workers, firefighters, foundry workers, and miners. In addition, suspect carbon monoxide poisoning whenever a patient has suffered burns in a poorly ventilated area. The affinity of carbon monoxide for hemoglobin is 240 times that of oxygen. Carbon monoxide inhalation results in a decrease in the blood's oxygen-carrying capacity and a decrease in oxygen dissociation from hemoglobin at the tissue level (i.e., the oxygen-hemoglobin dissociation curve shifts to the left). The signs and symptoms of intoxication are related to cellular hypoxia. In room air (21% oxygen), the half-life of carbon dioxide is 4 to 5 hr, whereas in 100% oxygen it is 60 to 90 min. Hyperbaric oxygen (100% oxygen at 2.5 atmospheres) will decrease the half-life of carbon monoxide to about 20 min.

History

The symptoms of carbon monoxide poisoning are protean and depend not only on the patient's carboxyhemoglobin level but also on his or her baseline medical condition and metabolic rate. Symptoms include headache, nausea, dizziness, dyspnea, fatigue, chest pain, or confusion. Determine the type and duration of carbon monoxide exposure as well as possible inhalation of other toxic fumes. Question the patient about occupational exposure or suicidal intent. Inquire if family members, coworkers, or pets have been sick with similar symptoms—particularly during the winter months. A smoking history is pertinent, as smokers may have chronically elevated carboxyhemoglobin levels of up to 12%. Underlying anemia or cardiac, pulmonary, or neurologic disease places a patient at greater risk. ECG changes and anginal symptoms have been observed with carboxyhemoglobin levels below 5% in patients with preexisting coronary artery disease. All women of child-bearing age should be questioned regarding pregnancy, because fetal hemoglobin will accumulate carboxyhemoglobin (CoHb) levels 10 to 15% higher than those measured in maternal blood.

Physical Examination

General. The patient's mental status correlates best with the degree of toxicity and can range from vague lethargy to frank coma.

Vital signs. Increased respiratory and pulse rates are generally present.

Skin. The cherry red color classically described in carbon monoxide poisonings is infrequently seen.

HEENT. Visual disturbances are common. Funduscopic exam occasionally exhibits flame-shaped retinal hemorrhages. An even more exact sign for carbon monoxide poisoning is the presence of red retinal veins. Note the presence of soot around the nose, lips, and mouth if the patient has suffered smoke inhalation. Look for signs of pharyngeal edema or thermal damage to the airway.

Neck. Listen for stridor (laryngeal edema due to thermal injury).

Lungs. Listen for rales or rhonchi (smoke inhalation).

Neurologic. Most findings are subtle in nature and pertain to poor memory, inability to concentrate, or apathy.

Diagnostic Tests

Carboxyhemoglobin Level

A CoHb level should be obtained in all patients with any history of smoke inhalation, exposure to methylene chloride, or flu-like illness in a setting where incomplete combustion (faulty heater) may produce exogenous carbon monoxide. Measured CoHb levels should always be extrapolated to the time of exposure by taking into account the duration of time since the exposure and the percentage of oxygen inhaled. Arterial and venous samples are equivalent. Clinical features correlate only roughly with CoHb levels. Reliance on CoHb levels alone will result in treatment errors. Death may occur at any of these levels, depending on the patient's baseline medical condition.

CoHb (%)	Findings
10–20	Headache, mild dyspnea on exertion, fatigue
20–30	Throbbing headache, weakness, nausea, flu-like symptoms
30–40	Dizziness, irritability, disturbed judgment, tachycardia, tachypnea
40–50	Coma, confusion, syncope on exertion
60–70	Coma, convulsions, respiratory failure
70+	Rapidly fatal coma

Other Tests

ABG. Routine PaO_2 measures only the oxygen tension and not the oxygen saturation or content; it can be inormal or high, despite a decreased saturation. Since the oxygen saturation on the ABG is a calculated value, it too can be misleading. Acidosis is a very ominous finding. Pulse oximetry can also give a false-normal reading.

CBC. Anemia will result in a greater degree of tissue hypoxia at a given carboxyhemoglobin level.

X-rays. A CXR should be obtained on all patients to rule out pulmonary edema.

ECG. All patients with carbon monoxide exposure should have a cardiogram to rule out myocardial ischemia.

Treatment

All patients should be placed on 100% oxygen to reverse tissue hypoxia and eliminate carbon monoxide from the blood. Oxygen not only improves tissue oxygenation but also aids in carbon monoxide elimination. In cases with respiratory depression or failure, the patient should be intubated and ventilated with 100% oxygen. Indirect laryngoscopy should be performed if thermal or toxic injury to the airway is suspected.

Hyperbaric oxygen (HBO) therapy is indicated for patients who are or were symptomatic. Indications for hyperbaric oxygen therapy following carbon monoxide exposure include

- Symptomatic patients with CoHb >20%;
- Comatose patients;
- Patients with neurologic impairment (even if already resolved);

- Pregnant patients with CoHb >10% or when fetal monitoring shows signs of distress;
- Patients with a history of unconsciousness after carbon monoxide exposure; and
- Patients with acute myocardial ischemia.

Admission Criteria

All symptomatic patients should be admitted.

Suggested Readings

Ginsberg MD: Carbon monoxide intoxication. Clinical features, neuropathology and mechanisms of injury. Clin Toxicol 1985;23: 281–288.

Ilano AL, Raffin TA: Management of carbon monoxide poisoning. Chest 1990;97:165–168.

7.9 ETHANOL, METHANOL, ISOPROPANOL, AND ETHYLENE GLYCOL POISONING

Description

Ethanol remains the most widely abused of all drugs, with ethanol dependency afflicting 5% of the American population. The clinical presentations of intoxication with ethanol, methanol, isopropanol, and ethylene glycol are very similar in the early stages. Ethanol's earliest effects are on the central nervous system (CNS), and while acting primarily as a CNS depressant, a paradoxical CNS stimulation may occur due to disinhibition (e.g., the patient is loud and offensive). Small historical clues and subtle physical findings can help to obtain laboratory analysis and to confirm ingestion of another alcohol so that significant morbidity and mortality will be avoided.

All these alcohols are rapidly absorbed from the GI tract. It is the metabolites of methanol (formaldehyde, formic acid) and ethylene glycol (glycolic acid, glyoxylic acid, oxalate, and formic acid) that are so toxic. Table 7.9.1. simplifies the task of determining which substance was ingested.

History

The history should focus on the type and amount of alcohol ingested as well as co-ingestions. A history of chronic alcohol or

Table 7.9.1
Alcohol Ingestion

Characteristic	Alcohol Type: Ethanol	Isopropanol	Methanol	Ethylene Glycol
Sources	Beer, whisky, cough syrup	Rubbing alcohol, solvents	Antifreeze, windshield washer fluid	Antifreeze
Signs and symptoms	CNS depression, ataxia, ethanol odor to breath	CNS depression without initial elation, ataxia, acetone odor to breath	Delayed-onset (8–24 hr) headache, blurred vision, retinal edema, CNS depression, no ethanol odor to breath, no initial CNS elation	No ethanol odor to breath; stages: 1–12 hr: CNS depression; <12–24 hr: cardiopulmonary depression; 24–72 hr: renal failure
Urine		Positive for ketones		Calcium dihydrate crystals (octahedral); may fluoresce under Wood's lamp
Anion gap metabolic acidosis	Nonexistent, except with AKA	Nonexistent	Profound	Moderate
Osmolal gap[a]	Moderate (50 mg/dL will give a 11-mOsm increase)	Moderate (50 mg/dL will give an 8-mOsm increase)	Profound (50 mg/dL will give a 16-mOsm increase)	Moderate (50 mg/dL will give a 7-mOsm increase)
Molecular weight	46	60	32	62

[a] Osmolal gap = Measured osmolality − Calculated osmolality

Calculated osmolality = 2(Sodium) + (Glucose/18) + (BUN/2.8)

Predicted concentration (mg/dL) = [(Osmolal gap)(Molecular weight of toxin)]/10

Note: A patient may have a significant methanol or ethylene glycol level (e.g., > 20 mg/dL) and have an insignificant osmolal gap. Treatment must be based on the history, clinical assessment, and presence of an anion gap acidosis.

drug use should be sought after. The past medical history and possibility of recent trauma need to be routinely ascertained.

Physical Examination

General. Note the mental status, slurred speech, and cerebellar dysfunction. Look for signs of trauma.

Vital signs. Hypotension is an ominous sign, often indicative of the severe metabolic acidosis of methanol poisoning. Tachypnea may be a sign of acidosis. Hypothermia is common with CNS depression.

HEENT. Check visual acuity (methanol). Note retinal edema, optic disk hyperemia, or dilated pupils seen with methanol ingestion. Miosis and nystagmus may be seen with isopropanol poisoning. Pharyngeal hyperemia may be prominent with isopropanol ingestion. Note an acetone odor (isopropanol) (Table 7.9.1). **Caution:** *The presence of alcohol on breath does not correlate with blood alcohol levels nor does it always account for a patient's mental status.*

Chest. Listen for rales and rhonchi (indicating possible underlying pneumonia or aspiration)

Abdomen. Check for guarding and look for signs of gastrointestinal bleeding.

Neurologic. Perform a complete examination with emphasis on cognitive and cerebellar functioning. *Serial examinations are necessary in the intoxicated patient—one exam is never enough!*

Diagnostic Tests

Osmolality

Serum osmolality assists in determining the osmol gap. The osmol gap is the measured value (normally 285 to 295 mOsm/kg), determined by the freezing point depression technique, compared with the calculated value:

$$\text{Calculated value} = 2(\text{Sodium}) + (\text{BUN}/2.8) + (\text{Glucose}/18) + (\text{Ethanol}/4.6)$$

If the difference between the measured and calculated value is greater than 10 mOsm/kg, an unmeasured osmotically active substance is said to be present. The most common substances in an alcoholic that increase the osmol gap (other than ethanol) are methanol, ethylene glycol, and isopropanol. However, *caution must be exercised when an osmol gap is absent;* because of the small amount of methanol and ethylene glycol that can cause toxicity (as little as 15 mL of methanol has been reported to cause death, and the toxic dose for ethylene glycol is 1 to 2 mL/kg) and the imprecision of the freezing point technique, a normal osmol gap does *not* exclude toxic levels of methanol or ethylene glycol.

Blood Ethanol Level

The clinical effects of a specific blood alcohol level are highly variable and depend on the patient's individual metabolism and prior drinking habits (e.g., alcoholics tolerate higher alcohol levels than abstainers or social drinkers). In the nontolerant patient who acutely consumes ethanol, there is an approximate relationship between the blood alcohol concentration and the degree of neurologic impairment; blood alcohol concentrations of 150 to 300 mg/dL ordinarily cause mental confusion, ataxia, disturbances in sensation and perception, and muscular incoordination. Lethal levels of ethanol vary considerably and are frequently much lower when sedative hypnotics or tranquilizers are coingested. For the typical 70 kg patient, 15 mL of absolute alcohol (1.5 oz of whiskey or a 12-oz beer) will increase the blood alcohol level by 25 mg/dL. *A level that is inappropriately low in a patient with a depressed mental status should prompt a search for alternative causes.* Some EDs employ breath tests (e.g., *Breathalyzer*) to rapidly estimate blood alcohol concentrations.

Level (mg/dL)	Clinical Findings in the Nontolerant Patient
0–100	Altered judgment, decreased inhibition
100–200*	Confusion, slurred speech, ataxia
200–300	Lethargy, altered equilibrium, stupor
300–400	Hypothermia, respiratory depression, coma
> 500	LD_{50} for death (from respiratory paralysis) in nonalcoholics

*A level ≥ 100 mg/dL is considered legally impaired (driving under the influence; DUI) in most states.

Other Tests

Toxicologies. Obtain methanol and ethylene glycol levels to verify ingestion and determine continuation of hemodialysis.

CBC. Check hematocrit and WBC count (hemoconcentration likely).

SMA. Look for electrolyte imbalances (e.g., hypokalemia, hypomagnesemia, and hypocalcemia) as well as hypoglycemia or hyperglycemia. *Hypoglycemia may be delayed for up to 6 hr after acute alcohol ingestion.*

ABG. Critical for assessment of acid-base status (both lactic and ketoacidosis can occur).

Urinalysis. Useful as outlined in Table 7.9.1.

CXR. Indicated when aspiration, CHF, infection, or chest trauma is suspected.

ECG. Required when ischemia, dysrhythmia (atrial fibrillation is the most frequent arrhythmia associated with ethanol ingestion; the so-called holiday heart), or an electrolyte imbalance is a consideration.

CT scan of the brain. Order in patients with significant head trauma in the setting of ethanol intoxication or in the intoxicated patient with new-onset seizures, focal neurologic deficit, or a degree of alteration of mental status out of proportion to the blood alcohol level.

Treatment

Supportive care (the ABCs) needs to be ensured in all intoxicated patients. Also exercise caution in positioning any intoxicated patient to prevent aspiration. Correct any fluid deficits; D_5NS is usually appropriate for the volume depleted in the acutely intoxicated patient. Hypoglycemia is not uncommon in the setting of alcohol intoxication, particularly with the chronic alcoholic. Check a lab stick and administer glucose as needed to any intoxicated patient with an altered mental status. Thiamine hydrochloride (100 mg IV or IM) needs to be included in the initial therapy for any patient with intoxication and/or altered mental status.

Isopropanol ingestion causes a ketonemia without acidosis and is not treated with ethanol. Hemodialysis is indicated only for uncorrectable hypotension, deteriorating vital signs, coma with severe underlying disease, or blood levels > 400 mg/dL. Rapid absorption precludes gut decontamination unless it is achievable within 1 hr postingestion. Supportive care is otherwise indicated for hypotension or gastrointestinal hemorrhage.

Alcoholic ketoacidosis typically befalls chronic alcoholics with malnutrition who binge drink. Treatment focuses on correcting volume deficits with crystalloid administration and reversing glycogen depletion by adding glucose to the solutions (e.g., a D_5NS run at 200 to 1000 mL/hr until the vital signs are normal and the volume deficit is corrected). Chronic ethanol use almost always results in magnesium deficiency, and repletion is necessary (2 g IV over 1 hr). Thiamine (100 mg IV) needs to be given at the onset of therapy. Hypokalemia likewise obligates correction (add 10 to 20 mEq/hr to intravenous fluids), once adequate renal function and output are verified.

For the most part, the treatments of ethylene glycol and methanol poisonings are similar. It is essential that therapy be instituted in an expedient manner, as both these poisonings are associated with irreversible damage. After securing the airway, correcting hypotension and hypoglycemia, and administering 100 mg of thiamine parenterally, specific measures need to be instituted. *Do not wait for a positive lab confirmation when you have a high suspicion for methylene or ethylene glycol ingestion (intoxication, acidosis, osmolar gap, low ethanol level).* Because the alcohols are rapidly absorbed, gastrointestinal decontamination usually plays a small role, unless the patient presents within 1 hr of ingestion. If the patient is acidotic ($pH < 7.2$), give sodium bicarbonate. Administer 2 mEq sodium bicarbonate as an IV bolus. Further correction is guided by frequent monitoring of arterial blood gases (attempt to normalize the pH) and electrolytes.

Since it is the metabolites of methanol and ethylene glycol that are toxic and not the parent compounds, begin ethanol therapy immediately for any patient when the history suggests a possible ingestion. Ethanol has a 100 times greater affinity for alcohol dehydrogenase (the enzyme responsible for the critical first step in the metabolism of methanol and ethylene glycol). Therefore, the goal of therapy is to saturate the enzyme system, which usually is achieved by maintaining a blood alcohol level of 100 to 150 mg/dL. Ethanol can be administered either orally or parenterally—give a loading dose of 1 g/kg. Dilute the absolute alcohol to a 10% solution (higher concentrations are irritating) with D_5W and give IV over 30 to 60 min, or administer as a 20% oral solution diluted in juice. Constant monitoring of the serum ethanol level is essential because of the wide variation in individual metabolism (chronic alcoholics will require higher infusion rates). The average maintenance infusion rate is 130 mg/kg/hr (approximately 1 mL/kg/hr of a 10% solution). If dialysis is required, the maintenance infusion should be increased to 250 to 300 mg/kg/hr. Dialysis is required for all patients who are symptomatic (i.e., those who have nausea, vomiting, abdominal pain, blurred vision, or an altered mental state), have a methanol or ethylene glycol level > 25 mg/dL, have a blood pH < 7.2, or have renal compromise.

Additional therapy for ethylene glycol toxicity includes pyridoxine (50 mg IV q 6 hr) and thiamine (100 mg IV q 6 hr). For methanol ingestions, add folic acid (50 mg IV q 4 hr) as well as thiamine (100 mg IV q 6 hr). Supplemental calcium is necessitated when symptomatic hypocalcemia (see section 6.5) accompanies ethylene glycol ingestion.

Admission Criteria

All patients with alcoholic ketoacidosis, or who are symptomatic from their ingestion of methanol, isopropanol, or ethylene glycol, need to be admitted. *Alcoholic patients with pneumonia, hepatitis, or significant head trauma,* i.e., loss of consciousness despite negative CT scan, usually justify admission because of their poor reliability and unwillingness to follow-up.

Patients who ingested methanol or ethylene glycol but are asymptomatic, are not acidotic, and have a serum level < 10 mg/dL can be safely discharged from the ED (however, if they are suicidal, they require a psychiatric evaluation; see section 19.2). Most intoxicated patients can be safely discharged from the ED after ensuring they have no underlying problem, they can tolerate fluids, they are sober, and they have reliable friends or family. Patients who are still intoxicated, however, cannot be relied on to make safe judgments (and may be a risk to themselves and others) and should not be permitted to leave the emergency department alone; if necessary, they should be restrained until sober (see section 19.2).

Suggested Readings

Duffens K, Marx JA: Alcoholic ketoacidosis—a review. J Emerg Med 1987;5:399–406.

Jacobsen D, McMartin KE: Methanol and ethylene glycol poisonings. Mechanism of toxicity, clinical course, diagnosis and treatment. Med Toxicol 1986;1:309–334.

Marco CA, Kelen GD: Acute intoxication. Emerg Med Clin North Am 1990;8(4):731–748.

7.10 WITHDRAWAL SYNDROMES

Ethanol Withdrawal

Description

Ethanol withdrawal usually requires up to 2 weeks of chronic alcohol ingestion, although shorter periods (as little as 4 days) have been reported. There is a wide spectrum of manifestations (e.g., anxiety, agitation, tremulousness, GI disturbances, autonomic disorders) that may culminate in seizures and/or delirium tremens. However, there is no predictable stepwise advance of clinical presentations. Four clinical conditions can be categorized as types of the *alcohol withdrawal syndrome* (AWS): *minor reactions* (anxiety, agitation, insomnia), *hallucinations* (range from disorders of perception to visual and auditory hallucinations), *withdrawal seizures* (ethanol withdrawal seizures or "rum fits" generally occur from 6 to 48 hr after the last drink and are usually short, nonfocal, and self-limiting; less than 5% progress to status epilepticus), and *delirium tremens* (a combination of autonomic hyperactivity, hallucinations, and convulsions).

History

A complete history can often suggest the diagnosis. Regular heavy drinkers are more likely to develop symptomatic withdrawal than binge drinkers. Autonomic nervous system stimulation accounts for most symptoms of ethanol withdrawal. Tremor, agitation, insomnia, nausea, vomiting, and headache are all frequent presenting complaints.

Physical Examination

General. Note any stigmata of alcoholism, such as spider angiomata, scleral icterus, gynecomastia, or ascites. The tremor associated with ethanol withdrawal may worsen on intentional motions. Look for signs of trauma.

Vital signs. Most patients are tachycardiac, often with hypertension and diaphoresis. Some may present with a low-grade fever.

HEENT. Conjunctival irritation is common. Highly adrenergic patients may have slightly dilated pupils. Nystagmus may be present.

Lungs. Check for rhonchi or other signs of pneumonia.

Cardiac. Binge drinking has been associated with atrial fibrillation. Cardiomyopathy has also been reported with chronic heavy ethanol intake.

Abdomen. Gastritis or pancreatitis can cause ileus.

Neurologic. Observe for hyperreflexia, hypertonia, ataxia, nystagmus, or asterixis. All findings should be nonfocal.

Treatment

The goals of treatment in the ED are to prevent progression to more serious states (e.g., withdrawal seizures, delirium tremens), alleviate symptoms, identify and treat any underlying disorders associated with chronic alcoholism, and attempt to connect the patient with long-term rehabilitation without causing dependence on a new substance.

Many chronic alcoholics are malnourished. All suspected alcoholics should receive 100 mg thiamine, dextrose, and multivitamins with folate intravenously. Most chronic ethanol abusers are dehydrated and will require intravenous hydration with crystalloid fluids such as D_5NS. Dextrose can be added. In addition, a preponderance of chronic alcoholics are magnesium deficient and will require 4 to 6 g IV of 10% solution dispensed over 3 to 4 hr.

Seizure precautions should be taken when withdrawal is suspected. Patients with the alcohol withdrawal syndrome will require tranquilization. Although barbiturates and other sedative hypnotics have been used in the past, benzodiazepines have become the mainstay of therapy. Diazepam can be given in 5-mg increments IV q 5 to 10 min until the desired effects and level of sedation are obtained. The dosage of diazepam required to treat withdrawal is highly variable. Frequent reassessment is necessary. Lorazepam is often chosen because of its reliable bioavailability, longer duration of action, and lack of active metabolites (unlike diazepam). The usual dose of lorazepam is 0.5 mg to 4.0 mg IV (depending on the severity of symptoms), with repeat doses every 15 to 30 min.

Phenothiazines (Thorazine) and butyrophenones (Haloperidol) should not be used in the management of ethanol withdrawal seizures, as they will not substitute for ethanol. Phenytoin has been shown in numerous studies to lack the efficacy of the benzodiazepines or barbiturates in preventing ethanol withdrawal seizures.

Status epilepticus should be managed as in any case with benzodiazepines and barbiturates. Large doses may be required. Prolonged seizure activity or altered mental status should always suggest the possibility of head injury or meningitis in the chronic alcoholic. CT scans are advisable when the diagnosis of ethanol withdrawal is in question or when focal neurologic findings are present on examination (see section 3.2).

Admission Criteria

Patients who are experiencing hallucinations, severe agitation, or marked tachycardia; who have a fever; who show frank psychosis; who are undergoing seizures; who show evidence of head injury or an altered mental status; or have severe electrolyte abnormalities or alcoholic ketoacidosis should be admitted. Patients with mild alcohol withdrawal syndrome may be discharged to a controlled environment after being observed for 4 to 6 hr without any deterioration in their vital signs and ensuring that there is no underlying medical problem.

Sedative Hypnotics Medication Withdrawal

Sedative hypnotics include benzodiazepines, barbiturates, meprobamate, ethchlorvynol (Placidyl), glutethimide (Doriden), and methaqualone. Withdrawal usually occurs when these substances are taken in 3 to 10 times the sedative dose for 1 to 2 months. Shorter-acting compounds will obviously cause withdrawal more quickly after cessation of therapy, and symptoms tend to resolve more rapidly. Seizures are usually more common from withdrawal of sedative hypnotics than from ethanol. Overall, the spectrum of hallucinations, autonomic hyperactivity, and convulsions described for ethanol withdrawal is similar to the clinical effects from withdrawal of all sedative hypnotics. Withdrawal from barbiturates can be more serious than withdrawal from other drugs of abuse and should be recognized as a potential medical emergency.

Patients should be admitted under the same criteria as used for ethanol withdrawal.

Opiate Withdrawal

Opiate withdrawal is generally not life threatening. Symptoms have been classified as "purposive" and "nonpurposive." Purposive symptoms are goal oriented and directed at obtaining more opiate. Symptoms include pleas, demands, and manipulative behavior that often includes mimicking of symptoms of physiologic opiate withdrawal. Nonpurposive withdrawal is physiologic. Signs and symptoms usually begin 8 to 12 hr after the last dose of heroin or morphine but may be delayed with longer-acting preparations such as methadone or propoxyphene. Lacrimation, rhinorrhea, yawning, and diaphoresis are frequently encountered first, increasing in intensity during the first 24 hr of withdrawal. Symptoms progress to include irritability, restlessness, dilated pupils, anorexia, and goose flesh. Nausea, vomiting, and diarrhea can be severe, and patients may develop tachycardia and mild elevations in blood pressure. With morphine and heroin, symptoms peak at 36 to 48 hr and may remain severe for 2 to 3 days. Effects usually subside after 5 to 10 days, or until the next dose.

All opiates cross-react and can be used to relieve withdrawal symptoms. Methadone is most frequently used to taper patients in detoxification clinics because of its long half-life. An oral dose of 40 mg of methadone daily should prevent nonpurposive withdrawal in addicted patients. Purposive withdrawal symptoms may continue at these doses of methadone, and patients complaining of withdrawal at these doses should be examined for physiologic signs. Methadone can be tapered over 1 to 2 weeks. In the ED setting, physiologic manifestations may be treated with methadone (10 mg IM) titrated as needed to control symptoms.

Amphetamine and Cocaine Withdrawal

Dependency on cocaine and amphetamines is largely psychological. Patients often relapse, especially with cocaine addiction, even after prolonged remissions. Physiologic withdrawal from sympathomimetics is subtle. Large daily users complain of fatigue, depression, excessive sleep, and irritability. Although they may be initially anorexic, most patients develop increased appetites several days after sympathomimetic binges. Patients detoxifying from sympathomimetics occasionally report paranoia, nausea, and vomiting.

Suggested Readings

Chiang WK, Goldfrank LR: Substance withdrawal. Emerg Med Clin North Am 1990;8:613–631.

Ozdemir V, Bremner NE, Naranjo CA: Treatment of alcohol withdrawal syndrome. Ann Med 1994;26:101–105.

Chapter 8

Allergy, Anaphylaxis, and Urticaria

DESCRIPTION

Anaphylaxis is a medical emergency that requires prompt and appropriate treatment. Initial symptoms can vary in severity from mild urticaria and pharyngeal edema to cardiovascular collapse and death. Anaphylaxis is characterized by an immediate, systemic, IgE-mediated reaction to a foreign substance in a previously sensitized individual. This reaction causes the release of chemical mediators from mast cells and basophils, resulting in vasodilation, bronchoconstriction, pruritus, bronchorrhea, and increased vascular permeability. An *anaphylactoid reaction* takes place when an offending agent causes the direct release of mediators without the involvement of IgE. Clinically, these two syndromes are indistinguishable.

The most common causes of anaphylaxis are drugs (penicillin, aspirin, NSAID), insect stings (Hymenoptera), food (shellfish, egg whites, peanuts), food additives (tartrazine, sulfites), radiocontrast material (iodinated contrast agents), complete proteins (streptokinase, insulin, toxoids, antiserum), and in some individuals, physical factors (exercise and cold). In addition, there have been increasing reports of life-threatening *angioedema* in patients taking ACE inhibitors (symptoms can occur from hours to years after the initiation of therapy).

HISTORY

If the patient is in extremis, do not dwell on the history—stabilize (see "Treatment," on page 307). If the patient is stable, gather data.

In patients who are stable, inquire about symptoms (onset,

quality, duration, and progression); generally, the more rapid the progression of symptoms, the more severe the reaction). Ask if the patient is aware of any exposure to offending agents ("the six I's": ingestion, injection, inhalation, infection, immunologic, idiopathic) and the route of exposure. The more direct access the agent has to the systemic circulation, the greater the risk of severe reaction, i.e., intravenous exposure is the most dangerous, followed by intramuscular, mucous membranes or GI tract, and skin exposures. Document any prior allergic reactions and the course of these reactions.

Early in the course of anaphylaxis, the patient may present with nonspecific symptoms, i.e., itching, a lump in the throat, or a "feeling of impending doom." Keep in mind that *apparently benign symptoms can progress to death within minutes.* The target organs of anaphylaxis are the skin (itching, burning, stinging, urticaria, facial swelling), respiratory tract (nasal congestion, sneezing, dysphagia, dyspnea, cough, chest tightness), cardiovascular (weakness, lightheadedness, palpitations, syncope), and gastrointestinal (abdominal pain, uterine cramping, diarrhea, nausea, vomiting).

PHYSICAL EXAMINATION

Warning: *There may be little objective findings initially; the onset of urticaria of the skin and mucous membranes can be subtle!*

General. The patient may appear flushed and anxious. Seizures and cardiopulmonary arrest represent a severe reaction.

Vital signs. Look for hypotension, tachypnea, and tachycardia, which signal a serious systemic reaction. Fever should not be part of the picture and, when present, suggests an infectious etiology or serum sickness.

Skin. *Urticaria* (edema of the upper dermis) appears as raised erythematous wheals that cover most of the body; they are very pruritic and may be painful. *Angioedema* (edema of the deeper dermis and subcutaneous tissue) appears as puffy, nonpitting, noninflammed areas of the skin or mucous membranes; it is generally painless, although the patient may describe tingling. It is most prominent about the face, lips, and hands. Look for diaphoresis.

HEENT. Look for conjunctivitis, tearing, chemosis, eyelid and perioral edema, rhinorrhea, mucosal edema, swelling of the tongue, and/or uvular edema (seen with angioedema secondary to ACE inhibitors). Document if patient can handle oral secretions (drooling).

Neck. Listen for stridor (laryngeal edema) and hoarseness.

Lungs. Note any wheezing (bronchoconstriction of lower airways) and intercostal and/or supraclavicular retractions (marked respiratory distress).

Heart. Check the rate (tachycardia common) and rhythm (dysrhythmias may occur with anaphylaxis).

Abdomen. Look for mild tenderness and hyperactive bowel sounds.

Extremities. Note if extremities cold, clammy, or cyanotic (shock).

DIAGNOSTIC TESTS

There is no role for diagnostic testing in the ED; life- threatening anaphylaxis must be identified by its signs and symptoms and addressed appropriately. Once the patient is stabilized, laboratory studies can be ordered as warranted by the symptoms or age, e.g., ECG if cardiac ischemia or arrhythmia is suspected.

DIFFERENTIAL DIAGNOSIS

Any entity presenting as respiratory or cardiovascular compromise can be confused with anaphylaxis, e.g., sepsis, cardiogenic shock, asthma, upper airway infection, and pulmonary embolus. In addition, the differential includes hereditary angioedema (a rare autosomal disorder characterized by repeated episodes of angioedema of the skin, upper airway, and gut), carcinoid syndrome (a neoplasm characterized by episodes of flushing and hypotension), scombroid fish poisoning (occurs after ingestion of spoiled tuna or mahi-mahi, resulting in urticaria, nausea, vomiting, headache, and dysphagia), Chinese restaurant syndrome (seen after ingestion of monosodium glutamate and remarkable for headache and burning chest pain), anxiety reactions (globus hystericus), and factitious (self-induced or Munchausen's) anaphylaxis.

SPECIFIC CAUSES

Penicillin

Penicillin is the most common cause of life-threatening anaphylaxis in the United States, accounting for 400 deaths a year. The incidence of true allergy to penicillin is around 1%, with severe reactions occurring in 0.04% of those treated. To put these numbers in perspective, if 100,000 patients were treated with penicillin, 1,000 could develop a reaction (usually urticaria); of these, 25 would go on to anaphylaxis. Of those 25, 1 has the potential to die.

The symptoms of anaphylaxis typically begin in the first 10 to 20 min after intravenous administration; thus a patient should be observed for 30 min after injection of penicillin. Cross-reactivity with cephalosporins occurs in 3 to 5% of penicillin-allergic patients, and cephalosporins are generally deemed safe to administer, *except* in patients with a history of severe or immediate allergic reaction to penicillin. Other antibiotics are less likely to cause anaphylaxis (although sulfonamides are associated with drug rash, serum sickness, and Steven's-Johnson syndrome). As a side note, patients with infectious mononucleosis or leukemia frequently develop a maculopapular rash after treatment with ampicillin.

Local Anesthetics

Immediate hypersensitivity to local anesthetics is rare. Although many patients may state they are allergic to Novocaine given to them by their dentist, realize that their reaction may not have been an allergic one (but merely the flushing and tachycardia seen with an inadvertent intravenous administration or had a vasovagal reaction). Local anesthetics are divided into two classes: the *esters* (procaine, tetracaine, and benzocaine), which are older and have been implicated in more allergic reactions, and the newer *amides* (lidocaine, mepivacaine, bupivacaine). If the anesthetic invoking allergy is identified as an ester, it is safe to use a local anesthetic from the amide class. In addition, many of the allergic reactions to amide anesthetics stem from the preservative methylparaben, which is used in multidose vials; therefore, one could substitute preservative-free intravenous lidocaine. Another option is to use diphenhydramine (Benadryl), which has anesthetic properties—take a 1 mL (50 mg) vial and dilute it with 4 mL of normal saline to produce a 1% solution.

Radiocontrast Agents

Of patients given contrast media, 5% develop an allergic reaction and 0.1% of these are severe. Patients who have endured a prior anaphylactoid reaction to radiocontrast media have a 50%

chance of reacting again on repeat exposure. Common allergies and a history of asthma may also place the patient at increased risk. Two alternatives for patients at risk are delaying the procedure for 12 hr and pretreating with steroids or to use the newer low-osmolarity contrast agents, which possess a significantly lower reaction rate (these agents are expensive but are useful in high-risk patients who require an emergent study with contrast).

Hymenoptera Stings

Insect stings from the order Hymenoptera (bee, wasp, yellow jacket, hornet, and fire ants) are the second most common cause of anaphylactic death in the United States. While 90% of insect stings occur in patients < 20 years old, 90% of the fatalities befall those > 20 years old. *There have been several reports associating acute myocardial infarction with acute allergic reactions to Hymenoptera stings!* Patients who experience an allergic reaction to insect stings should be referred to an allergist for immunotherapy.

Latex Allergy

In this age of universal precautions, the diagnosis of latex allergy has become more common. While many health care workers develop a nonimmune-mediated reaction to the stabilizers and antioxidants impregnated in surgical gloves, a significant number of individuals develop classic IgE hypersensitivity. Onset is often insidious, beginning with a hand dermatitis accompanied by pruritus, which can progress to full-blown anaphylaxis.

TREATMENT

All patients with suspected anaphylaxis should be triaged emergently to a room capable of resuscitation, placed on a cardiac monitor, and given supplemental oxygen (maintain $Po_2 > 60$ mm Hg or $O_2sat > 90\%$).

The first priority as in all emergencies is the *airway—it is mandatory to ensure airway patency.* Most deaths from anaphylaxis result from asphyxia due to laryngeal edema, bronchospasm, and/or mucous hypersecretion. *It is always better to intubate early than late,* as the anatomy can become rapidly distorted by impending laryngeal edema. If intubation is not possible, consider cricothyroidotomy or needle cricothyrotomy with percutaneous jet ventilation (see section 21.3). Patients with life-threatening ACE inhibitor–induced angioedema or hereditary angioedema may not respond to pharmacological measures (epinephrine, antihistamines, steroids) and will require aggressive airway management.

Epinephrine is the drug of choice in treating anaphylaxis; it both inhibits the release of mediators from mast cells and basophils and reverses bronchoconstriction and vasodilation. In patients who are normotensive, with mild or moderate symptoms, epinephrine is given as a 0.3- to 0.5-mL (0.01 mL/kg of a 1:1000 solution, up to 0.5 mL) dose SQ or IM (there is a risk of skin slough when given intramuscularly). Doses may be repeated every 10 to 20 min.

For patients *in extremis*—those with severe respiratory symptoms, or blood pressure less than 70 mm Hg—epinephrine should be administered intravenously to ensure adequate absorption. It is best to give intravenous epinephrine slowly in a dilute solution to avoid exacerbation of hypertension, tachycardia, chest pain, and ventricular arrhythmias. Make a 1:100,000 solution by diluting 0.1 mL of 1:1000 epinephrine with 9.9 mL of NS and infuse over 5 to 10 min.

While epinephrine can provoke cardiac ischemia in patients at risk (cardiac patients and the elderly), this should not preclude its use if upper airway obstruction is present or hypotension is unresponsive to volume infusion. The key to avoiding problems is to carefully monitor the patient's rhythm and blood pressure and titrate the drip as necessary. In the patient in extremis without intravenous access, give the epinephrine via the endotracheal tube (0.3 to 0.5 mg of a 1:10,000 solution) or inject 0.3 to 0.5 mg of a 1:10,000 solution into the rich plexus of veins under the tongue.

For patients who remain hypotensive after epinephrine, administer normal saline (up to 2 L). Because of increased vascular permeability, monitor for pulmonary edema. Patients on β-blockers are at an increased risk for more severe reactions (hypotension is usually profound and may occur with a relative bradycardia as well as increased bronchospasm) and may be refractory to the usual epinephrine doses. Additional measures to override the β-blocker effect include the use of higher doses of epinephrine, dopamine, norepinephrine infusion, or *glucagon*. Glucagon can be given as a single 1-mg in 1-mL dose or as an infusion of 1 mg in 100 mL of D_5W at 5 to 15 mL/min. The main side effects of glucagon are nausea and vomiting.

For bronchospasm, use nebulized *metaproterenol* (5%; 0.3 mL in 2.5 mL NS) or albuterol (0.5%; 0.5 mL in 2.5 mL NS). The doses of inhaled β-agonist can be repeated every 20 min. An additional inhalational therapy is ipratropium bromide (1 mg in 2.0 mL NS). It is best to avoid aminophylline, as it confers no additional benefit to β-agonist therapy.

Supplemental drugs for anaphylaxis include *corticosteroids* and *H1* or *H2 antagonists.* These drugs do *not* confer immediate clinical benefit, but instead they help to diminish or shorten the manifestations of anaphylaxis. Choices of corticosteroids include *methylprednisolone* (125 to 250 mg IV and *hydrocortisone* (250 to 1000 mg IV). Doses can be repeated in 6 hr. The usual H1 antagonist choice is *diphenhydramine* (1 mg/ kg IV or IM; the usual dose in adults is 50 mg; give intravenously in hypotensive patients). Some authors have found additional benefit by using the H2 antagonist *cimetidine* (300 mg IV, IM, or PO).

If the route of entry was an extremity, local measures can be attempted to decrease systemic absorption; these include the application of cold compresses and elevation of the extremity. For insect sting allergy (if seen within 1 hr), apply a tourniquet proximal to the site of the sting (do not leave on for longer than 10 min), inject aqueous epinephrine (0.15 mL SQ of 1:1000 solution) into the site of the sting to slow absorption, and remove the stinger (presence of a stinger usually means the culprit was a honey bee). *Do not grasp the stinger with forceps* (you risk contracting the venom sac and forcing more venom into body), *instead scrape the stinger in a side-to-side motion in a direction aimed away from the direction in which the stinger points.*

In patients with a food allergy, consider use of *activated charcoal* to decrease absorption.

ADMISSION CRITERIA

Disposition is based on the severity of the reaction, the patient's age and underlying physiological reserve, and the rapidity of resolution of symptoms. *Any patient with a life-threatening reaction,* i.e., shock or upper airway compromise, requires admission and observation for 24 hr, since delayed reactions and recurrence of symptoms can occur. *Patients who require repeat therapy,* i.e., more than two injections of epinephrine, *or show worsening of symptoms in the ED* should also be admitted. It is prudent to admit *elderly, debilitated, or cardiac patients who have experienced a systemic reaction. Patients with continuing life-threatening signs, those requiring intravenous epinephrine, and patients with β-blocker-accentuated anaphylaxis* should be admitted to a critical care bed.

DISCHARGE

Patients who respond rapidly to initial therapeutic measures and remain stable during a 3- to 4-hr observation period can be discharged home. Patients with systemic reactions should be placed on at least a 3- to 7-day course of corticosteroids (prednisone, 40 to 60 mg OD) and antihistamines (diphenhydramine or hydroxyzine; 25 to 50 mg q 6 hr for 72 hr). In addition, all patients should be referred to an allergy specialist and given a prescription for an epinephrine autoinjector (EpiPen or Ana-Kit).

Suggested Readings

Barna JS, Frable MA: Life-threatening angioedema. Otolaryngology 1990; 103:795–798.

Bochner BS, Lichtenstein LM: Anaphylaxis. N Engl J Med 1991;324: 1784–1789.

Chapter 9

Infectious Disease

9.1 MENINGITIS

Description

Infection of the meninges may result from *hematogenous dissemination* (bacteremia) through *direct inoculation* (iatrogenic dural defects following neurosurgery or lumbar puncture) or by *extension of parameningeal infections* (otitis media, sinusitis). In the United States, the primary etiologies of meningitis are bacterial and viral, with the majority of cases of bacterial meningitis in adults arising from *Streptococcus pneumoniae* or *Neisseria meningitidis* infection. The specific microbe responsible for bacterial meningitis depends on the patient's age and underlying medical status, with the definitive diagnosis being determined by *cerebrospinal fluid* (CSF) findings.

Clinically, it is helpful to separate meningitis into *bacterial* and *nonbacterial* causes. Classic bacterial meningitis displays a rapid onset (hours) without a prodromal period. Typically, viral meningitis is identified with a prodromal period (several days), with patients generally appearing less ill than patients afflicted with bacterial meningitis. In addition, both fungal and mycobacterial meningitides possess protracted onsets (weeks to months).

History

A brief and directed history and physical examination are indicated when meningitis is suspected. Consider meningitis in any patient who exhibits a combination of any of the following signs or symptoms: fever, chills, headache, myalgias/arthralgias, altered mental status, focal neurologic deficit, photophobia, nuchal rigidity, and seizures. Findings in the elderly are often subtle, such as altered mental status. Additional significant history includes the duration of symptoms, antecedent infection (particularly otitis media, sinusitis, upper or lower respiratory infection, pharyngitis), history of head trauma, epidemic exposure (family member, roommate, day-care center classmate, military training recruit), past medical history (immunocompromising systemic illnesses), and social history (alcoholism, drug use, homelessness).

Physical Examination

General. Evaluate overall appearance and level of consciousness.

Vital signs. Document fever, tachypnea, hypotension, and hypertension accompanying bradycardia *(Cushing's reflex)*.

HEENT. Examine for evidence of head trauma or surgery, papilledema, pupillary defects, or concurrent infections (otitis, pharyngitis, sinusitis).

Neck. Test for nuchal rigidity (*Brudzinski's sign:* passive flexion of the neck induces flexion of the thigh; *Kerning's sign:* flexion of the hip and straightening of the leg results in neck flexion and resistance in the leg). **Note:** *Absence of these findings does not rule out meningitis.*

Lungs. Auscultate for rhonchi, rales, and signs of consolidation.

Heart. Listen for murmurs.

Neurologic. Examine for focal deficits (cranial nerve, motor, sensory, cerebellar, reflex deficits). Carefully note mental status.

Skin. Inspect for petechiae (meningococcemia), purpura, and other characteristic lesions (herpes, leptospirosis).

Diagnostic Tests

Lumbar Puncture

A lumbar puncture (LP) is the cornerstone for establishing the diagnosis of meningitis. Culture the blood and administer intravenous antibiotics if any delay for LP is anticipated. Immediate LP is *relatively contraindicated* in the following scenarios:

- Signs of focality on physical exam;
- Suspected HIV disease;
- Evidence of increased intracranial pressure;
- Hemodynamic instability;
- Infection overlying puncture site; and
- Bleeding diathesis or liver disease (check coagulation studies and platelet count).

Obtain a CT scan of the head before doing an LP in the following circumstances:

- Focal neurologic deficit;
- Evidence of subarachnoid hemorrhage;
- Papilledema; and
- History of head trauma.

Record *opening pressure* with the legs straight once the needle is inserted. Ordinarily, CSF pressure varies from 5 to 19 cm H_2O, when the patient is in the lateral recumbent position. Normal CSF is clear and colorless. Cloudy CSF suggests infection, inflammation, or bleeding *(xanthochromia)*. To distinguish true CNS bleeding from blood resulting from a traumatic LP, request a cell count on tubes one and four. A persistent elevation of RBCs in tubes one and four favors a CSF bleed, while a decline in RBC counts from tube one to tube four indicates a traumatic tap.

Partially treated meningitis presents with variable CSF findings (Table 9.1.1). Collect three or four tubes of CSF for the following laboratory tests:

Tube 1 Gram stain and culture
Tube 2 Protein and glucose
Tube 3 Cell count and differential
Tube 4 Special studies as indicated (VDRL, India ink cryptococcal, antigen, CIE, etc.)

Note: The normal *CSF:serum glucose* ratio is 0.6. CSF glucose levels are regularly normal in aseptic meningitis, brain abscess, and subdural hematoma but are decreased with bacterial, fungal, and tuberculous meningitis.

Other Tests

Blood cultures. Obtain before initiation of antibiotics (identify offending organism 50 to 80% of the time).

Laboratory tests. Request a CBC and differential (leukocytosis commonly accompanies bacterial meningitis), platelets, SMA-7, PT, and PTT.

Countercurrent immunoelectrophoresis (CIE). Capable of identifying the presence of *S. pneumoniae, Haemophilus influenzae,* or *Neisseria* spp. on samples of blood, urine, or CSF.

Additional studies. Further testing such as x-rays of the chest, sinuses, or mastoids; urinalysis; and CT scan of the head may be necessary.

Table 9.1.1
CSF Findings in Meningitis

Result	Opening Pressure (mm H_2O)	Cell Count (cells/mm)	Glucose (mg/100 mL)	Protein (mg/dL)	Gram Stain
Normal	90–180	< 5 lymphs	50–75	15–40	–
Bacterial	200–350	0–5000 (> 80% PMN)	< 50	100–1000	+ for organism 80% of time
Viral meningitis	100–250	0–500 lymphs	50–75	50–100	–
Tuberculous meningitis	180–300	0–300 lymphs	< 40	100–200	+ for AFB stain 50% of time
Listeria meningitis	90–250	10–300 PMNs (monocytosis)	< 50	50–200	+ for organism 25% of time
Cryptococcal meningitis	180–300	10–500 pleocytosis	< 50	50–200	India ink

Specific Conditions

Immunosuppressed hosts are susceptible to a variety of bacterial organisms, either alone or in combination *(Listeria monocytogenes, Pseudomonas aeruginosa, Staphylococcus aureus, S. pneumoniae,* Gram-negative bacilli, streptococci, anaerobes, TB, *Actinobacter* spp., and coagulase-negative staphylococci), along with nonbacterial entities (cryptococcus, toxoplasmosis, herpes).

Patients with a *CSF shunt* have almost a 25% incidence of CNS infection. Implicated microbes include *Staphylococcus epidermidis, S. aureus,* streptococci, and mixed infections (including Gram-negative enteric organisms, diphtheroids, and *Bacillus* spp.).

Head trauma (skull fracture or facial trauma) patients are vulnerable to CNS disease when there is a CSF leak or communication of brain and or meninges with the external environment. Recurrent meningitis (especially with *S. pneumoniae* or *S. aureus*) should raise suspicion for CSF leak in any patient with prior head or facial trauma.

Postoperative neurosurgical patients are susceptible to nosocomial infections. Primary organisms implicated are Gram-negative enteric bacilli, *Pseudomonas* spp., *S. aureus, S. epidermidis,* and streptococci.

Elderly patients (those over 50 years old) have an increased risk of *L. monocytogenes,* Gram-negative enterics, *H. influenzae,* and tuberculosis.

HIV-infected adults are disposed to infection by *S. pneumoniae,* Enterobacteriaceae, *H. influenzae, L. monocytogenes, Pseudomonas* spp. as well as *Cryptococcus neoformans, Mycobacterium tuberculosis,* syphilis, and HIV aseptic meningitis.

Patients with *sickle cell disease* or *diabetes* are more prone to enteric Gram-negative meningitis.

Aseptic meningitis is a designation encompassing meningeal infections when a microbe cannot be readily identified. It includes viral etiologies (*enteroviruses,* particularly coxsackievirus, echovirus), bacterial causes (syphilis, *Treponema pallidum;* Lyme disease; *Rickettsia rickettsii),* and fungal and protozoan infections. Affected patients usually complain of an oppressive frontal or retroorbital headache. Herpes simplex is one of the few treatable viral CNS infections; it exhibits nonspecific symptoms (sudden headache, subtle behavioral changes).

Tuberculous meningitis typically follows an indolent, chronic course secondary to hematogenous spread or direct extension from a granuloma.

Treatment

Foremost, assess and stabilize the ABCs (establish intravenous access, provide supplemental oxygen, and initiate cardiac monitoring). Recognize *life-threatening* conditions that necessitate immediate treatment, such as *shock* (fluid therapy, pressors), *seizures* (anticonvulsant therapy), *cerebral edema* (hyperventilation, diuretics), and *head and neck trauma* (cervical spine immobilization).

An immediate LP is mandated (unless contraindications exist). If an LP must be delayed for a CT scan, perform blood cultures and start antibiotics first. The antibiotic regimen depends on the patient's age and immune status and the probable etiology. More than 90% of meningitis cases in adults arise from *pneumococcal* or *meningococcal* infection. However, *L. monocytogenes* is still a concern. In addition to giving antibiotics, provide supportive therapy (analgesia, antipyretics). Carefully, monitor intake and output (I&O) to avoid overhydration and subsequent worsening of cerebral edema.

Empirical therapy for 18- to 50-year-old *previously healthy adults* includes a third-generation cephalosporin (*cefotaxime,* 2.0 g IV q 4 hr, or *ceftriaxone,* 2.0 g IV q 12 hr) plus *ampicillin* (1.0 g IV q 6 hr) plus *rifampin* (600 mg PO once a day) in patients with *Neisseria* to eradicate the carrier state. Currently, there are no studies indicating any benefit of corticosteroid therapy in adults. Ampicillin is discontinued if *L. monocytogenes* is ruled out. In patients with a major penicillin allergy, use *chloramphenicol* (1.0 to 1.5 g IV q 6 hr) plus *trimethoprim-sulfamethoxazole* (TMP-SMX; 5.0 mg/kg SMX IV q 6 hr).

In *adults older than 50, alcoholics,* and *patients with debilitating comorbid medical illness* with suspected community-acquired meningitis, it is important to cover for *S. pneumoniae,* Enterobacteriaceae, *H. influenzae,* and *Listeria* spp. Use a third-generation cephalosporin (*cefotaxime,* 2.0 g IV q 4 hr, or *ceftriaxone,* 2.0 g IV q 12 hr) plus *ampicillin* (1.0 g IV q 6 hr). Provide *vancomycin* (1.0 g IV q 12 hr) for resistant *S. pneumoniae.* Patients with a severe penicillin allergy are treated as outlined above (chloramphenicol plus TMP-SMX).

In adult patients with a *ventriculoperitoneal or other CNS shunt* infection give *vancomycin* (1.0 g IV q 12 hr) plus *rifampin* (600 mg

PO once a day). If Gram-negative bacteria are seen on the Gram stain of the CSF, add a third-generation cephalosporin (*cefotaxime,* 2.0 g IV q 4 hr, or *ceftriaxone,* 2.0 g IV q 12 hr). Consult with neurosurgery; frequently, the shunt will need to be replaced.

For *HIV-1 infected* patients with suspected meningitis, use the regimen outlined above for adults older than 50. In addition, consider *amphotericin* (0.6 mg/kg IV once a day in 500 mL NS over 3 hr) for cryptococcal meningitis.

Offer *chemoprophylaxis* with *rifampin* (600 mg q 12 hr for 2 days) to individuals intimately exposed to patients with suspected *N. meningitidis* or *H. influenzae* infection. A single dose of a fluoroquinolone is also effective prophylactic therapy in patients unable to take rifampin.

Admission Criteria

All patients with suspected or proven bacterial meningitis require admission. In the event of a nondiagnostic LP, the procedure should be repeated in 8 to 12 hr. For patients with presumed viral meningitis and those who were started on antibiotics as an outpatient, the decision to use or withhold antibiotics can be very difficult, especially when the CSF values are nondiagnostic. Discuss subsequent therapy with the consultant.

Suggested Readings

Sanford JP, Gilbert DN, Sande MA: The Sanford guide to antimicrobial therapy. 25th ed. Dallas: Antimicrobial Inc., 1995.

Talan DA, Zibulewsky J: Relationship of clinical presentation to time for antibiotics for the emergency department management of suspected bacterial meningitis. Ann Emerg Med 1993;22:1738–1739.

9.2 LOWER RESPIRATORY TRACT INFECTIONS

Pneumonia

Description

Pneumonia is an inflammatory process of the lung parenchyma. Age and host defense mechanisms determine susceptibility and etiology. Most microbes gain access to the lungs via inhalation. *Community-acquired pneumonia,* contracted outside a hospital or nursing home, is often due to bacteria. *Atypical pneumonia* also takes place in a community setting, but it is secondary to viruses, mycoplasma, or chlamydia (TWAR). *Aspiration pneumonias* occur in patients with an impaired mental status or a swallowing disorder, which leads to aspiration of oropharyngeal contents.

History

Patients with pneumonia may present with any of the following clinical findings: *fever, chills, upper respiratory infection* (URI), *productive* (purulent, rust colored, bloody sputum) or *nonproductive cough* (*Mycoplasma pneumoniae, Pneumocystis carinii,* viral pneumonias), *dyspnea, chest or abdominal pain, diarrhea, tachycardia,* and/or *lethargy.* Establish the duration of the symptoms. An insidious course is often associated with mycobacterial, fungal, or anaerobic causes. Occupational and travel histories predispose the patient to unusual etiologies, for example, psittacosis (birds), coccidioidomycosis (Southwestern United States), Q fever, brucellosis, and anthrax (livestock). *Mycoplasma pneumonia* occurs in younger adults (18 to 45 years old) and is characterized by a gradual onset, along with a protracted, nonproductive cough. *Legionnaire's disease* tends to affect elderly patients and patients with underlying illness (DM, COPD). *True rigors* are often indicative of a bacterial pneumonia (especially pneumococcal). *Night sweats* are associated with chronic pneumonias (tuberculosis, fungal disease). Inquire about underlying diseases, sexual preference, and social history (intravenous drugs, smoking, alcohol, homelessness, recent stay in prison). Recent hospitalization or residence in a nursing home facility increases the risk for Gram-negative infection *(Pseudomonas, Klebsiella, E. coli)* (Table 9.2.1)

Table 9.2.1
Common Causative Organisms in Pneumonia

Young healthy adult	*S. pneumoniae, M. pneumoniae,* viral
Elderly	*S. pneumoniae,* influenza, *M. tuberculosis, Legionella,* Gram-negative bacilli
Seizures	Anaerobes (aspiration)
Alcoholism	*S. pneumoniae,* Gram-negative bacilli *(Klebsiella)*
Diabetes mellitus	Gram-negative bacilli, *M. tuberculosis*
Chronic lung disease	*S. pneumoniae, H. influenza,* Gram-negative bacilli
AIDS	*P. carinii, S. pneumoniae, H. influenzae, M. tuberculosis*

Physical Examination

General. Observe the appearance and degree of respiratory distress. Look for clues that suggest a noninfectious illness (DVT, PE) or cachexia/lymphadenopathy (malignancy, AIDS).

Vital signs. Note presence of tachypnea, fever (in the elderly, the fever may be unimpressive early in the course), hypothermia, or hypotension (sepsis). Record a rectal temperature.

HEENT. Examine the oropharynx, sinuses, and ears. Look for oral thrush (HIV).

Neck. Note cervical adenopathy.

Lungs. Auscultate for rales, rhonchi, and wheezes along with egophony (*E* to *I* changes). Palpate and percuss for fremitus and dullness.

Heart. Listen for murmurs (endocarditis).

Abdomen. Observe for an LUQ scar (splenectomy increases the risk of encapsulated bacteria infection).

Skin. Inspect for track marks, cyanosis, mottling, and diaphoresis.

Neurologic. Presence of an altered mental status mandates evaluation for meningitis or hypoxia.

Diagnostic Tests

CBC. Check for leukocytosis with a left shift. Leukopenia may be an ominous sign.

Sputum Gram stain and culture. Ensure an adequate, noncontaminated specimen (< 10 epithelial cells per low-powered field, with > 25 PMNs). The Gram stain is somewhat reliable for *S. pneumoniae* but frequently fails to detect common pathogens (mycoplasma, chlamydia). Direct fluorescent antibody testing assists in identifying *Legionella*, mycobacteria, and *Pneumocystis*. Sputum cultures are less useful than Gram stain (cultures are negative in 45 to 50% of patients with bacterial pneumonia) but are most useful for the diagnosis of tuberculosis, *Legionella*, and endemic fungi.

CXR. Findings vary with different organisms, although it is rarely possible to reach a specific diagnosis by x-ray alone. Besides corroborating the diagnosis and extent of pneumonia, CXR helps exclude other diagnoses (e.g., CHF). Radiographic changes occasionally lag behind clinical findings.

Blood cultures. Order when bacteremia or sepsis is suspected.

Pulse oximetry. Provides a rapid, noninvasive assessment of oxygenation.

ABG. Arterial blood gas may be required in severe cases. Calculate the alveolar-arterial (PAO_2–PaO_2) gradient (see section 2.2). Hypoxia is present in more than 80% of cases of *P. carinii* (PCP), along with an elevated PAO_2–PaO_2 gradient (>20 mm Hg).

SMA. Elevation of LDH occurs with PCP and *Legionella pneumoniae.* In addition, hyponatremia often accompanies *Legionella.* In patients with serious pneumonia that requires hospitalization, establish a renal function baseline (e.g., BUN, creatinine).

Additional tests. Order *cold agglutinin (M. pneumoniae)* and *gallium scan (Pneumocystis pneumoniae)* studies when clinically indicated. Also consider diagnostic thoracentesis when effusion is present.

Treatment

Acutely ill-appearing patients require prompt intravenous access, cardiac monitoring, pulse oximetry, and supplemental oxygen. Consider the need for intubation (see section 2.2). The microbe responsible for pneumonia differs among individual populations, and the choice of the appropriate regimen is based on the patient's age, presence of comorbid conditions (COPD, diabetes, alcohol abuse), and the setting where pneumonia was acquired (community, nursing home, recent hospital admission). Current guidelines from the American Thoracic Society classify patients into one of four categories.

1. *Empirical outpatient therapy for stable patients younger than 60 years with community-acquired infection.* Use a *macrolide* antibiotic: *erythromycin* (500 mg PO QID for 10 days), *azithromycin* (1.0 g PO day 1, then 500 mg PO once a day for 5 days), or *clarithromycin* (500 mg PO BID for 10 days). For patients allergic to or unable to tolerate a macrolide, substitute *doxycycline* (100 mg PO BID for 7 to 10 days). The most common infecting organisms in this group are *S. pneumoniae, M. pneumoniae* (primarily affecting adolescents and young adults), *Chlamydia pneumoniae,* and *H. influenzae.*
2. *Patients older than 60 years or younger than 60 years with serious underlying disease* (including smokers with COPD). Use com-

bination therapy; a second-generation cephalosporin (*cefaclor,* 500 mg PO TID, or *cefuroxime,* 250 mg PO BID for 10 days), TMP-SMX (*Bactrim DS* PO BID for 10 days), or *amoxicillin-clavulanic acid* (500 mg TID for 10 days) plus a *macrolide* (see above). The most likely etiologic agents (in order of frequency) are *S. pneumoniae,* viruses, *H. influenzae,* aerobic Gram-negative bacilli, *S. aureus,* and *Legionella* in elderly patients.

3. *Any age adult with community-acquired pneumonia who is ill enough to require hospitalization* (but not ICU level care). Recommended antibiotics regimens include a parenteral second- or third-generation cephalosporin (*cefuroxime,* 750 mg to 1.5 g IV q 8 hr; *cefotaxime,* 1 to 2 g IV q 8 hr; *or ceftriaxone,* 1 g IV q 12 hr) or a β-lactam/β-lactamase inhibitor (*ticarcillin clavulanate,* 3.1 g IV q 4 to 8 hr, or *ampicillin* and *sulbactam,* 1.5 to 3.0 g IV q 6 hr) plus a *macrolide* if *Legionella* suspected. *S. pneumoniae, H. influenzae,* polymicrobes (including anaerobes), aerobic Gram-negative bacilli, *Legionella, S. aureus, C. pneumoniae,* and viruses account for the majority of cases of community-acquired pneumonia that require hospitalization.
4. *For critically ill patients requiring hospitalization in an intensive care setting.* Use a *macrolide* antibiotic plus a third-generation cephalosporin with antipseudomonal activity (*ceftazidime,* 1 g IV q 8 hr, or *cefoperazone,* 2 to 4 g IV in divided doses q 12 hr), or other antipseudomonal agents such as *imipenem-cilastin* (500 to 1000 mg IV q 6 to 8 hr), or *ciprofloxacin* (400 mg IV q 12 hr). Note that treatment with ciprofloxacin or imipenem-cilastin alone is *not* sufficient coverage.

Aspiration pneumonia is common in patients with preexisting neurologic or esophageal disease, those with a history of ethanol or drug abuse, and those debilitated with an impaired mental status. Preferential involvement of the dependent portions of the lung is seen (posterior segment of the upper lobes, superior segments of the lower lobes). Frequently, anaerobes are the causative organism with an indolent clinical course. Sputum Gram stains and cultures are often unreliable. *Clindamycin* (450 to 900 mg IV q 8 hr) provides excellent empirical coverage against anaerobes. Aspiration pneumonia in a nursing home setting requires additional Gram-negative coverage: *cefotetan* (1 to 2 g IV q 12 hr) or a β-lactam/β-lactamase inhibitor (*ticarcillin clavu-*

lanate, 3.1 g IV q 4 to 8 hr, or *ampicillin* and *sulbactam,* 1.5 to 3.0 g IV q 6 hr).

Consider *PCP* in all *HIV patients* with fever and pulmonary complaints (cough, dyspnea). Order a CXR (diffuse or perihilar infiltrates, often, but not always, interstitial) along with a pulse oximetry reading when screening patients for PCP. Oral therapy is adequate for patients with mild disease (PaO_2 > 70 mm Hg, PAO_2–PaO_2 gradient < 35 mm Hg, LDH < 220 U/L). Severe disease obligates hospitalization along with parenteral therapy. The initial drug of choice is *TMP-SMX* (15 to 20 mg/kg/day TMP, PO divided into BID dosage). However, the combination of AIDS and TMP-SMX may induce severe side effects (hyperkalemia, rash, hepatitis, neutropenia). Alternative regimens include *TMP* (5 mg/kg PO q 6 hr) plus *dapsone* (50 mg PO BID), *clindamycin* (450 mg PO q 6 hr; or 600 mg IV q 6 hr) plus *primaquine* (15 mg PO once a day), or *atovaquone*(750 mg PO TID with food). Supplemental early use of *prednisone* (initiate dosing 15 to 30 min before antimicrobial administration) appears to lessen the risk of respiratory failure and death when PCP is associated with a PaO_2 < 70 mm Hg, and a PAO_2–PaO_2gradient > 35 mm Hg. Other frequent pulmonary infections occurring in AIDS patients include *tuberculosis* (follows a more fulminant course in AIDS patients), *bacterial pneumonia* (a high frequency of recurrent pneumonia is common with community-acquired microbes, including *S. pneumoniae, H. influenzae, Moraxella catarrhalis, M. pneumoniae,* and *Legionella*), and opportunistic infections *(Histoplasma capsulatum, Coccidioides immitis, Mycobacterium avium).*

Tuberculosis in AIDS patients is often multidrug resistant, and therapy should be initiated in conjunction with an infectious disease specialist, as should treatment for opportunistic infections. Therapy for bacterial pneumonia in AIDS patients is essentially the same as that for a normal host, although one may want to combine TMP-SMX with a macrolide antibiotic. The new macrolide *azithromycin* is particularly useful in HIV-infected patients because it does not interact with AZT, ddI, or terfenadine.

Admission Criteria

Although no hard guidelines exist concerning the need for hospitalization, the American Thoracic Society recommends that admission for patients with community-acquired pneumonia be *strongly considered when one or more of the following risk factors* are present:

- Age over 65 years old or social conditions that preclude safe outpatient care;
- Hospitalization within the past year for pneumonia or the need for mechanical ventilation;
- Significant comorbid illness (e.g., malnutrition, severe COPD, poorly controlled DM, CHF, chronic renal failure, liver disease, suspected aspiration pneumonia, altered mental status, post-splenectomy status, and chronic alcoholism);
- Presence of any of the following signs in adults: respiratory rate > 30/min, diastolic blood pressure < 60 mm Hg, systolic blood pressure < 90 mm Hg, temperature > 38.3°C (101°F), or suspected extrapulmonary sites of infection; and
- The following ancillary findings: WBC count < 4,000 mm^3 or > 30,000 mm^3, an absolute PMN count < 1,000 mm^3, PaO_2 < 60 or $PaCO_2$ > 50 on room air, a creatinine > 1.2 or BUN > 20, a hemoglobin < 9 or hematocrit < 30%, increased PT or PTT, decreased platelets (< 100,000 mm^3), presence of fibrin split products (> 1:40), or a CXR that reveals multilobe involvement, a cavitary lesion, or a pleural effusion.

In addition, *patients with any of the following clinical findings* should be considered intensive care unit candidates: respiratory rate > 30/min on admission, severe respiratory failure (PaO_2:FIO_2 ratio < 250), need for mechanical ventilation, CXR findings of bilateral or multilobar involvement, shock (systolic pressure < 90 mm Hg or diastolic pressure < 60 mm Hg), need for vasopressors, or oliguria (urine output < 20 mL/hr).

The four main predictors of serious disease in HIV-infected patients with suspected PCP pneumonia include (1) diffuse or perihilar infiltrates on CXR, (2) presence of mouth lesions, (3) lactate dehydrogenase > 220 U/L, and (4) erythrocyte sedimentation rate > 50 mm/hr. Furthermore, a PaO_2 < 70 mm Hg or PAO_2–PaO_2gradient > 35 mm Hg generally obligates admission.

Acute Bronchitis

Description

Acute bronchitis is an inflammatory condition of the tracheobronchial tree, resulting from respiratory infections with viruses (rhinovirus, coronavirus, influenza, adenovirus), *M. pneumoniae*, *C. pneumoniae*, and rarely *Bordetella pertussis*. *Mycoplasma* bronchitis is usually seen in young adults, occurring among close contacts and family members during summer and fall.

History

Bronchitis is characterized by cough with or without sputum production that is usually preceded by an upper respiratory infection. Sputum may be clear, purulent, or blood tinged. Fever may or may not be present. Patient may note a burning chest pain exacerbated by coughing. Bronchitis occurs more frequently and lasts longer in smokers.

Physical Examination

General. Toxic appearance is rare and if present suggests pneumonia or more severe illness.

Vital signs. Check for fever.

HEENT. Examine for signs of concomitant URI; presence of bullous myringitis suggests *Mycoplasma*.

Lungs. The lungs should be clear to auscultation and percussion.

Diagnostic Tests

CXR. Indicated when respiratory symptoms are accompanied by a temperature > 37.8°C (100.4°F), pulse > 100 bpm, and abnormal lung exam.

Sputum Gram stain. This may be helpful in identifying *H. influenzae* in patients with COPD. However, since most cases are viral, Gram stains are rarely necessary.

Treatment

The mainstay of treatment for acute bronchitis is supportive: cough expectorant, analgesia, and adequate hydration. For patients considered at high risk for pneumonia (smokers, COPD, CHF, cirrhosis, DM, patients with a tracheostomy, elderly) who present with increased cough and purulent sputum production, it is reasonable to start empirical treatment with antibiotics. Choices include *TMP-SMX* (Bactrim DS BID for 7 days), *macrolides* (*erythromycin,* 500 mg PO QID for 7 days; *azithromycin,*

500 mg PO day 1 then 250 mg PO daily for days 2 to 5; or *clarithromycin,* 500 mg PO BID for 7 days), or *tetracycline* (500 mg QID for 7 days). When a protracted course of acute bronchitis (> 3 weeks) occurs even in an otherwise healthy patient, antibiotic therapy is indicated. Smoking cessation should always be encouraged.

Tuberculosis

Description

After years of being kept in check in the United States, tuberculosis is on the rise (especially in urban settings), with emergence of resistant strains. Transmission is via aerosolized droplets. The majority of infected patients develop an asymptomatic, self-limited pneumonia, which heals with granuloma formation, scarring, and calcification. Only 15% of patients develop active disease, with most cases remaining dormant. Patients with impaired immunity (AIDS, DM, malnourishment, steroid therapy) exhibit an increased risk of active disease.

History

Active disease can affect several organ systems. The lungs are the most common target organ with four forms of pulmonary disease: *tuberculosis pneumonia, pleurisy, cavitary disease,* and *miliary disease.* Clinical manifestations of pulmonary tuberculosis are quite variable, often creating confusion in determining the diagnosis. Classical symptoms are *fever, night sweats, malaise, weight loss,* and *productive cough.* Pleuritic chest pain and hemoptysis occur with progressive disease. Lung involvement tends to be more extensive when an underlying HIV infection is present, along with a higher incidence of extrapulmonary manifestations of TB and combined infections (e.g., *M. avium).*

Physical Examination

General. Observe general appearance and presence of cachexia.
Vital signs. Check for fever.
HEENT. Note tracheal shift and lymph adenopathy.
Lungs. Listen for apical posttussive rales, tubular breath sounds, or decreased breath sounds.

Neurologic. Presence of cranial nerve palsies, altered mental status, or meningeal signs in patients suspected of harboring pulmonary TB should prompt a work-up for tuberculous meningitis.

Diagnostic Tests

CXR. Postprimary TB is more common in the apical segments of the upper lobes and superior segment of the lower lobes, with right upper lobe cavitation being classic. Additional x-ray findings include diffuse patchy densities, pleural effusion, hilar adenopathy, calcific and noncalcific granulomas, and miliary nodules (2- to 4-mm lesions) in the lower lobes.

Liver enzymes. Monitor liver enzymes for patients receiving antimicrobial therapy for TB.

Fluorescent antibody stain and Ziehl-Neelsen stain of the sputum. Assists in identifying acid-fast organisms. Confirm with cultures.

PPD. Cellular immunity measured by verifying skin sensitivity to PPD. However, false-negative reactions take place with systemic TB, overwhelming illness, and immunodeficiency.

Treatment

TB requires long-term therapy (6 months or longer), along with continuous medical supervision. Three- or four-drug therapy is usually needed, with the most commonly used agents being *isoniazid (INH), rifampin, pyrazinamide (PZA), streptomycin, and ethambutol.* Significant drug toxicity may arise (see Table 9.2.2).

Admission Criteria

Notify the public health department when you suspect TB infection. *Any patient suspected of recent TB infection ought to be isolated* (private room, negative pressure, accessibility of high-efficacy masks). Discuss the need for admission with the ID consultant. Admission is generally *indicated for the following patients: those with TB proceeding to respiratory compromise, those with significant hemoptysis, debilitated patients, those with adverse effects to chemotherapeutic agents, patients form whom you are unable to establish diagnosis* (arrange for bronchoscopy), and *those who have previously demon-*

Table 9.2.2
Drugs Used in the Treatment of Tuberculosis in Adults

Drug	Dosage	Adverse Effects
Isoniazid	5–10 mg/kg, up to 300 mg PO once a day	Hepatitis (more common in patients older than 35 and in alcoholics), peripheral neuritis, and seizures (seen with overdoses)
Rifampin	10–20 mg/kg up to 600 mg PO once a day	Orange discoloration of urine and secretions, hepatotoxicity, flu-like illness, and thrombocytopenia
Pyrazinamide	1.5 g PO once a day if < 50 kg; 2.0 g PO once a day if > 50 kg	Hepatotoxicity, rash, hyperuricemia, GI intolerance
Ethambutol	15 mg/kg PO once a day	Optic neuritis (color vision first affected), skin rash
Streptomycin	750 mg IM once a day if < 50 kg; 1.0 g IM once a day if > 50 kg	Ototoxicity (auditory and vestibular), nephrotoxicity

strated noncompliance. Some communities have instituted supervised intermittent outpatient therapy for TB.

Suggested Readings

American Thoracic Society: Guidelines for the initial management of adults with community-acquired pneumonia. Am Rev Respir Dis 1993;148:1418–1426.

Katz MH, Baron RB, Grady D: Risk stratification of ambulatory patients suspected of *Pneumocystis pneumonia.* Arch Intern Med 1991;151:105–110.

Mahmoudi A, Iseman MD: Pitfalls in the care of patients with tuberculosis. JAMA 1993;270:65–68.

9.3 CARDIAC INFECTIONS

Infective Endocarditis

Description

Endocarditis characterizes a microbial infection of the heart valves and/or endothelium. Initial manifestations are often vague, necessitating a high index of suspicion. Fever is the one universal finding. Occasionally, manifestations of embolic disease appear, such as stroke or splenic artery embolism with resultant infarction. Emboli tend to be small, and may cause infrequent but diagnostically useful findings *(Roth spots, Osler's nodes, Janeway lesions, subconjunctival hemorrhage).*

Patients with rheumatic heart disease, congenital heart disease, mitral valve prolapse, hypertrophic cardiomyopathy, and vascular grafts as well as intravenous drug abusers (IVDAs) are all at increased risk for *native valve endocarditis.* In addition, the presence of a prosthetic valve increases vulnerability to endocarditis. Staphylococci (both coagulase positive and coagulase negative) account for most cases of early (within 2 months of surgery) *prosthetic valve endocarditis,* while streptococci typically accompany late-onset infection.

Endocarditis can be further subclassified into acute and subacute forms. *Subacute bacterial endocarditis* (SBE) displays an insidious onset, overcoming previously damaged valves of the left side of the heart. Responsible organisms (streptococci viridans, enterococcus) tend to be less virulent. *Acute bacterial endocarditis* (ABE) exhibits a more fulminant course and is capable of infecting previously undamaged heart valves or endothelium. Responsible microbes include *S. aureus, S. pneumoniae. S. pyogenes,* and *N. meningitidis.*

Endocarditis associated with IVDA commonly strikes the right side of the heart (tricuspid valve) and is easily confused for pulmonary disease. While *S. aureus* is the most common etiologic agent, *Pseudomonas* and fungal infections (especially *Candida*) are capable of causing infection in IVDAs.

History

The clinical manifestations of infective endocarditis are protean and determined by the etiology of the microbe, whether the infection is superimposed on preexisting abnormal cardiac structures, and the source of the infecting organism. Constitutional symptoms (low-grade fever, weakness, myalgias, arthralgias, back pain, fatigue, anorexia, and weight loss) commonly accompany SBE infection.

In contrast, manifestations of ABE are usually more clear-cut with an abrupt onset of high fever, shaking chills, pleuritic chest pain, shortness of breath, and night sweats. Musculoskeletal complaints (i.e., back pain, diffuse myalgias, arthralgias) are also frequent with ABE.

Inquire about recent dental procedures, invasive gastrointestinal tests or genitourinary instrumentation, and recent bacterial infection as well as intravenous drug abuse.

Physical Examination

Vital signs. Assess for fever, tachypnea, tachycardia, or hypotension.

HEENT. Inspect fundi for Roth spots and mucosa for petechiae.

Neck. Examine for JVD, prominent V waves (tricuspid insufficiency), and nuchal rigidity.

Lungs. Listen for rales (CHF) or friction rub (pulmonary infarction secondary to emboli).

Heart. Despite presence in about 85% of cases of endocarditis, heart murmurs are not easily heard in the ED; the murmurs of tricuspid (more common in IVDAs) or pulmonic insufficiency are difficult to auscultate, while the murmurs of acute mitral regurgitation and aortic insufficiency tend to be brief and easily obscured. Stenotic murmurs rarely accompany endocarditis. In addition, it is difficult to judge a change in the intensity of a murmur in patients with prior valvular disease or prosthetic valves.

Abdomen. Check for hepatosplenomegaly and localized tenderness.

Extremities. Indicate presence of clubbing, cyanosis, or track marks. Gauge capillary refill.

Skin. Observe for appearance of pallor, petechiae, subungual splinter hemorrhages, Osler's nodes (painful raised nodules on fingers), or Janeway lesions (nontender red papules on palms and soles).

Neurologic. Note focal deficit or altered level of consciousness (arises from CNS emboli, mycotic aneurysm, brain abscess, or meningitis).

Diagnostic Tests

CBC. Note if leukocytosis with a left shift is present.

SMA. BUN and creatinine may be elevated in low-output failure or renal failure.

Urinalysis. Look for proteinuria, hematuria, or red cell casts.

PT. Elevated with DIC.

Blood cultures. Obtain three sets of blood cultures at 10-min intervals, if possible (preferably before antibiotic therapy). The recovery of the infecting organism depends on the volume of the blood cultured: at least 10 mL and preferably 20 mL should be collected with each sample.

ECG. May be abnormal due to coronary artery emboli or myocardial abscess.

CXR. May suggest septic embolization to lungs.

ESR. Frequently elevated.

Cardiac ultrasonography. Echocardiogram has assumed an increasing role in the diagnosis and treatment of infective endocarditis. Besides detecting vegetations > 5 mm in size, information concerning the degree of valvular destruction and its hemodynamic effects is obtained. However, a negative echo does *not* exclude the diagnosis of endocarditis.

Treatment

Provide basic life support and maintain hemodynamic stability. Urgent cardiac surgery is indicated in the following settings: (1) hemodynamic compromise, CHF, or valvular obstruction; (2) uncontrolled infection (fungal endocarditis, lack of effective antimicrobial agents); (3) unstable prosthetic valve; and (4) major embolization. Initiate antibiotic therapy for acutely ill patients immediately after obtaining blood cultures.

Native valve endocarditis. Empirically treat with *aqueous penicillin G* (10 to 20 million U/day continuous IV or divided q 4 hr) or ampicillin 3.0 g IV q 4 hr plus *nafcillin* 2.0 g IV q 4 hr and *gentamicin* (1 mg/kg IV q 8 hr, if normal renal function). An alternative regimen is *vancomycin* (1.0 g q 12 hr IV, up to 2 g/day) and *gentamicin* (1 mg/kg IV q 8 hr).

For *prosthetic valve endocarditis* the initial treatment is with *vancomycin* plus *gentamicin* and *ampicillin* as above. An alternate treatment uses a third-generation *cephalosporin* (cefotaxime, 12 g/day IV; ceftizoxime, 12 g/day IV; or ceftriaxone, 4 g/day) plus *vancomycin* and *gentamicin* as above.

Admission Criteria

All patients with suspected or proven endocarditis require admission for observation and treatment while awaiting culture results. Assume all IVDAs presenting with fever have endocarditis until proven otherwise.

Pericarditis

Description

The pericardium is a thin two-layer casing that envelops the heart. Normally, the pericardium contains only 20 to 50 mL of fluid. *Pericarditis* results from inflammation of the pericardium, with subsequent accumulation of pericardial fluid (effusion). The clinical presentation of pericarditis is highly variable and depends on the etiology and the speed and quantity of fluid accumulation (a rapid collection of 100 to 200 mL of fluid is capable of causing severe hemodynamic compromise, while a more insidious expansion of 1 to 2 L of an effusion may be associated with minimal consequences).

Pericarditis results from both *infectious* (bacterial, viral, fungal, parasitic, tuberculosis) and *noninfectious* (connective tissue disease, drug-related, malignancy, underlying cardiac disease) etiologies. However, in many cases, the exact cause remains ill-defined *(idiopathic pericarditis)*.

History

The cardinal symptom of pericarditis is *chest pain* (see section 1.4), typically described as sharp, pleuritic (aggravated by deep inspiration), and retrosternal. Pain frequently radiates to the left trapezius ridge and is aggravated by swallowing, coughing, and lying flat. Relief may be achieved by sitting up, leaning forward, and taking shallow breaths. Shortness of breath may occur.

Physical Examination

General. Note toxicity or cachexia.

Vital signs. Check for fever, tachycardia, and tachypnea. The presence of *pulsus paradoxus* (inspiratory decline in systolic blood pressure in inspiration of at least 10 mm Hg) implies cardiac tamponade.

Neck. Look for JVD and Kussmaul's sign (development of neck vein distention with inspiration).

Lungs. Auscultate for rales and rhonchi.

Heart. A *pericardial friction rub* (a scratchy, often triphasic, grating sound, best heard along left sternal border during expiration) is the fundamental sign of pericarditis. Distant heart sounds suggest pericardial effusion.

Abdomen. Examine for hepatomegaly or ascites.

Extremities. Observe for edema or cyanosis.

Diagnostic Tests

CBC. May show leukocytosis with a left shift.

ESR. Almost always elevated.

ECG. Often diagnostic for pericarditis. It is essential to distinguish the ECG findings of pericarditis from those of an AMI. Classically, the ST- and T-wave changes that accompany acute pericarditis include diffuse ST-segment elevation with upward concavity and absence of reciprocal ST-segment depression. With AMI, ST-segment elevation tends to be confined to anatomical leads that correspond with the coronary distribution and ST-segment depression is seen in the reciprocal leads. Moreover, an upward convexity of the ST segments occurs with AMI. In patients with pericarditis and an effusion, *low voltage of QRS* or *electrical alternans* may emerge.

Cardiac monitor. Commence continuous monitoring for associated dysrhythmia.

CXR. Usually normal in early acute pericarditis. Enlargement of the cardiac silhouette is a late finding, indicating a more chronic effusion of > 200 mL. An extremely large and chronic effusion appears as a water bottle–shaped heart.

Echocardiogram. An echocardiogram is indicated for all ED patients suspected of pericarditis.

CVP. May provide objective evidence of increased right-sided heart pressures (false-negative seen with hypovolemic patients).

Treatment

Life-threatening complications demand immediate treatment. *Cardiac tamponade* is a rare but life-threatening complication of a pericardial effusion. As little as 60 mL of additional fluid can cause significant disturbances. Besides pericarditis, nontraumatic causes of cardiac tamponade include iatrogenic complications (central line, pacemaker insertion) and incorrect use of thrombolytic therapy in a patient with pericarditis. Treatment demands emergent drainage of pericardial fluid. Temporizing measures include volume expansion and inotropic support (dopamine, norepinephrine). Hemodynamic deterioration requires an emergency *pericardiocentesis*(see section 21.2) or thoracic surgery (pericardial window).

Treat viral or idiopathic pericarditis with *antiinflammatory medications* (aspirin, 325 to 975 mg PO q 6 hr; ibuprofen 400 to 600 mg PO q 6 hr; or indomethacin 25 to 50 mg PO q 6 hr). *Corticosteroids* are reserved for patients who do not respond to antiinflammatory medications. Generally, oral anticoagulants must be discontinued (heparin is considered safer for patients who need anticoagulation).

Purulent pericarditis is due to a spread from a contagious infection, extension of intracardiac infection, hematogenous dissemination from a distant focus, or a surgical complication (open-heart surgery). Definitive diagnosis and treatment depend on the timely drainage of the pericardial fluid along with administration of antimicrobial therapy (*nafcillin,* 1.0 to 2.0 g IV q 4 hr, plus *gentamicin,* 3.0 to 5.0 mg/kg/day divided q 8 hr).

Pericarditis arising from systemic disease is best managed by treating the underlying disease (e.g., dialysis for uremic pericardial disease).

Admission Criteria

All patients with suspected pericardial effusion, underlying myocardial ischemia or infarction, or bacterial infection require admission to a monitored setting. It is prudent to discuss disposition of all patients with suspected pericarditis with the cardiology consultant and arrange admission for observation and/or echocardiography studies.

Suggested Readings

Molavi A. Endocarditis: Recognition, management, and prophylaxis. Cardiovasc Clin 1993;23:139–150.

Roberts R, Slovis CM: Endocarditis in intravenous drug abusers. Emerg Med Clin North Am 1990;8:655—682.

Sternbach GL: Pericarditis. Ann Emerg Med 1988;17:214—220.

9.4 SEXUALLY TRANSMITTED DISEASES

Description

Sexually transmitted diseases (STDs) cover infections secondary to bacteria (gonorrhea, chancroid), spirochetes (syphilis), *Chlamydia,* protozoa (trichomonas), and viruses (hepatitis B, AIDS, herpes simplex, papillomavirus). Furthermore, the incidence of sexually spread infectious diseases are on the upswing. Use a uniform approach when managing STDs (Table 9.4.1).

History

In addition to obtaining an appropriate history, ask about:

Presence of penile or vaginal discharge. If present, note how long it has existed as well as the quality and quantity.

Presence of ulcer(s). If present, ask whether they are painful or painless.

Presence of any associated testicular, pelvic, vaginal, abdominal, or rectal pain.

Presence of fever, chills, rash, or joint pain (disseminated gonorrhea).

For females, obstetric and menstrual history. Note any relation between menses and discharge.

Any immunocompromising illnesses.

Table 9.4.1
General Approach to Patients with Suspected STD

1. Obtain a complete history of the presenting problem. This covers the number of sexual partners, date of last sexual contact, sexual orientation, anatomic sites involved in sexual activity, method(s) of contraception (if any), and any previous history of sexually transmitted disease.
2. Symptoms and signs from various STDs tend to overlap, making it difficult to determine the etiologic agent based solely on the history and physical findings.
3. The presence of one STD increases the probability of accompanying STDs; always obtain a VDRL.
4. The results of ancillary tests to identify the specific etiologic agent are not always available to the ED physician and treatment frequently is directed against the most likely pathogen.
5. Treat sexual partner(s) when appropriate.
6. Report STDs to the health department when mandated.
7. Try to educate patients about preventative measures.

Allergies (important in determining medicines available to treat the patient).

Physical Examination

General. Assess the level of toxicity and mental status (neurosyphilis).

Vital signs. Check for fever, tachycardia, and orthostatic changes in blood pressure.

HEENT. Look for pharyngeal exudates, ulceration, and conjunctivitis (Reiter's syndrome).

Abdomen. Note right upper quadrant pain (perihepatitis), lower abdominal pain, and/or rebound tenderness.

Genital. Inspect external genitalia and urethra for lesions (ulcers, cysts, warts), erythema, strictures, and discharge. Also evaluate for inguinal adenopathy and *groove sign* (swelling above and below the inguinal ligament seen with LGV). In males, evaluate testes for tenderness, warmth, swelling, erythema, and/or masses.

Pelvic. Perform a speculum examination for females (inspect the cervix for inflammation and/or discharge) and a bimanual examination.

Rectal. Check for bloody stool, tenderness, purulent discharge, and rectal tone (decreased rectal tone is associated with frequent anal intercourse). In males, evaluate the prostate gland.

Skin. Note characteristic skin lesions (herpetic lesions, venereal warts). Look for pink papular lesions (disseminated GC).

Extremities. Inspect for any joint swelling or inflammation (tenosynovitis).

Diagnostic Tests

Gram stain. Examine Gram stain of urethral or cervical discharge for intracellular bacteria and PMNs (greater sensitivity in males).

Tzanck smear. A Giemsa-stained smear, prepared by scraping the base of a freshly unroofed vesicle, showing multinucleated giant cells is 90% sensitive for the diagnosis of *genital herpes.*

Cultures. Obtain cultures from the urethra or cervix when a discharge is present and from the pharynx and rectum when indicated. Employ Thayer-Martin media when gonorrhea is suspected. Newer techniques use a fluorescent antibody stain to detect *Chlamydia* infections and a polymerase-chain reaction assay that permits rapid detection of gonorrhea. Viral cultures for herpes should be reserved for patients in whom the diagnosis is in doubt or pregnant females. Draw blood cultures if systemic infection is suspected (disseminated gonorrhea). Cultures from joints (see section 9.6) generally show a low yield.

Venereal Disease Research Laboratory (VDRL) and rapid plasma reagent (RPR). Nontreponemal screening tests for syphilis (equally sensitive). Both tests may be falsely negative in early primary and late disease. A *fluorescent treponemal antibody absorption* (FTA-ABS) test (specific for treponemes) is indicated either to confirm the diagnosis of syphilis or to establish the diagnosis of tertiary syphilis. Once positive, the FTA-ABS remains so for life.

Darkfield examination. Examine a scraping from skin lesions for spirochetes.

HIV. The incidence of HIV in patients with STDs is increasing. In addition, the presence of HIV affects both the diagnosis and the treatment of STDs (especially syphilis).

Urinalysis. Positive test for leukocyte esterase together with absence of bacteria implies urethritis in males less than 25 years old.

Beta-hCG. Screen all women of child-bearing age (pregnancy affects both management and disposition).

CBC. Of limited value unless systemic infection is considered.

LP. Test CSF for VDRL in patients with suspected neurosyphilis or HIV+ patients with newly diagnosed syphilis.

Note: *The history, physical examination, and ordering of ancillary tests are fundamentally the same for all STDs.*

Specific Conditions

Gonorrhea

Gonorrhea results from the sexual transmission of *N. gonorrhoeae* (a Gram-negative intracellular diplococci) and may infect any mucosal surface. A variety of clinical syndromes take place, including *asymptomatic carrier state* (more common in women), *acute urethritis* (see section 11.3), *acute cervicitis* (copious, yellow vaginal discharge and friable, erythematous cervix), *pelvic inflammatory disease* (see section 10.3), *acute proctitis* (painful defecation, tenesmus, mucopurulent discharge, and bleeding in homosexual men and heterosexual females practicing anogenital intercourse), *pharyngeal gonorrhea* (exudative pharyngitis), and *disseminated gonococcemia* (arthritis-dermatitis syndrome).

Chlamydia trachomatis

C. trachomatis is an obligate intracellular bacterium responsible for the following syndromes: *cervicitis, acute urethral syndrome, pelvic inflammatory disease, Reiter's syndrome* (reactive arthritis, conjunctivitis, and urethritis), and *lymphogranuloma venereum* (chronic infection of the lymphatic system). Chlamydial infection may be difficult to distinguish from gonorrhea. In many cases, both infections are contracted simultaneously. However, there are a few distinctions between *Chlamydia* and gonorrhea: the urethral or cervical discharge secondary to *Chlamydia* tends to be scantier, thinner, and of mucoid quality, and there are no intracellular diplococci on Gram stain.

Syphilis

Syphilis is a venereal infection caused by the spirochete *T. pallidum.* The infection may be lifelong, passing through several stages after the incubation period. The *primary stage* is heralded by the appearance of a painless ulcerated *chancre* at the site of inoculation (penis, anus, vulva, lip). The chancre is characterized by a clean surface with rolled edges and an indurated, nonerythematous base. Chancres are highly infective, self-limited, and heal in 3 to 6 weeks.

Early *secondary syphilis,* characterized by the dissemination of infection, takes place after the resolution of the chancre. Features of this stage include systemic manifestations (malaise, anorexia, weight loss, fever, sore throat, arthralgias, generalized nontender adenopathy); a wide-spread erythematous rash (especially on the palms, soles); pustular, painless, dull grayish white patches on the buccal and genital mucosa; and wart-like lesions (condyloma lata) in the genital area. The skin and mucosal lesions are highly infectious (contain large numbers of treponemes) and may come and go repeatedly. Involvement of specific organs can occur, resulting in gastritis, nephritis, and asymptomatic meningitis. This stage is self-limited and is followed by a *latent* period. Late secondary or latent syphilis is clinically silent and noninfectious except via blood transfusion and transplacental spread.

Tertiary syphilis develops in only one-third of untreated patients (and may present 4 to 30 years after the primary infection). Features of this stage are protean, but three distinct clinical entities arise: *chronic granulomatous lesions* (gummata) of the liver, bone, and skin; *cardiovascular syphilis* (aortitis complicated by aortic aneurysm, aortic regurgitation, or obstruction of coronary ostia); and *neurologic disease* (meningovasculitis, tabes dorsalis, general paresis, or asymptomatic CSF abnormalities).

Chancroid

Chancroid is a painful genital ulceration caused by *Haemophilus ducreyi,* a Gram-negative bacillus that is difficult to grow in culture. The incubation period is 3 to 5 days. It has become increasingly common in the United States, particularly as focal epidemics associated with prostitution. Patients most commonly present with a painful, foul-smelling ulcer(s), that appears "superinfected." Chancroid must be differentiated from other genital ulcers (syphilis, herpes). Painful and suppurative unilateral inguinal adenopathy (buboes) appear ipsilateral to the side of the lesion. Women may not reveal external signs of infection. Balanitis and phimosis are frequent complications in males. A Gram stain of the exudate reveals fat Gram-negative rods.

Genital Herpes

Both herpes simplex virus type 2 (most commonly) and type 1 are causal agents of genital herpes infection. Lesions produced by these two types of viruses are clinically indistinguishable, and appear as the classic tender, grouped vesicles, pustules, or ulcers; but they may also manifest as nonspecific ulcers.

There are two main stages of infection. *Primary infection* takes place when an individual first seroconverts. Affected patients develop systemic signs and symptoms (fever, malaise, headache, lymphadenopathy) that can be severe and prolonged. The key initial clinical finding is multiple, discrete, bilateral vesicles and erosions on the external genitalia (penis, vulva). Painful, tender, bilateral inguinal adenopathy is also common. Female patients may complain of dysuria, vaginal discharge, urinary retention, and in some patients, lumbosacral radiculopathy. Lesions normally heal in 2 to 3 weeks. Up to 10% of patients with primary genital herpes may present with meningeal signs.

The episodes of *recurrent infection* are generally less severe; tightly clustered vesicles on erythematous bases are seen in the same anatomical location as the primary infection. A prodrome of tingling, burning, or itching sensation regularly occurs minutes to hours before an eruption. The lesions usually resolve in 1 week (the mean duration is 4 to 5 days).

Treatment

When treating *gonococcal infections* it is important to consider that (1) there is an almost 20% resistance rate nationally of *N. gonorrhoeae* to penicillin, (2) there is a high rate of coinfection with *C. trachomatis,* (3) the majority of patients with persistent symptoms are reinfected and not resistant to the antibiotic regimen, and (4) in pregnancy both quinolones and tetracycline are contraindicated (use a cephalosporin).

For *uncomplicated localized gonococcal infections* (urethral, endocervical, and rectal), treatment options include *ceftriaxone* (125 mg IM one time), *ciprofloxacin* (500 mg PO one time), *ofloxacin* (400 mg PO one time), or *cefixime* (400 mg PO one time) plus *doxycycline* (100 mg PO BID for 7 days) or *azithromycin* (1 g PO one time). Do not use doxycycline or ciprofloxacin in pregrant women.

Treatment for other infections is as follows:

Pharyngeal. Use the regimen for uncomplicated gonococcal infections above. (Spectinomycin has a high rate of failure.)

Conjunctivitis. Use ceftriaxone (1 g IM one time) plus saline irrigation of the infected eye.

Disseminated gonococcal infection. See section 9.6.

PID and salpingitis. See section 10.3.

Epididymitis. See section 11.3.

The following conditions warrant empirical treatment for *chlamydial infections:* nongonococcal urethritis, pelvic inflammatory disease, epididymitis in males less than 35 years old, proctitis in homosexual men, and men and women with known gonococcal infection. The preferred regimen for *urethritis, cervicitis, conjunctivitis,* or *proctitis* secondary to *Chlamydia* is *doxycycline* (100 mg PO BID for 7 days) or *azithromycin* (1 g PO one time). In *pregnancy,* give *erythromycin* (500 mg PO QID for 7 days). If erythromycin cannot be tolerated, employ amoxicillin (500 mg TID for 10 days). For *lymphogranuloma venereum,* a longer duration of therapy is required; *doxycycline* (100 mg PO BID for 21 days) is the treatment of choice. Patients with extensive lymphadenitis may require aspiration of buboes to prevent rupture. Patients with strictures and fistulas may require reconstructive surgery.

Primary, secondary, or latent syphilis infection of less than 1 year's duration is treated with long-acting *(benzathine) penicillin* (2.4 million units IM one time). An alternate therapy for penicillin-allergic patients is *tetracycline* or *erythromycin* (500 mg PO QID for 14 days). Successful treatment should result in a decline in the VDRL titer.

For *latent syphilis that has been present for more than 1 year, syphilis of indeterminate duration, or cardiovascular syphilis,* the treatment of choice is *benzathine penicillin* (2.4 million units IM weekly for 3 weeks). Alternate regimens include *tetracycline* or *erythromycin* (500 mg PO QID for 4 weeks). *Neurosyphilis* is treated with *aqueous penicillin G* (12 to 24 million units/daily as a continuous infusion or 2 to 4 million units q 4 hr IV for 10 to 14 days). Patients who state they are allergic to penicillin should be skin tested and desensitized if necessary. If outpatient compliance is ensured, treat with *procaine penicillin* (2.4 million units IM daily), followed by *probenecid* (500 mg PO q 6 hr for 10 to 14 days). Patients need follow-up evaluation.

Syphilis in pregnancy should be treated with penicillin in doses appropriate for the stage of the disease. If a pregnant patient states an allergy to penicillin, the US Public Health Service recommends hospitalization and desensitization. Offer HIV testing to all patients with syphilis because there is a high incidence of STDs in patients with HIV disease.

Treat *HIV+ patients* who also have primary syphilis with *benzathine penicillin* (2.4 million units IM once a week for 3 weeks). For patients beyond the primary stage perform an LP. A reactive CSF VDRL in an HIV-infected patient obligates treatment for neurosyphilis.

Therapy for *chancroid* is almost always empirical, as a culture medium is not commercially available. Treat patients with characteristic clinical findings with either *ceftriaxone* (250 mg IM one time), *erythromycin* (500 mg PO QID for 7 days), or *azithromycin* (1 g PO one time). An alternative is *ciprofloxacin* (500 mg PO BID for 3 days); it is contraindicated in pregnant or lactating females and patients less than 18 years old. Aspirate large, fluctuant nodes (buboes) to prevent rupture, but avoid incision and drainage.

For *primary herpes genitalis* treat with oral *acyclovir* (200 mg PO five times a day for 7 to 10 days or until clinical resolution occurs). For *rectal herpes infection* give *acyclovir* (400 mg PO five times a day for 10 days or until clinical resolution occurs). Treatment for *recurrent herpes* is helpful only if started at the beginning of the prodrome or within 2 days of the onset of lesions. Use *acyclovir* (200 mg five times a day for 5 days or 800 mg PO BID for 5 days). If the patient exhibits *sevère or disseminated disease,* hospitalize, ensure adequate hydration, and administer *acyclovir* (5 to 10 mg/kg IV q 8 hr; adjust the dose for renal insufficiency).

Therapy for concomitant *HIV infection and herpes* depends on the severity of the infection; when a mild disease is present, give *acyclovir* (400 mg PO three to five times a day until clinical resolution occurs). Patients with severe herpes and HIV require hospitalization along with the administration of *acyclovir* (5 to 10 mg/kg IV q 8 hr).

For *women in labor with herpes* consult OB-GYN (a C-section is frequently necessary). While the safety of acyclovir during pregnancy is not established, ongoing studies indicate that acyclovir should be given to women with life-threatening infections (disseminated disease with encephalitis, pneumonia, hepatitis). Topical therapy with acyclovir is not particularly effective.

Admission Criteria

Hospitalization is recommended for *all patients with significant complications of gonorrhea* (disseminated gonococcal infection, sepsis, endocarditis, meningitis, tuboovarian abscess). Disposition for PID secondary to *Chlamydia* is outlined in section 10.3.

Presence of neurosyphilis generally mandates hospitalization. *Patients with severe or disseminated herpes infection* require hospitalization, especially when host immunity is impaired. *Women with urinary retention and lumbosacral radiculopathy* must be hospitalized and given intravenous acyclovir, an indwelling Foley catheter, and parenteral analgesia.

Refer all patients with suspected or known STD to a venereal disease treatment center or private physician for follow-up. Follow state guidelines for reporting STDs. Attempt to get all sexual partners treated as well.

Suggested Reading

Centers for Disease Control and Prevention: 1993 STD treatment guidelines. MMWR 1993;42(RR-14):27–57.

Schmid GP: Approach to the patient with genital ulcer disease. Med Clin North Am1990;74:1559–1572.

Therapy for sexually transmitted diseases. Med Lett 1994;36:1–4.

9.5 SKIN AND SOFT TISSUE INFECTIONS

Description

Skin and soft tissue infections customarily start in areas of trauma or previous disease. Prognosis for infection depends on many factors, including type of injury, duration of injury, size of inoculum, presence of foreign material, and host immunity.

History

The important issues to address for any patient with a potential soft tissue infection include location, time of onset, history of trauma or surgery, associated symptoms (headache, fever, chills, myalgias, rigors), prior treatment, tetanus status, underlying medical problems (diabetes mellitus, AIDS, peripheral vascular disease, venectomy site postcoronary artery grafting, cancer, inflammatory bowel disease, use of corticosteroids or cytotoxic drugs), history of alcohol abuse or intravenous drug abuse, and allergies (can affect medications available for treatment).

Physical Examination

General. Note presence of toxicity and mental status.

Vital signs. Fever, tachycardia, tachypnea, and orthostatic pressure changes signal systemic involvement.

Skin. Examine for erythema, tenderness, heat, and swelling. Look for local breaks (Tinea pedis, wounds, and cutaneous ulcers). Red streaks indicate *lymphangitis.* Fluctuance suggests abscess formation, while crepitus implies a gas-forming infection of the deeper tissues. Characterize discharges (amount, appearance, odor).

HEENT. Note any redness, swelling, or tenderness of the face (it is important to separate eyelids and examine the patient for orbital disease). Note any cranial nerve involvement (restriction of eye movement suggests orbital cellulitis). Check for signs of otitis media, sinus infection, dental, or oropharyngeal infection (can have contiguous spread to skin).

Neck. Determine if swelling, adenopathy, or meningeal signs are present.

Heart. Note any murmurs (underlying valvular disease or endocarditis); see section 9.3.

Rectal. Inspect for erythema, fissures, and tenderness (suggest perianal or ischiorectal abscess).

Extremities. Ensure neurovascular status (particularly important if injury or deeper infection is suspected). A *paronychia* is an infection localized to the nail fold.

Diagnostic Testing

CBC. Usually not helpful; may be elevated (leukocytosis) with a left shift.

Blood cultures. Indicated if patient appears toxic.

Gram stain. Consider for any discharge.

Cultures of purulent material. Generally not needed for folliculitis or cutaneous abscesses unless the patient is acutely ill or immunosuppressed. In diabetics and patients with underlying immune deficiency, consider anaerobic as well as aerobic cultures.

Needle aspiration. The diagnostic yield by aspirating the edge of a cellulitis has a low yield. If you are unsure whether an abscess is present, aspirate the area to confirm the presence of pus.

Antistreptolysin-O (ASLO) titer. Possibly can help in diagnosis of strep infections.

Wood's light examination. Assists in making the diagnosis of *erythrasma* (caused by *Corynebacterium minutissimum*) and fungal disease (taenia).

Radiological studies. Useful if a gas-forming organism, underlying osteomyelitis, or foreign body is suspected. Also indicated if a fracture or joint space violation is considered (e.g., bite wound). CT scanning is indicated for patients with suspected orbital infections.

Specific Conditions

Cellulitis

Cellulitis typically arises from infection by *S. aureus* or *group A β-hemolytic streptococci* and is characterized by redness (blanching erythema), warmth, and tenderness of involved skin (may be localized or widely disseminated). Gram-negative bacteria *(E. coli, Pseudomonas, Klebsiella,* and *Enterobacter)* can cause cellulitis in patients with underlying illness (DM, PVD) or IVDA. Specific types of cellulitis include the following.

Lymphangitis. Lymphangitis is an infection of the lymphatic vessels, typically involving an extremity. Both group A streptococci (more common) and *S. aureus* can be the causative organism. It is characterized by red, tender streaking of the skin overlying the inflamed lymphatic channels along with lymphadenopathy.

Erysipelas. Erysipelas (St. Anthony's fire) typically results from group A streptococci infection, causing a painful, superficial cellulitis. Margins of the lesions tend to be raised and sharply demarcated from the adjacent skin. Classically, the site of predilection was the face, but distribution patterns have changed and now the lower extremities are the predominant location. Systemic symptoms (pain, chills, fever, malaise, rigors) are common.

Erysipeloid. Erysipeloid, following infection with *Erysipelothrix rhusiopathiae,* appears as a purplish colored cellulitis on the hands and/or fingers. It is most common in fishers or meat handlers.

Erythrasma. Erythrasma is a chronic superficial infection of the skin caused by *C. minutissimum* (glows under Wood's light). The intertriginous areas (groin, axilla, toes, inframammary folds) are most commonly affected. Inspection reveals a well-demarcated brownish red patch.

Vibrio vulnificus. Vibrio vulnificus follows exposure to saltwater and results in a rapidly spreading cellulitis that usually appears on the extremities. Many of the affected patients have underlying liver disease.

Gas-Forming Infections. Gas-forming infections follow colonization with either Gram-negative organisms or combinations of anaerobic bacteria and Gram-negative organisms. They are commonly associated with DM, IVDA, ischemia, trauma, or surgery of the abdomen or perineum. While *Clostridium tetani* (see section 9.8) is frequently associated with deeper gas-containing infections, *Enterobacter, Pseudomonas,* anaerobic streptococci, and *Bacteroides* are all capable of producing gas under appropriate conditions. The hallmark of these infections is the presence of subcutaneous gas either discovered by palpation or appearing on x-ray.

Pyoderma Gangrenosum. Pyoderma gangrenosum occurs in patients with underlying inflammatory bowel disease, rheumatoid arthritis, and leukemia. It typically manifests as small pustules, papules, or hemorrhagic blisters that enlarge and develop into ulcers with edematous, dusky, overhanging borders with surrounding erythema.

Other Conditions. For *periorbital cellulitis,* see section 14.2. For *toxic shock syndrome,* see section 9.8.

Bites

The most common sources of bites are dogs (80% of reported bites), cats, and humans. The chief complication is infection or damage to underlying tendons, nerves, vessels, joints, and bone. Despite a common mechanism of injury, bites from different species have unique etiologies, and clinical and treatment implications. Most dog bites produce crush type wounds, while cat bites are associated with deep puncture injuries. Human bites most commonly result from altercation (fight bites) or an amorous encounter. Human and cat bites are more prone to bacterial infections than dog bites.

The most common agent of infection in *dog and cat bites* is *Pasteurella multocida,* a small Gram-negative coccobacillus harbored in the animal's mouth. *P. multocida* infection develops 24 to 48 hr after the bite and manifests principally as a cellulitis at the site of injury (e.g., redness, swelling, discharge, and lymphadenopathy). Systemic complaints (fever, chills, prostration) may accompany local infection. Dog and cat bites are also capable of transmitting *Capnocytophagia canimorsus* (DF-2), a pleomorphic, Gram-negative bacillus that has recently been implicated as the microbe that provokes fulminant sepsis (25% mortality rate) in people with impaired immunity (especially asplenia). Skin flora of the victim, mainly staphylococci and streptococci, are the usual etiologic organisms responsible for delayed infections (> 24 hr). However, up to 50% of animal bite wounds reveal multiple pathologic organisms. A cat bite or scratch may also produce *cat-scratch disease,* a self-limited, painful regional lymphadenitis.

Human bites are a serious problem. Patients are often reluctant to admit being bit (a familiar scenario is when a closed fist strikes another person's mouth) and a high degree of suspicion is necessary whenever treating injuries to the hand, scalp, or genitalia. Early infections following human bites are typically due to mixed aerobic and anaerobic flora. *Eikenella corrodens,* an anaerobic Gram-negative rod, is particular to human bites. Transmission of hepatitis B is a well-established complication of human bites, although there have been no reported cases of AIDS transmission via human bite. An innocuous-appearing bite injury can rapidly deteriorate to a fulminant infection (especially when the bite involves the hand).

Abscess

Cutaneous abscesses are localized collections of pus, arising from the blockage of secretions from the superficial exocrine glands (apocrine, sebaceous), Bartholin's (vulvovaginal) gland, or mucus glands of the rectum or breast duct tissue. The responsible organism is determined by the neighboring flora of the area of the body in which the abscess is located. *Anaerobic abscesses* are associated with infection of mucosal surfaces (mouth, rectum), whereas abscesses following skin trauma contain aerobic organisms *(S. aureus, Streptococcus). N. gonorrhea* might be isolated from abscesses of the perineum—particularly *Bartholin's cyst abscess*—and from periurethral abscesses. In addition, drainage from congenital cysts and sinuses may get impeded, leading to infection and outgrowth of an abscess (e.g., *pilonidal cysts*). Presence of a foreign body leads to slowly healing or recurrent abscesses. Intravenous drug users are particularly prone to abscesses from skin infections (skin popping). Infections may also occur in accessory structures such as hair follicles *(folliculitis)*. A *carbuncle* is a complex of deep interconnecting abscesses extending into the subcutaneous tissues. *Hidradenitis suppurativa* involves recurrent apocrine gland abscesses (especially axillary and inguinal).

Typically, the patient complains of pain, redness, and warmth, along with localized swelling. Although the abscess tends to be tender and fluctuant on palpation, the underlying muscle and tissue should not be. Presence of intense discomfort on manipulation of deeper tissues implies a more serious infection *(necrotizing fascitis, gas gangrene)*. Perirectal abscesses are frequently deceiving (can be more widespread than they initially appear) and are easily missed on physical examination.

Treatment

Depending on the type of infection, therapy may include both medical and surgical intervention, requiring the use of antibiotics, antitoxins, débridement, hyperbaric oxygen, or other agents. Ensure that the patient's tetanus status is current (see section 9.8). Provide adequate analgesia (see Chapter 17).

The type and route of antibiotic administration are determined by what is considered the most likely pathogen as well as the extent of infection and the patient's overall condition. *Mild to moderate cellulitis or lymphangitis* in an immunocompetent, nontoxic patient can be treated as an outpatient with antibiotics directed against both staphylococci and streptococci. Choose *dicloxacillin* (250 to 500 mg PO q 6 hr for 10 days), *amoxicillin-clavulanate* (250 to 500 mg PO q 6 hr), *cephalexin* (250 to 500 mg PO q 6 hr for 10 days), *cefadroxil* (1 to 2 g PO once a day for 10 days), or *erythromycin* (250 to 500 mg PO q 6 hr for 10 days). Additional supportive measures include immobilization of the affected extremity, elevation, warm moist heat packs, and sufficient analgesia.

Patients with *cellulitis who appear toxic* (without underlying illness) require basic supportive measures in addition to intravenous antibiotics. The primary choice of antibiotics is either a penicillinase-resistant synthetic penicillin (nafcillin, 1.0 to 2.0 g IV q 4 to 6 hr) or a first-generation cephalosporin (*cefazolin,* 1 to 2 g IV q 8 hr). Alternatives include *clindamycin* and *vancomycin* (1 g IV q 12 hr).

For *erysipelas,* the preferred agent is *penicillin* (2 to 20 million units a day IV, divided and given q 4 hr or q 6 hr). An alternative is *erythromycin* for penicillin-allergic patients.

For *diabetics* or *immunocompromised patients with cellulitis* (particularly cellulitis involving the foot), suspect a polymicrobial infection. Prompt surgical consultation is essential if *necrotizing cellulitis, gas-forming cellulitis,* or *streptococcal myonecrosis* is considered. If the infection is severe and/or the patient appears toxic, use *impinem-cilastin* (500 mg IV q 6 hr), *ticarcillin-clavulanate* (3.1 g IV q 6 hr), *piperacillin-tazobactam* (3.375 g IV q 6 hr), or a *penicillinase-resistant penicillin* plus *aminoglycoside* (or *aztreonam*) plus *clindamycin* (600 mg IV q 8 hr).

Treatment for *bites* is predicated on the type of wound, the severity, its anatomic location, and how old the wound is. Certain general measures apply to all bite wounds: cleanse and irrigate the wound using a 19-gauge catheter and normal saline; explore the wound for damaged tissue (from crushing or tearing) and foreign material; check for damaged tendons, joints, bones, or blood vessels; and débride devitalized tissue (for facial injuries with a significant quantity of devitalized tissue, consult plastic surgery). The hand is at particularly high risk for tendon or nerve damage. Extremity wounds should be elevated and immobilized. Assess all patients for possible rabies prophylaxis (section 9.8).

Decisions about *primary closure for bites* depend on the individual case. Generally, render primary closure only for cosmetically important wounds determined to be low risk for infection, e.g., animal bites less than 12 hr old; bites to the face, scalp, trunk or proximal extremity; and large, clean lacerations that can be easily cleansed.

High-risk criteria for infection from bites include cat bites and scratch wounds; all human bites (although a potentially disfiguring facial bite < 12 hr old can be considered for closure); any bite > 12 hr old; puncture or crush wounds; and bites to the hand, wrist or foot. Patients who are at high risk for infection include those older than 50 years, diabetics, alcoholics, and those with altered immune status or PVD. Keep in mind that delayed closure can be performed in 3 to 5 days.

Antibiotics are indicated for *infected animal and human bites.* Use a parenteral agent for treating serious infected human, cat, and dog bites—either a second- or third-generation cephalosporin such as *cefoxitin, cefuroxime, or ceftriaxone* or *ampicillin-sulbactam* or *ticarcillin-clavulanate.* The necessity of antibiotic prophylaxis is not clear. Consider *prophylactic antibiotics* in patients with high-risk criteria, those with prosthetic or diseased heart valves or joints, and patients who do not have a functioning spleen. *Amoxicillin-clavulanate* (250 to 500 mg PO TID for 5 days) serves as an ideal agent for human, cat, and dog bite prophylaxis. First-generation cephalosporins alone are not always adequate for animal bites, while human bites require a penicillinase-resisting agent because of high incidence of β-lactamsae-producing bacteria.

Always consider the possibility of deeper involvement or more serious infection when managing an *abscess.* While *I&D* is a simple procedure, and necessary to adequately treat any abscess, it is generally *not* appropriate to perform the procedure in the ED in the following situations: *perirectal, ischiorectal, or periurethral abscess;* involvement of the *danger triangle of face* (the area demarcated by corners of mouth inferiorly and glabella superiorly); *periorbital abscess; deep underlying foreign body;* and abscesses in close proximity to significant neurovascular channels (vascular aneurysms, particularly in the neck region, may be mistaken for an abscess) or tendons. Attempt aspiration first if the abscess is questionable. Employ a #11 blade to incise the abscess (incise along skin lines) at the point of maximal bulging. Ensure an adequate incision size (1 to 2 cm); a simple stab wound is generally wanting. Break loculations with a Mayo scissors or hemostats. Débride necrotic material. Irrigate and loosely pack the cavity with iodoform gauze or similar material (special packing devices may be employed, e.g., a Word catheter).

Pretreatment with *antibiotics for abscess* is suggested for patients who are immunocompromised, septic, have a prosthetic valve or joint, or have rheumatic or valvular heart disease. A first-generation cephalosporin (*cefazolin,* 1.0 g IV) or a combination of amoxicillin and β-lactamase inhibitor (*ampicillin* plus *sulbactam,* 1.5 to 3.0 g IV) is usually adequate (given IV 30 min before the procedure; consider repeating as an oral dose 6 hr later). If one is concerned about Gram-negative organisms (abscesses in the abdominal, genitourinary region), the American Heart Association recommends endocarditis prophylaxis *ampicillin* (2.0 g IV) plus *gentamicin* (1.5 mg/kg IV; not to exceed 80 mg) 30 min before the procedure, repeating the regimen 8 hr later. The necessity of treating otherwise healthy patients is unclear.

Admission Criteria

The necessity of admission for parenteral therapy is *predicated on the patient's degree of toxicity* (admit patients who appear systemically ill), *immune status* (patients who are immunocompromised require a lower threshold to admit), and *potential compliance* (need to ensure patient will be able to follow outpatient regimen).

In addition to the general criteria for admission, it is prudent to consider admission for *all human bites to the hand that are clearly infected with violation of the joint capsule or tendon.* If there is any doubt, a surgical specialist ought to be consulted.

Admit *patients with abscesses in high-risk areas* (triangle of the face; perirectal, ischiorectal, or periurethral; orbital; or those located near vital structures).

All patients who are discharged require follow-up in 24 hr.

Suggested Readings

Chisolm CD, Howell JM, eds.: Soft tissue emergencies. Emerg Med Clin North Am 1992;10:655–861.

Trott A. Wounds and lacerations. St. Louis: Mosby, 1991.

Weber DJ, Hansen AR: Infections resulting from animal bites. Infect Dis Clin North Am 1991:5:663–678.

9.6 BONE AND JOINT INFECTIONS

Description

Septic arthritis is a bacterial infection involving the synovium and joint space, while *osteomyelitis* arises from inflammation and infection of bone. In general, infections of joints and bones share a common etiology, developing in one of three ways: *hematogenous dissemination* (commonly affecting long bones and vertebra), *contiguous extension* (frequently appearing in the femur, tibia, skull, and mandible), or *direct inoculation* as a result of trauma or surgery. Many patients who acquire infections of the skeletal system suffer impaired immunity (cancer, AIDS, steroid therapy), display vascular insufficiency (PVD, diabetes, sickle cell anemia, neuropathy), or exhibit preexisting joint disease (rheumatoid arthritis, prosthetic joint).

Suspect underlying *osteomyelitis* in any patient complaining of oppressive, localized bone pain that is accompanied by an obvious soft tissue infection, especially when subsequent to surgery or trauma. In descending order, the most commonly implicated pathogens in adults with osteomyelitis are *S. aureus, Streptococcus* spp., Gram-negative bacilli, and *S. epidermidis.* Hematogenous osteomyelitis is classified as either *acute* (characterized by systemic illness followed by localized bone pain, often without radiographic evidence of infection, with a duration of < 10 days), *subacute* (lack of systemic signs, radiographic bony changes at presentation, and duration > 10 days), or *chronic* (systemic symptoms are variable, bony radiological changes are present, and there is a history of previous infection).

Septic arthritis ordinarily (90%) presents as an acute, single-joint (monoarticular) arthritis, although a polyarticular septic arthritis may appear in the elderly and chronically ill. The etiology can be divided into gonococcal or nongonococcal causes.

Gonococcal arthritis results from hematogenous dissemination of *N. gonorrhea,* frequently affecting the wrist, although the knees and hands are also commonly involved. *A single septic joint in a young person is gonococcal arthritis until proven otherwise.* Usually, there is an accompanying skin rash (papular, petechial, pustular, necrotic, or hemorrhagic skin lesions) that is confined to the extremities as well as an extensor tenosynovitis of the wrist, hands, or feet.

Nongonococcal bacterial arthritis regularly results from infection with *S. aureus* (50%), *S. epidermis, Streptococcus* spp., Gram-negative bacilli, or *M. tuberculosis.* Nongonococcal arthritis prevails in large weight-bearing joints, striking the knee 50% of the time, followed (in descending order of frequency) by the hip, shoulder and elbow. Patients customarily complain of extreme pain that is exacerbated with joint movement and, when a weight-bearing joint is affected, a limp.

Septic arthritis affects atypical sites in IVDAs, e.g., the *sacroiliac joint, sternoclavicular articulations,* and *pubic symphysis.* Furthermore, the following conditions are associated with unique bacterial infections:

Infection in patients with peripheral vascular disease. A particularly common problem in diabetics (especially involving the foot). Infections are frequently polymicrobial, including anaerobes, and often require surgical débridement. Healing is generally poor.

Parenteral drug abusers. Potential additional pathogens include *P. aeruginosa,* and *Serratia marcescens.*

Sickle cell disease. Salmonella infections occur at a much higher rate.

Hemodialysis patients. M. tuberculosis may be implicated in bone and joint infections (the ribs and thoracic vertebrae are common sites).

Infection after stepping on a nail. Puncture wounds to the forefoot secondary to a nail (particularly if wearing sneakers) are at risk for *Pseudomonas osteomyelitis* or septic arthritis.

History

Determine the site of infection and whether the symptoms have remained localized or are spreading (migratory). Inquire about the duration of symptoms and their onset (sudden or gradual).

Ask about trauma or known injury to affected area. Question the patient about any recent urinary tract infection, manipulation, or surgery (increases risk for Gram-negative bacilli infection of vertebra). Establish the presence of associated symptoms (myalgias, rash, fever, weight loss). Ascertain if any underlying medical disorders coexist (diabetes, sickle cell disease, inflammatory bowel disease, collagen-vascular disorders, PVD, hepatitis, AIDS). Verify medications, social history (alcoholism, IVDA), and allergies. Ask about sexual history (prior history of venereal disease; last menstrual period, vaginal or urethral discharge in females).

Physical Examination

General. Note the level of toxicity.

Vital signs. Fever may be absent (present only 50% of the time with septic arthritis, and 75 to 80% of the time with acute osteomyelitis).

HEENT. Look for conjunctivitis, iritis (seen in Reiter's syndrome and certain arthropathies), and pharyngitis (gonorrhea).

Chest. Auscultate the heart and lungs for murmurs, and/or pleural or pericardial friction rubs (possibly indicate systemic infection or inflammatory disorder). Inspect the sternoclavicular joints in IVDAs.

Abdomen. Check the liver for tenderness or enlargement (Fitz-Hugh-Curtis).

Genitourinary. Investigate for clues to venereal disease, e.g., urethral discharge.

Musculoskeletal. Examine for swelling, erythema, warmth, tenderness, joint effusions, and limitation (both passive and active) of extremity movement. Patient may "hold" joint in a characteristic position to maximize comfort (hip involvement is notable for flexion, abduction, and external rotation posture). Palpate for spinal tenderness, including the sacroiliac joints when indicated.

Skin. Observe for distinctive rashes (erythema marginatum occurs with acute rheumatic fever, while pustular or vesicular lesions with darker necrotic centers imply gonococcemia), overlying ulcers, sinus tracts (underlying infection), or needle tracks.

Diagnostic Tests

Arthrocentesis. Synovial fluid examination is the definitive study for diagnosing septic arthritis. Joint fluid is aspirated and analyzed for cell count, crystal analysis, glucose and protein levels, Gram stain and culture and sensitivity. However, a negative Gram stain of synovial fluid does *not* rule out infectious arthritis. Arthrocentesis of the hip joint or prosthetic joints are best left to a consultant.

WBC count and ESR. Nonspecific tests that ordinarily will not differentiate inflammatory from infectious disease processes. The ESR is elevated in most cases.

Cultures. Positive in less than 50% of cases of skeletal infection. Microbiological diagnosis is often contingent on bone aspiration and culture.

Plain radiographs. Radiographic evidence of osteomyelitis typically lags behind symptoms by 7 to 10 days. Look for evidence of bone destruction such as demineralization of bone or appearance of punched-out lesions. In the spine, early findings include joint space narrowing and vertebral wedging. Classic radiographic changes include periosteal reaction accompanied by *involucrum* (outgrowth of new bone) and *sequestrum* formation (necrosed bone separates from adjacent bone). In cases of suspected septic arthritis, evaluate for soft-tissue swelling, joint effusions, and preexisting joint disease.

Bone scan. Although very sensitive for osteomyelitis, it frequently cannot distinguish bone infection from more superficial soft tissue infections.

CT scan and MRI. MRI imaging is superior to CT scan for displaying soft tissues and bone marrow.

Differential Diagnosis

Rheumatoid arthritis, gout, pseudogout, traumatic hemarthrosis, rheumatic fever, and arthritis secondary to systemic diseases (e.g., hepatitis, lupus erythematosus, Lyme disease).

Treatment

Orthopedic and/or surgical consultation is necessary, as the drainage of purulent collections is often necessary. Spinal infections may obligate stabilization procedures.

Initiate antibiotic therapy as soon as possible, based on the synovial fluid Gram stain. If you are unable to identify the organism, treat the most likely organism. For suspected *gonococcal arthritis* prescribe *ceftriaxone* (1 g IV or IM daily) or *ceftizoxime or cefotaxime* (1 g IV q 8 hr). For patients allergic to β-lactam therapy, substitute *spectinomycin* (2 g IM q 12 hr). Parenteral therapy should be continued for 24 to 48 hr after symptoms resolve. This can be followed outpatient oral therapy with *cefixime* (400 mg PO BID) or *ciprofloxacin* (500 mg PO BID); the duration of antimicrobial therapy is generally 7 to 10 days. For *nongonococcal septic arthritis* use *nafcillin* (8 to 12 g IV per day, divided into four to six doses). In patients who are immunocompromised employ *nafcillin* plus *gentamicin* (3 to 5 mg/kg/day divided q 8 hr; adjust the dose for renal function). For IVDAs with septic arthritis, cover with *vancomycin* (30 to 40 mg/kg/day in four divided doses) plus gentamicin.

Empiric therapy for *osteomyelitis* is predicated on the route of infection (hematogenous versus direct inoculation) and the host's condition (sickle cell disease, IVDA). For suspected *S. aureus infection,* treat with *nafcillin* (2 g IV q 4 hr) with or without an *aminoglycoside.* For sickle cell patients initiate therapy with *nafcillin* plus *ampicillin or chloramphenicol,* while patients with impaired immunity (DM, AIDS) or vascular insufficiency (especially infections involving the foot) require broad coverage with an *aminoglycoside* plus *clindamycin* (1.2 to 2.7 g/day IV in two to three doses), *imipenem* (alone; 500 mg IV q 6 hr), or a *quinolone* plus *clindamycin* (600 mg IV q 8 hr; discuss with consultant).

Admission Criteria

All patients with septic arthritis and acute osteomyelitis will require admission for parenteral antibiotics and consultation for surgical drainage and/or débridement.

Suggested Readings

Brancos MA, Peris P, Miro JM, et al.: Septic arthritis in heroin addicts. Sem Arthritis Rheum 1991;21:81–87.

Esterhai JL, ed.: Orthopedic infection. Orthop Clin North Am 1991; 22:363–549.

Middleton DB: Infectious arthritis.Prim Care 1993;20:943–953.

9.7 ACQUIRED IMMUNODEFICIENCY SYNDROME (AIDS)

See particular sections for specific infectious-related complications of AIDS.

9.8 SELECTED INFECTIOUS EMERGENCIES

Botulism

Botulism is an acute paralytic condition caused by a preformed neurotoxin of *Clostridium botulinum.* There are approximately 10 cases of botulism annually in the United States. Most cases are related to the ingestion of contaminated, improperly canned foods. A gastrointestinal prodrome (nausea, vomiting, abdominal cramps, constipation, or diarrhea occurring 12 to 36 hr after ingestion) precedes the classic flaccid paralysis.

The toxin interferes with the release of acetylcholine at the neuromuscular junction, resulting in a progressive descending muscle paralysis (especially of the cranial nerves) that dominates the clinical picture. Other symptoms include difficulty swallowing and chewing food, diplopia, blurry vision, and a generalized symmetric motor weakness of the extremities. Loss of pupillary reflexes is an early finding. Death typically results from respiratory paralysis.

The differential diagnosis covers any cause of acute weakness, such as Guillian-Barré syndrome, myasthenia gravis, Lambert-Eaton syndrome, tick paralysis, periodic paralysis, shellfish poisoning, and drug-induced disorders (pesticides, aminoglycosides, lithium). Diagnosis is established by proof of the toxin in serum, gastric contents, stool, and/or ingested food or the finding of spores in the wound or stool.

Management of botulism is primarily supportive, with careful monitoring of the patient's respiratory status, together with providing parenteral hydration while swallowing difficulties persist (to avoid aspiration). Gastric lavage and saline catharsis may facilitate removal of the spores and toxin from the gut. Administration of antitoxin binds free toxin in the serum but has no influence on already paralyzed muscle. Antibiotics are generally not helpful. If botulism is suspected, notify either the state health department, local poison center, or contact the Centers for Disease Control and Prevention (404–639-3670) for assistance in procuring the antitoxin and performing necessary assays.

Lyme Disease

Lyme disease is a multisystem infection caused by the spirochete *Borrelia burgdorferi* and transmitted by the deer tick. Originally described in New England, it has now been reported in most of the United States, with three major endemic areas (southern New England, New York, and the mid-Atlantic States; much of Wisconsin and Minnesota; and the coastal and wooded areas of California and Oregon). Three stages of infection are recognized.

Stage 1

The first stage is characterized by a distinctive rash, *erythema migrans* (EM), which begins as a red macule or papule at the site of the bite (approximately 1 week later), and expands over days to weeks to form a large, round (at least 5 mm) annular lesion with central clearing. There is also a flu-like illness associated with fatigue, malaise, headache, fever, and myalgias as well as regional or generalized lymphadenopathy. About 20% of patients lack the typical skin findings or the rash goes unnoticed.

Stage 2

The second stage is a disseminated phase of infection, with CNS and/or cardiac manifestations, e.g., headache, meningeal irritation, meningoencephalitis, facial nerve palsy (Bell's palsy), radiculoneuropathy, and cardiac AV block.

Stage 3

In the third stage, articular manifestations develop in as many as 80% of patients with Lyme disease who remain untreated. Initially, brief attacks of pain and/or swelling occurs in large joints (especially the knees). About 10% of affected patients develop a chronic arthritis.

Stage 2 generally follows stage 1 by weeks or months, and stage 3 succeeds stage 2 by months or years, but any one of the stages may fail to appear or overlap one another.

A diagnosis is based on compatible clinical findings in a patient with possible tick contact in an endemic area. Current laboratory methods generally serve only as imperfect adjuncts. Early Lyme disease is treated with oral antibiotics: *doxycycline* (100 mg PO BID) or *amoxicillin* (500 mg PO TID) for pregnant or lactating women or patients who cannot tolerate doxycycline. Antibiotics are given for 10 to 30 days. Employ intravenous antibiotics (ceftriaxone 2 g IV once a day for 14 to 21 days) for Lyme disease–related carditis, neurologic manifestations, and arthritis. Remove the tick if found. Patients presenting with suspected Lyme disease together with a prolonged PR interval (>0.30 sec) or a high degree AV block require hospitalization (a temporary pacemaker may be required). Prophylactic antibiotics are not recommended by the American College of Rheumatology.

Percutaneous Exposure to Blood and Body Fluids

Blood and body fluids from all patients are potentially hazardous, representing an occupational danger to health care workers. Routes of exposure include percutaneous (most frequently from needlestick recapping, also seen with lacerations and bites), mucous membranes (splash to eyes or mouth) or cutaneous (exposure to skin with breaks in integument). The chance of contracting hepatitis B from a noted contaminated source is about 26% per parenteral exposure, while the risk of HIV infection is 1 in 300 after a single parenteral exposure from a known HIV+ source.

Foremost, determine the risk of infection by establishing the infectivity of the source and address the donor's hepatitis and HIV status. Treat open, contaminated wounds as warranted. Check immune status to hepatitis B in previously vaccinated persons. Ask all employees to file an incident report.

An unvaccinated patient at is at high risk for contracting hepatitis B if the source is known to be positive for hepatitis B or is from high-risk group such as an IVDA, dialysis patient, or male homosexual; for patients presenting in first 48 hr, offer *hepatitis B immunoglobulin* (IgHB; 0.06 mL/kg up to 5 mL in adults) and the first dose of recombinant hepatitis vaccine (2 μg IM). If the donor's hepatitis status is unknown, draw blood for HBsAg and HBsAb and refer for 2 more vaccinations at 1 and 6 months. The decision to prescribe IgHB therapy to victims of an unlikely hepatitis exposure (the source is unknown or considered low risk) needs to be individualized and discussed with the patient. Recommend vaccination to all health care workers lacking a previous history of hepatitis or immunity. For vaccinated patients exposed to known or high risk sources of hepatitis B, check their antibody status (titers > 10 SRU by RIA imply immunity). There is controversy as to the best revaccination policy for transient-responding health workers (whether to proceed as if the patient were unvaccinated or just recommend a booster).

Offer HIV testing to both the donor and the recipient (document preexposure HIV status), obtaining permission from both individuals as indicated, along with providing counseling and follow-up. Exact regulations vary from state to state and from hospital to hospital. Bear in mind the possibility that the source may be HIV+; individuals may test negative for the antibody early in the course of the disease. When the source is HIV+ or of unknown HIV status and refuses to be tested, advise the exposed patient to repeat HIV testing at 3, 6, and 12 months and to refrain from any activities that could possibly transmit the virus until his or her status is clarified. The issue of *zidovudine* (AZT) prophylaxis following significant HIV exposure is both controversial and complex. A recent case-controlled series reported by the CDC suggests it may have some benefit. Explanation of the possible short-term (headache, myalgias, and fatigue) and long-term (blood dyscrasias) side effects of the medication is important. The present dosage used is 200 mg q 4 hr for the first 72 hr and then 500 to 600 mg/day for 25 days, in divided doses q 4 to 8 hr. All patients need follow-up.

Rabies

Rabies is an almost uniformly fatal infection of the central nervous system caused by a RNA rhabdovirus transmitted via percutaneous exposure (bites or contact with an open wound, scratch, or abrasion) to saliva from infected wildlife, including skunks, bats, raccoons, cows, dogs, foxes, and cats. Rodents and rabbits have never been implicated as carriers. Rabid animals often display abnormal behavior such as agitation, unprovoked attacks, feeble barking, drooling, impaired locomotion, and convulsions. If left untreated, the risk of contracting rabies from an infected animal ranges from 5 to 20%. Once it gains entrance to the body, the virus spreads along the peripheral nerves to the CNS, resulting in encephalomyelitis. The incubation period is variable (2 weeks to 1 year).

Determine the species of the animal involved, the date and time of occurrence, whether the attack was provoked or unprovoked, and the ownership and vaccination status of the animal (if possible). Note the location and depth of the wound. Initial symptoms include pain and tingling at the inoculation site, followed by extreme agitation, altered mental status, muscle spasms, and opisthotonus, along with subsequent severe spasm of the larynx and pharynx, exacerbated by swallowing attempts, giving rise to hydrophobia. Seizures may take place. Ultimately, a flaccid paralysis with apnea ensues, with the patient lapsing into a coma.

Diagnosis in the animal is confirmed by histopathological examination of the brain (looking for Negri bodies). Postexposure management of bitten people includes thorough cleaning of the bite and passive immunization with *human rabies immunoglobulin* (administer 20 IU/kg, half of the dose should be infiltrated into the wound if possible, with the remaining half being given at a different site IM). Begin an immediate course of *human diploid cell rabies vaccine* (hDCV), given as a 1-mL IM injection in the deltoid, repeated on days 3, 7, 14, and 28 (for a total of five doses).

Rocky Mountain Spotted Fever

Rickettsia rickettsii is the causative agent of Rocky Mountain spotted fever (RMSF), which is transmitted by the bites of several species of ticks. Infection is *not* limited to the Rocky Mountain region and is endemic to the south Atlantic belt as well as the

Southwestern states. Infection induces a diffuse vasculitis, which is accompanied by rash, fever, and edema (nonpitting). If left untreated, encephalitis, myocarditis, pneumonitis, disseminated intravascular coagulation, gangrene, and death (20 to 50%) ensue. After an incubation period of 2 to 14 days, high fever, headache, rigors, photophobia, nausea, vomiting, diarrhea, and generalized myalgias abruptly emerge. A characteristic pink macular rash evolves to dark red petechiae, which appears first on the wrists and ankles; then spreads centrally to involve the arms, legs, and trunk; and somewhat later affects the palms and soles. However, the rash is absent in 15% of cases, and the classic triad of headache, fever, and rash is seen in only 60% of cases. Consider meningococcemia, *S. aureus* septicemia, typhus, leptospirosis, viral exanthems (measles, varicella, rubella, enterovirus), drug reaction, and immune complex vasculitis in the differential diagnosis. Diagnosis is based on clinical findings; *do not wait* for serological confirmation. Prompt antibiotic therapy with *tetracycline* (0.5 to 1.0 g IV q 12 hr) or *chloramphenicol* (50 mg/kg/day IV) is essential. Some patients require therapy for shock (see section 1.2). Remove the tick if found.

Tetanus

C. tetani, the causative agent of tetanus, is a Gram-positive, anaerobic, spore-bearing bacillus that produces a powerful exotoxin (tetanospasmin) that prevents feedback inhibition of neural discharges, resulting in severe skeletal muscle hypertonicity. *C. tetani* is ubiquitous (soil, dust, water), with infection resulting when spores encounter the proper tissue milieu in which to germinate. "Tetanus-prone" wounds include those that are heavily contaminated by soil or feces, crush type injuries, puncture wounds, burns, ischemic tissue, and delayed presentation of skin trauma (> 24 hr). However, one-third of patients who contract tetanus in the United States (about 60 cases per year) have no obvious wound or a wound that is considered trivial by the patient. Groups at higher risk for tetanus include the elderly (older women more so than elderly men since many men were vaccinated during military service), immigrants from countries where tetanus prophylaxis is not mandated, and IVDAs (especially "skin poppers"). There are three forms of tetanus disease: *generalized* (the most common form), *cephalic* (rare, follows otitis media or injuries to head and face), and *neonatal* (most prevalent in developing countries, typically arising from contamination of the umbilical stump).

After an incubation period of 3 to 21 days (the incubation period is inversely proportional to the distance between the site of injury and the CNS), muscle spasm develops. Patients may initially complain of trismus of the jaw (lockjaw), dysphagia, and oppressive pain at the site of injury. The disease proceeds to generalized muscle spasm, which is most pronounced in the neck and back, resulting in opisthotonus. Painful muscle spasms are frequently triggered by sensory stimuli, e.g., loud noises. Disturbances of the autonomic nervous system (e.g., fluctuations in the blood pressure, tachycardia, hyperpyrexia, and cardiac arrhythmias) are common. The diagnosis is based on the history and clinical findings. There are no diagnostic laboratory findings. Consider oral infections or abscess, rabies, strychnine poisoning, phenothiazine reaction (dystonia) or overdose, black widow spider bite, narcotic withdrawal, hypocalcemic tetany, epilepsy, and hyperventilation in the differential diagnosis.

The primary goals of emergency management are (1) neutralization of unbound toxin (*tetanus immune globulin,* 3000 to 6000 units IM), (2) removal of source of infection (surgical débridement of tissue along with concomitant administration of antibiotics, e.g., *penicillin G,* 1 million units IV q 6 hr; or metronidazole, 500 mg IV q 6 hr in penicillin-allergic patients; see Table 9.8.1), (3) relief of muscle spasm (give *diazepam,* 5 to 10 mg IV), and (4) respiratory support (endotracheal intubation or tracheostomy may be required to protect against laryngospasm and aspiration). Patients must be admitted to an ICU setting, where

Table 9.8.1
Guide to Tetanus Prophylaxis for Adults

History of Tetanus Immunization	Nontetanus-Prone Wounds[a]		Tetanus-Prone Wounds	
	TIG	Td	TIG	Td
Unknown or less than three doses	No	Yes	Yes	Yes
Three or more doses	No	No[b]	No	No[c]

[a] Dose of tetanus immunoglobulin (TIG) is 250 units IM, and dose of tetanus-diphtheria toxoid (td) is 0.5 mL IM.
[b] Yes if > 10 years after last dose.
[c] Yes if > 5 years after last dose.

external stimuli can be minimized. Sedation, paralysis, and mechanical ventilation are frequently essential.

Tetanus in the United States occurs almost exclusively in nonimmunized or partially immunized patients and can be completely prevented through proper vaccination.

Toxic Shock Syndrome

Toxic shock syndrome (TSS) is a multisystem disease that arises from the exotoxin of certain staphylococcal species and an increasingly recognized association with toxins mediated by group A streptococci organisms. TSS due to *S. aureus* was formerly identified primarily in the setting of menstruating females using tampons but is now recognized to occur with equal or greater frequency in females outside the cycle of menses. Microbes responsible for TSS can be cultured from several sites, the nasopharynx, vagina, rectum, and all types of wounds (including those resulting from surgical procedures). TSS is a clinical diagnosis based on the findings of fever; a generalized blanching, macular rash that later desquamates; hypotension; and involvement of three other systems—e.g., GI (vomiting or diarrhea at onset), muscular (severe myalgias or CPK more than five times normal), mucous membranes (vaginal, oropharyngeal, or conjunctiva hyperemia), respiratory (development of adult respiratory distress syndrome), renal (BUN or creatinine two times normal or > 5 WBC/HPF in absence of a UTI), hepatic (bilirubin or transaminase levels more than two times normal), hematologic (falling hematocrit, thrombocytopenia, or coagulopathy), and CNS (disoriented or altered consciousness without focal neurologic signs).

TSS caused by group A β-hemolytic streptococci shares traits of both a *necrotizing fascitis* (i.e., oppressive pain in the affected extremity, soft tissue swelling, and erythema that rapidly progresses to vesicle and bullae formation and necrosis) and TSS (shock, myositis, renal failure, ARDS, coagulopathy, delirium). However, the disseminated skin rash that desquamates and commonly appears in staphylococci-related TSS is lacking in toxic streptococci cases. Also, bacteremia, frequently absent in staphylococci toxic shock, occurs in at least 50% of cases of streptococci-induced TSS.

Early and extensive surgical débridement of affected tissue, removal of tampons, and drainage of abscesses are essential to survival. Provide supportive care, ensure adequate ventilation and oxygenation, restore fluid volume, and maintain blood pressure with pressors if necessary. Administer antibiotics covering both staphylococci and streptococci (*nafcillin,* 1.0 to 2.0 g IV q 4 hr; or cefazolin, 1 g IV q 6 hr).

Suggested Readings

Critchley EM, Mitchell JD: Human botulism. Br J Hosp Med 1990; 43:290–292.

Go GW. Baraff LJ, Schriger DL: Management guidelines for health care workers exposed to blood and body fluids. Ann Emerg Med 1991;20:1341–1350.

Grouleau G: Tetanus. Emerg Med Clin North Am 1992;10:351–360.

Grouleau G: Rabies. Emerg Med Clin North Am 1992;10:361–368.

Spach DH, Lilies WC, Campbell GL, et al.: Tick-borne diseases in the United States. N Engl J Med 1993;329:936–947.

Starausbaugh LJ: Toxic shock syndrome: Are you recognizing its changing presentations? Postgrad Med 1993;94(6):107–118.

9.9 SEPSIS

Description

Septic shock results from a systemic infection—most commonly Gram-negative rods *(E. coli, Klebsiella, Proteus, Pseudomonas)* but also Gram-positive cocci *(Staphylococcus, Streptococcus),* anaerobes, *Rickettsia,* parasites, and fungi—which overwhelms the body's defenses through the release of complex inflammatory mediators. The definitive diagnosis of sepsis depends on the demonstration of microbes from bacteriological cultures, but successful management depends on rapid recognition of acutely ill patients and prompt treatment. Sepsis is of concern in any patient presenting with fever and systemic illness, especially when accompanied by hypotension or delirium. The most frequent sites of infection are the respiratory tract, genitourinary system, GI organs (especially biliary tract), and skin, but identification of the source of sepsis may not be possible in the ED.

History

Determine the patient's *chief complaint* (e.g., fever, chills, weakness, dyspnea, rigors, altered mental status), abruptness of onset, and duration of symptoms. In addition, establish the patient's *underlying medical status* and any *recent hospitalization* or *surgery* (including dental work), *residence* (community living versus nursing home care), *medications* (use of antipyretics may suppress fever, intake of antibiotics may negate blood cultures, and corticosteroids or cytotoxic agents may mask signs and symptoms of infection), *allergies* (influences choice of antimicrobials), *travel history* (particularly to areas endemic for Rocky Mountain spotted fever, malaria, and babesiosis), and *occupation* (exposure to animal transmitted infections). Conditions increasing the probability of sepsis include underlying heart disease, splenectomized patients (prone to overwhelming infection by encapsulated organisms), presence of prosthetic devices or indwelling catheters (e.g., Hickman, Groshong, Foley), inflammatory bowel disease, cirrhosis, recent bowel or genitourinary manipulation or surgery (increased risk of Gram-negative and anaerobic infection), peripartum females (including recent abortion, premature rupture of membranes, C-section), homosexual men (chance of AIDS, hepatitis, and other illnesses increased), IVDAs, alcoholics, AIDS, and other immunocompromising diseases (e.g., diabetes, cancer) and the elderly (65 years and older).

Physical Examination

Note: *It is essential to completely disrobe the patient or subtle clues may be missed.*

General. Document overall appearance. Note whether the patient is chronically ill (cachexia, malnourished) or acutely toxic.

Vital signs. Obtain *rectal temperature* (both hyperthermia and hypothermia are important clues), *tachycardia* (may result from dehydration or physiologic response to sepsis), *blood pressure* (do not rely solely on blood pressure to diagnose septic shock; early on, blood pressure may be normal), and *respiratory rate* (tachypnea may be an early sign of sepsis).

Skin. Carefully inspect the skin, looking for distinctive rashes (e.g., meningococcemia, Rocky Mountain spotted fever) and evidence of skin or soft tissue infection (including decubiti). Also note presence of jaundice (RBC destruction or liver failure), petechiae (DIC, thrombocytopenia), cyanosis (inadequate oxygenation), and skin temperature (whether warm and dry, or cool and clammy). Examine skin surrounding indwelling intravascular catheters for signs of infection.

HEENT. Search for signs of underlying infection, i.e., sinus tenderness, unilateral nasal drainage, chronic ear infections, mastoiditis, pharyngitis, oral ulcers, abscesses, gingivitis or conjunctiva or retinal findings.

Neck. Check for meningismus, lymphadenopathy, and thyroid enlargement or tenderness.

Chest. Listen for localized or diffuse crackles, rubs, and/or rhonchi (in elderly dehydrated patients with early pneumonia, the lungs often sound initially clear).

Heart. Auscultate for murmurs or rubs (lack of a murmur does not exclude diagnosis of endocarditis).

Abdomen. Examine for abdominal tenderness, rebound, distention, masses, or absent bowel sounds (findings may be subtle in the elderly or immunocompromised). Assess for flank tenderness.

Rectal and pelvic. Inspect for urethral or pelvic discharge as well as rectal, pelvic or prostatic tenderness. Test the stool for blood (GI bleed is possible complication of sepsis).

Extremities. Observe for joint or muscle tenderness, swelling, or crepitus, and note bony pain and evidence of phlebitis or IVDA.

Neurologic. Recognize changes in mental status (may be the first sign of sepsis, especially in the elderly).

Diagnostic Tests

CBC with differential. Leukocytosis with a left shift, toxic granules, and Döhle bodies all occur with sepsis. Overwhelming infection may also produce a profound neutropenia (presence of neutropenia signifies a poor prognosis). Hematocrit may be increased secondary to volume depletion.

PT, PTT, platelets, and fibrin split products. Thrombocytopenia may result from DIC (sepsis most common cause of DIC) or occur as an isolated finding.

Serum electrolytes. A decreased bicarbonate level with an increased anion gap suggests lactic acidosis. Elevation of serum potassium concomitant with a decreased serum sodium level implies adrenal insufficiency.

Biochemical profile. Altered by sepsis; establish baseline values. Hyperglycemia may signal uncontrolled infection in diabetic.

Arterial blood gases. *Respiratory alkalosis* ($P_{CO_2} \leq 30$ mm Hg) is one of the earliest findings of sepsis. Respiratory acidosis suggests impending respiratory failure. Presence of hypoxemia and metabolic acidosis signals overwhelming infection.

Microbiology. All patients with suspected sepsis require three sets of blood cultures (10 mL, 10 min apart). Gram stain and culture all possible sites of infection (e.g., urine, wounds, sputum).

Radiological studies. Obtain a CXR as part of diagnostic workup. A CT exam of the abdomen and pelvis may assist in localization of abscesses.

ECG. Inspect for evidence of ischemia.

Treatment

A two-pronged approach is advocated in treating septic shock. First, eradicate the nidus of infection with *antibiotics, surgical drainage,* or both. If unable to identify an obvious focus of infection, collect cultures and immediately start empirical antibiotic therapy, directing treatment at the most likely pathogen(s) (see section 9.10). Broad-spectrum antibiotic coverage is provided by combination therapy, e.g., *nafcillin* (1 g IV q 6 hr) or *vancomycin* (500 mg IV q 6 hr) plus *gentamicin* (3 to 5 mg/kg day IV in three divided doses, adjusting the dose for renal insufficiency) plus *clindamycin* (600 to 900 mg IV q 6 to 8 hr). While antibiotics are capable of controlling the systemic spread of infection, they will not eradicate a focal abscess. Therefore, surgical consultation is mandated for questionable deep abscess, infected prosthesis (valvular, orthopedic, graft) or intravascular catheter, and/or infarcted bowel. In complicated cases, consult an ID specialist.

Second, *support cardiopulmonary function.* Diligently monitor vital signs, and mental status along with additional hemodynamic parameters, e.g., pulse oximetry, cardiac monitors, intraarterial line, automatic blood pressure cuffs, Foley catheter for urine output, and central venous pressure when appropriate. Provide supplemental oxygen to all septic patients, with intubation and mechanical ventilation performed as indicated (see section 2.2). Cardiovascular assistance is conveyed by rapid and adequate fluid administration, along with vasopressors as needed (see section 1.2).

Admission Criteria

All patients with suspected septic shock obligate admission to a critical care unit, often requiring an invasive Swan-Ganz catheter to guide therapy.

Suggested Readings

Harris RL, Musher, DM, Bloom K, et al.: Manifestations of sepsis. Arch Intern Med 1987;147:1895–1906.

Parillo JE: Pathogenic mechanisms of septic shock. N Engl J Med 1993;328:1471–1477.

Chapter 10

Obstetrics and Gynecology

10.1 ECTOPIC PREGNANCY

Description

Ectopic pregnancy is the consequence of the implantation of a fertilized ovum in an extrauterine site. The vast majority occur within the patient's fallopian tubes. Almost half of ectopic pregnancies are misdiagnosed on initial evaluation. Both the incidence and the prevalence of ectopic pregnancies in the United States continue to rise each year.

History

Always consider the possibility of ectopic pregnancy in any female of child-bearing age presenting with abdominal pain and/or vaginal bleeding. Verify dates and characteristics of their last normal menstrual period. Document history of previous pregnancies, abortions, and deliveries. Inquire about risk factors for ectopic pregnancy (Table 10.1.1). Also ask the patient if she is taking ovulation-inducing agents (they increase the risk of combined intrauterine and extrauterine pregnancy).

Atypical histories are frequent, with few patients actually presenting with the classic picture of ectopic pregnancy (amenorrhea, followed by pelvic pain, and adnexal mass enlargement). Initial symptoms may mimic those of early pregnancy (nausea, vomiting, breast tenderness). Up to 25% of women with ectopic pregnancies report a normal menstrual history. The amount, timing, and character of bleeding should not obviate the possibility of ectopic pregnancy. Consider suspect any self-reported pregnancy status.

Table 10.1.1
Risk Factors for Ectopic Pregnancy

History of pelvic inflammatory disease
History of previous ectopic or tubal surgery
History of infertility (hormonal therapy or in vitro fertilization)
Previous abdominal or pelvic surgery
Use of intrauterine device

Eventually, the ectopic pregnancy outgrows its blood supply. The characterization of pain is highly variable, depending on the site of implantation and the amount of trophoblastic tissue formed. Classically, there is a rapid onset of oppressive, unilateral pain. Pain may radiate to the shoulder, secondary to hemoperitoneum, inducing irritation of the diaphragm (Kehr's sign). Syncope occurs in up to 20% of cases.

Physical Examination

General. The presence of pallor, clamminess, and restlessness all can signal *hypovolemic shock.* Shock occurs in about 20% of patients and implies > 1000 mL of blood loss.

Vital signs. Check rectal temperature, pulse, and blood pressure, including orthostatics. **Note:** *Vital signs can be deceiving with ectopic pregnancy; some patients may not mount a tachycardiac response to significant hypovolemia.*

Abdomen. Palpate for localized lower abdominal tenderness, rebound, or masses.

Pelvic. Check for vaginal bleeding and softening or blue coloration of the cervix. Inspect the internal os to determine if it is open or closed. Evaluate the uterus for size and tenderness. Palpate the adnexa carefully for tenderness or masses. The cul-de-sac may feel doughy and distended.

Diagnostic Tests

Laboratory Tests

Order a stat CBC and blood typing (including Rh) in all pregnant females with suspected ectopic pregnancy.

Pregnancy Testing

Human chorionic gonadotropin (hCG) levels become detectable in the blood and urine 2 to 5 days after implantation; a negative pregnancy test virtually rules out an intrauterine and an ectopic pregnancy (false-negative rate < 1%). While not always immediately available, *quantitative hCG levels* can be invaluable in distinguishing an ectopic from an intrauterine pregnancy. In normal pregnancy, the hCG levels double approximately every 2 days in early pregnancy (peaking at 100,000 mIU/L at 11 weeks gestation age) but rise more slowly in an ectopic pregnancy. Failure of the hCG to double every 48 hr suggests an abnormal pregnancy. Quantitative hCG levels can also be used in combination with sonography. *Serum progesterone,* a product of the corpus luteum, remains at a fairly constant level (> 25 nanograms/mL) during the first 10 weeks of pregnancy. Low levels (< 5 ng/mL) are associated with either a nonviable or an ectopic pregnancy. Levels between 5 and 25 ng/mL are indeterminate, and additional studies are needed.

Sonogram

Ultrasonography effectively excludes an ectopic pregnancy if an intrauterine pregnancy is demonstrated (except for the rare heterotopic pregnancy). An *intrauterine gestational sac* is the earliest sign of pregnancy seen on ultrasound, appearing at 4 to 5 weeks with *transvaginal sonography* (TVS) versus 5 to 6 weeks with *transabdominal sonography* (TAS). Unfortunately, 20% of ectopic pregnancies present with a *pseudogestational sac* (lacks a fetal pole), which confuses the picture. Absence of a gestational sac suggests an ectopic pregnancy or an intrauterine pregnancy too small to be seen on sonography. A gestational sac generally becomes visible on TVS when the quantitative hCG level is > 1500 mIU/L; while for TAS, the level usually exceeds 6500 mIU/L. Fetal heart activity is not present until 7 weeks. Other findings that suggest an ectopic pregnancy include an adnexal mass and fluid in the cul-de-sac.

Culdocentesis

Culdocentesis is most appropriate for the stable patient with suspected hemoperitoneum but may not be indicated for the critically ill, unstable patient who requires immediate diagnostic laparoscopy or laparotomy. It is contraindicated when pelvic examination reveals a retroverted uterus or a mass in the cul-de-sac. The high incidence of both false-positive (bleeding ovarian cysts) and false-negative findings (unruptured ectopic pregnancies) and the advances and availability of ultrasonography have contributed to its decline in popularity.

Treatment

Consult OB-GYN once the diagnosis of ectopic pregnancy is considered. All unstable patients require immediate resuscitative measures, while arrangements are made for laparoscopy or laparotomy. The management of the stable patient is more controversial. In some centers, pharmacologic therapy, e.g., methotrexate, is used to ablate an unruptured, small ectopic pregnancy. In addition, some consultants may elect to admit a stable patient for observation, and follow the hCG levels (spontaneous tubal abortion is a possibility in patients with declining hCG levels).

Admission Criteria

All patients with a documented ectopic pregnancy require admission for OB-GYN management. In addition, it is prudent to admit for observation *all patients in whom the diagnosis cannot be excluded.* Some consultants may elect to manage the reliable, stable patient as an outpatient with serial hCG levels and ultrasonography. Such decisions need to be documented, with clear delineation of future responsibility. The patient should be instructed to seek immediate medical attention for worsening of symptoms.

Suggested Readings

Abbot JT, Emmans SR, Lowenstein SR: Ectopic pregnancy: ten common pitfalls in diagnosis. Am J Emerg Med 1990;8:515–522.

Carson SA, Buster SE. Ectopic pregnancy. N Engl J Med 1993;329: 1174–1179.

Ramoska EA, Saccheti, AD, Nepp M: Reliability of patient history in determining possibility of pregnancy. Ann Emerg Med 1988;18:48–50.

10.2 EMERGENCY DELIVERY

Description

Although the need for emergency delivery outside a hospital obstetric unit is relatively rare, there must be a calm and orderly approach to the evaluation of these patients as well as established policies for transfer or delivery. The Consolidated Omnibus Budget Reconciliation (COBRA) prohibits the transfer of women in "active labor" unless the harm in transfer is less than that of remaining in the hospital. *Active labor,* by definition occurs when delivery is imminent, there is inadequate time to effect safe transfer to another hospital before delivery, or a transfer may pose a threat of the health and safety of the patient or unborn child. It is essential that all transfers are arranged physician to physician. Failure to adhere to these policies results in severe financial penalties to both the physician and hospital.

History

Obtain a focused history. Establish the chief complaint, past medical and surgical history, allergies, and present medications. Ask questions relevant to the pregnancy, including gravidity, parity, estimated date of confinement, and pregnancy-related difficulties. Also ask (1) if and when the membranes ruptured ("bloody show"); (2) about the frequency, duration, and intensity of the contractions; and (3) whether the patient has an uncontrollable urge to bear down.

Physical Examination

A purposeful examination of the obstetric patient will determine whether the patient is in true labor and, if so, how far labor has progressed. The initial evaluation consists of (1) determining maternal vital signs and fetal heart sounds, (2) determining the frequency and intensity of contractions, and (3) inspecting the perineum. Any woman who is beyond 20 weeks of gestation and presents in active labor or with complications of pregnancy (e.g., vaginal discharge or bleeding) should first undergo an aseptic speculum examination to check for fluid, blood, or meconium. Any fluid in the vaginal vault requires testing to rule out amniotic fluid leakage—amniotic fluid is alkaline (pH 7.0 to 7.5) and will turn nitrazine paper blue, whereas vaginal fluid tends to be acidic (pH 4.5 to 5.5). Also check the fluid for *ferning,* another indication of leakage, on a glass slide. If vaginal bleeding is present, *do not* insert the speculum any farther and transport the patient to the operating room for a *double setup* (see section 10.5). The presenting part and degree of dilation are determined by the speculum examination.

Treatment

Unless delivery is imminent (the mother presents fully dilated, perineum bulging, and/or fetal parts apparent on the perineal verge, *crowning*), the pregnant patient should be transported expeditiously to *labor and delivery*. No attempt should be made to stop the natural progression of fetal descent. However, if the patient is pushing excessively, she should be encouraged to cease bearing down (advocate breathing rapidly through the mouth, *panting*). Attempt to record fetal vital signs every 5 min during the second stage of labor. The normal fetal heart rate is 120 to 160 bpm. If fetal tachycardia or bradycardia is detected, the mother should be given oxygen and an intravenous fluid challenge and be positioned in the left lateral decubitus position. Bradycardia following contractions (30 sec after) are considered "late decelerations" and are an ominous sign. Consider possible causes of fetal distress, including cord prolapse and placental abruption. Urgent delivery or cesarean section may be required.

If the membranes are intact, there is generally no reason to rupture them artificially until actual delivery. Once full dilatation has been established and the baby's head descends, imminent delivery can be anticipated by bulging of the perineum and the appearance of the fetal scalp at the introitus. At this point, a controlled delivery is important in preventing both fetal and maternal injury. Three stages occur with spontaneous vaginal deliveries—delivery of the head, delivery of the shoulders, and delivery of the body and legs. A *Ritgen's maneuver,* gentle pressure applied to the perineum with one hand, while the other hand is placed on the head of the infant to control speed of the delivery, facilitates delivery of the head, and lessens the chance of peripartum trauma. The role of episiotomy is controversial.

The majority of women will deliver spontaneously if left alone.

When presented with a precipitous delivery, focus your attention on the baby and the ABCs rather than on the cord and placenta. Suction the infant's nose and mouth quickly once the head is delivered and before delivery of the thorax and the initial vital breath happens. Clamp and cut the cord, and give the baby to an assistant to dry off. Quickly ensure adequate respirations and survey the infant for congenital abnormalities. Spontaneously breathing babies ought to be dried off, wrapped in a warm blanket, and placed on the mother's abdomen or under a radiant warmer.

Generally, the placenta will deliver naturally (20 to 30 min following birth of the neonate). Only when there is large, ongoing bleeding that does not stop after delivery are special measures to deliver the retained placenta necessary. Excessive traction on the umbilical cord may provoke uterine inversion. Infusion of *oxytocin* (20 U of oxytocin in 1 L of NS at a rate of 100 to 500 mL/hr) may help minimize postpartum blood loss. Cautiously monitor the mother's vital signs. Improper dosing of oxytocin can lead to uterine rupture as well as seizures and coma.

Special Considerations

Meconium Staining

If a thick pea soup material appears during crowning, stop the delivery with the infant's head on the perineum (ask the mother not to push), and thoroughly suction the baby's nose, mouth, and pharynx before the thorax is delivered to try to prevent aspiration of meconium. Upon delivery, intubate the infant with largest endotracheal tube that is feasible and suction under direct laryngoscopy.

Preterm Delivery

Emergency deliveries frequently involve preterm infants. Although small in size, becuase of the increased fragility of the infant (particularly the intracranial blood vessels), it is still imperative to deliver the neonate in a controlled manner. Avoid artificial rupture of the membranes if possible and permit an "en cul" (membranes intact) delivery.

Breech Presentation

There is an increased propensity to breech presentation in premature infants. Although the procedure of choice is delivery by cesarean section, this is regularly not possible in an emergency. In any breech delivery, difficulty should be anticipated; an episiotomy should be performed. Allow the breech infant to deliver spontaneously, at least until the level of the umbilicus. Place a warm towel on the baby's lower back and buttocks and gently rotate the shoulders into the anterior-posterior plane. The posterior shoulder is delivered first by raising the infant's entire body. Reversing the procedure should deliver the anterior shoulder.

Application of suprapubic pressure by an assistant helps maintain flexion of the baby's head. As the neck emerges, place a finger over the baby's maxilla or gently into the baby's mouth, flexing the head for delivery and avoiding entrapment.

Prolapsed Cord

Umbilical cord prolapse is an obstetric emergency. Palpate the cord for presence of pulsations (fetal viability); if pulsations are not felt, assess fetal heart tones. If the baby is dead, there is no need for emergent c-section. For a viable fetus, it is essential to manually elevate the presenting parts away from the cord by inserting a hand in the vagina and pushing up. Do not attempt to reposition the cord! Place the patient in the Trendelenburg or knee-chest position, administer oxygen and intravenous fluids, and transport to the operating room for cesarean section with the examiner's hand in position until the c-section is completed.

Uterine Inversion

A potentially disastrous complication of an overzealous delivery is *uterine inversion,* whereby the uterus protrudes through the cervix; depending on the degree of inversion, the uterus can extend through the vagina. Shock can rapidly ensue. If oxytocic agents are being given, they must be stopped immediately and the uterus repositioned at once. The inverted uterus is placed in the palm of the hand and pushed upward, without attempting to remove the placenta.

Perimortem Salvage and Postmortem Cesarean

In the event a pregnant woman presents in cardiac arrest, a stat c-section may be attempted after 4 min of unsuccessful CPR if fetal viability is possible (survival is unlikely if the gestational age is < 28 weeks). When performing a perimortem cesarean section, continue aggressive CPR. Using a scalpel and sterile technique, make a vertical midline incision through the abdominal cavity to expose the uterus. Next, use scissors to make a vertical incision in the uterus (classical approach), placing one finger inside the uterus to protect the fetus. Strive to avoid injuring the maternal bladder and bowel. Remove the fetus and placenta. Control bleeding with clamps and direct pressure. Continue CPR and close in the operating room if the patient stabilizes.

Suggested Readings

Brunette DD, Sterner SP: Prehospital and emergency department delivery: a review of eight years experience. Ann Emerg Med 1989;18: 1116–1118.

Gianopoulos JG: Emergency complications of labor and delivery. Emerg Med Clin North Am 1994;12:201–217.

10.3 PELVIC INFLAMMATORY DISEASE

Description

Pelvic inflammatory disease (PID), also known as salpingo-oophoritis, is the most common serious infection among reproductive-age women in the United States. *Neisseria gonorrhoeae* (25 to 50%) and *Chlamydia trachomatis* (25 to 61%) are the major identifiable pathogens. However, other microorganisms are also indicated, with current thinking proposing that PID is a polymicrobial infection.

Short-term complications include tuboovarian abscess or perihepatitis (Fitz-Hugh-Curtis syndrome), while chronic pelvic pain, scarring of the fallopian tubes, dyspareunia, infertility, ectopic pregnancy, pelvic adhesions, or recurrent episodes of PID comprise the long-term sequelae.

History

Symptoms of PID are protean, with no sign or complaint being specific. Inquire about (1) the level of sexual activity, (2) the number of partners in the last 2 to 3 months, (3) first day of the last menstrual period (onset of pain with PID often coincides with the start of menstrual flow), (4) any abnormal bleeding (see section 10.5), (5) use and type of contraception, (6) dyspareunia and/or rectal pain during defecation, and (7) any recent surgical and gynecological procedures.

Physical Examination

General. Note if the patient appears toxic.

Vital signs. Evaluate for fever and orthostatic changes.

Skin. Note the presence or absence of rash.

HEENT. Look for pharyngeal injection or exudate.

Abdomen. Palpate for peritoneal signs (involuntary guarding, rebound tenderness), masses, and voluntary abdominal tenderness. Suprapubic tenderness and bilateral lower quadrant tenderness are most common, with right upper quadrant tenderness implying perihepatitis (Fitz-Hugh-Curtis syndrome).

Pelvic. Note labial or vaginal lesions; vaginal discharge (describe the color, quantity, and texture); cervical motion tenderness or lesions; uterine size, texture, and tenderness; adnexal masses or tenderness; and rectal masses or tenderness.

Diagnostic Tests

Laboratory tests. CBC, urinalysis, urine culture, β-hCG, ESR, VDRL, endocervical Gram stain, and cultures for gonorrhea and *Chlamydia* should be obtained.

Sonogram. An adjunct to the pelvic examination. Helpful findings that support the diagnosis of PID include adnexal enlargement or a tuboovarian abscess. Suggestive clues include an increase in uterine size, adnexal adherence, and fluid in the cul-de-sac.

Diagnosis

The classical signs of PID (fever, adnexal tenderness, purulent vaginal discharge, a pelvic mass, and an elevated white blood cell count and ESR) are more common with gonococcal infection. Nongonococcal PID (*Chlamydia* in particular) tends to follow a more indolent course. Anaerobic infections are more prevalent in older patients, those with IUDs, or women who have had a recent gynecological procedure. The appearance of many of the signs and symptoms of PID is variable, and definitive diagnosis often calls for laparoscopy (Table 10.3.1). The following criteria assist the clinician in making the tentative diagnosis of PID. All three should be present:

1. Lower abdominal tenderness;
2. Cervical tenderness with motion; and
3. Adnexal tenderness.

Presence of at least one of the following additional criteria is required:

1. WBC count > 10,500;
2. Temperature > 38.0°C (100.4°F);
3. Culdocentesis yielding purulent drainage;
4. ESR >15 mm/hr;
5. Gram stain of endocervical discharge that displays > 5 WBCs/oil immersion field;

Table 10.3.1
Differential Diagnosis of PID

Gynecological system
Ectopic pregnancy
Endometritis
Endometriosis
Tuboovarian abscess
Abortion (threatened, septic)
Intrauterine pregnancy
Dysmenorrhea
Ovarian cyst
Mittelschmerz syndrome
Ruptured follicle
Adnexal torsion
Gastrointestinal tract
Appendicitis
Diverticulitis
Inflammatory bowel disease
Gastroenteritis
Constipation
Irritable bowel syndrome
Urinary tract
Pyelonephritis
Cystitis
Urethritis

6. Gram stain of endocervical discharge that exhibits intracellular Gram-negative diplococci;
7. Endocervical discharge that is positive for monoclonal antibody to *C. trachomatis;* or
8. An inflammatory mass on bimanual examination or ultrasonography.

Treatment

CDC Regimens for Inpatient Treatment of PID

Recommended Regimen A: cefoxitin (2 g IV q 6 hr), cefotetan (2 g IV q 12 hr), or other cephalosporin, such as ceftizoxime, cefotaxime, or ceftriaxone, at an equivalent dose and frequency plus doxycycline (100 mg PO or IV q 12 hr).

Recommended Regimen B: clindamycin (900 mg IV q 8 hr) plus gentamicin (loading dose of 2 mg/kg IV followed by a maintenance dose of 1.5 mg/kg IV q 8 hr).

CDC Regimens for Outpatient Treatment of PID

Ceftriaxone (250 mg IM), cefoxitin (2 g IM), or other third-generation cephalosporin, such as ceftizoxime or cefotaxime, plus probenecid (1 g PO) plus doxycycline (100 mg PO BID for 14 days). A recent alternative is ofloxacin (400 mg PO BID) plus either clindamycin (450 mg PO BID) or metronidazole (500 mg PO BID for 14 days).

Admission Criteria

Appearance of any of the following criteria is a clear justification for admission: patients who appear toxic, have a temperature > 39.0°C, have suspected tuboovarian or pelvic abscess, have nausea and vomiting severe enough to preclude oral therapy and hydration, fail to improve with 48 to 72 hr of outpatient therapy, have evidence of the spread of infection outside pelvis (Fitz-Hugh-Curtis syndrome), are pregnant, have peritonitis, have an unclear diagnosis, have an IUD, or are nulligravidas. Since effective treatment is essential to prevent late sequelae (sterility, ectopic pregnancy), it is advisable to admit *all patients with PID* for intravenous therapy.

Suggested Reading

McCormick WM. Pelvic inflammatory disease. N Engl J Med 1994;330: 115–121.

10.4 SEXUAL ASSAULT

Description

Sexual assault (*rape* is a legal term) is defined differently in various municipalities. ED physicians and caregivers should be well versed with laws pertaining to sexual assault in their jurisdiction. *Rape is an act of violence* where there is nonconsensual vaginal, anal, or oral contact executed by the offender's penis or hand or a foreign body. Most sexual assault victims are female (> 95%). Sexual assault is a terrifying experience for the victims; they often fear for their life. To provide good medical care, the ED staff must be compassionate and nonjudgmental toward all victims. A nurse, social service worker, or counselor (preferably of the same sex) should remain with the victim throughout the ED stay.

History

While it is essential to gather pertinent information to fully evaluate the extent of injuries, *do not* attempt to obtain unnecessary, frivolous information from the victim, as this may adversely affect subsequent criminal proceedings. It is reasonable, however, to ask about the time of assault, description of the assailant, number of assailants, the nature of the physical abuse (use of weapons and restraints), and which body cavities were penetrated (oral, anal, or vaginal penetration). Ask the patient if he or she bathed, urinated, defecated, or douched since the assault, as this may alter the presence of evidence. A general gynecological history should include last menstrual period, current pregnancy, most recent consensual sexual activity, contraceptive use, and prior history of sexually transmitted disease. Record drug allergies and any general medical problems.

Physical Examination

General. Note the patient's appearance (disheveled, agitated, bloody). All clothing should be labeled and saved as evidence. Inspect the patient's entire body for evidence of injury.

Skin. Look for bruises and lacerations.

Abdomen. Palpate for masses and tenderness, particularly in the left upper quadrant (splenic rupture or hematoma). Also consider the possibility of exploitation with a foreign body and the possibility of penetration into the peritoneal cavity.

Pelvic. Examine the external genitalia for ecchymosis, dried semen, laceration, or perineal injuries. On internal examination, note any recent mucosal tears or trauma to the hymenal ring. In addition, inspect for small abrasions or telangiectasias in the posterior fourchette or distal vagina as well as engorgement or erythema of the labia or clitoris. Use only saline for lubrication of speculum, since commercial lubricants (e.g., K-Y jelly) may alter results. Determine the size and tenderness of the uterus and surrounding structures. **Note:** *The absence of genital injury* does not *imply consent by the victim.*

Rectal. Perform if clinically indicated to find any tenderness or lacerations.

Extremities. In addition to examining for tenderness, lacerations, bruising, and crepitus, look for any evidence of physical restraint (rope or leather marks) and search under the fingernails for hair or skin fragments.

Diagnostic Tests

Note: If the patient is reluctant to have specimens gathered, explain that this *does not* obligate him or her to prosecute, but it will allow collection of important evidence if the patient were to change his or her mind.

Rape kits. Most hospitals have a prepackaged rape kit with equipment for and directions on sample collection and maintenance of the chain of evidence. If no kit is available, smears of material from the vagina, cervix, anus, and mouth are made, labeled, and air dried. The swabs are placed in tubes, labeled, and air dried.

Normal saline wet mount. Smears of the cervix and the vaginal and anal vaults are examined to establish if sperm are present. Motile sperm persist in the vagina for 8 hr postintercourse and up to 2 to 3 days in the cervical mucus. Nonmotile sperm can remain in the vagina or rectum for up to 24 hr and endure for up to 17 days in the cervical mucus.

Pap smear. May provide later identification of sperm by the laboratory.

Acid phosphatase strips. Can be tested immediately or saved. Semen will fluoresce under a Wood's light.

Pubic hair sampling and material scraped from fingernails. Pubic hair combing and fingernail samples should be placed in appropriately marked envelopes. Pubic hair from the victim must also be plucked. Inform the patient of this need; ask if the patient would rather do this himself or herself.

Cultures. May obtain for gonorrhea and *Chlamydia,* although many physicians prefer to treat patients prophylactically. Also obtain samples for *Trichomonas* and bacterial vaginosis (see section 10.6), as these are relatively common sequelae to rape.

Laboratory tests. Baseline labs should include β-hCG and VDRL. HIV testing should be offered.

Photographs. Any film or photographs taken (with the consent of the patient) should be labeled with the patient's name and the date, given to the police, and placed in the record.

Treatment

Management of serious injuries assumes precedence over the sexual assault examination. Provide reassurance and support. Many hospitals have a multidisciplinary team or support personnel for victims of sexual assault. One of the most important and therapeutic functions of the staff is simply to listen.

Discuss the options of pregnancy prophylaxis. If the patient is not currently pregnant and wishes to prevent any possible pregnancy, she should be offered the option of a "morning-after" pill if seen within 72 hr. The currently recommended regimen is two *Ovral* (0.5 mg norgestrel plus 0.05 ethinyl estradiol per pill) repeated 12 hr later.

The CDC estimate for the risk of acquiring gonorrhea from sexual assault is 6 to 12%; *Chlamydia,* 4 to 17%; syphilis, 0.5 to 3%; and HIV, < 1%. STD prophylaxis comprises ceftriaxone (250 mg IM), metronidazole (2 g PO as a single dose), and either doxycycline (100 mg BID for 7 days) or azithromycin (1 g PO as one-time dose).

Save any potential evidence. Underwear and soiled, torn, or bloody clothing should be clearly marked and set aside as evidence. Some EDs have Polaroid cameras to document lacerations and other bodily injuries. **Note:** *The chart is a legal document and in many cases may be the only evidence available.* Be sure to review the chain of evidence policy before your evaluation.

Remember tetanus and hepatitis B prophylaxis, if indicated. The patient should be seen within 6 weeks for follow-up testing, i.e., pregnancy, VDRL, hepatitis B, and HIV, if she or he desires. Ensure ongoing emotional and psychological support for the patient.

Suggested Readings

Gostin LO. HIV testing, counseling, and prophylaxis after sexual assault. JAMA 1994;271:1436–1438.

Hampton HL: Current concepts. Care of the woman who has been raped. N Engl J Med 1995;332:234–237.

10.5 VAGINAL BLEEDING

History

All women of child-bearing age who complain of vaginal bleeding should be considered pregnant until proven otherwise. Pregnancy cannot be excluded solely on the basis of personal, sexual or menstrual history. Sources of vaginal bleeding include the vagina, cervix, and uterus. Pertinent historical information includes (1) presence of *early pregnancy symptoms* (fatigue, morning nausea, breast tenderness) or knowledge of a recent *positive pregnancy test;* (2) *gravidity, parity,* and *date of last menstrual period* (LMP); and (3) *characterization of current bleeding episode.* For current bleeding, find out when the bleeding started, how long it has lasted, and whether it is *cyclic* (time of normal period) or *noncyclic* (out of phase with the normal period). Inquire about the color and character of the bleeding or discharge or passage of any tissue. The number and type of pads or tampons used over the last 24 hr roughly estimates the flow rate. Compare this episode with the patient's normal periods (complete with dates, duration, amount of flow). Remember, there is marked individual variability with menstrual cycles.

Ask about accompanying *abdominal or pelvic pain,* specifically about the duration, progression, and location of the pain. The time association of the onset of pain and bleeding may help determine the etiology (Table 10.5.1). For example, patients with an ectopic pregnancy often develop pain before the onset of bleeding, whereas those undergoing a spontaneous abortion generally bleed before they experience the pain.

Ask if the *patient is sexually active* and what *means of contraception* is used. If the patient is using birth control pills (BCP), find out for how long and if she takes them regularly or sporadically.

Table 10.5.1
Causes of Vaginal Bleeding

- Pregnant or nonpregnant patient
  - Minor trauma
  - Cervicitis or cervical erosions
  - Polyps or tumors (invasive cervical cancer, endometrial polyp or cancer, submucosal leiomyomata)
  - Blood dyscrasias
  - Urethral or rectal bleeding
  - Dysfunctional uterine bleeding
- Pregnant patient
  - First- and second-trimester bleeding
    - Spontaneous abortion
    - Ectopic pregnancy
    - Uterine rupture
    - Hydatidiform mole
  - Third-trimester bleeding
    - Placenta previa
    - Abruptio placenta
    - Labor (bloody show)

Determine the history of any *systemic disease* such as diabetes mellitus, endocrine disorders, bleeding dyscrasias, or immunocompromising illnesses. Document *medication use* (including NSAIDs) and *allergies.* Also ask about *recreational drug use, smoking,* and *alcohol abuse.* In the *review of systems* ask about symptoms that suggest volume depletion (e.g., weakness, early fatigability, vomiting, postural dizziness, chest pain or shortness of breath), infection (fever, chills, vaginal discharge), or previous bleeding problems (nosebleeds, prolonged bleeding after dental extraction).

Physical Examination

Note: *The physical findings in patients with vaginal bleeding during pregnancy do not follow any particular pattern.* They change according to the gestational age of the pregnancy, the presence and degree of tubal distention, the amount of bleeding, and whether tubal or uterine rupture has occurred.

General. Look for signs of hypovolemia (patient apprehensive, skin pale or clammy) as well as evidence of clotting disorders (bruising, or petechiae).

Vital signs. Check for tachycardia, fever, and orthostatic changes.

Abdomen

The abdominal examination in most cases of vaginal bleeding is normal (except with intraperitoneal or massive intrauterine bleeding, such as a ruptured ectopic pregnancy, uterine rupture, or placental abruption). Findings may include rebound pain, guarding, or abdominal or uterine tenderness. If the patient appears pregnant, estimate fetal age by measuring fundal height (the top of the symphysis pubis corresponds to 12 weeks; the level of the umbilicus, 20 weeks; and the tip of the xiphoid, 36 weeks of pregnancy). Also check for fetal heart tones (will not be positive until after 8 to 10 weeks).

Pelvic

The pelvic examination should include visualization of the labia and vagina, noting evidence of lacerations, inflammation, or masses. The cervix should be examined for lacerations, inflammation, bleeding, or visible tissue. Assess the color and consistency of the cervix; the nonpregnant cervix is firm to the touch and pink in color, while a bluish (Chadwick's sign), soft cervix (Hegar's sign) is consistent with pregnancy. Note whether the internal os is open or closed.

Since there exists a potential for precipitating harm, pregnant patients beyond the 20th week of pregnancy with vaginal bleeding should not *undergo a bimanual examination, unless appropriate resources are accessible for emergent delivery or surgical intervention.* Perform a bimanual exam to check uterine size, location, and tenderness as well as consistency and presence of irregularity. Check for pain on cervical motion and palpate the adnexa for tenderness and masses (e.g., the ovaries should not be palpable in postmenopausal women; therefore, any mass perceived in this region is abnormal). Note any bulging or fullness of the cul-de-sac (indicating fluid, blood, or pus). Finally, examine the rectum and urethra to assess possible alternative sources of bleeding.

Diagnostic Tests

Laboratory Tests

The only mandatory laboratory test is a urine or blood qualitative hCG level. When physical findings or symptoms imply a significant blood loss, obtain a *CBC* along with a type (including *Rh*) and *cross-match.* Trends tend to be more helpful than isolated values, since compensatory mechanisms may mask initial blood loss. When the initial hematocrit is low (< 30), consider either a severe acute bleed or an acute bleeding episode superimposed on chronic anemia. In patients with major blood loss, questionable coagulopathy, or the possibility of retained products of conception or abruptio placenta obtain clotting studies and fibrin split products (FSPs) to rule out disseminated intravascular coagulation (see section 13.3).

Other Tests

Sonogram. Ultrasonography is the most useful diagnostic adjunct at any stage of pregnancy and is beneficial in identifying potential gynecological pathology. Transvaginal ultrasound provides superior images of the intrauterine contents, fallopian tubes, ovaries, and cul-de-sac. **Note:** *Placenta previa is a potential contraindication to vaginal ultrasound.*

Culdocentesis. See Chapter 21.

Special Considerations

Vaginal Bleeding in Nonpregnant Female

Bleeding in nonpregnant females results from infection, hormonal imbalance, hematological abnormality, anatomical (uterine) irregularity, trauma (including insertion of foreign bodies), and malignancy. The first step is to ensure hemodynamic stability; if the patient demonstrates symptoms or signs of significant blood loss, treat as *hypovolemic shock* (see section 1.2). Once assured that the patient does not have a life-threatening process, strive to locate the source. If blood is not advancing from the os, carefully examine the surrounding areas (vagina, vulva, and anus). Obtain a clean-catch urine to exclude hematuria.

In nonpregnant females with vaginal bleeding, establish when in the menstrual cycle the bleeding is taking place. Normally, the menstrual cycle is every 21 to 40 days, with menses typically lasting 2 to 8 days. The heaviest flow occurs in the first 2 days. The average blood loss is normally 40 mL. Profuse bleeding coinciding with the menstrual period is labeled *menorrhagia* (seen with anatomic abnormalities of the uterus and hormonal imbalances). Bleeding that occurs between normal menstrual cycles is termed *metrorrhagia* (etiology most likely anatomic or systemic disturbance); while vaginal bleeding that is both excessive and irregular at the time of menses (there is no normal cyclic bleeding) is termed *menometrorrhagia* (any etiology possible).

Gonococcal and nongonococcal infection may provoke cyclic and noncyclic vaginal bleeding (obtain cultures; see section 9.4). If bleeding is timed regularly to the midcycle, the most likely etiology is hormonal.

Young patients who have just reached menarche, near-menopausal females, and women with underlying diabetes or thyroid disease frequently experience anovulatory or breakthrough bleeding. This type of bleeding is also referred to as *dysfunctional uterine bleeding (DUB)*. However, the diagnosis of DUB must not be concluded until other causes (infection, malignancy, trauma) are ruled out.

For women in their main child-bearing years (16 to 40 years old), the most frequent cause is *polycystic ovary disease* (Stein-Leventhal syndrome); this disease is distinguished by obesity, excessive or abnormal body hair growth, and enlarged ovaries on bimanual examination. A similar pattern is experienced by women starting birth control pills (if there are no other problems, they should be encouraged to complete the cycle of birth control pills and follow-up with their gynecologist).

Uterine abnormalities, such as *leiomyomata* (fibroids) may be responsible for heavy cyclical bleeding; on pelvic examination, the uterus may appear enlarged or irregular. *In any postmenopausal patient, one is obligated to rule out a uterine (endometrial) malignancy when uterine bleeding transpires.*

Patients may also bleed following a conization procedure (usually within 14 days). Bleeding in this situation is best controlled by suturing any lacerations.

Vaginal Bleeding in Early Pregnancy

For *ectopic pregnancy,* see section 10.2.

Minor Cervical Trauma. The most benign form of vaginal bleeding during the first two trimesters is due to normal cervical changes that accompany pregnancy. Exposed cervical epithelium is friable and bleeds easily when traumatized by any manipulation, including a Pap smear or sexual intercourse. Patients usually give a history of spotting bright red blood following intercourse or other mechanical manipulation. Management includes obtaining a Pap smear (if one has not been recently performed), applying gentle pressure locally to the bleeding site, and cautioning the patient to avoid all possible trauma to the cervix for at least 5 to 7 days. **Note:** *All patients with evidence of trauma should be carefully questioned about the possibility of abuse or battering.*

Spontaneous Abortion. Spontaneous abortions probably complicate greater than 20% of pregnancies. The vast majority of spontaneous abortions will occur in the first 12 weeks of pregnancy. Spontaneous abortions are classified as *threatened, inevitable, incomplete, complete,* and *missed.* Risk factors for spontaneous abortions include increased age, presence of a chronic-debilitating disease or a chronic occult genital tract infection (e.g., *Chlamydia*), history of smoking, and use of cocaine.

Threatened abortion is defined by vaginal bleeding in conjunction with a closed cervix and no loss of fetal tissue. Uterine contractions may accompany the bleeding, indicating a much higher risk for completing the abortion. Management is expectant, including bed rest, abstinence from coitus, IUD removal (if present), and administration of Rh-immune globulin if the patient is Rh−.

An *inevitable abortion* is characterized by the presence of ruptured membranes and/or a dilated cervix. The patient may complain of uterine contractions (cramping) or ballooning of the lower uterine segment. Therapy comprises admission for uterine evacuation and curettage, adminstration of Rh-immune globulin if the patient is Rh− and facilitation of the grieving process.

An *incomplete abortion* is distinguished by the presence of the products of conception. On examination, the physician typically finds a dilated cervix, tissue in the os or vagina, and relatively heavy bleeding. Patients may complain of uterine cramping. The treatment plan for incomplete abortions is virtually the same as that for inevitable abortions: Most patients will require admission for curettage to remove retained products of conception.

The term *complete abortion* implies the passage of the entire conceptus. Certain complete abortions are associated with a closed cervix and a normal uterine size, while at other times the cervical os may still be open. The fetus and placental tissue may be found in the vaginal vault or brought in by the patient. Because of these disparate presentations, making the diagnosis of a complete abortion can be difficult on clinical grounds alone. Management decisions need to be made in conjunction with the OB-GYN consultant.

In *missed abortion,* the pregnancy has terminated, but the products of conception have not yet passed and have been present for at least 4 weeks. Typically, the patient will report that abdominal swelling has discontinued and breast changes have receded. Often patients will complain of a prune juice–colored discharge.

Gestational Trophoblastic Disease. Gestational trophoblastic disease (GTN) is a general term for a spectrum of proliferate abnormalities of the trophoblastic tissue. Three entities are represented: *hydatidiform mole* (benign form), *invasive mole* (locally invasive), and *choriocarcinoma* (malignant form). Dark red vaginal bleeding in the first trimester is the most common symptom. Additional associated symptoms include an absence of fetal heart tones, uterine size larger than expected for gestational age, and abdominal pain. Some patients develop hyperemesis, clinical hyperthyroidism, or preeclampsia (see section 1.7) in the first trimester. Ancillary studies demonstrate an elevated quantitative β-hCG level (> 1,000,000 IU/L in many cases) that is inconsistent with dates and multiple echoes on sonography without the normal gestational sac.

Bleeding in Late Pregnancy

Cervical Effacement. Cervical effacement (bloody show) is characterized by a pink mucous discharge from the cervix that precedes labor from hours to weeks. If the mother is in active labor, maternal monitoring and fetal monitoring are all that is required while arrangements are made for delivery.

Placenta Previa. Placenta previa is defined by an implantation of any part of the placenta in the lower uterine segment that covers (partially or totally) the internal os, thereby obstructing the descent of the fetus. If not recognized before delivery, severe hemorrhage results. Placenta previa is associated with advanced maternal age, previous c-section, malposition of the fetus, multiparity, and multiple gestation. The hallmark of placenta previa is *painless hemorrhage* after 28 weeks gestation. The best way to diagnose placenta previa is by ultrasound. Proper management of placenta previa depends on the stage of the patient's pregnancy and the amount and persistence of hemorrhage. Avoid vaginal or rectal examination when placenta previa is suspected. Immediate obstetric consultation is required.

Uterine Rupture. Uterine rupture may occur spontaneously or as a result of trauma (which may appear incidental) or overstimulation by oxytocin or prolonged labor. Generally, this transpires in a patient who has had a previous c-section or other operative procedure of the uterus (myomectomy). This is a *life-threatening condition to both the mother and the baby*. Vaginal bleeding may be scant (concealed in peritoneal cavity) or heavy. Typically, severe pain precedes the rupture; pain may subside once rupture occurs. When the symptoms of shock in later pregnancy are out of proportion to external blood loss, suspect concealed hemorrhage (e.g., uterine rupture or abruptio placenta). These patients need immediate surgical intervention.

Abruptio Placenta. Abruption placenta refers to the premature separation of a normally implanted placenta from the uterine cavity. Predisposing factors to placental abruption include maternal hypertension, external trauma, polyhydramnios, multiparity, cocaine abuse, and maternal alcohol consumption. The diagnosis of abruptio placenta is based on clinical findings. Classically, abruptio placenta presents with dark red, painful bleeding. However, the amount of vaginal bleeding varies from scant to profuse, with the blood being a darker red than that from placenta previa. An especially risky scenario is when abruption presents with a concealed hemorrhage, increasing the morbidity and mortality for both the mother and the fetus. Abdominal pain typically accompanies the bleeding, ranging from mild abdominal cramping to backache to oppressive continuous abdominal distress. Pain may occur without bleeding. On physical examination, the uterus is tender, with an increased tone noted between contractions. Unless placenta previa is ruled out, the vaginal examination should be deferred to the OB-GYN consultant, where it can be done under a double setup with provisions for stat c-section instantly accessible. Ultrasound is diagnostic for abruptio placenta only 25 to 40% of the time. An additional complication is *consumptive coagulopathy*. The main objective of the emergency physician is to suspect abruption, anticipate a hemorrhagic emergency, and provide attentive monitoring for both the mother and the baby. Immediate obstetric consultation is essential.

Treatment

Nonpregnant females presenting with stable vital signs and absence of severe anemia (Hgb 7 mg/100 mL) can be managed as outpatients. Consult with the gynecologist before the initiation of hormonal therapy. Patients with a pelvic or vaginal infection should be treated as outlined in section 9.4. Postmenopausal females with vaginal bleeding require an endometrial curettage. Timely follow-up with a suitable gynecologist is imperative. Hormonal therapy is best withheld in postmenopausal patients until the diagnosis of endometrial carcinoma is excluded.

Emergency department evaluation and treatment of first- and second-trimester mothers depend on the patient's hemodynamic stability, determination of fetal viability, gestational age, and amount of maternal blood loss. Spontaneous abortion can sensitize Rh− women; therefore, *all pregnant females with vaginal bleeding require Rh determination,* with administration of *RhoGAM* when indicated (50 mg IM is considered adequate for first-trimester bleeding problems and 300 mg IM is suggested for later bleeding if the patient is seen within 96 hr). Furthermore, any abortion (whether spontaneous or therapeutic) may proceed to a *septic abortion.* A septic abortion is associated with fever and signs of pelvic or generalized peritonitis. The definitive management of a spontaneous abortion depends on the type and is generally left to the expertise of the OB-GYN consultant.

Remember, the best treatment for the fetus is to stabilize the mother. Due to physiological changes, the mother can lose up to 30% of her intracellular volume before manifesting signs of shock. Volume loss may be concealed (i.e., retroperitoneal or uteroplacental). Place pregnant females in distress in the left lateral decubitus position. Fetal well-being is the most accurate indicator of adequate resuscitation (normal fetal heart tones are between 120 and 160 bpm). All pregnant females with a potentially viable fetus (> 20 to 24 weeks) who present with vaginal bleeding necessitate fetal heart monitoring and obstetrical consultation.

Admission Criteria

Patients with the following conditions require admission:

- Hemodynamic instability and vaginal bleeding;
- Severe trauma requiring surgical repair;
- Spontaneous abortion (except threatened abortions and some complete abortions);
- Suspected ectopic pregnancy;
- Uterine rupture;
- Active labor;
- Placenta previa; and
- Abruptio placenta.

All patients discharged from the ED should receive clear instructions and early gynecologic referral.

Suggested Readings

Grant J, Hyslop M: Underutilization of Rh prophylaxis in the emergency department: a retrospective survey. Ann Emerg Med 1992;21:181–183.

Rulin MC, et al.: The reliability of ultrasonography in the management of spontaneous abortion, clinically thought to be complete: a prospective study. Am J Obstet Gynecol 1993;1768:12–18.

Turner LM: Vaginal bleeding during pregnancy. Emerg Med Clin North Am 1994;12:45–54.

10.6 VAGINITIS

Description

Vaginal discharge is a common gynecological complaint encountered in the ED setting. Unfortunately, both physicians and patients consider the term *vaginitis* to refer to any discomfort or irritation in the vulvovaginal area. Gynecologists generally reserve the term for any "vaginal inflammation associated with colonization by microorganisms." The three most common causes of vaginitis are (1) *Candida* spp.; (2) *Trichomonas vaginalis;* and (3) a poorly understood clinical entity known as bacterial vaginosis, caused by *Gardnerella* (previously *H. vaginalis*) and other anerobes.

History

Obtain a focused history, asking about the chief and related complaints (pruritus, pain, discharge). Evaluate the quantity and quality of discharge and the presence of any odor. Questions should also be asked about any previous episodes of vulvovaginal disease. Other essential points to cover include past medical history (particularly diabetes or AIDS), obstetric and gynecological history (gravity, parity, LMP, birth control, whether partner is symptomatic), current or recent medications (especially use of antibiotics), allergies, and personal hygiene (i.e., douching, feminine hygiene products).

Physical Examination

General. Check if the patient looks toxic.

Abdomen. Check for abdominal tenderness.

Pelvic. Begin by inspecting the external genitalia, noting presence of skin lesions and/or vaginal discharge. Document the amount, color, consistency, and the location of any vaginal fluid. Rule out retained foreign body (tampon). Obtain specimens (including a cervical gonococcal and *Chlamydia* cultures) for microscopic examination and culture. Finally, perform a bimanual examination noting uterine size, cervical motion tenderness, and presence or absence of adnexal masses.

Rectal. Examine around the anus and rectum carefully for any defects that suggest rectovaginal fistula (associated with a fecal-appearing discharge in vaginal vault).

Diagnostic Tests

Unfortunately, the history and physical examination are usually limited in establishing the etiology of vaginosis. Thus laboratory adjuncts are necessary.

Bedside tests. Inspect the vaginal discharge: test the pH (nitrazine paper) and conduct a "whiff test" (add 10% potassium hydroxide to a sample of discharge and note the odor).

Saline wet mount. Collect the discharge on a cotton swab and then either deposit it in a test tube with a drop of saline or smear it onto two slides. If the slide method is employed, one drop of saline is placed on one slide, and 10% potassium hydroxide (KOH) on another. The wet-mount specimen is then viewed under a microscope (both low and high powers) for *trichomonads* (ovoid or pear-shaped protozoa that are motile via a flagella), *clue cells* (sloughed epithelial cells that have a stippled appearance secondary to adherent bacteria), *hyphae* and *spores* of vaginal candidiasis, and WBCs.

KOH wet mount. KOH will dissolve all cellular elements except the pseudohyphae of *candidiasis.*

Cultures. Results for *Candida* and *Trichomonas* rarely add to management decisions (not available for 48 hr); however, cultures for gonorrhea and *Chlamydia* need to be performed if the history and physical findings are suggestive.

Blood tests: Obtain a VDRL on all patients with STDs.

Treatment

Trichomonas generally results from sexual transmission, suggesting the possibility of a concomitant STD infection (see section 9.4) (Table 10.6.1). The usual treatment is *metronidazole* (2 g PO as a single dose or 500 mg PO BID for 7 days). Avoid metronidazole in the first trimester of pregnancy (unfortunately there is no curative alternative therapy). *Clotrimazole* suppositories (100 mg intravaginally HS for 7 days) or vinegar douches may serve as a temporizing measure. After the first trimester, prescribe a 2-g single-dose regimen. Treat sexual partners of patients with *Trichomonas,* using a 2-g single-dose or 500 mg PO BID for 7 days. Warn patients of a disulfiram-like reaction (i.e., nausea, vomiting, flushing) that can occur if alcohol is ingested while taking metronidazole (avoid alcohol at least 1 to 2 days posttreatment).

Bacterial vaginosis, or nonspecific vaginitis, is also treated with

Table 10.6.1
Special Considerations

Characteristic	Normal	Bacterial Vaginosis	*Trichomonas vaginalis*	*Candida*
Common symptoms	None	Malodorous discharge, pruritus, exacerbated with intercourse	Excessive discharge, malodorous, vulvar pruritus, dyspareunia, dysuria	Itching, burning, discharge, dysuria, dyspareunia
Appearance of discharge	Whitish, flocculent	Profuse, homogenous, whitish gray, frothy 10% of time	Yellow, green, frothy (10% of cases), increased, malodorous	White, curdy "cottage cheese–like," sometimes increased
Appearance of vagina or vulva	Normal	Normal to minimal inflammation	Cervical and vaginal erythema, subepithelial abscesses, may see punctate or petechial lesions (strawberry cervix)	Erythema of vagina or vulva, edema of vulva
pH	3.8–4.2	> 4.5	> 4.5	≤ 4.5
Amine odor (KOH whiff test)	Absent	Positive (fishy or putrid smell)	Positive or negative	Negative
Microscopic	Epithelial cells, lactobacilli	Clue cells, no WBCs	Trichomonads (motile, flagellated protozoa), WBCs	Budding yeast, hyphae, pseudohyphae seen with KOH prep

metronidazole (500 mg PO BID for 7 days or 2 g as a single dose). Alternatives to metronidazole include *clindamycin* (300 mg PO BID for 7 days), *clindamycin vaginal cream* (2%; one applicator intravaginally daily for 7 days), or *metronidazole gel* (0.75%; one 5-g applicator intravaginally two times a day for 5 days). Heed same precautions for use in pregnancy and consumption of alcohol outlined for *Trichomonas.*

Most yeast infections (candidiasis) can be treated with one of the *imidazole* creams: *butoconazole* 2% cream (5 g; HS for 3 days), *clotrimazole* 1% cream (5 g for 7 days), *miconazole* 2% cream (5 g daily for 7 days), *miconazole* (200-mg suppositories daily for 3 days), or topical *Triazole terconazole* 0.8% cream (5 g for 3 days). In pregnancy, it is acceptable to use one of the topical creams (clotrimazole, miconazole). The distinction in cure rates is negligible between the different creams and suppositories. In patients with recurrent (at least three episodes a year) and/or refractory candidiasis, consider the possibility of undiagnosed diabetes mellitus or HIV (candidiasis may be the initial symptom of HIV in 25% of women). For severe or refractory cases of candidiasis fluconazole (150 mg PO one time; currently *not* FDA approved and *not* safe for pregnancy) is an alternative.

Admission Criteria

Generally, patients with vulvovaginitis do not require admission. Possible exceptions are *those with severe infection accompanied by urinary retention, fever, and/or severe pain; and those with a concomitant STD that causes an overwhelming infection* (especially in the immunocompromised patient). All patients should receive follow-up appointments within 1 week to assess progress and follow-up cultures and/or VDRL.

Suggested Readings

Lossick J: Trichomoniasis: trends in diagnosis and management. Am J Obstet Gynecol 1991;165(4):1217–1221.

Horowitz B: Mycotic vulvovaginitis: a broad overview. Am J Obstet Gynecol 1991;165(4):1188–1191.

Thomason J: Bacterial vaginosis: current review with indications for asymptomatic therapy. Am J Obstet Gynecol 1991;165(4):1210–1215.

Chapter 11

Urology

11.1 ACUTE URINARY RETENTION

Description

Acute urinary retention is much more common in males because of *benign prostatic hypertrophy* (BPH). However, the etiologies are diverse, and retention may result from an interaction among several causes (e.g., the previously asymptomatic older male with moderate benign prostatic hypertrophy who takes a "cold" tablet). An episode of infection, bleeding, or overdistention of the bladder is the usual precipitating event.

History

Patients usually complain of urinary hesitancy, decreased force and caliber of the stream, straining to void, and a sensation of incomplete emptying. Inability to void results in the development of agonizing suprapubic pain. Additional historical information includes constitutional symptoms like bone pain and weight (carcinoma), a history of venereal diseases (stricture), previous urinary tract surgery, and presence of neurologic symptoms such as visual disturbance or paresthesias (multiple sclerosis) or pain and paresthesias associated with a cord lesion (Table 11.1.1).

Physical Examination

Vital signs. Check for fever.

Abdomen. The degree of retention can be assessed by careful examination of the suprapubic region. The bladder is typically percussible or palpable when it contains more than 150 mL of urine.

Genitourinary. Inspect external genitalia; note if the penis is cir-

Table 11.1.1
Etiology of Acute Urinary Retention

Penis
Phimosis
Paraphimosis
Meatal stenosis
Foreign body
Urethra
Foreign body
Urethritis
Stricture or stenosis
Prostate
Benign prostatic hypertrophy
Carcinoma
Prostatitis
Infection
Herpes simplex
Herpes zoster
Neurologic
Spinal cord syndromes
Spinal shock
Diabetes mellitus
Multiple sclerosis
Landry-Guillain-Barré
Drugs
Anticholinergics
Antihistamines
Tricyclic antidepressants
Alpha-stimulators
Amphetamines
Cold tablets
Psychogenic

cumcised or not. Look for *phimosis, paraphimosis, or meatal stenosis.* In addition, document any signs of herpetic infection (e.g., erythematous papules, grouped vesicles, pustules).

Rectal. Note prostate size and consistency (although the gland size does not correlate with degree of obstruction). Assess rectal tone.

Neurologic. The bladder shares innervation with the same spinal cord segments as the lower extremities. Evaluate the muscle strength, reflexes, and sensation of the legs to determine if there is any suggestion of neurologic compromise.

Diagnostic Tests

Urinalysis. Check for presence of pyuria (infection) and hematuria (infection, tumor, calculi).

SMA. Renal function should be assessed.

Treatment

The initial treatment of choice is to place a Foley catheter. However, this may prove difficult. Helpful suggestions include employing liberal lubrication and topical anesthesia with 2% lidocaine jelly, using a large-caliber catheter (e.g., 22 French) when the passage of a standard-size Foley catheter (a 16 or 18 French) is not possible (the stiffness of the heavier catheter may help to separate the hypertrophied lobes seen with BPH), using a coudé catheter when repeated attempts with a Foley catheter are unsuccessful (the coudé catheter is passed with the curved tip directed superiorly).

If attempts at placing catheters fail, the next step is to use of dilators, filiforms, and followers or to insert a percutaneous suprapubic tube (contraindicated if there is a history of prior surgical procedures in this area because of possible bowel adhesion). Customarily this is performed by the urologic consultant.

Complications of relieving the obstruction include *postobstructive diuresis* (continual diuresis of greater than 200 mL/hr resulting in fluid and electrolyte disturbances), *hemorrhage* (secondary to bladder mucosal disruption; if major, monitor and irrigate the bladder), and *hypotension* (the most common mechanism is a vasovagal reaction following the rapid drainage of large amounts of urine, typically >1 L).

If more than 700 mL of urine is retained, it is probably best to leave the Foley catheter in place and allow catheter drainage to continue for a few days to permit recovery of detrusor tone.

You can discuss the use of *finasteride* (5-α reductase) or *terazosin* (α1 antagonist) with the urologic consultant in cases of BPH.

Admission Criteria

Indications for admission include *to relieve the urinary retention, findings consistent with spinal cord compression,* and *patients with significant complications* such as postobstructive diuresis or significant hemorrhage.

Note: *Stable patients can be managed on an outpatient basis.* The patient is sent home with Foley catheter in place and a leg bag with instructions for urologic follow-up in 24 to 48 hr. The use of antibiotics should be discussed with the consultant.

Suggested Readings

Harwood-Nuss AL, Holland RW: Genitourinary disease. In Rosen P, Barkin RM, eds, Emergency medicine: concepts and clinical practice, 3rd ed. St. Louis: CV Mosby, 1992:1878–1910.

Petterson NE, Ross SN, Miller HC: Common urologic emergencies. Emerg Med Rep 1994;15:147–158.

11.2 URINARY TRACT INFECTIONS

Description

Urinary tract infections (UTIs) are among the most common infectious entities encountered in the ED. Infection generally follows inoculation and colonization of the lower urinary tract (urethra, bladder) by viable bacteria from the patient's own bowel flora. Coliform bacteria are responsible for the vast majority of infections, with *E. coli* accounting for most cases of community-acquired, noncomplicated UTIs. *Staphylococcus saprophyticus* is responsible for 10 to 15% of infections and is the second most common cause of infection in sexually active females. Inoculation frequently follows instrumentation or sexual intercourse. However, presence of further risk factors, such as an indwelling Foley catheter, obstruction (urinary tract abnormality or stone), vesicoureteral reflux, intrinsic renal disease, pregnancy, or immunosuppression (elderly, chronic disease, alcohol or drug abuse, diabetes mellitus, AIDS, sickle cell disease) increases the susceptibility to infection. Males are at greater risk for UTI when they practice rectal intercourse or are uncircumcised.

Urinary tract infections are often characterized in terms of the involved urinary structures. *Urethritis* (see section 11.3) and *cystitis* (an infection of the bladder) are considered "lower tract" infections, while *pyelonephritis* is an "upper tract" infection whereby bacteria produce infection and inflammation of the renal parenchyma.

Repeated episodes of UTI are usually secondary to recurrent infections (reinfection often with a new pathogen), rather than a relapse of chronic infection. A UTI associated with a medical, neurologic, or structural problem is referred to as a *complicated*

UTI and may result in a persistent or relapsing infection. Most cases of complicated UTI are caused by *E. coli,* but other uropathogens such as *Klebsiella, Enterobacter, Pseudomonas,* and *Serratia* species need to be considered. *Asymptomatic bacteriuria*—presence of a significant number (generally > 10^5) of colony-forming units (CFUs) on culture—occurs frequently in the elderly but is consequential in pregnant patients and those with underlying immunosuppression.

History

Symptoms that suggest a lower tract urinary infection include urinary frequency; urgency; dysuria; suprapubic discomfort; malodorous, cloudy, or bloody urine; and incontinence. Consider acute pyelonephritis (PN)when voiding symptoms are accompanied by back or flank pain (referred pain from kidneys) along with a temperature elevation. Patients with pyelonephritis may also complain of GI symptoms (nausea, vomiting, diarrhea). There is often an overlap between the symptoms of a lower urinary tract and an upper urinary tract infection, with subclinical pyelonephritis manifesting lower tract symptoms even though it is an upper tract infection. Fever higher than 38°C (101°F) and the presence of WBC casts in the urine favor the diagnosis of PN.

Physical Examination

General. Patients with pyelonephritis frequently appear quite ill. Alteration in mental status (including coma) implies possible septic shock (see section 9.9).

Vital signs. Temperature may be elevated to 40°C (103°F) or higher and is often the most dependable finding to distinguish upper from lower tract infection.

Abdomen. Palpate the abdomen for suprapubic and/or flank tenderness.

Genitourinary. Important to carefully examine the vulvovaginal region and pelvis in females and urethra, testicles, epididymis, and prostate in males to detect alternative causes of symptoms.

Diagnostic Tests

Urinalysis and Culture

The diagnosis of UTI requires the collection of a urine specimen. Midstream voided "clean catch" urine yields an accurate specimen when properly performed. Bladder catheterization is indicated in patients who cannot void spontaneously; are too ill, immobilized, or obese to cooperate; or who present with vaginal bleeding or discharge.

Since the causative organisms and their antimicrobial susceptibility are so predictable in women with acute cystitis, an abbreviated lab work-up with empirical treatment is safe, appropriate, and cost-effective. For patients with characteristic symptoms, the diagnosis can be corroborated if pyuria is exhibited by hematocytometer (> 8 to 10 WBC/mm^3 is significant), by Gram stain (presence of bacteria) of unspun urine, or by urine dipstick (positive leukocyte esterase reaction). Hematuria is seen in up to 50% of women with cystitis.

Urine cultures are not a requirement in healthy women of child-bearing age who are not pregnant. Cultures are generally reserved for patients who present with signs and symptoms of a urinary tract infection and are at risk for pyelonephritis, bacteremia, or urosepsis (including those with known structural abnormalities); males; pregnant women; patients who have recently completed a course of antibiotics; patients whose symptoms have persisted for more than 1 week; patients who have had a UTI within 6 weeks; diabetics; immunocompromised patients; patients on dialysis; patients older than 50 years; and those with a neurogenic bladder, chronic indwelling Foley catheter, or history of GU instrumentaion.

Classically, a colony count ≥ 100,000 CFUs in a clean catch specimen implied infection, but recent work has suggested that any patient with dysuria or pyuria and a urine culture colony count > 10^2 CFUs obligates treatment. If urine cultures are negative in the presence of pyuria, consider gonococcal or chlamydial urethritis (see section 11.3).

Other Tests

Blood studies. A WBC count with differential and blood cultures are indicated in ill patients. Also consider ordering a serum creatinine and a BUN to assess renal function in complicated UTIs or patients with pyelonephritis.

Imaging studies. If fever and other symptoms fail to resolve in 72 hr despite appropriate studies, consider ultrasound or computed tomography to detect possible obstruction, congenital abnormality, or perinephric abscess.

Treatment

Most uncomplicated UTIs respond to a 3-day regimen of antibiotics (as effective as a 7-day course, but causes fewer side effects). Single-dose therapy (trimethoprim-sulfamethoxazole, or TMP-SMX, 4 tablets double-strength) may be used in healthy young females, but the failure rate is higher than that of the 3-day course. In fact, lack of response to a 3-day course of therapy implies presence of either a complicated urinary tract infection or pyelonephritis. A 7-day regimen is indicated for diabetics, those with symptoms that have persisted for more than 1 week, those with a history of recent UTI (past 6 weeks), females who use a diaphragm, pregnant females (fluoroquinolones are not approved for pregnancy; *do not* use sulfonamides if the patient is near term), and patients older than 65 years. For uncomplicated lower urinary tract infections, TMP-SMX (1 tablet double-strength BID for 3 days) is the best choice. Fluoroquinolones (ciprofloxacin, 250 mg PO BID, or norfloxacin, 400 mg PO BID) are also highly effective and are often preferred in complicated UTIs.

The recommended therapeutic regimen for *pyelonephritis* is dictated by the patient's overall health and clinical status. Nontoxic, previously healthy young females without persistent symptoms can be treated as an outpatient with amoxicillin-clavulanate or one of the fluoroquinolones for 10 to 14 days. Patients who look toxic or have underlying medical illnesses should be hospitalized and recieve a parenteral regimen for 24 to 48 hr:

- *Ciprofloxacin* (400 mg IV q 12 hr);
- *Cefotaxime* (2.0 g IV q 4 hr);
- *Ceftriaxone* (2.0 g IV once a day);
- *Amoxicillin/sulbactam* (3.0 g IV q 4 hr); or
- *Gentamicin* (loading dose of 2.0 mg/kg IV, then maintenance dose of 1.5 mg/kg, if normal renal function) plus *ampicillin* (1.0 g IV q 6 hr).

Asymptomatic bacteriuria obligates treatment in pregnant women, diabetics, immunocompromised patients, and patients who have undergone a urologic procedure. Asymptomatic bacteriuria is common in the elderly, but advanced age alone is not an indication for treatment.

Admission Criteria

Admission is indicated in *any patient with a complicated UTI or pyelonephritis who is toxic, displays hemodynamic instability or severe dehydration, is unable to take oral medication, or has an immunosuppressive or complicating illness.* Also admit *pregnant females with upper tract infections.*

Patients discharged with pyelonephritis require close follow-up, within 24 hr. Any worsening of their condition necessitates immediate return to the emergency department. Patients with a pending urine culture or those not responding to therapy in 3 days should be referred for follow-up.

Suggested Readings

Forland M: Urinary tract infection: how has its management changed? Postgrad Med 1993;93:71–86.

Stamm WE, Hooton TM: Management of urinary tract infections in adults. N Engl J Med 1993;329:1328–1334.

11.3 INFECTIONS OF THE MALE GENITOURINARY SYSTEM

Description

Genitourinary symptoms in the male are typically due to inflammation and/or infection of the *urethra, epididymis, testicles,* or *prostate gland.*

History

Many males with genitourinary infection present with pain as the chief complaint (whether dysuria or pain localized to the penis, testicles, prostate, or suprapubic region). Urologic pain typically is poorly localized and often out of proportion to physical findings. Other frequent complaints include urethral discharge, change in urinary habits (frequency, urgency, hesitancy, nocturia, or inability to void), or abnormal urine color (cloudy, hematuria). Presence of fever, flank pain, or GI symptoms (nausea, vomiting) implies systemic infection. The past medical history should include previous episodes of genitourinary disease (including STDs and prior infections), recent urologic surgery or procedures, medical problems (diabetes, sickle cell disease, bleeding disorders), and medications (especially potentially nephrotoxic drugs such as nonsteroidal antiinflammatories) and allergies.

Physical Examination

General. A general physical assessment should be done along with a detailed examination of the genitalia.

Vital signs. Fever, hypertension, or hypotension implies systemic illness.

Genitourinary. A careful examination of the penis, foreskin, urethral meatus, and scrotum (swelling, masses, tenderness, gangrene) is essential.

Rectal. In addition to evaluating the prostate (size, consistency, tenderness, nodularity), inspect the perineal region and assess rectal tone.

Diagnostic Tests

Laboratory (urinalysis, blood studies, cultures of discharge) and radiological studies are determined by the presenting complaint and clinical findings.

Special Considerations

Urethritis

Generally sexually acquired, urethritis manifests as a urethral discharge and/or dysuria. Suspect urethritis when pyuria is present only in the initially voided urine (document with leukocyte esterase strip) but desists beyond midstream. Urethritis can be classified as gonococcal or nongonococcal. *Gonococcal urethritis* is characterized by the abrupt onset of purulent urethral discharge, dysuria, and pruritus. Analyze a Gram stain of the discharge for Gram-negative intracellular diplococci and obtain gonococcal and chlamydial cultures. Primary treatment for gonococcal urethritis is either *ceftriaxone* (125 mg IM) or various oral regimens (*ciprofloxacin,* 500 mg PO one time; *ofloxacin,* 400 mg PO one time; or *cefixime,* 400 mg PO one time).

Presumptive treatment of *Chlamydia trachomatis* is indicated, based on the high rate of co-infection of *Chlamydia* with gonorrhea. Therefore, one of the above treatment protocols for gonorrhea is coupled with one of the following antibiotics: *doxycycline* (100 mg PO BID for 7 days) or *azithromycin* (1 g PO one time).

Nongonococcal urethritis (NGU) is usually caused by either *C. trachomatis* or *Ureaplasma urealyticum.* The discharge tends to be clear or milky and is more prominent in the morning. The patient has minimal complaints of dysuria and pruritus. Clinical criteria do not accurately distinguish NGU from gonococcal urethritis. The diagnosis is implied by the presence of inflammatory cells on a urethral smear (> 4 PMNs) in the absence of *Neisseria gonorrhea. Chlamydia* culture or antibody tests may also be helpful (see section 9.4). Testing for syphilis (VDRL or RPR) should also be performed. Primary treatment options for NGU include doxycycline (100 mg PO BID for 7 days), azithromycin (1.0 g PO once), or ofloxacin (300 mg PO BID for 7 days). Due to the high incidence of coexisting gonococcal urethritis, therapy for *N. gonorrhea* should be instituted as well. Sexual contacts need to be treated. Failure of therapy may be due to several reasons: noncompliance with medication (the most common reason), failure to treat sexual partner(s), acquiring a "new" infection from another source, infection due to trichomoniasis, or urethritis resulting from insertion of foreign body.

Complications of urethritis in males include progression of the infection to epididymitis, orchitis, or prostatitis. Chronic urethral strictures occur in 2 to 5% of patients.

Acute Epididymitis

Most cases of acute epididymitis arise from an infectious etiology. Under the age of 40, this is primarily a sexually transmitted disease, with the pathogens responsible for urethritis (gonorrhea and *Chlamydia*) being the most likely offenders. Over the age of 40, epididymitis is usually the result of infection by coliform organisms *(E. coli)* and is associated with UTIs and prostatitis.

Clinically, the patient presents with a gradual onset of scrotal or groin pain that intensifies over hours to days. The patient may also complain of dysuria or a urethral discharge (particularly in the setting of the STD form). On physical examination, the patient may appear toxic and be febrile. Initially, scrotal swelling, erythema, and tenderness are noted, and the epididymis may be distinguishable from the testis on examination. Later, infection and congestion of the testis occurs, making it difficult to differentiate the testis from the epididymis, and the patient may present with one enlarged, tender mass (epididymoorchitis). Laboratory studies often reveal a leukocytosis with a left shift. Urinalysis may or may not reveal evidence of a bacterial infection. Urethral swabs and urine cultures should be obtained, but they should not guide initial diagnosis or therapy. Obtain a VDRL when epididymitis is sexually acquired. Torsion of the testis (most prevalent in 12- to 18-year-old males and rare after age 30), testicular tumor (one of the most common malignancies in young men), hydrocele, and varicocele should be considered in the differential diagnosis. Doppler ultrasound and radionuclide scans may be helpful in making this differentiation.

The treatment is directly related to the presumed etiology. For the sexually transmitted form, antibiotic therapy is similar to that for urethritis. For a presumed coliform infection, treatment for a UTI should be instituted. Adjuncts to antibiotic therapy include bed rest until pain free, scrotal support, ice to the involved area, and analgesics. Consider admission for older patients with suspected anatomic abnormalities of the GU system, patients suspected of harboring an abscess, and patients who appear toxic.

Prostatitis

Prostatic inflammation can be secondary to acute and chronic bacterial infections of as well as have nonbacterial origins. *Prostatodynia* is a catch-all phrase used to describe a condition where a patient presents with symptoms of prostatitis, but the prostate is actually normal. Acute prostatitis is usually caused by Gram-negative rods (especially *E. coli*) and is characterized by perineal, suprapubic, or low back pain, accompanied by dysuria.

Patients may appear quite toxic, while the prostate is warm, and swollen, and tender to touch. Be gentle when palpating the prostate to avoid hematogenous bacterial dissemination. A urinalysis will reveal pyuria and bacteriuria, with urine cultures defining the offending organism. Hospitalization should be considered for toxic patients and those exhibiting urinary retention (temporary catheterization may be necessary).

One must be aggressive in the treatment of acute prostatitis and treat long enough to ensure elimination of bacteria from the gland. For inpatients, ampicillin (1 g IV q 6 hr) with gentamicin (1 mg/kg IV q 8 hr if normal renal function) provides reliable coverage. Outpatient therapy consists of TMP-SMX (2 tablets BID) or a quinolone (e.g., ciprofloxacin, 500 to 750 mg BID) for 10 to 14 days. Supportive care incorporates adequate hydration, an analgesic, an antipyretic, cold packs to the perineum, and sitz baths. It is important to differentiate chronic from acute bacterial prostatitis, because chronic bacterial prostatitis requires several weeks to months of therapy with TMP-SMX or a quinolone.

The usual picture of chronic bacterial prostatitis is one of a relapsing series of episodes characterized by dysuria, tenesmus, and perineal and low back discomfort. Examination may be unremarkable, even of the prostate. While the midstream urinalysis is frequently normal, prostatic massage may demonstrate leukocytes (> 10/HPF). Chronic nonbacterial prostatitis is characterized by the same symptoms as that of chronic bacterial prostatitis but no organism is cultured from the urine or prostatic secretions. Speculation exists concerning the roles of *C. trachomatis, Ureaplasma,* and *Mycoplasma* as the causative agents in this entity. For that reason, empiric antibiotic treatment (doxycycline, 100 mg PO BID for 14 days, or erythromycin, 500 mg PO QID for 14 days) has been used with occasional success. In other instances, nonsteroidal antiinflammatory drugs provide relief.

Fournier's Gangrene

Fournier's gangrene is a fulminant, life-threatening polymicrobial (Gram-negative bacilli, anaerobes, *S. aureus,* and β-hemolytic streptococcus) infection of the scrotum, perineum, and penis. Typically, the affected patient is elderly, diabetic, and debilitated. While early clinical findings may be vague, infection rapidly advances into a progressive necrosis of the scrotal skin, with involvement of the subcutaneous tissue, fascia, and/or muscle. Patients appear toxic and in severe distress. Clinical findings include a foul-smelling, "dishwater" pus from the perineal area, crepitus of involved tissue, and advancing erythema and edema. Treatment comprises basic resuscitative measures (airway management, fluids), initiation of broad-spectrum antibiotic coverage (often triple antibiotics: *ampicillin* plus *clindamycin* plus *gentamicin* or *imipenem-cilastatin*), and prompt surgical consultation for radical debridement. Hyperbaric oxygen may serve an adjunctive role after incision, débridement, and drainage.

Suggested Readings

Moul JW: Prostatitis: sorting out the different causes. Postgrad Med 1993;94:191–201.

Reid DL, Goldman GE: Genitourinary infections. Top Emerg Med 1991; 13:55–65.

11.4 RENAL CALCULI

Description

Kidney stones affect 2 to 5% of the population at some time during their life (70% of cases affect 20- to 50-year-olds), with men being affected three times more often than women. There is a 70 to 80% recurrence rate. Approximately 80% of renal stones are composed of *calcium-containing crystals* (calcium oxalate is the most common pure substance stone). Hyperexcretion of calcium (idiopathic hypercalciuria) is the major factor in stone production. *Uric acid stones* (responsible for 10% of all stones) are radiolucent and are found in patients with increased uric acid secretion (gout, myeloproliferative disorders) and an acidic urine (pH 5.5). *Magnesium, ammonium,* and *phosphate* (*triple phosphate* or *struvite*) constitute about 15% of stones and occur in the setting of a persistently alkaline urine due to the presence of urea-splitting organisms *(Proteus, Klebsiella)*.

Ureteral stones ordinarily obstruct at the narrowest points of the ureter, including the kidney calyces, ureteropelvic junction, pelvic brim (where the ureter crosses the iliac vessels), and the uterovesicular junction. The size of the stone is critical in determining its potential for spontaneous passage. Whereas 80% of stones less than 5 mm will pass, only 5% of stones larger than 8 mm will do so (when estimating stone size remember that the x-ray image is magnified; actual stone mass is 80% of that on the film).

History

Patients with renal colic typically present with a sudden onset of pain, which often awakens them from sleep. Pain and related symptoms often vary according to the anatomic location of the stone as it transverses the genitourinary tract, commonly commencing in the flank (implies obstruction at ureteropelvic junction or proximal ureter) and shifting to the lower abdomen (stone located at ureter near the pelvic brim). Urinary urgency occurs when the stone passes to the ureterovesical junction, and the pain radiates to the testicle in males and labia in females. Acute episodes of colicky pain may wax and wane, with a dull ache persisting in the flank or back area. Additional complaints include nausea and vomiting, along with irritative voiding symptoms (frequency, urgency, dysuria). Gross hematuria is a primary symptom in up to 33% of patients and may precede the pain. The presence of chills and/or fever suggests infection.

Inquire about a history of sickle cell disease, analgesic abuse (increased risk of papillary necrosis), recurrent UTIs, and previous episodes of colic or hematuria. Certain medications (antacids, calcium supplements, high-dose vitamin C, thiazides, and allopurinol) increase the propensity for stone formation. The differential diagnosis includes renal colic secondary to bleeding from a renal tumor or papillary necrosis (Table 11.4.1).

Physical Examination

General. The patient will appear agitated and in obvious distress (often appearing pale or diaphoretic) and will be constantly moving about in an unsuccessful attempt to find a comfortable position. This is unlike the patient with peritonitis, who avoids movement.

Vital signs. The pulse rate, respiratory rate, and blood pressure may be elevated due to pain and anxiety. Fever implies possible infection.

Abdomen. The abdominal examination may reveal hypoactive bowel sounds and flank or CVA tenderness. Particularly in patients > 50 years, examine for possible aortic abdominal aneurysm (see section 1.9).

Table 11.4.1
Differential Diagnosis of Renal Colic

Acute intermittent flank pain
- Renal calculus
- Renal tumor (particularly after hemorrhage)
- Papillary necrosis
- Obstructing blood clots
- Ureteropelvic obstruction (especially from extrinsic compression)

Acute constant flank pain
- Aortic aneurysm dissection
- Renal artery embolus
- Renal vein thrombosis

Gradual onset, constant flank pain
- Pyelonephritis
- Perinephric Abscess

Diagnostic Tests

Laboratory Tests

Routine blood tests are usually not helpful or necessary in the acute management of renal colic. Reserve blood studies for the patient in whom admission is anticipated. However, if a CBC is performed, a leukocytosis may occur in the absence of infection due to demargination associated with pain. An elevated WBC count (> 15,000/mm^3) and/or a slight shift to the left coupled with a fever obligates investigation for an infection; consider the possibility of a renal abscess.

Obtain a creatinine and BUN in patients at risk for contrast-induced nephropathy (i.e., patients > 50 years old; those with known renal disease, diabetes, or multiple myeloma; and patients who are severely dehydrated).

Other Tests

Urinalysis. Provides much useful information. Hematuria is noted in approximately 85% of kidney stones. Absence suggests possible complete ureteral obstruction. If the diagnosis is suspected but the urinalysis is negative, one should repeat the U/A or proceed to an intravenous pyelogram (IVP).

Plain x-rays. Approximately 80% of renal stones are radiopaque and would, therefore, be expected to be seen on the KUB. However, there are drawbacks to a KUB: it will not identify radiopaque renal calculi < 2 mm in size or radiolucent causes of renal colic (uric acid stones, blood clots, or sloughed papillae) and it fails to diagnose the degree of ureteral obstruction.

Contrast studies. The IVP is the radiographic procedure of choice in the ED evaluation of renal colic. The IVP allows the physician to identify the stone as the cause of an obstruction, to measure the size of the stone, and to identify the location and degree of obstruction. Contraindications to the performance of an IVP include a history of contrast allergy (see chapter 8), renal insufficiency, and pregnancy. In these instances ultrasonography may be performed. Use of nonionic contrast material is generally safer. If necessary, patients at risk of an anaphylactoid reaction (e.g., asthmatics) can be premedicated with steroids and antihistamines.

Ultrasound. Demonstrates significant abdominal and pelvic pathology, along with hydroureter, but is not as sensitive in confirming small stones as is the IVP.

Special Considerations

The differential diagnosis of flank pain is extensive. *However, the diagnosis of abdominal aortic aneurysm (AAA) or iliac aneurysm must be considered in any patient over 50 years of age with sudden onset of abdominal, back, or groin pain.* Flank pain may also result from gastrointestinal, gynecological, respiratory, cardiac, and musculoskeletal disorders.

Treatment

Management involves providing sufficient *analgesia* and *hydration.* Traditionally, prompt relief of pain has been provided by *opioid analgesics* (see chapter 17). Recently, the role of *nonsteroidal antiinflammatory drugs* (NSAIDs) in treating renal colic has expanded. In particular, the use of *ketorolac* (30 mg IM or IV) has become popular. Indomethacin suppositories are also effective. *Antiemetics* may be administered to control nausea. In the absence of clinical dehydration, fluids should be provided in maintenance amounts only.

Admission Criteria

Admit *patients with obstruction, infection, intractable pain or vomiting, a solitary or transplanted kidney, a stone diameter greater than 6 mm that is not moving clinically or radiologically, or intrinsic renal disease.* The majority of patients with renal colic may be managed as outpatients. Provide sufficient analgesics and antiemetics along with instructions to strain the urine and save the stone. Arrange follow-up care with a urologist.

Suggested Readings

Coe FL: The pathogenesis and treatment of kidney stones. N Engl J Med 1992;327:1141–1145.

Larsen LS. The use of intravenous ketorolac for the treatment of renal colic in the emergency department. Am J Emerg Med 1993;11: 197–201.

11.5 MISCELLANEOUS UROLOGIC EMERGENCIES

Balanitis

Balanitis is either an *inflammation* or *irritation* of the foreskin and/or glans of the penis. The foreskin exhibits redness and swelling, accumulating smegma. Balanitis is usually a consequence of poor personal hygiene, with an increased incidence in diabetics and males with indwelling catheters. Local care, e.g., tepid baths, cleaning the foreskin and glans with a mild antiseptic soap, and application of a topical antibiotic or antifungal ointment (bacitracin, neomycin-polymyxin, clotrimazole), is generally adequate. If permitted to progress untreated, *phimosis* can ensue.

Phimosis and Paraphimosis

Phimosis arises when stenosis of the uncircumcised foreskin prevents proximal retraction over the glans. If it is severe enough to hinder urine flow a *dorsal slit procedure* may be inevitable. Normally, this is performed by the urologic consultant. However, if the ED physician is adequately trained, and a urologist is not readily available, a dorsal midline incision of the foreskin may be necessary, following adequate anesthesia and preparation of the skin. A hemostat is advanced and secured under the foreskin (taking care to avoid the glans or urethra). Next, the hemostat is closed, crushing the underlying foreskin; then the incision is made (usually with a scissors) through the devitalized tissue. To prevent postincision bleeding, secure the edges with 4-0 absorbable suture. This is only a temporizing measure (the patient is left with a "beagle-eared" deformity) and obligates urology follow-up for a formal circumcision.

Paraphimosis occurs when the foreskin is left retracted behind the glans, resulting in engorgement and edema of the glans and leading to vascular compromise and tissue necrosis if untreated. Paraphimosis typically results from failure to replace the foreskin after urethral catheterization. Attempt manual reduction of the foreskin; if the patient is catheterized, the catheter is removed, and replaced later. Encircle the glans with a gloved index and thumb, and squeeze the glans to reduce the amount of edema. Next, stabilize the glans with the second and third fingers of both gloved hands and simultaneously exert gentle downward pressure over the glans with the thumbs, while gently pulling the foreskin forward. Difficult reductions may be facilitated by applying a topical anesthetic lubricant to the undersurface of the foreskin or invaginating the thumb portion of a glove filled with cold water with the paraphimotic penis (hold in place 5 to 10 min to alleviate edema). When attempts at manual reduction fail, a urology consult is necessary for an emergent circumcision or a dorsal slit procedure.

Penile Fracture

Penile fracture transpires when an erect penis is suddenly bent, inducing a rupture of the capsule of the corpus cavernosum. The patient reports hearing a sharp sound (such as a snap or crack), which is followed by severe pain, detumescence, and penile swelling and ecchymosis. Urology consultation is required.

Priapism

Priapism is defined as a persistent, painful erection, unrelated to sexual activity or excitement. Causes of priapism include sickle cell disease, leukemia, medications (antipsychotics, antihypertensives, anticoagulants, topical cocaine), and injection of vasoactive substances (papaverine, phentolamine) into the corpus cavernosum. Patients complain of an agonizing erection often accompanied by an inability to void. If allowed to continue, irreversible ischemia and fibrosis of the penis can occur. Supportive care should be offered while awaiting urologic consultation; these measures include sedation, hydration, analgesia, and supplemental oxygen. β-agonist therapy (terbutaline, 0.25 mg SQ or 5.0 mg PO) may be helpful.

Nondeflating Urinary Catheter

A frustrating problem for the emergency physician arises when a self-retaining balloon to a Foley catheter will not deflate. The usual cause is a defect in the valve of the inflating lumen catheter. The simplest solution involves cutting off the adapter plug from the inflating channel. If this fails, insert the firm end of a CVP guide wire into the inflating channel and attempt to pop the balloon. Alternatives include overinflating the balloon and injecting erosive substances into the inflation port to try to dissolve the balloon. The problem with these techniques is that they can fragment the balloon (leaving pieces in the bladder) or induce a chemical cystitis. When simple measures fail, it is best to involve a urologist.

Suggested Readings

Peterson NE, Rous SN, Miller HC: Common urologic emergencies: a logical and practical approach to rapid diagnosis and treatment. Emerg Med Rep 1994;15:147–158.

Zbaraschuk I, Berger RE, Hedges JR: Genitourinary procedures. In Roberts JR, Hedges JR, eds.: Clinical procedures in emergency medicine, 2nd ed. Philadelphia: WB Saunders, 1991:867–888.

Chapter 12

Renal

12.1 ACUTE RENAL FAILURE

Description

Acute renal failure (ARF) is characterized by an abrupt decline in renal function that leads to an accumulation of nitrogenous waste products, proceeding to a rising serum creatinine and urea nitrogen, electrolyte imbalances, acid-base disturbances, and volume overload. ARF may be classified into three broad categories: prerenal, intrarenal, and postrenal. *Prerenal* is due to a decrease in effective renal perfusion (volume contraction, hypotension, severe heart failure).

Intrarenal results from toxic, immunologic, systemic, or iatrogenic disorders that involve the renal blood vessels, glomeruli, tubules, and/or renal parenchyma (acute tubular necrosis, vasculitis, glomerulonephritis, acute interstitial nephritis, uric acid deposition, myeloma).

Postrenal, also known as obstructive nephropathy, is the blockage of urine outflow from either the upper or the lower urinary tract (ureteral obstruction: clot, calculus, tumor, sloughed papillae, external compression; bladder outlet obstruction: benign prostatic hypertrophy, carcinoma, calculus, clot, renal stricture).

Chronic renal failure (CRF) is suggested by the development of a progressive azotemia over weeks to months, accompanied by anemia, hypertension, renal osteodystrophy, neurologic manifestations (lethargy, myoclonus, asterixis, peripheral neuropathy), an active urinary sediment (broad casts > 3 WBCs in width), and the appearance of bilateral small kidneys on imaging studies. An increase in kidney size in the presence of chronic renal failure implies polycystic disease, diabetic renal disease, scleroderma, or amyloidosis as the cause.

History

The initial symptoms of ARF are mainly influenced by the underlying illness or toxin. A prerenal etiology is suggested when the symptoms are consistent with volume loss (dizziness, syncope, persistent vomiting, diarrhea, excessive diuretic use). Ask about potentially nephrotoxic medications (nonsteroidal antiinflammatory drugs, diuretics, antibiotics, lithium, ACE inhibitors, chemotherapeutic agents), recent events (upper respiratory infection, exposure to radiocontrast material, trauma, surgery), and underlying systemic illnesses (hypertension, diabetes, lupus, TTP, hemolytic-uremic syndrome, scleroderma).

Patients may also report a decrease in urine output. While oliguria (< 100 mL/day or < 20 mL/hr) is disturbing, a normal urine output (>500 mL/day) or polyuria (> 3 L/day) can occur with ARF.

In the review of systems, inquire about symptoms compatible with fluid overload, GI disturbance, or altered mental status. The constellation of symptoms (fatigue, weakness, anorexia, nausea, abnormal taste, hiccoughs, muscle cramping, dyspnea) that evolves with prolonged severe renal insufficiency is called *uremia.* As uremia advances, patients may develop pruritus, chest pain (pericarditis), easy bruisability (coagulopathy, platelet dysfunction), and paresthesias (neuropathy).

Physical Examination

General. Does patient appear chronically ill, cachectic, or in extremis?

Vital signs. Check pulse, blood pressure, respiratory rate, and temperature. Specifically look for signs of volume depletion (poor skin turgor, dry mucous membranes, orthostatic changes) or overload.

HEENT. Examine pupils and fundi carefully (look for chronic changes of diabetes or hypertension).

Neck. Inspect for jugular venous distention and hepatojugular reflux.

Lungs. Auscultate for rales or wheezes.

Heart. Listen for murmurs and gallops, an S_3, friction rub, and distant heart sounds.

Abdomen. Note distention, fluid wave, and enlarged liver. Palpate for masses and tenderness. Auscultate for bowel sounds and renal bruits (renal artery stenosis). Percuss for bladder distention as well as CVA tenderness.

Rectal. Test stool for blood. Palpate prostate size and consistency, and check for a mass.

Pelvic and genital. Examine for masses, tenderness, stricture, and phimosis.

Neurologic. Document changes in mental status, weakness, asterixis, or focal neurologic signs.

Extremities. Note edema, cyanosis, rash (vasculitis), muscle tenderness (rhabdomyolysis), joint swelling, or sclerodactyly.

Diagnostic Tests

ABG. Provides a rapid assessment of acid-base status and oxygenation.

SMA. Order electrolytes (hyperkalemia, hypermagnesemia, hyperphosphatemia, hypocalcemia, and decreased bicarbonate are most common electrolyte abnormalities seen with renal failure), creatinine (the level in a patient with previously normal renal function and total renal failure will rise by only 1 to 2 mg/dL per day), and BUN (less specific for renal disease than creatinine). The BUN:creatinine ratio is typically elevated (> 20:1) in cases of preneal azotemia.

CBC. Check WBCs and differential (eosinophilia is associated with interstitial nephritis), hematocrit (often decreased), and platelets.

PT and PTT. Check for coagulation defects.

ECG. Inspect for ischemic changes, decreased voltage (pericardial effusion), and evidence of hyperkalemia and/or left ventricular hypertrophy.

X-rays. Verify cardiac size on CXR and look for pulmonary congestion, infiltrates, or effusion. Note bony changes. A KUB may display kidney size, retroperitoneal disease, or radiopaque stone.

Ultrasound. Useful for evaluating kidney size, renal obstruction, and pericardial effusion.

Intravenous pyelography. May be helpful when an obstruction is suspected. Exercise caution in patients susceptible to renal failure, as contrast may precipitate nephropathy.

CT scan. May help delineate intraabdominal causes of obstruction. It is the technique of choice for visualizing ureteral obstruction at the level of the bony pelvis.

Urinalysis. Check for hematuria, proteinuria, and active sediment (RBC or WBC casts, eosinophils, oval fat bodies). Obtain sodium and creatinine levels before use of diuretic agents to help differentiate prerenal azotemia from acute tubular necrosis (ATN) (Table 12.1.1).

Treatment

The foremost priority in any patient with suspected ARF is to identify and treat potentially life-threatening complications: *hyperkalemia* (see section 6.9), *CHF* (see section 1.6), *encephalopathy* (see section 3.1), *pericarditis* (see section 9.3), and *severe metabolic acidosis* (pH < 7.2). Following adequate stabilization, seek the cause of ARF.

Prerenal azotemia is generally the most straightforward problem to correct—replenish the intravascular volume with normal saline (NS) boluses of 250 to 500 mL. Avoid supplemental potassium or lactated Ringer's) until adequate urine output is established and potassium levels have been determined.

Next, exclude bladder outlet obstruction by passing a Foley catheter. If a Foley catheter is already in place, ensure free flow by flushing the catheter with 20 to 30 mL of NS. However, the clear passage of a Foley catheter excludes only lower urinary tract obstruction, and further diagnostic studies are needed to rule out an upper tract obstruction.

Frequently, it is not feasible to determine the precise parenchymal etiology of ARF in the ED. Supplemental measures

Table 12.1.1
Prerenal Versus ATN[a]

Test	Prerenal	ATN
BUN:creatinine ratio	> 20:1	< 15:1
Urine osmolality (mOsm/kg)	> 500	< 350 (isosthenuria)
Urinary casts	Normal or pigmented	Hyaline cast; granular sediment
Urinary sodium (mEq/L)	< 20	> 40
Fractional excretion of sodium[b]	< 1%	> 2%

[a]Prior administration of diuretics or osmotic diuresis (mannitol, glycosuria, bicarbonaturia, and ketonuria) may interfere with renal tubular reabsorption of sodium and water and thus alter these urinary chemical indices.

[b]Fractional excretion of sodium = (urine sodium/plasma sodium) ÷ (urine creatinine/plasma creatinine) × 100.

include adjusting and avoiding the use of certain medications (potassium supplements, NSAIDs, aminoglycosides) and agents (contrast material) that may worsen the status of patients with impaired renal function and trying to restore normal urine output. Nonoliguric ARF has a better prognosis than oliguric ARF. Consider using high-dose loop diuretics (*furosemide,* 2 to 6 mg/kg up to 400 mg IV), *mannitol* (12.5 to 25 g IV), and/or *renal dose dopamine* (1 to 3 μg/kg/min) if there is no response to volume infusion.

Fluid overload in patients with CRF is treated with high-dose loop diuretics, intravenous nitroglycerin, and the use of sorbitol to create diarrhea and fluid loss from the GI tract.

Indications for emergent *dialysis* (hemodialysis and, if not available, peritoneal dialysis) include the following:

- Intractable volume overload;
- Symptomatic hyperkalemia not amenable to conservative measures;
- Severe metabolic acidosis unresponsive to bicarbonate (HCO_3 < 10 mEq/L);
- Certain drug intoxications;
- CNS disturbances such as encephalopathy and seizure;
- Bleeding diathesis; and
- Uremic pericarditis.

The major complications associated with dialysis are *hypotension, dialysis disequilibrium syndrome* (nausea, vomiting, muscle cramping, CNS disturbances), *bleeding, infection,* and *air embolus* (especially with use of temporary subclavian catheters).

Admission Criteria

All patients with new-onset ARF or serious complications secondary to uremia obligate admission. Consider transfer, if dialysis is necessary but not available. Consult a nephrologist to assist in management.

Suggested Readings

Anderson RJ: Prevention and management of acute renal failure. Hosp Pract 1993;28:61–68.

Sacchetti A, Harris R, Patel K, et al.: Emergency presentation of renal dialysis patients. J Emerg Med 1991;9:141–144.

12.2 RHABDOMYOLYSIS

Description

Rhabdomyolysis arises from injury or ischemia of skeletal muscle with subsequent release of muscle cell contents into the extracellular fluid. Myoglobin, a cellular component of muscle is nephrotoxic. Causes of rhabdomyolysis include trauma (including iatrogenic compression injuries), toxins (alcohol, cocaine, PCP), and seizures. Frequently, the source of rhabdomyolysis is multifactorial.

History

The clinical presentation is variable. Classically, patients complain of myalgias, weakness, and a dark urine, but this triad occurs in only a minority. Inquire about possible trauma, extreme physical activity, environmental or occupational exposures, drug ingestion (alcohol, cocaine, amphetamines, combination of lovastatin and gemfibrozil), and preexisting medical problems (especially seizures or muscular or metabolic illness). Unfortunately, many of these patients are poor historians, making it necessary to question observers or prehospital providers.

Physical Examination

General. Note agitation and level of consciousness.

Vital signs. Check a rectal temperature; note pulse, blood pressure, and respiratory rate.

HEENT. Inspect for signs of trauma. Note pupil size and reactivity.

Neck. Note stiffness or thyromegaly.

Lungs. Listen for rales or rhonchi (consider aspiration).

Heart. Determine rate, rhythm, and murmurs.

Abdomen. Auscultate bowel sounds. Palpate for tenderness and masses.

Neurologic. Perform as complete an examination as possible. Note mental status, check for nystagmus and sensory loss. Examine muscle tone and strength. The flaccid paralysis associated with crush injuries generally fails to correspond with dermatomal sensory loss.

Extremities. Rule out compartment syndrome (see section 16.4). Note any deformity, tenderness, swelling, crepitus, discoloration, or open wounds.

Diagnostic Tests

ABG. Check for acidosis and oxygenation.

SMA. Check electrolytes, BUN, creatinine, calcium, phosphorous, uric acid, and albumin. Hyperkalemia, hypocalcemia, hyperuricemia, and hyperphosphatemia are the most common metabolic abnormalities. Note the anion gap (usually increased).

CPK. Classically markedly elevated, usually more than five times normal. Despite accompanying increases in the CPK-MB, the relative ratio of CPK-MB:CPK should remain < 5%. Expect CPK levels to decline in 24 hr; failure to decrease implies a possible compartment syndrome.

CBC. Check hematocrit and platelets.

PT and PTT. Suspect DIC when PT is increased.

X-rays. Dictated by history and physical examination.

Urinalysis. Characteristically, the urine dipstick tests heme positive, with few or no RBCs being detected on microscopic examination. Nevertheless, a negative test for blood on the urine dipstick *does not* rule out rhabdomyolysis (up to 20% of patients with rhabdomyolysis will have a negative dipstick for heme). Both myoglobinuria and hemoglobinuria create a positive test for blood on a urine dipstick and a lack of RBCs found on urine microscopy. However, with hemoglobin by-products, the plasma is pink; while with myoglobin breakdown, the plasma appears clear.

Myoglobin. May be measured quantitatively in both the serum and the urine. Unfortunately, myoglobin is rapidly cleared from the serum (elimination half-life 1 to 3 hr), and, therefore, is not a sensitive test for rhabdomyolysis.

Special Considerations

Complications include metabolic imbalances (hyperkalemia, hyperuricemia, hyperphosphatemia, and hypocalcemia), DIC, compartment syndrome (not always obvious on admission), and acute renal failure.

Treatment

As for all emergencies, first secure the ABCs. Aggressively hydrate the patient with intravenous crystalloids, striving to maintain a urine output > 200 mL/hr. Once euvolemia is achieved, consider administration of mannitol (0.5 mg/kg) to improve diuresis. Administer bicarbonate until the urinary pH > 7.0 (pay careful attention to serum pH, electrolytes, and calcium). Although hypocalcemia is a common associated finding, it rarely requires treatment. Further therapeutic measures include eliminating the toxin if present, controlling excessive muscle exertion (use sedation, anticonvulsants, and intubation along with pharmacologic paralysis if necessary), fasciotomy for compartment syndrome (see section 16.4), and stabilizing the body temperature. Consider hemodialysis in refractory cases.

Admission Criteria

Admit *all patients with suspected rhabdomyolysis.*

Suggested Readings

Better OS, Stein JH: Early management of shock and prophylaxis of acute renal failure in traumatic rhabdomyolysis. N Engl J Med 1990;322: 825–829.

Welch RD, Todd K, Krause GS: Incidence of cocaine-associated rhabdomyolysis. Ann Emerg Med 1991;20:154–157.

Chapter 13

Hematology

13.1 BLOOD TRANSFUSION

Blood Products

Red Cell Components

Red cell components are obtained from *whole blood* and *packed red blood cells* (PRBCs). Whole blood contains both cellular elements (*red blood cells, platelets, leukocytes*) and plasma. Although *fresh whole blood* is optimal for replacement in the actively bleeding patient, its use is limited because of problems with availability and storage; thus PRBCs are normally used.

The typical 300-mL unit of PRBCs displays a hematocrit of 65 to 80%; as a rule, 1 unit of PRBCs raises the hematocrit in the adult by three points. PRBCs alone are not sufficient for volume restoration, but they can be combined with normal saline (mixing lactated Ringer's, which contains calcium, with blood products may cause coagulation). The drawbacks of PRBC transfusion include exposure to antigens, limited concentrations of clotting factors (especially V and VIII) and platelets, lack of functional granulocytes, and thermal insult unless the product is adequately warmed (banked blood is stored at 4°C). The use of *leukocyte-poor RBCs* or *washed RBCs* may prevent nonhemolytic transfusion reactions in previously sensitized patients.

Platelets

The necessity for platelet transfusion is based on both the platelet count and the clinical condition. The risk of spontaneous hemorrhage is high when platelet counts are $< 5{,}000/mm^3$. The likelihood of bleeding with platelet counts of 5,000 to $10{,}000/mm^3$ is increased when associated with trauma, ulceration, or an invasive procedure. For platelet counts in the range of 10,000 to 50,000/mm^3, the risk of bleeding is variable. Hemorrhage due to platelet deficiency is unlikely with counts > 50,000/mm^3. Platelets are stored in plasma (about 50 mL) and have a short shelf life (< 3 days).

Each 50-mL pack raises the platelet count by 5,000 to 10,000/mm^3. The goal of platelet supplementation is to increase the platelet count to the 50,000/mm^3 range (about 1 platelet pack/10 kg); for the average-size patient 5 to 6 units usually suffice.

Fresh Frozen Plasma

Fresh frozen plasma (FFP) consists of all the blood coagulation factors (including labile factors V and VIII) and is packaged in 200- to 250-mL units. By definition 1 mL of FFP contains 1 unit of factor activity. FFP, like packed RBCs, must be typed and crossmatched (for ABO compatibility). The indications for giving FFP are not clear-cut but generally include the presence of coagulopathy and when massive PRBCs transfusions are required (give 1 unit of FFP for every 5 units of PRBCs).

Cryoprecipitate

Cryoprecipitate is prepared from plasma and contains large quantities of *factor VIII* (80 to 120 units), *fibrinogen* (200 to 300 mg), and *von Willebrand's factor* (vWF; 80 units). Cryoprecipitate is principally employed in the treatment of mild hemophilia A, von Willebrand's disease (vWD), hypofibrinogenemia (seen with DIC and dilutional coagulopathies), or bleeding from thrombolytic therapy. Factor VIII concentrates are favored over cryoprecipitate for the management of hemophilia A because of their lower risk of disease transmission.

Indications for RBC Transfusion

The decision to transfuse a patient ought to conform to a rational plan. Transfusion practices vary throughout the country, and no single numerical value can be applied to guide all transfusions. Essential factors to consider are that rapid bleeding may produce a critical blood loss without a change in the hematocrit and the truism that the ability to tolerate a significant blood loss depends on both age and underlying physiologic status (impaired with chronic disease, especially CAD). Furthermore, patients with chronic anemias may better endure lower hematocrits. RBC transfusion is generally indicated when anemia is associated with signs of continuing blood loss or tissue hypoperfusion (anginal-type chest pain, ischemic ECG changes, altered mental status, high output congestive heart failure, peripheral ischemia). An additional consideration for transfusion is the actively hemorrhaging patient who has already endured a blood loss of > 15% of his or her estimated blood volume (see Table 4.1.1). Base transfusion decisions on the patient's clinical condition.

In emergent cases, order *type-specific* blood (usually obtainable in 5 min). In life-threatening situations when a blood sample is unavailable, use type O blood (use Rh− in women of childbearing age).

The individual hanging the blood must be responsible for following blood bank guidelines, ensuring that the proper patient is receiving the blood, and checking the blood unit identification. When transfusing blood in the ED:

- Infuse via a large-bore (18-gauge or larger) intravenous catheter;
- Use a standard blood set or Y-type large-bore tubing if blood is to be reconstituted;
- Mix PRBCs with normal saline to infuse at a faster rate, and use a pressure infusor, if necessary;
- Employ micropore filters to prevent the infusion of platelets, fibrin, and leukocyte fragments; and
- Use blood warming systems when large transfusions (> 5 units) are given.

Infusion time should not exceed 4 hr for 1 unit (keep each portion refrigerated until used) or be interrupted for > 30 min, to minimize the risk of bacterial infection or hemolysis. *Monitor the patient closely during the first 5 to 10 min of infusion.* Frequently recheck vital signs.

Special Considerations

Transfusion Reaction

When faced with an adverse reaction to a blood transfusion, i.e., fever, chills, back pain, occipital headache, diaphoresis, or shortness of breath, *terminate* the transfusion *without delay,* keep the intravenous line patent with saline, and recheck the patient's and blood unit's identification. Major *life-threatening* reactions include *acute hemolytic reaction* (ABO incompatibility) as well as *anaphylaxis* (usually IgA incompatibility). Both these reactions can be rapidly fatal. Anaphylaxis may cause death either from laryngospasm, bronchospasm, or cardiovascular collapse (see chapter 8), while an acute hemolytic reaction typically proceeds to renal failure and/or acute DIC. Less serious responses to transfusions include urticaria and a febrile leukoagglutinin reaction.

Examine the patient, confirming vital signs. Note flushing, wheezing, and "oozing" from intravenous sites. Check a urine and a plasma specimen for color. Free Hgb turns a distinctive reddish brown. After stopping the transfusion, return the unit along with a posttransfusion match specimen (and urine sample) to the blood bank. For anaphylaxis, follow the guidelines delineated in chapter 8: epinephrine (3 to 5 mL—0.3 to 0.5 mg—of a 1:10,000 solution by slow IVp, if in frank shock, or 0.3 mL—0.3 mg—of a 1:1000 solution SQ, with repeat doses q 15 min as needed) with normal saline (500 mL bolus), high flow oxygen via a face mask, diphenhydramine (50 mg slow IVp), and hydrocortisone (250 mg IVp). *Intubate early if the airway is jeopardized.*

For a presumed acute hemolytic reaction, administer a fluid bolus normal saline (500 mL IV), trying to maintain a urine output > 100 mL/hr. Sustain the urine flow with either mannitol (12.5 to 25 g IV over 5 min) or furosemide (40 to 80 mg by slow IV). Draw the patient's blood for repeat cross-match, Coombs test, free Hgb, CBC, RBC morphology, renal function tests, electrolytes, and coagulation screen (check for DIC). Also, check serum bilirubin and haptoglobin levels for evidence of hemolysis. If oliguria persists despite adequate fluid resuscitation and appropriate diuretic therapy, suspect acute renal failure (see section 12.1).

Fluid Overload

If pulmonary edema occurs, discontinue the transfusion (or slow it down if it is essential) and provide furosemide (40 mg IV); a higher dose may be required for patients already receiving a diuretic or who have renal insufficiency.

Infections

Current screening routines (including testing for VDRL, hepatitis B surface antigen, hepatitis B core antibody, hepatitis C antibody, HIV, HTLV−, and alanine aminotransferase as a marker for non-A, non-B hepatitis) have notably lessened the incidence of, but have not eliminated, the transmission of infectious disease via blood transfusions. The chance of contracting HIV from transfused blood is now estimated at 1 in 40,000, while the risk of serum hepatitis is 1 in 1,000. Rare diseases that may be transmitted include cytomegalovirus, malaria, brucellosis, Chagas disease, toxoplasmosis, and Epstein-Barr virus.

Suggested Readings

Development Task Force of the College of American Pathologists: Practice parameter for the use of fresh-frozen plasma, cryoprecipitate, and platelets. JAMA 1994;271:777–781.

Silberstein LE, Kruskall MS, Stehling LC, et al.: Strategies for review of transfusion practices. JAMA 1989;262:1993–1999.

13.2 SICKLE CELL CRISIS

Description

Sickle cell anemia (SCA) is a hereditary anemia that results from an abnormal β-hemoglobin molecule (valine is substituted for glutamic acid), forming *hemoglobin S.* Sickle cell crisis occurs when an individual homozygous for the sickle cell gene is exposed to an adverse state (hypoxia, dehydration), causing the cell to take on a sickle shape, with subsequent occlusion of small vessels. Long-standing sickle cell anemia eventually leads to chronic multisystem disease. Sickle cell–like illness also occurs when a hemoglobin S gene is paired with another abnormal hemoglobin molecule, e.g., *hemoglobin C, hemoglobin D,* or thalassemia, but this tends to cause a less severe disease. Patients who are heterozygous for hemoglobin S (hemoglobin AS disease affects 10% of African-Americans) are ordinarily asymptomatic but may develop problems when placed under severe stress (oxygen deprivation).

History

Familiarity can breed mistakes, and every patient with sickle cell crisis deserves a comprehensive assessment, no matter how well you think you know him or her! The history assists in determining not only what type of crisis the patient is undergoing but also the possible reason for the problem. There are four varieties of crisis in patients with SCA: thrombosis, hyperhemolysis, aplastic anemia, and splenic pooling. Most patients with a sickle cell crisis present to the ED complaining of pain secondary to vaso-occlusion. The pain tends to follow a repetitious pattern from one painful crisis to the next. However, note that sometimes the discomfort of a different acute process (acute surgical abdomen) may masquerade as a painful crisis. Patients may also develop acute neurologic symptoms (aphasia, hemiplegia, cranial nerve palsies, seizures) as well as cough, dyspnea, or chest pain. At times, it may be difficult to distinguish vaso-occlusive complications (pulmonary infarction) from an infectious process. In addition, pallor, syncope, or weakness may signal a hemolytic crisis or characterize a nonspecific manifestation of infection or vaso-occlusion. Inquire about possible triggering events (infection, cold exposure, dehydration, pregnancy) and ask questions concerning prior surgeries, transfusions, medications (folate), allergies, and immunizations (especially pneumococcal vaccine status).

Physical Examination

Vital signs. Temperature elevation may accompany vaso-occlusive crisis (usually low grade); however, elevations > 38.4°C (101°F) should prompt a search for infection. Check for hypotension or orthostatic changes, tachypnea (pain, pulmonary infarction, infection), and tachycardia (pain, fever, sepsis).

HEENT. Look for icterus, retinopathy and signs of infection (pharyngitis, sinusitis).

Neck. Assess for meningismus.

Lungs. Examine for rales, pleural rubs, decreased breath sounds, dullness to percussion, and splinting.

Heart. Auscultate for gallop, murmurs, and rub.

Abdomen. While guarding may be present with a vaso-occlusive crisis, appearance of peritoneal signs implies an "acute" abdomen. Check for Murphy's sign (cholelithiasis) along with CVA tenderness.

Rectal. Inspect for perirectal abscess.

Genitourinary. Investigate for priapism in males and consider ectopic pregnancy or PID in females with abdominal pain.

Extremities. Examine for hot swollen joints (septic arthritis), point tenderness of bones (osteomyelitis), abscesses, and phlebitis.

Neurological. Perform a thorough examination.

Diagnostic Tests

CBC. Check the *hematocrit* and order a *reticulocyte count* (try to obtain the patient's old records to compare previous values). Typical ranges for the hematocrit in patients with sickle cell disease are 17.0 to 29.0%, while reticulocyte counts tend to run from 5.0 to 30%. A reticulocyte count of < 3.0% is suspicious for aplastic crisis. The WBC count is frequently elevated (15,000/mm^3 range); nevertheless, if a left shift is present, consider the possibility of infection.

Urinalysis. Check for UTI. Hematuria is not uncommon with sickle cell trait. Decreased concentrating ability (hyposthenuria) with a fixed specific gravity of approximately 1.010 is associated with sickle cell disease.

SMA. Order when dehydration or renal function compromise is suspected.

Pulse oximeter. Noninvasive screening for patients with respiratory complaints. However, it may be inaccurate in patients with severe anemia or when oxygen saturation levels are < 93%.

ABGs. Indicated in patients with respiratory distress.

X-rays. Warranted when pulmonary signs or symptoms are present. Bone films may be indicated when localized bone pain or new joint swelling develops, but they often fail to distinguish infarction from infection.

Ultrasound. Helpful in diagnosing cholecystitis or ectopic pregnancy.

CT scan. Indicated when CNS signs or symptoms are present.

Treatment

First rule out life-threatening conditions: acute surgical abdomen (see section 5.1), serious infection (see chapter 9), CVA (see section 3.3), or aplastic crisis. Transfusion therapy is frequently required for CVA, aplastic crisis, priapism, women in active labor, or when major surgery is anticipated. One should check the blood to be transfused to ensure it is not sickle trait and attempt to raise the patient's hemoglobin A concentration to 70%.

The most common problem afflicting the sickle cell patient is *pain* from a vaso-occlusive crisis. Unfortunately, prejudicial judgments are often made in treating these patients, and they are frequently viewed as manipulative and addiction prone. Lacking objective criteria, the pain of sickle cell crisis is repeatedly dismissed. However, *treatment of pain should be prompt,* and it is best to develop a protocol to decrease the widespread variability of both medication and admission decisions. Intravenous rehydration is indicated only if the patient is clinically dehydrated (otherwise encourage oral repletion), likewise supplemental oxygen has no proven benefit except in the hypoxic patient.

Satisfactory relief of pain is the cornerstone of the treatment of a vaso-occlusive painful crisis; approach the pain of sickle cell crisis as one would discomfort in a cancer patient. *Morphine* (given as a 5- to 10-mg IV bolus) followed by a morphine drip (5 to 10 mg/hr) has been successfully employed. Unless observation rooms are available, limit treatment time in the ED to 6 to 8 hr before deciding to admit the patient. While intramuscular meperidine may be preferred by the patient, it has the following drawbacks: a short duration of action (2 to 3 hr), possibly toxic metabolites (normeperidine is a CNS excitant), and the inconveniences of intramuscular injections (pain, induration, and abscess formation of skin). Various other regimens, including oral therapy have been proposed (see chapter 17). Morphine sulfate (60 mg PO followed by doses of 30 mg q 30 min) is quite adequate. Following a temperature recording opiate analgesia can be supplemented with NSAIDs such as ibuprofen (800 mg q 6 hr). No matter what drug is chosen, it is important for the emergency physicians to be consistent in dealing with sickle cell patients and to understand the pharmacology of the medications used.

Admission Criteria

Admission is *clearly indicated for life-threatening conditions*—CVA, aplastic crisis, and serious infection. *Patients with pulmonary complaints who are hypoxic* obligate consideration for ICU-level care. In additional, *patients with vaso-occlusive pain crises who do not respond to ED protocols for pain within a predetermined time* (usually 6 to 8 hr) require admission.

Patients who are discharged should be supplied with clear follow-up instructions. It is unwise to discharge these patients with potent analgesics, since this may encourage drug dependency. Acetaminophen and codeine should suffice. All patients with SCA should receive folate (5 mg per day).

Suggested Readings

Francis RB, Johnson CS: Vascular occlusion in sickle cell disease: current concepts and unanswered questions. Blood 1991;77:1405–1412.

Serjeant GR, Ceular CD, Lethbridge R, et al.: The painful crisis of homozygous sickle cell disease: clinical features. Br J Hematol 1994;87: 586–591.

13.3 BLEEDING DISORDERS

Description

Satisfactory hemostasis relies on the proper integrity and interaction of the blood vessels, platelets, and clotting factors. Three sequential events need to take place: (1) a vascular reaction (blood vessels constrict with injury), (2) formation of a platelet plug, and (3) activation of the coagulation cascade (a series of enzymatic reactions). Problems arise when there is a disturbance in any of these functions: increased capillary fragility, a defect in platelet number or function, or difficulty in the formation of the fibrin clot (coagulation). Vessel or platelet abnormalities are characterized by skin or mucosal bleeding (easy bruisability, purpura, petechiae, epistaxis, bleeding gums, menorrhagia, GI bleeds); while coagulopathies manifest as recurrent, delayed, or prolonged bleeding from wounds or visceral organs along with formation of hematoma and/or hemarthrosis.

History

Establish the *type and site(s) of bleeding* (bruising of skin, epistaxis, prolonged bleeding following dental extraction, menorrhagia, GI bleed, hematuria, hemorrhage into joints or muscles), the *cause of bleeding* (trauma, surgery or spontaneous), the *onset* (immediately following trauma or surgery or delayed for hours or days), and the *pattern of bleeding* (antecedent episodes or first-time event). Inquire about recent illnesses, complications associated with surgery (tonsillectomy, tooth extraction), prior bleeding problems (including need for transfusion, menstrual history, and family history of coagulation disorders), past medical history (especially liver, renal, collagen-vascular, and oncologic diseases), medications (aspirin, NSAIDs, thiazide diuretics, quinidine, quinine, estrogen, corticosteroids, antibiotics, phenytoin, warfarin), and social history (alcohol, IVDA). Also ask about symptoms that may indicate an underlying problem (headache, syncope, dyspnea, melena, abdominal pain, weight loss, fever).

Physical Examination

The major purpose of the physical examination is to determine the severity of the blood loss and whether a single site or multiple sites are implicated. **Remember:** *Hemorrhage may be concealed (in chest, abdominal cavity, or pelvis).* A secondary objective of the examination is to carefully search for clues that may suggest an underlying illness.

General. Observe the overall appearance (malnourished, cachexia). Assess mental status and inspect for generalized lymphadenopathy (infection, malignancy, AIDS).

Vital signs. Check for hypotension (including orthostatics) and fever (rectal temperature). **Note:** *The presence of fever with petechiae is sepsis until proven otherwise.*

HEENT. Inspect the mucosal surfaces for gingival bleeding and epistaxis. Examine fundi for retinal hemorrhages. Check for scleral icterus.

Neck. Examine for soft tissue swelling and listen for stridor.

Lungs. Auscultate for rales or wheezes (pulmonary hemorrhage).

Abdomen. Examine for hepatomegaly and splenomegaly (platelet sequestration, myeloproliferative disorders, lymphoma) and look for dilation of superficial veins (caput medusa), gynecomastia, and ascites (fluid wave, shifting dullness) found with cirrhosis.

Pelvic. Determine the presence and location of vaginal bleeding.

Rectal. Check for hemorrhoids (portal hypertension) and occult blood.

Extremities. Note prolonged bleeding from wounds and intravenous sites. Assess joints (especially knees, elbows, wrist, ankles, and shoulder) for swelling and range of motion (hemarthrosis) and evaluate large muscle groups (such as the thigh) for distention or tenderness (deep hematoma). The presence of palmar erythema suggests chronic liver disease

Neurologic. Document focal deficits.

Skin. Carefully examine the skin for *petechiae* (dot hemorrhages that do not blanch), *purpura* (red or purplish lesions), *ecchymosis* (expansive bruising), *necrosis* (warfarin), *telangiectasias, angiomas,* and *jaundice.* Confluent petechiae imply a greater risk for hemorrhage than scattered petechiae. Likewise, note any petechiae appearing subsequent to the placement of a tourniquet.

Diagnostic Tests

The following tests are usually readily available in the ED and are essential in the diagnosis and management of patients with a bleeding disorder: *CBC with platelet count, peripheral smear, prothrombin time (PT), activated partial thromboplastin time (aPTT),* and *thrombin time.* While not ordinarily performed in the ED, the availability of a bleeding time test may be helpful. *Normal PT, aPTT, and bleeding times do not eliminate the possibility of a significant bleeding disorder!*

CBC. Order hemoglobin and hematocrit in all patients with abnormal bleeding to judge the extent of blood loss. Also request a manual platelet count (normal count is 250,000/mm^3, ranging from 150,000 to 350,000/mm^3); some automated platelet counters tend to be imprecise when platelet counts are < 50,000/mm^3 or the WBC count is > 100,000/mm^3.

PT. Screens the extrinsic and common pathways for satisfactory clotting: factors I (fibrin), II (thrombin), V, VII, and X. Elevations take place with liver disease, vitamin K deficiency, warfarin use, and DIC. Traditionally, the prothrombin time was calculated by comparing a control sample with a test specimen (normal values being 11 to 15 sec). Recent recommendations from the World Health Organization advise the use of international normalized ratios (INRs) for reporting the PT. This method is considered to be a more reliable parameter, with current guidelines recommending that patients be maintained at an INR between 2.0 and 3.0 for almost all conditions, except mechanical prosthetic valves (keep INR levels at 2.5 to 3.0). Isolated prolongation of the PT by 2 to 3 sec is unlikely to cause excessive bleeding alone. Artificial increases of the PT may result from underfilling of the test tube or extreme polycythemia.

aPTT. Measures clotting ability of the intrinsic pathway (normal is < 38 sec). Prolongation occurs with a deficiency of any of the coagulation factors (except VII and XIII) and with the presence of circulating anticoagulant (heparin, lupus anticoagulant). The aPTT is particularly useful for monitoring heparin therapy, although the PT level is also frequently prolonged in patients receiving therapeutic heparin. Isolated prolongation of the aPTT can occur due to improper collection (incomplete filling of the citrate tube [blue top] or drawing the blood sample from a previously heparinized line). *Lupus anticoagulant* is rarely associated with lupus, despite the name, and more commonly causes thrombosis not bleeding problems.

Peripheral blood smear. Obtained via a fingerstick (anticoagulants distort platelet morphology). Helpful in estimating platelet counts; exhibits disrupted RBCs (schistocytes) that result from a hemolytic process (DIC, hemolytic-uremic syndrome, or TTP).

Bone marrow aspiration. Discuss with the hematologist, as he or she may want a sample before transfusion therapy is begun.

Thrombin time. Measures the time necessary to convert fibrinogen to a fibrin clot. Aberrant results correlate with abnormal or deficient fibrinogen, the presence of heparin, or the presence of fibrin-degradation products. The normal range is 18 to 20 sec.

Fibrin-degradation products. Even though it may not be immediately available, an extra blue top tube (for FDP only) of blood should be drawn to document the presence of these small peptides when DIC or primary fibrinolysis is suspected. Recent work has validated that the *D-dimer* is the most sensitive and specific marker for intravascular coagulation.

Renal function tests. Order BUN and creatinine if renal pathology is suspected (hemolytic uremic syndrome, renal failure).

Liver function tests. Important when liver failure is thought to be the cause of the bleeding problem.

Urinalysis. Examine for blood and/or RBC casts.

CT scan. Essential to rule out CNS bleed. Also invaluable in evaluating the retroperitoneum for bleeding and the extremities for hematoma or hemarthroses.

Special Considerations

Platelet Disorders

Thrombocytopenia is generally a consequence of decreased bone marrow production of platelets, increased peripheral destruction of platelets, or dilutional effects associated with massive PRBC transfusion. Petechiae, bruising, and mucous membrane bleeding are the hallmarks of thrombocytopenia. In general, bleeding due to a platelet deficiency is unlikely if the platelet count is > 50,000/mm^3. A platelet count < *5,000/mm^3* predisposes to spontaneous hemorrhage; while platelet counts ranging from *5,000 to 10,000/mm^3* display a high probability of bleeding when combined with trauma, invasive procedures, or ulcerations. The risk of bleeding is variable when counts are *10,000 to 50,000/mm^3*. Serious disorders associated with thrombocytopenia include the following.

Idiopathic Thrombocytopenic Anemia. Idiopathic thrombocytopenic anemia (ITP) is a prototypical autoimmune-mediated disorder where antibodies are formed against the patient's own platelets. A chronic form appears in adults (most prevalent in women between 20 and 50 years old), often complicating preexisting defective immune states (SLE, Hodgkin's, HIV).

ITP is regularly characterized by an insidious onset with frequent exacerbations and remissions. Life-threatening events are rare (< 1% of cases), with the typical presenting complaint being epistaxis, oral bleeding, menorrhagia, hematuria, hematochezia, or skin lesions (purpura, petechiae). Generally, the patient appears well, with a key physical finding being a *normal spleen size.* The defining laboratory study is the platelet count, which may be as low as < 10,000/mm^3) but usually ranges from 20,000 to 80,000/mm^3. CBC values tend to be normal, apart from the decreased platelet count, although 10% of patients may have an associated hemolytic anemia (Evans's syndrome).

In the absence of severe hemorrhage, the timing and necessity of therapeutic modalities used in the management of ITP need to be discussed with the hematology consultant (corticosteroids, intravenous immunoglobulin, splenectomy). Any drugs that may aggravate bleeding (i.e., aspirin) must be discontinued. Prophylactic platelet transfusions *are not* indicated (the infused platelets are rapidly destroyed and may provoke antibody formation).

Thrombotic Thrombocytopenic Purpura. Thrombotic thrombocytopenic purpura (TTP) is an uncommon, potentially fatal syndrome, characterized by the clinical pentad of (1) microangiopathic hemolytic anemia, (2) thrombocytopenia, (3) neurologic abnormalities, (4) fever, and (5) renal dysfunction. The etiology remains unknown, but TTP occurs primarily in adults between 20 and 50 years old (with a slight female predominance). There are increasing reports of TTP being encountered in AIDS patients.

Presenting complaints tend to be related to bleeding complications (bruising, anemia) or neurologic abnormalities (headache, confusion, seizures, coma). Additional clinical symptoms include abdominal pain, nausea, vomiting, arthralgias, malaise, and weakness. These patients appear ill and are usually febrile. Laboratory findings include hemolytic anemia (red cell fragmentation) along with thrombocytopenia (may be < 20,000/mm^3). LDH levels tend to be markedly increased. Renal involvement manifests as hematuria, abnormal urinary sediment (RBC casts), and aberrant renal function studies. Life-threatening complications may arise from the formation of micro thrombi, which can embolize to the heart, brain, and abdom inal organs.

Emergent hematology consultation is critical so prompt treatment (administration of FFP, steroids, and plasmapheresis) can be instituted.

Sepsis. Sepsis may give rise to thrombocytopenia even in the absence of other evidence of DIC. It is believed that an endotoxin leads to platelet sequestration in the capillary circulation. *The combination of fever and petechiae is presumed sepsis until proven otherwise.* Organisms reported to have a direct toxic effect on platelets include Gram-negative bacteria *(Haemophilus influenza, Neisseria meningitides),* Gram-positive bacteria (both *Staphylococcus* and *Streptococcus* spp.), and *Rickettsia rickettsi.*

Treatment is geared toward the underlying infection. Platelet counts < 50,000/mm^3 often reflect DIC and have a poorer prognosis.

Drug-Induced Thrombocytopenia. Drug-induced thrombocytopenia is capable of causing severely depressed platelet counts, stemming from either a decrease in bone marrow production (alcohol, heparin, chloramphenicol, amrinone), or immune-mediated destruction (quinine, thiazide diuretics, gold, sulfonamides, cephalothin). Aspirin interferes with both platelet function and coagulation. The clinical manifestations of drug-induced thrombocytopenia are similar to the bleeding complications encountered in other forms of thrombocytopenia.

In most patients with drug-induced thrombocytopenia, rapid recovery of platelet function occurs within 7 to 10 days of discontinuing the offending agent. In patients with severe thrombocytopenia that results in bleeding complications, a short course of prednisone may be beneficial. Reserve platelet transfusions for critical or life-threatening hemorrhage.

Primary Coagulation Disorder

Disorders of the clotting process are represented by an abnormal PT, aPTT, or both. These disorders may be congenital (hemophilia A and B, and von Willebrand's disease) or acquired (vitamin K deficiency, liver disease, anticoagulant therapy or overdose) (Table 13.3.1). Bleeding secondary to coagulation defects may be lethal, so prompt identification and treatment of the defect are imperative. Adequate therapy depends on knowledge of the level of factor in the recipient's plasma.

Von Willebrand's Disease. Von Willebrand's disease is the most common congenital disorder of hemostasis, transmitted via an autosomal dominant pattern (seen in both men and women). Coagulation problems arise from deficiency or dysfunction of *von Willebrand factor* (mediates platelet adhesion). The degree of clinical bleeding is highly variable, with the majority of cases resulting in mild, mucosal bleeding (epistaxis, gingival bleeding, menorrhagia). Life-threatening episodes (GI bleeding, intracranial) are possible. Patients with severe disease display a prolonged aPTT.

Hemophilia A and B. Hemophilia A (*classic hemophilia,* low levels of factor VIII activity, 85% of hemophiliacs) and hemophilia B (*Christmas disease,* low levels of factor IX activity, 14% of hemophiliacs) are hereditary diseases that show an X-linked recessive pattern of inheritance. More than 20,000 American males are affected. Clinically, hemophilia A and B are indistinguishable. Patients render a history of life-long soft tissue bleeding with easy bruisability and hemarthroses as well as spontaneous hematuria, melena, and excessive bleeding after dental extraction. Intracranial hemorrhage (ICH) is the leading cause of death in hemophiliacs. It is important to determine the patient's factor level. Hemophiliacs with a factor

Table 13.3.1
Laboratory Studies of Common Bleeding Disorders

Condition	PT (sec)	aPTT (sec)	Platelet Count (k/mL)	TT (sec)
Normal	11.5–13.5	25–35	150–350	18–20
Thrombocytopenia (ITP, TTP drug-induced)	Normal	Normal	< 50,000 with severe disease	Normal
Hemophilia A	Normal	> 35 when factor VIII level is < 15%	Normal	Normal
Von Willebrand's disease	Normal	Variable, can be increased	Normal	Normal
Vitamin K deficiency, excessive Coumadin				
Early	ca. 16	ca. 32	Normal	Normal
Late	> 25	ca. 58	Normal	Normal
Heparin				
Small	Normal	> 35	Normal	Normal
Large	ca. 18	> 100	Normal	Slightly increased
Liver disease				
Early	ca. 18	> 35	Low normal	Normal
Late	>25	> 55	< 50,000	Moderately increased
Dilutional coagulopathy				
Mild	ca. 16	> 35	Low normal	Normal
Severe	> 25	> 80	< 50,000	Moderately increased
DIC				
Mild	Normal	Normal	Low normal	Slightly increased
Severe	> 25	> 80	< 50,000	Greatly increased

level ≤ 1% have *severe disease* (frequent spontaneous bleeding episodes), those in the 1 to 5% range have *moderate disease* (bleeding episodes customarily provoked), and those with levels of 6 to 25% have *mild disease* (bleeding associated with significant trauma). Patients with a factor activity level > 5% pose little risk for spontaneous bleeding. The platelet count, fibrinogen level, and PT should be normal, but the aPTT is inclined to be prolonged if the patient has $< 15\%$ factor activity.

Warfarin. Warfarin interferes with activation of vitamin K–dependent factors (II, VII, IX, and X). The most serious complications are intracranial, pericardial, gastrointestinal, retroperitoneal, and spinal cord bleeding. Many drugs (aspirin, NSAIDs, cimetidine, dipyridamole, quinidine, tricyclic antidepressants, cephalosporins, sulfonamides, INH, metronidazole) are capable of potentiating the effects of warfarin. However, there is no increased association between age and risk of bleeding. Warfarin therapy prolongs both the PT and the aPTT. Oral anticoagulants may also cause a skin necrosis.

Heparin. Heparin binds to antithrombin III and heparin cofactor II and accelerates their inhibition of thrombin and factors XIIa, XIa, IXa, and Xa. Both the aPTT and the PT are prolonged. Heparin may also induce thrombocytopenia. The severe form, which is antibody-mediated, may be fatal. Patients on heparin must be monitored with platelet counts. Heparin should be discontinued if the platelet count falls below 50,000/mm^3. The major side effect of heparin is bleeding from sites of trauma or surgery as well as internally. The heparin metabolism rate is dose dependent.

Vitamin K Deficiency. Vitamin K deficiency results in a prolonged prothrombin time when vitamin K–dependent factors (II, VII, IX, and X) fall below 30% of normal (the aPTT is also prolonged but to a lesser extent). Vitamin K deficiency is associated with poor diet, malabsorption, and ingestion of broad-spectrum antibiotics that suppress colonic flora. There are no specific clinical features to distinguish vitamin K deficiency from hepatic coagulopathy, and differentiation is possible by measuring levels of non–vitamin K–dependent factors, obtaining a thrombin time, and judging the response to supplemental vitamin K.

Combined Platelet and Coagulation Disorders

Liver Disease. Liver disease is capable of inducing abnormalities of both platelets and clotting factors. The liver is the site of synthesis of all coagulation factors, except factor VIII. Because of its rapid turnover, factor VII is the first to decline. Conversely, fibrinogen levels generally remain unaffected unless the liver disease is very severe. Coagulation disorders develop when liver function declines to < 15% of normal activity level, giving rise to bleeding at any site, with oozing from venipuncture sites. Laboratory test abnormalities in liver disease include prolonged PT, aPTT, and TT and a modest decrease in platelets, and elevated levels of fibrin-degradation products.

Dilutional Coagulopathy. Dilutional coagulopathy is most prevalent in trauma patients undergoing massive transfusions (more than the body's blood volume within 24 hr). Banked blood stored for longer than 10 days becomes depleted of functioning platelets, factor VIII, and factor V. The result may be iatrogenic thrombocytopenia, prolongation of PT and aPTT, and consequential bleeding problems.

Disseminated Intravascular Coagulation. Disseminated intravascular coagulation (DIC) is a succession of hematological derangements, resulting from a number of serious illnesses (sepsis, burns, severe soft tissue injuries, heat stroke, obstetric complications, malignancies, major hemolytic transfusion reactions). The exact clinical course and specific management depend on the underlying etiology. However, the basic underlying problem arises from inappropriate and unregulated activation of the coagulation system, which promptly leads to a consumption of platelets and coagulation factors as well as fibrinolysis. Hemorrhage and thrombosis take place simultaneously. Bleeding usually dominates the clinical picture and may occur at any site (spontaneous bleeding and oozing from venipuncture, catheter, or sites of injury are especially distinctive for DIC). Characteristic lab findings include prolongation of PT, aPTT, and TT; a decrease in the levels of platelets and fibrinogen; fragmentation of RBCs (schistocytes); and an elevation of fibrin-degradation products (FDPs). Recent work has recognized the fibrin-degradation product *D-dimer* as being both a specific and a sensitive marker for intravascular coagulation. A subacute form of DIC is associated with malignancies, manifesting as a recurrent venous thrombosis *(Trousseau's syndrome)*.

Treatment

The two basic situations that demand immediate attention are (1) ongoing blood loss leading to hypovolemia and ensuing shock and (2) hemorrhage into a critical organ (especially intracranial hemorrhage). Quickly institute general supportive measures (see section 1.2). After initial stabilization, control external active bleeding by applying local pressure.

Patients with identifiable disorders may require replacement of a specific clotting factor, platelets, FFP or RBCs (see section 13.1). Transfuse only the components the patient needs. Consult a hematologist when specific factor replacement is necessary.

Primary Platelet Disorders

Treatment of primary platelet disorders is focused on identifying and treating the underlying problem (discontinuing the offending agent, chemotherapy). Generally, platelet transfusions (see section 13.1) are avoided unless the situation is life-threatening (in TTP, platelet therapy may actually be detrimental). Supplemental measures include use of corticosteroids, immunosuppressive agents, and plasmapheresis.

Primary Coagulation Defects

Treatment of primary coagulation defects depends on the particular deficiency.

Von Willebrand's Disease. Bleeding associated with vWD is generally mild, requiring no specific treatment other than avoidance of aspirin and related products. Specific therapy is based on the subtype of vWD identified. *Desmopressin* (DDAVP; 0.3 mg/kg in saline infusion over 20 to 30 min IV or, if the problem is minor, spray 150 mg per nostril) is usually sufficient for type I disease, while *cryoprecipitate* (1 unit raises vWF levels approximately 3%; 10 to 15 are units typically required) or *humate P* (25 to 50 U/kg IV) may be necessary for bleeding complications associated with type II disease. **Note:** *DDAVP is contraindicated in type II disease as it may give rise to thrombocytopenia.* Exercise caution using DDAVP in patients with coronary artery disease.

Hemophilia. The mainstay of treatment for hemophilia is intravenous replacement of factor deficiencies. Factor replacement is essential when a hemophiliac presents with a severe headache, altered mental status, or significant trauma and before any invasive diagnostic procedure. Replacement ought to be with *specific factor concentrate* (avoid cryoprecipitate and plasma unless the specific factor is not available and a life-threatening situation exists, since there is an increased risk of disease transmission). For hemophilia A this is accomplished with the recently developed, disease-free, recombinant *factor VIII products* (New York Blood Center FVIII-SD, American Red Cross method M). Hemophilia B is managed with hepatitis-free *factor IX concentrate* (Konyne 80, Mononine).

The number of units of factor replacement the hemophilia A patient needs is governed by the (1) type of hemophilia, (2) patient's factor level, (3) type of injury or medical condition, (4) presence of inhibiting antibodies, and (5) patient's weight. Each unit of factor VIII per kilogram increases the level 2%. **Note:** *In emergency situations* (CNS, GI, retroperitoneal, paratracheal bleeding, major trauma, hemorrhage from noncompressible region) *assume the hemophiliac has a 0 factor VIII activity level and administer 40 to 50 U/kg, followed by a continuous infusion of 5 to 10 U/kg/hr.* Order *factor VIII concentrate* (20 to 25 U/kg IV bolus) for hemarthrosis, intramuscular hematoma, epistaxis, gross hematuria, and actively bleeding wounds.

The principles guiding factor replacement of hemophilia B are similar to those for hemophilia A, but the amount of factor IX required is twice that of factor VIII (each unit of factor IX per kilogram will raise the level by 1%). However, the half-life of factor VIII is 8 to 12 hr, while that of factor IX is 18 to 24 hr, requiring more transfusions of factor VIII.

A major problem in the treatment of hemophilia is the development of inhibitors (occurs in up to 15% of hemophiliacs); consult a hematologist for specific management of these patients. Treat hemarthrosis with factor replacement and joint immobilization for 2 to 3 days. Limit all invasive procedures (arthrocentesis) and avoid intramuscular injections and the use of aspirin and aspirin-like drugs in all hemophiliacs. Desmopressin acetate (DDAVP; 0.3 mg/kg) may useful in patients with minor bleeding problems secondary to hemophilia A. **However,** *DDAVP is incapable of substituting for factor-replacement therapy in patients with life-threatening bleeding, severe factor VIII deficiency, or factor IX deficiency.*

Note: *Most of these patients have an established hematologist who can supply essential information.* For more information, contact the National Hemophilia Foundation at 212–219–8180.

Excessive Oral Anticoagulation. For excessive oral anticoagulation accompanied by active bleeding, obtain intravenous access and administer *plasma* or *FFP* (2 units initially). When further reversal of oral anticoagulants is necessary, *vitamin K* (10 to 15 mg) may be given orally for nonemergent conditions and parenterally for life-threatening conditions. There is a risk of hematoma formation with an intramuscular injection and an anaphylactoid reaction with intravenous administration (give an intravenous dose at a rate ≤ 5 mg/min). Vitamin K can also be given subcutaneously in the standard 10- to 15-mg dose. Minor problems may require only temporary discontinuation of the medication.

Excessive Heparin Therapy. Heparin has a short half-life (approximately 1.5 hr), and most patients can be treated by simply discontinuing the infusion. For serious complications, give *protamine sulfate* slowly via an intravenous route (1 mg neutralizes 100 units of heparin). Estimate the dose based on the half-life of heparin and the elapsed time since the last dose of heparin. Protomine can itself interfere with coagulation if given in excessive amounts.

Vitamin K Deficiency. Treat vitamin K deficiency as described under "Excessive Oral Anticoagulation." Vitamin K replacement should be continued for 3 days, with correction of laboratory abnormalities being apparent in 12 to 24 hr.

Mixed Disorders

The management of mixed (platelet and coagulation factor) disorders depends on the cause.

Bleeding secondary to liver disease. Patients with severe liver disease are usually unresponsive to vitamin K, although these patients should still receive empiric parenteral vitamin K. Replacement therapy with FFP is essential when bleeding is serious (for severe coagulopathy administer an initial dose of 10 to 15 mL/kg of FFP, with repeat doses as necessary every 6 hr). Give platelets as needed.

Dilutional coagulopathy. Can be avoided by the administration of

1 unit of FFP for every 5 units of packed RBCs and/or 8 to 12 platelet units for every 10 units of PRBCs transfused.

DIC. Successful management of DIC depends on recognition and treatment of the underlying cause (antibiotics for sepsis, delivery or D&C of the OB-GYN patient). The hemorrhagic diathesis of DIC may require repletion of coagulation factors (FFP, platelets, or cryoprecipitate; see section 13.1). The role of heparin in the treatment of DIC is controversial, and should be discussed with the hematology consultant.

Iatrogenic Bleeding

Treat iatrogenic bleeding secondary to the administration of *thrombolytic agents* by first applying local pressure to any external bleeding sites. Avoid invasive procedures. If serious or life-threatening bleeding is suspected, discontinue the thrombolytic agent. FFP may be necessary to replace depleted fibrinogen. Use of *aminocaproic acid* (an inhibitor of fibrinolysis) should be initiated only after hematological consultation.

Admission Criteria

Disposition decisions need to be individualized, relying on the type of bleeding disorder and the patient's overall status and reliability for follow-up. *All patients with life-threatening bleeding* (CNS bleed, severe GI bleed, TTP) will require admission to a monitored bed. *The patient with a newly diagnosed bleeding disorder* generally requires admission for a diagnostic work-up and management, unless the disorder is obviously benign or chronic and *not* associated with serious problems.

Suggested Readings

Bussey HI: Reliance on prothrombin time ratios causes significant errors in anticoagulation therapy. Arch Intern Med 1992;152:278–284.

Kitchens CS: Approach to the bleeding patient. Hematol Oncol Clin North Am 1992;6:983–989.

Rutherford CJ, Frenkel EP: Thrombocytopenia: issues in diagnosis and therapy. Med Clin North Am 1994;78:555–575.

Chapter 14

Ophthalmology

14.1 GENERAL CONSIDERATIONS

Description

It is the task of the emergency physician to determine if a true eye emergency exists, what immediate treatment is needed, and the timeliness of ophthalmologic referral.

Triage

The following *emergent conditions* need immediate attention:

Chemical burns; and
Acute visual loss that could possibly be secondary to central retinal artery occlusion.

The following *immediate ophthalmology referrals* need to be seen within 1 hr:

Lacerated or ruptured globe; and
Acute angle-closure glaucoma.

The following conditions are *urgent referrals,* which need to be seen within several hours, but the sooner the better:

Hyphema;
Orbital cellulitis;
Retinal detachment;
Vitreous hemorrhage;
Corneal ulcer;
Intraocular foreign body;
Central retinal vein occlusion;
Full-thickness or medial eyelid lacerations; and
Suppurative iritis.

The following conditions require *referral to ophthalmologist* in 24 to 48 hr:

Diffuse keratitis;
Nonsuppurative or recurrent iritis;
Scleritis;
Corneal rust ring;
Unresponsive conjunctivitis;
Persistent blepharitis; and
Symptomatic hordeolum or chalazion.

History

The history is as essential with eye emergencies as with any other emergency. Patients commonly complain of a red eye, a painful eye, discharge from the eye, or visual loss. These are not mutually exclusive conditions. Inquire about previous eye problems (including refractive errors) and eye surgery. Verify the patient's overall health, medications (including over-the-counter products), allergies, and tetanus status.

Physical Examination

Visual acuity. *This is the vital sign of the eye and must be tested in all patients with eye complaints.* (In chemical burns, visual acuity testing is initially deferred until irrigation is complete.) Visual acuity carries both diagnostic and prognostic significance. Glasses should be worn to establish the best visual acuity. If there is a question of refractive error, a card with pinholes is employed (improvement implies a refractive problem). Traditionally, a Snellen chart is read at 20 feet. If the patient is unable to read the largest letter of the Snellen chart, then the clinician assesses best visual acuity by using set parameters (can count fingers at a certain distance, can discern hand motion, has light perception, or has complete visual loss).

Pupils. Examine with a pen light, noting discrepancies in size or shape. Evaluate optic nerve function by the *swinging flashlight test* (shift light from eye to eye without pausing). If the pupil fails to respond to direct light but constricts when the other eye is illuminated, an afferent nerve defect exists (*Marcus-Gunn* pupil).

Extraocular movements. Record the position of the eyes and their ability to follow cardinal fields of gaze.

External examination of lids, lashes, conjunctiva, and cornea. Check for symmetry, swelling, discharge, edema, erythema, hemorrhage, foreign bodies, and lacerations. Palpate the orbital rim for tenderness, step off, and subcutaneous air. Also evert the upper lid when looking for foreign bodies (place a cotton-tipped swab below the orbital rim, grasp the eyelashes, and flip the eyelid over the applicator stick). Determine where the conjunctival injection is most intense (perilimbal or peripherally). Evaluate corneal clarity.

Ophthalmoscopy. Test for a red reflex (a clear retinal image requires a transparent cornea, clear lens, and clear vitreous medium). Examine the optic disk (color, presence of elevation, cup:disk ratio), retinal vessels (nicking, emboli), and macula (hemorrhages, exudates) and inspect for peripheral retinal tears, lesions, detachments, or hemorrhages.

Slit-lamp examination. The slit lamp is a binocular microscope that affords excellent visualization of the anterior aspect of the eye. Start with a broad beam of white light and scan the conjunctival and corneal surfaces. Next, narrow the light ray and direct it at an angle to visualize the anterior chamber (look for cell and flare; resembles a movie projector light in a smoky room). The slit lamp is also helpful in removing foreign bodies.

Tonometry. Despite newer (tonopens) and more accurate (applanation tonometers) methods of measuring eye pressure, the Schiötz tonometer is still the instrument of choice in many EDs to record *intraocular eye pressure* (IOP). Place the patient in a supine position and instill a drop of topical anesthetic to the eye. Retract the lids with thumb and forefinger (avoid excessive pressure on the globe). The IOP is proportional to the extent that a fixed weight depresses the surface of the globe (correlate the reading on the scale to a conversion chart, noting that each weight has an independent scale. *Do not* use tonometers in any patients with a suspected ruptured globe or infection.

Fluorescein. A water-soluble dye available in dry strips that highlights defects of the cornea *(abrasions, burns, herpetic involvement)* when viewed under cobalt lighting. Moisten the strip before application (apply to the lower tarsal conjunctiva).

Treatment

Topical anesthetics. The two most commonly used are *proparacaine* 0.5% and *tetracaine* 0.5%. The complete relief of pain with instillation of topical anesthetic indicates superficial disease (conjunctiva or cornea). Never prescribe for home use (it may delay wound healing and add to the vulnerability of the eye).

Topical antibiotics. Used to treat purulent conjunctival discharges and applied prophylactically for corneal abrasion. Agents include *sulfacetamide, gentamicin,* and *erythromycin* (available only as an ointment). Drops are usually preferred because they do not interfere with vision, but instillation is required every 2 to 3 hr while awake for the first 48 hr. Ointments last longer (4 to 6 hr) and are advocated for overnight use.

Mydriatic and cycloplegic agents. Topical agents (red-top bottles) employed to dilate the pupil for examination and to alleviate the pain and photophobia seen with iritis. *Tropicamide* 1% is a short-acting agent (30 to 120 min) used for funduscopy, while *cyclopentolate* (duration of 6 to 24 hr) and *homatropine* (10- to 48-hr half-life) are used to prevent painful reactive ciliary spasm (iritis, large corneal abrasions). Avoid using these in the head injured patient (might obscure developing neurologic signs) and in patients with a history of narrow-angle glaucoma.

Topical corticosteroids. *Do not* prescribe from the ED without consulting an ophthalmologist. Inappropriate use could lead to worsening infection, glaucoma, and cataracts.

Suggested Readings

Sklar DP: Topical anesthesia of the eye as a diagnostic test. Ann Emerg Med 1989;18:1209–1211.

Strong N: Ocular emergencies. Practitioner 1988;232:174–178.

14.2 RED EYE

History

Determine if there is any subjective visual impairment, photophobia, pain, or discharge. Establish rapidity of onset and if one or both eyes are involved (Table 14.2.1).

Table 14.2.1
Nontraumatic Causes of Red Eye

Characteristic	Conjunctivitis	Iritis	Corneal Infection	Acute Glaucoma
Incidence	Very common	Common	Common	Uncommon
Pain	None to mild	Moderate	Moderate to severe	Severe
Photophobia	No	Yes	No	Yes
Visual acuity	No effect	Slight blurring	Blurring common	Marked blurring
Injection	Diffuse	Circumcorneal	Diffuse	Diffuse
Pupil size	Normal	Small, irregular	Normal	Midsize, dilated
Anterior chamber	Normal	Cell and flare, normal depth	Possible hypopyon, normal depth	Absent
Cornea	Clear	Clear	Change in clarity	Steamy
Discharge	Watery to purulent	None	Watery to purulent	None
Intraocular pressure	Normal[a]	Normal	Normal[a]	Elevated

[a]Should not be measured unless the diagnosis is in doubt.

Physical Examination

A red eye with decreased vision warrants a detailed eye examination. If the etiology is unclear, check IOP. Pain with consensual light reflex suggests iritis.

Special Considerations

Conjunctivitis

Conjunctivitis is the most prevalent etiology of red eye. Bacterial conjunctivitis is depicted by the classic sticky eye that is worse upon awakening. In sexually active patients, consider gonococcal (copious purulent discharge together with red swollen eyelids and chemosis) and chlamydial infections. Viral conjunctivitis typically takes place in epidemics in young adults. Symptoms that suggest a viral etiology include bilateral watery discharge accompanied by preauricular lymphadenopathy. The main features of allergic conjunctivitis are itching, tearing, and seasonal variation.

Iritis

Iritis describes a medley of ailments that cause inflammation of the anterior segment of the eye. Patients with iritis exhibit ocular pain, headache, photophobia, and blurred vision. Gross inspection of the eye exhibits a poorly reactive pupil with a ciliary flush (hyperemia of the vessels surrounding the pupil). Slit-lamp examination of the anterior chamber reveals cell and flare.

Suppurative Iritis

Suppurative iritis usually occurs secondary to penetrating trauma. Infection is capable of spreading to adjacent areas (paranasal sinuses) and provoking systemic illness. *Hypopyon* (an aggregation of WBCs in the anterior chamber) may accompany suppurative iritis. Nonsuppurative iritis is associated with a variety of systemic diseases (sarcoid, inflammatory bowel disease, ankylosing spondylitis, etc.).

Herpes

Herpes is the most common infectious cause of visual loss in the United States. Herpetic eye involvement is seen with both primary infection and secondary reactivation. Symptoms vary from mild irritation and foreign body sensation to severe pain with photophobia. Herpes zoster involving the fifth nerve may present with characteristic skin lesions. Involvement of the eye is suggested by lesions on the tip of the nose (nasociliary nerver). Fluorescein staining reveals diffuse punctate corneal uptake or the pathognomonic branching or dendritic pattern.

Orbital Infections

It is essential to distinguish *preseptal cellulitis* (infection confined to eyelid) from *orbital cellulitis* (infection extends posterior to the orbital septum). Preseptal cellulitis exhibits lid swelling, erythema, and tenderness of the eyelid, whereas the hallmark of orbital cellulitis is pain on eye motion, restriction of eye motion (ophthalmoplegia), and proptosis. Severe infection may manifest as an afferent pupillary defect and visual impairment in addition to fever and malaise. Immediate diagnosis is essential to prevent life-threatening complications such as *cavernous sinus thrombosis, meningitis,* and *brain abscess.* Orbital infections commonly arise from sinus infections. Computed tomography (CT) scanning is essential in defining the extent of orbital involvement.

Acute Narrow-Angle Glaucoma

Acute narrow-angle glaucoma is an ophthalmological emergency characterized by a sudden rise in IOP ($>$ 35 mm Hg) associated with a narrowing of the anterior chamber (the iris "bows" anteriorly, blocking the drainage of trabecula and causing the pressure in the posterior chamber to be higher than the pressure in the anterior chamber). Patients with narrow-angle glaucoma generally appear sick and complain of headache, deep ocular pain, photophobia, diminished vision (may relate seeing rings or halos surrounding light), nausea, and vomiting. Determine the triggering event (dilation of pupil with sympathomimetic or anticholinergic drug, going into a dark place like a movie theater). On examination the cornea is hazy, semidilated, and fixed, with impairment of visual acuity. There is ciliary injection with conjunctival edema. An accurate estimate of anterior chamber depth is key (shine a pen light parallel to the surface of the iris from the lateral side; if the anterior chamber is shallow, a shadow is cast on the medial, or nasal, portion of the iris near the pupil).

Ultraviolet Keratitis

Ultraviolet keratitis occurs in patients who are exposed to high or prolonged doses of uv light (welders, sun lamp users, skiers). Symptoms may not begin until 2 to 6 hr after exposure. Pain is frequently intense, with conjunctival injection and diffuse punctate fluorescein staining being seen on examination.

Corneal Ulcers

Corneal ulcers are a sight-threatening condition characterized by a stromal infiltrate with an overlying corneal defect. Clinically, a dense, white opacity surfaces on the cornea, in the setting of a red eye along with pain, foreign body sensation, and blurring of vision. Corneal scrapings (obtained by the eye consultant) are necessary for the diagnosis.

Contact Lenses

Contact lenses are capable of producing mechanical damage, hypersensitivity reactions, and hypoxia of the cornea *(contact lens overwear syndrome)*. In addition, unusual infections such as *Acanthamoeba keratitis* are associated with contact lens use.

Eyelid Infections

A *hordeolum* (sty) is an abscess of the lid glands or hair follicles. *Blepharitis* (commonly due to a staph infection superimposed on seborrhea) is an inflammation of the eyelid margins that causes crusting and scaling. Patients complain of eye irritation accompanied by a gritty sensation. A *chalazion* is a chronic inflammatory reaction that involves the secretory glands of the eyelids, manifesting as eye pain, tenderness, and a lid nodule. It is best visualized on eversion of the lid.

Treatment

Conjunctivitis. In practice it is difficult to distinguish bacterial from viral conjunctivitis. Therefore, treatment is the same, namely topical antibiotic therapy (sulfacetamide) and warm compresses. For conjunctivitis secondary to *Neisseria gonorrhea,* admission with the initiation of parental antibiotics (ceftriaxone) is required. Treatment for allergic conjunctivitis is basically supportive, with cool compresses and topical antihistamines. Any case of conjunctivitis not responding to routine care in 48 hr must be reevaluated by an ophthalmologist.

Iritis. Treatment is geared toward relief of pain from ciliary spasm by use of cycloplegics. Ophthalmology consultation and follow up are essential to diagnose the underlying condition and prevent complications.

Herpes. Treatment involves topical antiviral agents initiated after consultation with an ophthalmologist.

Orbital infections. Immediate consultation with an ophthalmologist and/or otolaryngologist is essential. Hospitalization with early administration of antibiotics is indicated for orbital cellulitis.

Narrow-angle glaucoma. Definitive treatment is surgical, and therefore, urgent ophthalmology referral is indicated. Temporizing measures are directed toward lowering the IOP. This is accomplished initially with *acetazolamide* (500 mg IV) and/or *timolol* 0.5% (2 drops topically). Additional medications include osmotic agents (*mannitol,* 1 to 2 g/kg IV; *glycerol,* 1 mL/kg of a 50% solution PO) and topical *pilocarpine* 1 to 2% (2 drops q 15 min two to three times).

Ultraviolet keratitis. Treatment includes a cycloplegic agent, topical antibiotics, and patching (if both eyes are involved, patch the worse eye). Narcotic analgesics are often necessary for initial pain relief.

Corneal ulcers. Urgent ophthalmologic evaluation for determination of specific antibiotic therapy (fortified topical antibiotics and intravenous antibiotics) is obligatory.

Contact lens complications. The first step is removal of the contact lens. If the patient reports relief of symptoms with lens removal and has normal pupillary reflexes, then the problem is usually not urgent. Instruct the patient not to wear the lenses until cleared by an eye doctor. However, if vision is markedly reduced or a corneal ulcer is present, urgent referral to ophthalmologist is indicated.

Eyelid infections. Treatment of a hordeolum consists of warm compresses five to six times daily along with topical antibiotics. If spontaneous drainage has not occurred despite 1 week of local therapy, then elective referral for surgical drainage is indicated. Blepharitis is treated with topical antibiotics and daily scrubs (with mild shampoo) of lashes and lids.

Admission Criteria

The decision to admit should be made on an individual basis in consultation with an ophthalmologist. Generally, the following conditions require admission: *gonococcal conjunctivitis, orbital cellulitis, corneal ulcers, narrow-angle glaucoma, and perferation of the globe.*

Suggested Readings

Brown MM: The red eye. Curr Concepts Ophthamol 1995;3:9–15.

Schein OD: Contact lens abrasions and the nonophthalmologist. Am J Emerg Med 1993;11:606.

Snyder RW, Glasser DB: Antibiotic therapy for ocular infection. West J Med 1994;161:579–584.

14.3 ACUTE VISUAL LOSS

History

A sudden visual loss should be considered an eye emergency until proven otherwise. Initial history focuses on patient's customary visual acuity, if one or both eyes are affected, abruptness or time course of visual loss, and type of vision loss (peripheral, central, blurred). Inquire about associated symptoms (pain, weakness, nausea) as well as existing medical problems (diabetes, AIDS). Suspect intracranial pathology in patients complaining of diplopia (Table 14.3.1).

Physical Examination

Rule out a refractive error first (pinhole testing) and record the best corrected vision. Visual field testing is necessary when the patient complains of visual loss. Binocular visual loss is usually associated with central nervous system disturbance and warrants a careful neurologic examination.

Miscellaneous causes include *CNS abnormalities* (CVA; pituitary tumor or hemorrhage; CNS insult from ischemia, anoxia, or tumor affecting the cortex), *toxins* (methanol, quinine, ergot derivatives, lead, arsenic, salicylate, mercury), *functional visual loss* (conversion reactions, malingering), and *papilledema* (secondary to hypertension, intracerebral bleed, CNS tumor, pseudotumor cerebri) in which loss of vision is a late finding. *Transient bilateral loss* may be associated with cardiac arrhythmias, vertebrobasilar insufficiency, migraine, and hypotension.

Diagnostic Tests

Tonometry. Measure intraocular pressures if glaucoma is suspected.

ESR. Usually markedly elevated (> 80) with temporal arteritis but may be normal in 10% of patients.

Collagen vascular studies and VDRL. May be indicated in work-up of optic neuritis.

Ultrasound. May be needed to evaluate for retinal detachment if the fundus cannot be visualized.

Toxicological studies. Indicated if a toxicological etiology is suspected. Tests include methanol, salicylate, lead, arsenic, mercury levels, and serum osmolality.

Table 14.3.1
Causes of Nontraumatic Unilateral Visual Loss

Disorder	Pain	Fundus	Pupil	Other Clues
Central retinal artery occlusion	No	Pale with cherry red macula	Normal	Abrupt onset; usually older patient
Central retinal vein occlusion	No	"Blood and thunder"	Normal	Patient usually has underlying atherosclerosis, diabetes, or blood dyscrasias
Iritis	Yes	Normal	Small	Ciliary flush
Narrow-angle glaucoma	Yes	Normal	Fixed, dilated	Steamy cornea; patient appears ill
Retinal detachment	No	Can be diagnostic or unremarkable	Afferent pupillary defect if extensive	Scintillations, floaters
Vitreous hemorrhage	No	Obscured	If hemorrhage extensive, afferent defect and a decreased red reflex	Flashes of light; cannot see into eye; in absence of trauma seen in diabetics
Optic neuritis	Pain on eye movement	Blurred disk	Afferent defect	Scotomata; possible toxins

Diffuse retinopathy	No		Hemorrhages; afferent defect; exudates; cotton wool spots	Patients usually have underlying disease (AIDS, diabetes)
Migraine	Cephalgia	Normal	Normal	Transient eye symptoms (last 5–30 min); prior history; scintillations
Temporal arteritis	Cephalgia	Normal or pale and swollen	Normal	Elderly patient; elevated ESR; weakness or arthralgias
Amaurosis fugax	No	Normal	Normal	Symptoms transient; carotid or heart disease
Cataract	No	Normal; decreased red reflex	Normal	Gradual onset; opacity of lens
Endophthalmitis	Yes	Often obscured	Normal; decreased red reflex if hypopyon present	Look for history of eye trauma, eye surgery, or systemic infection
Refractive error	No	Normal	Normal	Gradual onset; improves with pinhole

Head CT scan or MRI. Order when intracerebral pathology is a consideration.

Special Considerations

Central Retinal Artery

Artery occlusion is an ophthalmologic emergency that requires immediate attention. It is characterized by a sudden, unilateral, painless loss of vision. In older patients, the usual etiology is embolic. Visual acuity is regularly $< 20/200$. The pupil of the affected eye does not react to direct light stimulus but maintains a normal consensual reflex. Ophthalmoscopic inspection reveals a pale retina ("milky") except for the fovea, which shows through as a cherry red spot.

Central Retinal Vein Occlusion

Retinal vein occlusion is associated with a painless monocular visual loss. Typically, the patient is elderly with underlying hypertension or diabetes mellitus. Visual loss is more gradual than with central retinal artery occlusion. Examination of the anterior segment of the eye is unrevealing. Funduscopic examination is diagnostic, exhibiting multiple hemorrhages of various sizes and shapes around the disk, which have been aptly termed "blood and thunder."

Retinal Detachment

Suspect retinal detachment in patients complaining of the sudden onset of lightning flashes or sparks followed by visual loss. Retinal detachment is associated with trauma, myopia, and recent eye surgery. Although peripheral lesions are often difficult to detect in the ED, retinal detachment that is extensive enough to impair vision usually is apparent on funduscopic inspection (the involved retina appears gray with white folds).

Optic Neuritis

Optic neuritis is associated with several conditions that affect the optic nerve. Patients complain of reduced visual acuity, pain on eye movement, and central scotoma. Examination displays an afferent pupil defect, a Marcus Gunn pupil, blurring of the optic disk margin, and a pale optic disk. Optic neuritis is differentiated from papilledema in that papilledema is usually bilateral with minimal visual loss and more pronounced retinal changes.

Other Considerations

Temporal arteritis. Primarily a disease of the elderly (> 60 years old). Diagnostic features include jaw claudication, tenderness over the temporal artery, and an elevated sedimentation rate.

AIDS. Sudden loss of vision in AIDS patients usually arises from cytomegalovirus (CMV) or toxoplasmosis infection. CMV retinopathy presents as a painless loss of vision, distinguished by multiple areas of white retinal opacification and retinal hemorrhages. Toxoplasmosis is identified by large yellow-red chorioretinal lesions.

Toxins. There is a large group of organic chemicals that affect vision. The most commonly implicated substances are *methanol, digitalis, quinine, ethambutol, ergot derivatives,* and *salicylates.*

Functional loss of vision (conversion reaction or malingering). Always a diagnosis of exclusion and should be made only by an ophthalmologist. It can be suspected in patients with normal direct and consensual reflexes.

Treatment

Central retinal artery occlusion obligates immediate consultation and treatment. If occlusion persists beyond 1 hr, irreversible damage occurs. Temporizing therapy in the ED is directed at efforts to dislodge the embolus and increase arteriolar blood flow. Measures that might be tried while awaiting arrival of the ophthalmologist include intermittent digital massage (apply firm pressure to the globe with the fingertips for 15 sec and then release for 15 sec, repeating for a total of 5 min), inhalation of carbon dioxide–rich gas (a mixture of 95% oxygen and 5% carbon dioxide), or breathing into a paper bag for 5 min. Definitive treatment of central retinal vein occlusion is controversial and ought to be instituted by the eye specialist.

The only effective treatment for *retinal detachment* is surgical. Place the patient at bed rest with both eyes patched until he or she can be seen by an ophthalmologist.

Specific management of *optic neuritis* is based on the etiology.

The treatment of temporal arteritis involves immediate steroid therapy once the diagnosis is suspected.

Management of *AIDS-related retinopathy* needs to take place under the coordinated care of an ophthalmologist and infectious disease specialist. *Ganciclovir* is prescribed for CMV retinopathy and *pyrimethamine* plus *clindamycin* for toxoplasmosis.

Therapy for *visual loss due to toxins* depends on the specific toxin involved. Methanol toxicity requires emergent hospitalization for ethanol loading and dialysis (see section 7.9).

Admission Criteria

All admission decisions need to be made on an individual basis and in consultation with the ophthalmologist. However, these conditions generally warrant admission: *central retinal artery or vein occlusion, retinal tear and/or detachment, temporal arteritis with visual impairments, and visual loss secondary to toxins.*

Suggested Readings

Brown GC: Sudden unilateral visual loss. Curr Concepts Ophthalmol 1995;3:52–57.

Charley JA, Allaman C, Edler AW: Sudden bilateral visual loss. Curr Concepts Ophthalmol 1995;3:58–60.

14.4 EYE TRAUMA

Description

Damage to the eye may result from penetrating or blunt trauma. Injuries from sharp objects are known as *lacerations* and range from confined puncture wounds of the eyelid to cuts transecting the globe. Blunt trauma (fist, ball) runs the gamut from orbital fractures to eyelid ecchymosis ("black eye"), subconjunctival hemorrhages, corneal abrasion, hyphema, lens subluxation or dislocation, and severe scleral or corneal disruption (better known as a *ruptured globe*). Any eye injury that traverses the full thickness of the sclera or cornea and intrudes the intraocular cavity is classified as a *perforation.*

History

Obtain a detailed description of how the eye was injured and subsequent symptoms. Inquire about treatment before arrival in the ED. Previous eye problems (including eye glass wear), general medical history, allergies, medications, and tetanus status need to be noted. *Any patient presenting with a history of eye pain after using a hammer, chisel, injection device, or high-speed machine is assumed to have an intraocular foreign body until proven differently.*

Physical Examination

Given the proximity of the eye to the airway, face, neck, and intracranial space, a complete evaluation of vital signs, the face, and neurologic function is indicated with significant orbital trauma (see section 4.1).

Once stabilization is ensured, attention may be directed to the eye. Verify visual acuity. Periorbital edema may interfere with the eye exam, requiring the physician to retract the eyelid (an unfolded paper clip bent at a right angle serves as a makeshift lid retractor). If active bleeding is occurring beneath the eyelids, assume a major penetrating injury of the globe and avoid further manipulation of the eye. Other findings that suggest a perforating eye injury include flattening and collapse of the anterior chamber, protrusion of the pigmented uveal tissue or jelly-like vitreous, and a misshapen pupil. In addition, subconjunctival hemorrhage (bloody chemosis) and hyphema may signal occult rupture of the globe.

Once a laceration or rupture of the globe is suspected, cover the affected eye with a plastic or metal shield until the patient can be seen by an ophthalmologist. Check for eye muscle entrapment. *Do not* instill any drops or perform tonometry on an eye suspected of being perforated.

Diagnostic Tests

Radiological studies are indicated when there is significant blunt trauma to the orbit or an intraocular foreign body is suspected. A CT scan is superior to plain films and is better at defining damage to intraocular, bony, and orbital structures and at locating ocular foreign bodies.

Special Considerations

Chemical Burns

A chemical burn is a true eye emergency. *Begin irrigation at once;* any delay worsens the prognosis. Do not wait for sterile solutions; use tap water if necessary. If pain or blepharospasm limits cooperation, employ topical anesthetics and parental narcotic analgesia.

Irrigate with at least 1 L of solution for acid burns and 2 L or more for alkali burns (monitor eye pH; the normal range is 7.3 to 7.7). A nasal cannula for oxygen connected to intravenous tubing will allow irrigation of both eyes simultaneously. After irrigation, sweep the fornices of the eye with a cotton-tipped applicator to remove any solid particles or debris.

Alkali agents (ammonia, lye) are especially damaging, causing a liquefaction necrosis with rapid penetration into the eye tissues. *Acids* (car battery explosions) produce a coagulation necrosis, precipitating proteins on the surface of the eye. Ocular chemical burns are graded on the extent of damage to the cornea and conjunctiva. Moderate or severe burns result in widespread tissue ischemia with blanching of the conjunctiva and diffuse corneal opacification.

Corneal Abrasion

A corneal abrasion is a localized traumatic disruption of the corneal epithelium. Typically, the injury is secondary to a fingernail, twig, or foreign body. Patients present with a painful, tearing red eye, along with complaints of photophobia and foreign body sensation. Diagnosis is confirmed with fluorescein staining of the eye viewed under a cobalt blue light. The pattern of fluorescein uptake provides a clue to the type of foreign body (fine vertical scratches on the upper half of the cornea suggest a foreign body entrapped under the upper lid, whereas fluorescein uptake localized to the lower half of the cornea usually is the consequence of a direct blow). The *Seidel* test, helps detect perforations of the anterior chamber (instill fluorescein and observe for a central zone of blue or green flowing from the site of perforation). Carefully inspect the surrounding eye structures to detect accompanying injuries (corneal lacerations, hyphema, iritis) or retained foreign bodies.

Treatment of corneal abrasions comprises irrigation of the eye along with removal of loose foreign bodies. For large lacerations or those demonstrating signs of iritis (cell and flare), instill a short-acting cycloplegic (cyclopentolate or homatropine) to thwart painful ciliary spasm. Eye patching is traditionally used, but recent work questions efficacy (caution patients with a patched eye against driving). Recheck the patient in 24 hr; corneal abrasions that fail to heal in 72 hr or become more painful need urgent ophthalmologic consultation.

Other Foreign Bodies

Suspect an ocular foreign body in any patient complaining of eye pain or foreign body sensation, especially if he or she had been hammering, chiseling, or working with high-speed machine tools. If possible, determine the type of material the patient was working with. Visualization of conjunctival or corneal foreign bodies is assisted by magnification loupes or a slit lamp. In cases where there is suspicion of deeply penetrating foreign bodies, radiographic studies with plain radiographs, CT scan, or ultrasound is required.

For superficial foreign bodies of the conjunctiva and cornea, initially try to remove with irrigation. If this is unsuccessful, anesthetize the eye and attempt manual removal by gently wiping with a moistened cotton swab. For foreign bodies resistant to these measures, attempt removal with a 25-gauge needle stabilized on a cotton-tipped applicator or tuberculin syringe. This is best done under slit-lamp guidance. Although the cornea is more resilient than one would think, *any foreign body below Bowman's membrane* (the layer beneath the epithelium) *necessitates removal by an ophthalmologist.*

Following removal of the foreign body, fluorescein stain the eye. Metallic foreign bodies present for > 12 hr frequently develop a "rust ring" that requires removal with a needle or burr. Place a protective eye shield over the affected eye in cases of suspected anterior chamber perforation until the patient can be seen by the ophthalmologist. Confirm tetanus immunization.

Hyphema

Hyphema denotes bleeding into the anterior chamber of the eye. The triad of decreased vision, ocular pain, and headache following eye trauma suggests traumatic hyphema. Hospitalization depends on the size of the hyphema as well as the patient's reliability. Specific therapy is initiated by the ophthalmologist with the goal of preventing complications such as rebleeding, glaucoma, and staining of the cornea. Patients with sickle cell disease and hyphema pose a special problem because red blood cells tend to undergo sickling in the anterior chamber. Place a protective eye shield over the affected eye until the patient can be seen by the ophthalmologist.

Orbital Fractures

Orbital fractures can occur as isolated fractures of the orbital rim, floor, or medial wall or extend to involve the adjacent zygoma, maxilla, and skull.

Blow-out fractures typically result from the impaction of the orbit by a rounded object that is slightly larger than the orbital rim. The orbital margin is left intact, but the resultant increase in intraocular pressure causes a fracture of the weaker orbital floor. Clinical findings consistent with a blow-out fracture include periorbital bruising; crepitus in surrounding tissues (air from sinuses); impairment of sensation on the ipsilateral cheek, nose, and medial lip (involvement of infraorbital branch of trigeminal nerve); diplopia on upward gaze (entrapment of inferior rectus or inferior oblique muscle); and enophthalmos or retraction of the globe on the affected side. Radiological findings characteristic of a blow-out fracture include clouding of the ipsilateral maxillary sinus, disruption of the inferior orbital floor, and intraorbital free air. The Waters view best demonstrates the orbital floor and maxillary sinus. CT scans provide better definition of the orbital fractures than plain films. Discuss early management with the consultant. Many patients do not require surgery and can be managed conservatively (cold compresses to swelling, prophylactic antibiotics, and avoidance of forceful blowing of the nose).

Orbital roof fractures arise from blunt or penetrating trauma. The most serious consequence is when the fracture extends through the cribriform plate, violating the dura. Presence of clear fluid drainage from the nose (rhinorrhea) that increases with coughing or straining implies a CSF leak (perform a halo test; see section 4.2; test for glucose with a lab stick). Optic nerve injury also occurs. Fractures of the orbital roof can usually be seen on plain radiographs (Waters view), but CT scanning provides better bone definition. Neurosurgical evaluation may be necessary (craniotomy may be required). Discuss the use of prophylactic antibiotics with the consultant.

Medial wall fractures follow blows to the orbit or nose. Frequently, the thin lateral wall of the ethmoid sinus is fractured, resulting in orbital emphysema. Additional signs of medial wall fractures include widening of the intercanthal distance and a limitation of lateral gaze. Damage to the nasolacrimal drainage system may also occur. CT scanning is recommended when there is suspicion of muscle entrapment.

A *tripod fracture* classically comprises breaks at three points: (1) the frontozygomatic arch at the suture line, (2) the zygomatic-maxillary suture and (3) the zygomatic arch near the body of the zygoma. Facial swelling may obscure certain clinical findings, but examine for flattening of the cheek along with a step-off on palpation of the intraorbital rim. Check for trismus resulting from impingement of the temporomandibular joint by the depressed zygomatic arch. Special radiographic views ("bucket handle" view) allow the complete visualization of the fracture. The patient should be admitted for open reduction and fixation. Reduction is usually delayed for a few days to allow the swelling to subside.

Lid Lacerations

The overriding concern in evaluating eyelid lacerations is to rule out any underlying ocular damage. First establish the integrity of the globe and verify visual acuity. General principles of wound repair apply to eyelid lacerations, including assessing the depth of the wound, exploring for foreign bodies, and irrigation. Because of the generous blood supply to the lid, little if any debridement is indicated. Lacerations of the eyelid margin, full-thickness lacerations (involving all three layers), those involving the tarsal plate, and lacerations of the medial fifth of the lid (potential damage to the lacrimal duct system) are best left to the ophthalmologist or plastic surgeon (there is a risk of notching with subsequent corneal exposure and corneal ulceration).

Admission Criteria

The decision to admit should be made on an individual basis in consultation with an ophthalmologist. Generally, the following conditions obligate admission: *lacerated or ruptured globe, chemical burns with corneal opacification, lens dislocation, orbital hemorrhage, retinal injury, orbital fractures that require operative repair, and exten-*

sive hyphema. Reliable adults with a small hyphema may be treated with bed rest at home after consultation with an ophthalmologist.

Suggested Readings

Kirkpatrick JNP: No eye pad for corneal abrasion. Eye 1993;7:468–470.

Shingleton BJ: Eye injuries. N Engl J Med 1991;325(6):408–413.

Wilson TW, Nelson LB, Jeffers JB, et al.: Outpatient management of traumatic microhyphemas. Ann Ophthalmol 1990;22:366–368.

Chapter 15

ENT

15.1 DIZZINESS AND VERTIGO

Description

A common yet vexing problem in the ED is the chief complaint of "dizziness." A thorough history and an extensive physical examination are required to arrive at the correct diagnosis and rule out serious pathology. The sense of balance and position in space is maintained by the interaction of the visual, proprioceptive, and vestibular systems. When the visual and proprioceptive mechanisms malfunction, a patient may complain of disequilibrium (dizziness, lightheadedness). Only when the vestibular system is affected will a sense of spinning or motion be felt (vertigo).

History

The initial objective is to determine whether the patient is experiencing *vertigo* or *disequilibrium.* Have the patient describe in his or her own words what symptoms are being experienced; tell the patient not to use the word *dizzy.* Patients with vertigo relate a sensation of motion, which ranges from spinning to subtle tilting or propulsion.

Once vertigo is established, determine the duration and frequency of symptoms and any exacerbating factors such as movement or head position. Equally important are associated symptoms such as nausea, vomiting, tinnitus, hearing loss, headache, or other neurologic complaints (diplopia, slurred speech, numbness). The history can offer hints of peripheral or central origin. Central vertigo lacks the intensity and sporadic nature of peripheral vertigo. Inquire about previous infections, illness, trauma, alcoholism, and medication usage. Also, certain drugs are associated with nystagmus (phenytoin, carbamazepine, alcohol, PCP).

Physical Examination

HEENT

Examine the eyes for an abnormal pupillary response and papilledema. Search the ear canal and tympanic membrane for wax or foreign bodies, and look for signs of infection. Perform corneal reflex and *fistula* tests (nystagmus and vertigo are induced by exerting mild positive pressure in the ear canal with pneumatic otoscopy). Screen for hearing loss (conductive versus sensorineural). The *Rinne test* employs a tuning fork and compares hearing through bone conduction versus air conduction. With hearing loss present, the tuning fork sounds loudest on the mastoid process when there is a conductive problem. With the *Weber test,* the tuning fork is placed in the midline of the forehead, and the patient is asked to indicate in which ear, if any, the sound is the loudest. If one ear has a sensorineural deficit, the sound will localize to the better cochlea. If a conductive loss is present on one side, the sound lateralizes to the affected side.

Neurologic

A thorough neurologic examination is critical in refining the differential diagnosis. Special attention should be paid to all the cranial nerves. Test extremity strength and sensation (especially proprioceptive sense). Assess cerebellar function by observing gait, rapid alternating movements, and finger-to-nose pointing. A positive *Romberg test* (steadiness with eyes open, but loss of balance with eyes closed) indicates vestibular or proprioceptive disease. Cerebellar dysfunction causes ataxia whether the eyes are open or closed.

Examine for *nystagmus.* The slow component of nystagmus is regulated by the vestibular system. The fast, corrective movement is regulated by the cortex. The direction of the nystagmus is always determined by the direction of the fast component. A few beats of nystagmus are normally present at extreme horizontal gaze. Pathologic nystagmus occurs with the eyes in a forward position or in association with symptoms. Examination of the direction of the nystagmus and changes with movement or fixation helps determine whether the vertigo is peripheral or central.

Peripheral vestibular disease (outside the CNS) results in nystagmus toward the normal ear and is worsened when the gaze is directed toward the normal ear. Nystagmus is suppressed when the gaze is directed toward the impaired ear or is fixed. Subdued lighting helps bring out peripheral nystagmus due to impaired fixation. Peripheral nystagmus may be horizontal or rotational but is never vertical.

Central vestibular disease (cerebellum and brainstem) exhibits nystagmus that changes direction with position and is difficult to suppress. The nystagmus is often associated with minimal symptoms. Vertical nystagmus is always central and may be due to drugs like phenytoin, barbiturate, alcohol, and phencyclidine.

If spontaneous nystagmus is absent, try *Hallpike (Nylen-Barany) testing* to elicit a response. This maneuver is performed by rapidly moving a patient from a sitting to a supine position with his or her head extending over the bed; observe for 20 sec and note the direction of nystagmus. This is performed three times with the head straight and turned to either side. Positional nystagmus of peripheral origin exhibits a rotational component, a latency period, a brief duration, and fatigability (Table 15.1.1).

Other Exams

Vital signs. Test for orthostatic blood pressure changes. Confirm blood pressure in both arms (a systolic blood pressure differ-

Table 15.1.1
Peripheral Versus Central Vertigo

Feature	Peripheral	Central
Occurrence	Episodic	May be constant
Type of nystagmus	Rotatory or horizontal (never vertical)	Any direction (may change directions)
Laterality of nystagmus	Bilateral	May be unilateral
Symptom severity (nausea, vomiting)	Proportional to nystagmus	May be disproportionate to nystagmus
Hearing loss, tinnitus	Possible	No
Other neurologic signs	No	Abnormalities frequent in adjacent cranial nerves
Effect of visual fixation	Nystagmus suppressed	Nystagmus enhanced
Position testing		
Latency	Short (3–20 sec)	Long
Duration	Transient	Sustained
Fatigability	Fatigable	Nonfatigable

ence > 20 mm Hg may indicate subclavian steal syndrome or aortic dissection).

Cardiovascular. Listen for arrhythmias, evidence of valvular disease, and bruits.

Diagnostic Tests

No laboratory test is immediately required for peripheral vertigo; audiometric testing and electronystagmography can be obtained in follow-up with a consultant.

CBC. Check for anemia or leucocytosis (suggests infection).
Serum glucose. Check for hypoglycemia.
ECG. Note significant dysrhythmias.
Radiology. When central vertigo is suspected, order an emergent head CT scan or MRI.
VDRL. Syphilis serology is useful diagnostically only in recurrent, difficult cases.

Special Considerations

Dysequilibrium

Causes of disequilibrium include hypoglycemia, uncontrolled hypertension and hematological disorders (anemia). In addition, patients with attacks of anxiety or hyperventilation frequently list dizziness or vertigo among their complaints. Multiple sensory deficits (decreased visual acuity, neuropathy) may result in a vague sense of dizziness (especially in elderly patients exposed to poor lighting or unfamiliar surroundings or who take sedatives). Diffuse cerebral anoxia due to postural hypotension, arrhythmias, or other cardiovascular etiologies often presents as lightheadedness or faintness (see section 1.3). Motor weakness ought to be distinguished from disequilibrium.

Peripheral Vertigo

Peripheral vertigo implies a problem that is isolated to the membranous labyrinth and the vestibular nerve. Approximately 80% of cases of vertigo seen in the ED have a peripheral origin.

Benign positional vertigo occurs when the patient changes position or moves his or her head. Symptoms last for only 10 to 20 sec and do not recur if the patient remains stationary. *Hallpike testing* reveals typical peripheral nystagmus. There is no associated hearing loss or other neurologic symptoms.

Vestibular neuronitis commonly follows a viral illness, developing over a 24- to 48-hr period, and persists for 4 to 5 days. Symptoms are exacerbated with head movement, but hearing remains unaffected.

Ménière's disease is seen in the elderly and is characterized by attacks of vertigo lasting up to several hours, fluctuating hearing loss, tinnitus, and fullness in one ear. Many other diseases are commonly misdiagnosed as Ménière's (vertigo lasting less than 20 m or greater than 24 hr is not Ménière's disease).

Labyrinthitis is caused by an extension of chronic otitis media or ototoxic ingestion (aminoglycosides, salicylates, diuretics, phenytoin). Like vestibular neuronitis, the vertigo lasts for days, but it is differentiated by the presence of hearing loss.

Miscellaneous causes include motion sickness, syphilis, cholesteatoma, and a foreign body in the ear canal.

Central Vertigo

Central vertigo implies a disorder of the vestibular nuclei in the brainstem and their connections with the cerebellum. Suspect central vertigo when the patient exhibits concomitant cranial nerve involvement or limb ataxia.

Cerebellar hemorrhage must be the primary diagnostic consideration in any patient who presents to the ED with the acute onset of vertigo and ataxia. Severe headache, nausea, or vomiting may accompany these symptoms. Cerebellar hemorrhage is a true neurosurgical emergency, necessitating emergent evacuation of the clot. Cerebellar infarction presents similarly but does not demand immediate neurosurgical intervention.

The most notable of the *cerebellopontine angle tumors* are acoustic neuromas, which initially cause a peripheral vertigo that progresses to a central disease. Early symptoms include tinnitus and hearing loss along with vertigo or subtle ataxia. Suspect the diagnosis when associated cerebellar or other cranial nerve dysfunction (decreased corneal reflex, facial weakness) turns up.

Vascular etiologies are associated with temporary or persistent episodes of central vertigo. *Vertebrobasilar insufficiency* causes transient vertigo that is associated with other brainstem symptoms such as diplopia, slurred speech, facial numbness, and hemiparesis. A *TIA* of the labyrinth produces nonpositional vertigo, which lasts for minutes in older patients. An occlusion of the posterior inferior cerebellar artery results in *lateral medullary syndrome,* also known as *Wallenberg's syndrome.* This disorder is characterized by vertigo, nausea, vomiting, Horner's syndrome, and ipsilateral loss of pinprick and temperature of the face accompanied by contralateral loss of pinprick and temperature sensation of the body. The patient may also demonstrate ataxia, falling to the side of the lesion. Severe hypertension (diastolic > 120 mm Hg) is capable of provoking arterial spasm with decreased labyrinthine blood flow and consequent vertigo.

Postconcussive vertigo is a common, inadequately understood disorder that follows even minor head trauma. Symptoms may not appear for days to weeks subsequent to the injury and can last for months. Fractures of the temporal bone (longitudinal or transverse) can cause vertigo along with otorrhea, hemotympanum, or CSF leak into the nasopharynx. Sudden hearing loss, tinnitus, and vertigo following barotrauma (flying, diving, or even forcefully blowing nose) may indicate a perilymph fistula.

Miscellaneous causes include subclavian steal syndrome, multiple sclerosis, basilar migraine, neoplasm, complex partial seizures, Ramsey-Hunt syndrome (see section 15.5), and cervical strain.

Treatment

For central vertigo, treatment is based on the specific diagnosis (consider immediate surgery for cerebellar hemorrhage). Peripheral vertigo is treated symptomatically. Acute attacks are controlled with medications designed for sedation, anticholinergic effects, or nausea control. Intravenous diazepam (5 to 10 mg) effectively stops acute vertigo by acting centrally. Anticholinergic drugs such as atropine (0.5 mg IV or SQ) or a scopolamine patch control symptoms well. Antihistamines with anticholinergic properties such as meclizine (25 to 50 mg PO q 12 hr) and diphenhydramine (50 mg PO q 6 hr) are also useful. Finally, hydroxyzine (50 mg PO q 6 hr) and promethazine (12.5 to 25 mg PO or PR q 6 hr) are examples of drugs that provide both antiemetic and anticholinergic effects.

Patients with multiple sensory deficits or ill-defined dizziness will be made worse by the administration of the above medications. Treatment includes withdrawal of any sedatives and increasing ambient light.

Admission Criteria

The following cases should be admitted: *all surgical causes of vertigo* (including all patients with suspected CNS etiology and/or cranial fracture), *suspected new-onset vertebrobasilar insufficiency, and acute suppurative labyrinthitis. Patients with debilitating symptoms of peripheral vertigo,* such as profuse vomiting and inability to walk, should also be admitted.

All patients with vertigo who are treated as outpatients require follow-up by a neurologist or otolaryngologist.

Suggested Readings

Cohen NL: The dizzy patient: update on vestibular disorders. Med Clin North Am 1991;75:1251–1260.

Froehling DA: Does this patient have a serious form of vertigo? JAMA 1994;271:385–388.

15.2 SINUSITIS

Description

Sinusitis is an inflammation of one or more of the paranasal sinuses. The four pairs of paranasal sinuses *(ethmoid, maxillary, frontal, and sphenoid)* are normally filled with air cells lined by respiratory mucosa (Table 15.2.1). Mucus accumulating in the sinus drains into the nasal cavity through openings called ostia. Impedance to this flow can lead to stasis and subsequent bacterial overgrowth. Obstruction of the ostium can occur from either local mucosal swelling or mechanical obstruction. The most common cause of local swelling is viral rhinitis. Other causes include allergic rhinitis, trauma, and exposure to environmental agents

Table 15.2.1
Symptoms of Infected Sinuses

Infected Sinus	Symptoms
Maxillary sinus	Pain over the cheekbone or upper teeth (maxillary sinusitis can masquerade as a toothache)
Frontal sinus	Severe frontal headache
Ethmoid	Periorbital or medial canthal pain
Sphenoid	Deep-seated headache at the occiput, vertex of the skull, or behind the eye; isolated sphenoid sinusitis is rare

(smoke, barotrauma). Mechanical obstruction may result from nasal polyps, deviated septum, foreign bodies, or nasal packings.

Common causative pathogens of *acute sinusitis* include the following: *Streptococcus pneumoniae, Haemophilus influenzae, Moraxella catarrhalis, Staphylococcus aureus,* and other streptococci. *Chronic sinusitis* is generally caused by anaerobic streptococci, *Bacteroides* species, and *S. aureus.*

History

The onset of acute sinusitis often follows viral rhinitis, and it may be difficult to distinguish between the two. However, viral URI symptoms that persist beyond 7 days should be considered suspicious for sinusitis. The most common symptoms are headache, facial pain and/or pressure, and nasal congestion (discharge may be clear or purulent). Infection of a specific sinus will usually give a characteristic pain pattern, with the pain worsening on straining or bending forward.

Chronic sinusitis often presents as a constellation of vague symptoms. Ask about underlying disorders that increase the risk for sinusitis (AIDS, DM). Certain drug ingestions can cause symptoms that mimic sinusitis (reserpine, prazosin, cocaine). In addition, some patients abuse over-the-counter topical nasal decongestants and develop *rhinitis medicamentosa.*

Physical Examination

Vital signs. Note any fever (although a fever is not required to make the diagnosis).

HEENT. Examine for percussion tenderness over the affected sinus(es) and on the maxillary teeth (10% of cases of maxillary sinusitis evolve from dental root infection). Examine the nasal cavity for polyps or discharge. Examine the pharynx for postnasal drainage.

Lung. Rule out lower respiratory infection.

Neurologic. Funduscopic and neurologic examination are vital to eliminate other causes of headache.

Note: *Despite the reported poor accuracy of individual signs and symptoms in diagnosing sinusitis, combinations of findings prove most useful in establishing a tentative diagnosis.* The composite clinical picture of maxillary toothache, a poor response to nasal decongestants, abnormal transillumination, and purulent nasal discharge by history and by physical examination has a high predictability for sinusitis when all five findings are present and virtually rules out sinusitis when none is present.

Diagnostic Tests

Laboratory tests. Blood tests are of little help in the nontoxic patient.

Transillumination. May be helpful when taken in context with other findings.

Radiology. A single Water's view is usually as good as a four-view sinus series in confirming the diagnosis of sinusitis (air-fluid levels, mucosal thickening > 5 mm). Use plain films only when the diagnosis is in question, not if there is already strong evidence that indicates infection. CT scan is more specific for sinusitis but is generally not cost-effective, thus it should be reserved to rule out suspected contiguous spread in patients at risk.

Special Considerations

Complications arising from sinusitis can include the following.

Osteomyelitis. Associated with frontal sinusitis. Clinically, one finds a doughy edema of the forehead *(Pott's puffy tumor)*. A coexisting brain abscess must be ruled out.

Orbital cellulitis. See section 14.2.

Cavernous sinus thrombophlebitis. Results from retrograde spread of infection along venous channels. Clinical findings include high fever; toxicity; lid edema; proptosis; chemosis; and third, fourth, and sixth cranial nerve palsies. Fundi exhibit venous engorgement and papilledema.

Epidural abscess, subdural empyema, brain abscess, or meningitis. Associated with frontal or ethmoid sinusitis.

Treatment

Initial antibiotic treatment is begun with *amoxicillin* or *trimethoprim-sulfamethoxazole*. Failure to respond within 5 days mandates a switch to either *cefaclor, cefuroxime axetil,* or *amoxicillin-clavulanate potassium*. The length of therapy is usually 10 days.

Vasoconstrictive sprays such as *phenylephrine hydrochloride* (Neo-Synephrine) or *oxymetazoline hydrochloride* (Afrin) assist drainage. These drugs are to be used for only 3 to 4 days (there is a potential for rebound edema with longer usage).

Oral α-agonists supplement vasoconstriction of sinus mucosa that is unaffected by topical agents; *phenylephrine-phenylpropanolamine hydrochloride* plus *guaifenesin* and *pseudoephedrine hydrochloride* are often used. Antihistamines are generally not helpful in acute sinusitis.

Admission Criteria

Patients with any of the aforementioned complications, with acute frontal or sphenoid sinusitis, with diabetes or immunosupression, or with sinusitis that does not respond to oral antibiotics should be admitted.

Suggested Readings

Oppenheimer RW: Sinusitis: how to recognize and treat it. Postgrad Med 1992;91:281–286, 289–292.

Williams JW, Simel DL: Does this patient have sinusitis? Diagnosing acute sinusitis by history and physical examination. JAMA 1993;270: 1242–1246.

15.3 EPISTAXIS

Description

The nose receives a rich vascular supply derived from both internal and external carotid arteries. When treating epistaxis, you must determine whether the bleeding source is in the anterior or posterior nasal cavity. *Anterior bleeds* account for 90% of all nosebleeds; they are easily visualized (within 1 cm of the nasal vestibule) and are located at the site of anastomosis of several vessels on the anterior septum *(Kiesselbach's plexus or Little's area)*. The remaining 10% of nosebleeds are *posterior bleeds,* usually occurring posterior to the inferior turbinate, and cannot be visualized with a nasal speculum.

The preponderance of nasal bleeds (especially anterior bleeds) are due to local disturbances (desiccation of mucous membranes; viral, bacterial, or allergic rhinitis; overuse of topical decongestants; insufflational use of tobacco, or cocaine). Additional etiologies include trauma (nose picking, external blows) and systemic disorders (atherosclerosis, severe hypertension, coagulopathies, platelet disorders).

History

To determine the site (anterior versus posterior) and cause of epistaxis, ask about the *onset* (spontaneous, trauma) and *duration* (resolved with pressure, continuous) of the bleed. Determine from where (front of nose, back of throat) and from which naris (nares) the blood was initially noted. Anterior nose bleeds are more likely to commence with blood coming out of one nostril, while posterior epistaxis is associated with bleeding from both nares as well as hemorrhage down the back of the throat.

Ask about prior history of nosebleeds (frequency, severity, and treatment required). Also ascertain if there is a history of hypertension, coagulopathy, or easy bruising. Find out if the patient has been taking oral anticoagulants or drugs with antiplatelet effects. Inquire about illicit drug use (cocaine, amphetamine) and route (insufflational).

Note: *Bleeding from the respiratory or GI tract can masquerade as epistaxis; conversely, epistaxis can present as a GI bleed or hemoptysis.*

Physical Examination

General. If the patient appears hemodynamically stable, examine the patient while he or she is sitting up and leaning forward so blood flows from the nose.

Vital signs. Ensure that there is no airway compromise. Check pulse, blood pressure, and orthostatics.

Skin. Inspect for rashes, pallor, ecchymosis, purpura, and petechiae.

Once the primary examination is completed, examine the *nose and oral cavity.*

Diagnostic Tests

Patients with only recurrent short, but bothersome, nosebleeds do not require laboratory studies if the history and physical examination do not suggest systemic disease. *CBC, platelet count, protime, prothrombin time,* and *bleeding time* are indicated for persistent bleeding, recurrent severe nosebleeds, use of anticoagulants, and clinical suspicion for underlying bleeding disorder. *Type and cross* when blood loss is significant.

Radiologic studies are indicated if significant facial trauma is involved.

Treatment

The key to successful management of epistaxis in the ED is sufficient preparation and determining the site of bleeding (Table 15.3.1). Have the patient pinch his or her nose. Both the physician and patient should be gowned, with the ED physician also complying with universal blood precautions (gloves, gown, goggles or face shield).

Examine the nasal cavity and septum by inserting a nasal speculum into the vestibule and spreading the speculum in an inferior to superior direction (*do not* spread laterally). Remove any clots with suction or forceps. Search for a bleeding site, a prominent vessel or a scab on the septal mucosa, before inserting medication in the nose. Failure to locate a bleeding site implies either bleeding from a nonvisualized site (superior or posterior) or diffuse bleeding from a coagulation disorder.

Gauze or cotton pledgets soaked with a topical vasoconstrictor and anesthetic may then be inserted into the nares. Choices include 4% *lidocaine* with 1:1000 *epi,* 4% *lidocaine* with 0.5 to 1.0% *phenylephrine,* or 4% cocaine (limit to 4 mL of 4% solution and avoid use in the elderly and patients with known cardiovascular disease). Pledgets are left in the nares for 5 min. Localized, controlled anterior bleeding sites can be *cauterized* with *silver nitrate sticks.*

Table 15.3.1
Essential Supplies for Examination and Treatment of Epistaxis

Light source (headlight or head mirror with light bulb)
ENT chair
Nasal speculum
Emesis basin
Gauze, 4 × 4
Tongue depressor
Bayonet forceps
Topical vasoconstrictor and anesthetic
Cotton pledgets
Suction setup (Frazier tips)
Silver nitrate cautery sticks
Vaseline gauze packing (½ × 72 inches)
Antibiotic ointment
Gelfoam
Commercial balloon catheters
Nasal tampons
Foley catheter

If the bleeding is uncontrollable or a site is not available for cautery, insert an anterior packing. If the patient is uncomfortable or extremely anxious, provide systemic analgesia (morphine, 5 to 10 mg IV). Apply an antibacterial ointment to the Vaseline-impregnated gauze and carefully layer (in an accordion-like fashion), so that every nook and cranny is filled. Both the leading and tail ends of the gauze are left outside the nares. Since the packing acts as a foreign body occluding the sinuses, prescribe a systemic antibiotic (amoxicillin, cephalosporin, erythromycin, or trimethoprim-sulfisoxazole). A nasal tampon serves as an alternative to an anterior nasal packing.

If the bleeding persists despite an anterior pack or if a posterior bleed is suspected, either use a formal posterior gauze nasal pack or employ an inflatable balloon device. Insert a Foley catheter with a 30-mL balloon into the nasopharynx, cutting off the tip of the catheter. Inflate the balloon with 10 to 15 mL of saline or water, and retract until the balloon wedges in the posterior nasal cavity. Commercial balloon devices are also inserted via the nares (after adequate lubrication), until the posterior balloon reaches the nasopharynx. Once adequately positioned, inflate the posterior balloon with 5 to 8 mL of water or saline, adjust the device forward, and then fill the anterior balloon with 10 to 20 mL of fluid. Confirm the location of the devices.

Absorbable hemostatic agents *(Avitene, Oxycel, Gelfoam)* are beneficial in cases of diffuse epistaxis secondary to hemostatic disorders. Refractory bleeding may require surgical intervention (arterial ligation, embolization).

Note: *Epistaxis from a nasal fracture usually ceases spontaneously.* Always check for a septal hematoma, which requires incision and drainage.

Admission Criteria

Admit *patients who require hemodynamic resuscitation, and those with epistaxis secondary to coagulation disorders. All patients with posterior packings* (associated with hypoxemia and hypoventilation) require admission.

Patients with anterior epistaxis can be discharged once bleeding is controlled and they have been observed for 30 to 60 min (safeguard against rebleed). Patients with an anterior pack need a follow-up in 24 hr.

Suggested Readings

Josephson GD, Foley FA, Stierna P: Practical management of epistaxis. Med Clin North Am 1991;75(6):1311–1320.

Randall DA, Freeman SB: Management of anterior and posterior epistaxis. Am Fam Physician 1991;43:2007–2014.

15.4 SORE THROAT

Description

Viral and streptococcal infections account for most cases of pharyngitis. Group A β-hemolytic *Streptococcus* is the organism of greatest concern, because it can lead to *rheumatic fever* and *glomerulonephritis* (the latter is not preventable even with appropriate antibiotics). Other offending organisms include non-group A strep, *Corynebacterium, Neisseria gonorrhea, Chlamydia trachomatis, Mycoplasma, Candida,* and a variety of viruses (especially Epstein-Barr). Except for group A β-hemolytic *Streptococcus* and *N. gonorrhea* (a concern in the sexually active population), these microbes do not generally mandate antibiotic therapy.

History

Historically, most patients with "strep" throat complain of an abrupt onset of sore throat, fever, and tender anterior cervical adenopathy. A scarlatiniform rash may appear 2 to 3 days later. It is important to note (1) the time course of symptoms, (2) the presence of fever, (3) the presence of associated symptoms, (4) possible contacts with known cases, (5) the presence of underlying immunosuppression, and (6) sexual practices (oral sex). Ascertain past medical history (DM, AIDS, cancer, rheumatic fever, valvular heart disease), medications, allergies, and immunization history (DPT status).

Physical Examination

General. Listen for alteration of voice (hoarseness, muffling) and assess the patient's ability to handle his or her secretions (drooling).

Vital signs. Check temperature and respiratory rate.

HEENT. Inspect for pharyngeal injection, erythema, and exudate. Palpate for enlarged and tender cervical nodes. Examine the oral pharynx for a lacy white exudate and gingivitis associated with necrotic tonsillar ulcers (necrotizing pharyngitis due to *Fusobacterium* infection). If possible, directly visualize the epiglottis.

Abdomen. Check for splenomegaly (infectious mononucleosis).

Skin. Look for a bright erythematous rash with a sandpaper feel and Pasta's lines *(scarlet fever).*

Diagnostic Tests

Throat culture. The diagnostic standard for group A β-hemolytic pharyngitis. Results are usually obtainable in 24 to 48 hr. Antibiotic therapy can be delayed for up to 9 days after the onset of symptoms and still protect from rheumatic fever. A partially treated strep infection may a yield false-negative culture result. Culture for gonococcal infection (Thayer-Martin media) in the appropriate clinical setting.

Rapid strep screen. Results are generally available in 30 min. Sensitivity ranges from 60 to 95%, with approximately 95% specificity (strep carriers will test positive). Perform a throat culture if the rapid test is negative.

Blood tests. Epstein-Barr-related mononucleosis is associated with lymphocytosis ($> 4500/mm^3$), atypical lymphs (>10%), and a positive heterophile antibody (Monospot) test.

Radiology. Indicated when diagnosis of epiglottitis or retropharyngeal abscess is considered.

Special Considerations

Peritonsillar Abscess

Peritonsillar abscess (Quinsy) is a suppurative complication of pharyngitis that is characterized by the clinical findings of a fluctuant mass (arising from the superior pole of the tonsillar crypt), uvular displacement from the midline (to contralateral side), and prominent unilateral cervical adenopathy. Patients complain of throat and unilateral ear pain along with dysphagia and trismus. *Peritonsillar cellulitis* presents in a similar fashion, but there is an absence of a fluctuant mass and a lack of uvular displacement. To confirm the diagnosis, anesthetize with lidocaine jelly or anesthetic spray and palpate the tonsil for fluctuance or aspirate. Treatment of abscess consists of incision and drainage, after ensuring adequate exposure and anesthesia.

Epiglottitis

Epiglottitis, an acute inflammation involving the epiglottis and supraglottic structures, is becoming an increasingly recognized problem in adults. It is usually caused by infection (*H. influenzae,* streptococci, staphylococci, anaerobes). Onset may be gradual (2 to 3 days). Indirect visualization of the epiglottis (appears as a red, swollen structure protruding above the posterior base of the tongue) may be attempted, but only after preparations are made to intubate and provide a surgical airway if necessary. Diagnostic adjuncts include x-ray imaging (portable lateral neck x-ray performed in the ED).

Uvulitis

Uvulitis (Quincke's disease) manifests as swelling and erythema of the uvula and soft palate caused by infection, trauma, or angioedema. Symptoms include alteration of the voice and a "fullness" in the back of the throat. The uvula often resembles a big white grape.

Ludwig's Angina

Ludwig's angina (a cellulitis of the floor of the mouth) is the most frequent cause of a "bull neck," a prominent swelling of the submandibular area accompanied by the elevation and posterior displacement of the tongue due to sublingual edema. Infection can result in upper airway obstruction (see section 2.1).

Treatment

Render symptomatic therapy (analgesia, throat lozenges, saline gargles, anesthetic mouth spray). Dexamethasone (10 mg IM) may provide symptomatic relief in patients with severe inflammation of the pharynx.

Treat strep culture– or rapid antigen–positive patients with *penicillin VK* (250 mg PO QID for 10 days), *penicillin VK* (500 mg PO BID for 10 days), or *benzathine penicillin G* (LM) (a single dose, 600,000 units IM for patients < 30 kg, and 1,200,000 units IM for patients > 30 kg). Erythromycin (250 mg PO QID or 333 mg PO TID for 10 days) has historically been the drug of choice in penicillin-allergic patients. In cases of treatment failure or recurrence of group A β-hemolytic strep pharyngitis (persistent symptoms and positive cultures despite penicillin therapy), consider alternative treatment with a cephalosporin (cefadroxil, 1 g BID for 5 days).

Some clinicians believe that early use of antibiotics results in quick relief of symptoms. Others feel that this does not justify the risk of inappropriate use of antibiotics. Either approach is acceptable, provided a throat culture is used.

In the absence of a rapid antigen test, patients who should probably be empirically started on antibiotics include those

With a previous positive culture who were noncompliant with recommended therapy;
With a scarlatiniform rash;
Who are immunosuppressed;
With a past history of rheumatic fever (especially rheumatic endocarditis);
Who partially self-treated themselves with antibiotics; and
Who are in close contact with children (teachers, day care workers).

Treat gonococcal pharyngitis with *ceftriaxone* (125 mg IM). Pharyngeal candidiasis is treated with oral *nystatin suspension* (500,000 units three to five times a day for 10 to 14 days), *clotrimazole troches* (10 mg troches three to five times a day for 10 to 14 days), *ketoconazole* (200 mg PO BID for 5 to 7 days), or *fluconazole* (200 mg PO stat dose, then 50 to 100 mg a day).

The definitive treatment for a Quinsy abscess is I&D (a consultant may help decide if this can be done in the ED under local anesthesia or if admission for general anesthesia is required). Once the airway is secured, initiate parenteral antibiotic therapy with aqueous penicillin G (10 to 20 million units/day IV) or clindamycin (600 to 900 mg IV q 6 hr).

The key to management of adult epiglottitis is to recognize the diagnosis early and to be prepared to secure the airway. If airway compromise appears imminent, then oral intubation is essential; provisions should be on hand for surgical or needle cricothyrotomy. It is advisable to notify the airway team (anesthesiologist, ENT) to help manage the airway. Antibiotic coverage is provided by *cefuroxime* (50 mg/kg IV q 8 hr), *cefotaxime* (50 mg/kg IV q 8 hr), or *ceftriaxone* (50 mg/kg IV q day).

Treatment of Quincke's disease depends on the presumed etiology. If infection is suspected, start a course of antibiotics (cover for *H. influenzae*) after obtaining appropriate cultures (blood, throat). For allergic etiologies, treat as for anaphylaxis (see chapter 8): epinephrine (0.3 to 0.5 mL SQ), diphenhydramine (50 mg IV), cimetidine (300 mg slow IVp), along with hydrocortisone (180 mg IV). Close monitoring of vital signs is imperative. Be prepared to manage the airway.

Antibiotic therapy for Ludwig's angina includes *high-dose aqueous penicillin* (24 million units/day IV) or *cefoxitin* (2.0 g IV q 8 hr). Surgical drainage is sometimes necessary, but hospitalization is essential to ensure airway maintenance.

Admission Criteria

The following patients require admission: *patients with peritonsillar abscess, those with potential airway compromise* (epiglottitis, Ludwig's angina, retropharyngeal abscess), *those who are systemically toxic* (especially if immunocompromised), and *those who are unable to swallow liquids or who are markedly dehydrated.*

Suggested Readings

Dort JC, Frohlich AM: Acute epiglottitis in adults: diagnosis and treatment in 43 patients. J Otolaryngol 1994;23:281–285.

Maharaj D: Management of peritonsillar abscess. J Otolaryngol 1991;105:743–745.

O'Brien JF, Meade JL, Falk JL: Dexamethasone as adjuvant therapy for severe acute pharyngitis. Ann Emerg Med 1993;22:212–215.

Vukmir RB: Adult and pediatric pharyngitis: a review. J Emerg Med 1992;10:607–616.

15.5 EARACHE

Description

Most cases of earache (otalgia) seen in the ED result from an inflammatory process in the middle or external ear. However, at times the pain is referred to the ear from a secondary source (Table 15.5.1).

History

Normally, the chief complaint focuses on ear pain. Inquire about the onset (insidious, barotrauma, trauma, thermal injury), duration (acute infection present < 3 weeks), and location (unilateral or bilateral; inside or outside the ear) of the pain. Ask for a description of the pain (sharp, dull, throbbing, pressure) and in-

Table 15.5.1
Causes of Pain with Earache

Common causes of primary otalgia	
External ear pain	Otitis externa, furunculosis, impacted cerumen, perichondritis, Herpes zoster (Ramsay-Hunt), foreign bodies, frostbite
Middle ear pain	Acute otitis media, serous otitis, acute mastoiditis, bullous myringitis, tympanic membrane perforation, cholesteatoma, barotrauma
Common causes of referred ear pain	Sinus infection, infection of the nasopharynx, impaction or infection of molar teeth, temporomandibular joint (TMJ) dysfunction, peritonsillar infection, neoplasm of tongue or larynx, elongated styloid process, cervical spine disease or injury

quire about exacerbating factors (biting, chewing). Discharge (otorrhea) from the ear canal is associated with both otitis media with perforation and otitis externa (malignant otitis externa). Additional symptoms include fever, nausea, vomiting, disturbances in hearing, dizziness, or vertigo). Pain, fever, and hearing loss are the classic presenting complaints of otitis media. Acute otitis media is often preceded by an upper respiratory illness. Ascertain if there is a history of ear problems, head or neck surgery, and underlying immunocompromising illnesses (DM, AIDS); ask about medications and allergies.

Physical Examination

Vital signs. Check for fever (more common with otitis media than otitis externa).

HEENT. Examine the external ear (auricle) and surrounding structures (preauricular, mastoid process, temporomandibular joint, oral pharynx, neck) for tenderness, erythema, and swelling (adenopathy). The pain of external otitis is significantly increased by pulling on the external ear or applying pressure on the tragus. Next, inspect the ear canal (discharge, foreign body) and tympanic membrane (erythema, retraction, bulging, perforation). Mobility of the tympanic membrane is tested with pneumatic otoscopy; lack of mobility is the most sensitive sign of otitis media. Cholesteatoma appears as a white ball or cyst in the middle ear. Test hearing acuity by whispered voice and a vibrating tuning fork (Weber, Rinne). It is imperative to evaluate cranial nerve function (particularly CN VII) when malignant external otitis is suspected.

Diagnostic Tests

CBC. Generally not indicated unless a systemic infection is suspected.

Serum glucose. Order when underlying diabetes is suspected in a patient with infection.

Imaging studies. Necessary with suspicion that infection has spread beyond the ear.

Special Considerations

Acute Otitis Media

Acute otitis media (AOM) is a suppurative affliction arising from the blockage of the eustachian tube with subsequent accumulation of fluid in the middle ear. Bacteria may than gain access to the middle ear via the pharynx or dissemination from a neighboring structure. The most common pathogens encountered are *Streptococcus pneumonia, H. influenza,* group A *S. pyogenes,* and *Moraxella catarrhalis* (formerly *Branhamella catarrhalis*). If left untreated, AOM can infect the surrounding bone (mastoiditis, temporal bone osteomyelitis) and cranial vault (sinus thrombophlebitis; extradural, subdural, or intracranial abscesses; meningitis). In addition, local complications may occur, including perforation of the tympanic membrane (especially the posteroinferior aspect), conductive and sensorineural hearing loss, chronic suppurative otitis media, cholesteatoma formation, labyrinthitis, and facial nerve paralysis.

Other Considerations

Serous otitis media. Noninfectious middle ear effusions.

Bullous myringitis. Characterized by severe ear pain associated with one or more vesicles or blebs on the tympanic membrane. Although associated with *Mycoplasma pneumoniae,* recent studies reveal that the etiology is similar to that found in AOM.

Otitis externa. Also called swimmer's ear. Identified by inflammation of the ear canal and auricle, customarily caused by exposure to moisture (swimming), trauma, or dermatitis. Customarily, patients have discomfort of the affected ear, but fever should be absent. *Pseudomonas aeruginosa* and *S. pyogenes* are the most common etiologies.

Malignant otitis externa (MOE). A rare, necrotizing infection of the external ear that can lead to cranial nerve neuropathies, meningitis, mastoiditis, osteomyelitis of the temporal bone, and death (20% mortality rate). Seen especially in elderly diabetics. Patients suffering from MOE complain of severe, excruciating pain of the ear along with a purulent discharge. Up to 25% of instances of MOE are bilateral.

Herpes zoster oticus (Ramsay Hunt syndrome). A herpetic infection of the geniculate ganglion that manifests as vesicles or blisters on the external ear, tympanic membrane, and face or scalp. It is associated with oppressive ear pain, cranial nerve neuropathies, facial paralysis, hearing loss, and vertigo.

Treatment

Therapy is directed toward the underlying cause. Supplemental analgesics should be provided as needed.

Treatment of uncomplicated otitis media is generally straightforward; amoxicillin (250 to 500 mg PO TID for 10 days) remains the drug of choice. Alternative antibiotic regimens for patients who either fail to respond to amoxicillin or with documented allergy include amoxicillin-clavulanic acid (250 mg PO TID for 10 days), TMP-SMX (1 double-strength tab PO BID for 10 days), cefaclor (250 to 500 mg PO TID for 10 days), or erythromycin (250 to 500 mg PO QID for 10 days). The value of decongestants is unclear.

Treatment of otitis externa involves suctioning of debris from the ear canal, irrigating gently with warmed saline (if the tympanic membrane is intact), and instilling antibiotic drops (corticosporin otic solution or suspension, 2% acetic acid solution, or gentamycin ophthalmic solution, 2 to 4 gtt in ear canal QID for 7 days). If severe edema of the external canal is present, the use of commercial ear wicks (leaving in place for 2 to 3 days) is beneficial. Systemic antibiotics are rarely indicated for simple otitis externa but should be considered in the presence of cellulitis (either a first-generation cephalosporin or ciprofloxacin). It may be appropriate to treat diabetics with early external otitis with oral ciprofloxacin (500 mg BID for 7 to 10 days). Topical anesthetic drops *(Auralgan otic)* may help alleviate pain.

Management of acute malignant otitis externa requires parenteral antibiotics (*imipenem cilastatin,* 0.5 g IV q 6 hr, or *ciprofloxacin,* 400 mg IV q 12 hr) along with emergent ENT consultation (surgical debridement may be called for).

Admission Criteria

Admission is indicated *when sepsis, mastoiditis, intracranial involvement,* or *malignant external otitis externa accompanies ear pain. Patients with an acute tympanic membrane perforation* (especially when associated with hearing loss or vertigo) necessitate emergent ENT consultation. Follow-up should be arranged to ensure that the infection has resolved and hearing is restored.

Suggested Readings

Celin SE: Bacteriology of acute otitis media in adults, JAMA 1991;266: 2249–2253.

Rubin J, Yu VL: Malignant external otitis: insights into pathogenesis, clinical manifestations, diagnosis and therapy. Am J Med 1988;85:391–398.

Chapter 16

Basic Orthopedics

16.1 FRACTURES

Description

A *fracture* is a break in the continuity of a bone. For appropriate treatment and communication with consultants, a fracture must be described properly. The following terms describe fractures and the alignment of bony fragments at the fracture site. Several terms may apply to any single injury.

Angulated. The angle formed by the bony fragments; described by the direction of the apex of this angle, although if distally located, described by the direction of the distal fragment.

Avulsion. A small piece of bone is pulled out of the cortex by a ligamentous attachment.

Closed. No violation of tissues overlying the fracture site.

Comminuted. Three or more bony fragments.

Compression. Compaction of bone trabeculae due to a compressive force.

Displacement. The degree to which the ends of the bony fragments are offset.

Impacted. One of the fragments is driven into the opposite fragments.

Location. Proximal, midshaft, distal, etc.

Oblique. Fracture line is oblique to the long axis of the bone.

Open. Any communication with the surface; may vary from a puncture wound to complete avulsion of overlying tissues. Grade I, $<$ 1-cm lesion; grade II, 1- to 10-cm lesion; grade III, $>$ 10-cm lesion; grade IIIa, severe soft tissue injury; grade IIIb, bone exposed; and grade IIIc, vascular injury.

Overriding. An overlap of the ends of the bony fragments.

Pathologic. Fracture due to underlying disease process but not necessarily associated with any recognized trauma.

Spiral. Fracture line traverses the shaft in more than one plane.

Stress. Fracture caused by repetitive stress rather than single acute event.

Transverse. Fracture line is perpendicular to the long axis of the bone.

History

Determine the mechanism of injury (attempt to establish the exact position of the affected extremity at the time of injury); any previous injury to the affected area; and any associated symptoms, especially those that suggest neurovascular compromise. Ask about the patient's occupation, dominant hand, and past medical history. Document the tetanus status for all patients with open fractures.

Physical Examination

General. Note the presence of multiple trauma or any associated injuries. Remove clothing for exposure. Remove any jewelry to avoid tourniquet effect. Always examine the joint above and the joint below the area of injury.

Specific. Note any signs of fracture such as tenderness, deformity, ecchymosis, crepitus, or swelling. Check pulses. Perform a careful motor and sensory exam. Note integrity of skin overlying suspected fracture site.

Diagnostic Tests

Radiologic studies are indicated for any suspected fracture, dislocation, or subluxation. A minimum of two views in different planes (anteroposterior and lateral) is required. These views should include the joints above and below the level of injury and demonstrate the trabeculae pattern of the bone. Oblique films and other views may be required. Bone scan, tomograms, or computed tomography (CT) may be required in certain cases. **Note:** *The diagnosis should be based primarily on the history and physical examination and then confirmed with radiographic and other adjunctive studies.*

Special Considerations

Complications associated with fracture injuries include the following:

- Nonunion or malunion;
- Avascular necrosis (AVN);
- Compartment syndrome;
- Osteomyelitis (with open fractures);
- Fat embolus; and
- Reflex sympathetic dystrophy.

Treatment

Reduction of the fracture should be performed if necessary and should be immediate if the distal pulse is absent. Apply longitudinal traction in the long axis of the bone, reduplicate the direction of injury, and correct the displacement.

Open reduction. Indications include the following: closed reduction that is impossible or cannot be maintained, open fractures, displaced articular fractures, and associated vascular injuries.

Immobilization. Splinting is often initially preferred to full cast because a noncircumferential splint allows for continued swelling and causes less pain.

Open fracture. A true orthopedic emergency. Administer intravenous antibiotics early, generally a first-generation cephalosporin to cover staphylococcal and streptococcal organisms (e.g., cephalothin, 1 g IV q 6 to 8 hr). Provide tetanus immunization as needed for a contaminated wound. Do not attempt to cover the exposed bone with tissue; use a sterile, normal saline–soaked dressing. Definitive debridement, irrigation, and reduction take place in the operating room. Early orthopedic consultation should be obtained.

Admission Criteria

Patients with open fractures; fractures requiring open reduction with internal fixation; fractures of the femur, hip, pelvis, or spine; neurovascular insufficiency; or compartment syndrome require admission. Outpatient management includes splinting, analgesia, ice, elevation, and orthopedic follow-up. Discharge instructions must include symptoms and signs of compartment syndrome.

Suggested Readings

Gustilo RB, Merkow RL, Templeman D: Current concepts review: the management of open fractures. J Bone J Surg 1990;2:299–303.

Heckman JD: Fractures: emergency care and complications. Clin Symp 1991;3:2–32.

16.2. DISLOCATIONS

Description

A dislocation is the complete loss of continuity between two opposing articular surfaces. A subluxation is a partial loss of continuity between such surfaces. These injuries are described by the relationship of the distal articulating surface to the proximal articulating surface of the involved joint. For example, with an anterior shoulder dislocation, the humeral head (distal articulating surface) is displaced anteriorly in relation to the glenoid (proximal articulating surface). See Table 16.2.1 for descriptions of dislocations.

History

Establish the mechanism (isolated or multiple trauma) of injury and ask about any previous injury to the involved joint. Check for any symptoms of neurovascular injury.

Physical Examination

Always examine the extremity or area above and below the involved joint. Diagnose any associated injuries. Document neurovascular status before and after reduction.

Diagnostic Tests

Radiographs are useful to rule out fracture with displacement or dislocation with associated fracture. Additional views may be necessary, such as a scapular Y view with a shoulder dislocation. Reduction should not be delayed by x-rays in patients with neurovascular compromise or severe pain.

Treatment

For *reduction* make sure that there is adequate analgesia (using narcotics such as morphine, meperidine, or fentanyl) and muscle re-

Table 16.2.1
Dislocations of Major Joints

Dislocation	Mechanism	Clinical Findings	Comments and Complications
Anterior shoulder	Fall on abducted and externally rotated upper extremity	Loss of deltoid contour; shoulder held still in slight abduction	Axillary nerve injury; Hill-Sachs deformity
Posterior shoulder	Forceful abduction and internal rotation	Full posterior shoulder; shoulder adducted and internally rotated; passive or active external rotation not possible	Often misdiagnosed initially; usually associated with seizure or electrical shock
Posterior elbow	Fall on outstretched hand with arm held in extension.	Elbow held in moderate flexion; prominent olecranon process	High incidence of neurovascular compromise; median, radial, or ulnar injury; brachial artery injury; compartment syndrome
Posterior hip	Frequently, knee striking dashboard	Affected leg shortened with hip internally rotated and adducted	AVN of femoral head sciatic nerve injury
Knee	Extensive force required	Grossly unstable knee; may spontaneously reduce	Popliteal artery injury; misdiagnosed due to spontaneous reduction
Ankle	Posterior: forced plantar flexion; anterior: forced dorsiflexion	Obvious deformity; unable to bear weight	Usually associated fractures

laxation (using benzodiazepines such as diazepam or midazolam). Alternative medications include nitrous oxide and ketamine.

Apply slow, steady traction; many methods have been described (refer to comprehensive textbooks for details). Immobilize the area immediately after successful reduction. Postreduction films are always necessary.

If reduction is unsuccessful, interposed soft tissue may be responsible.

Orthopedic consultation is necessary if you are unable to reduce the dislocation (hip dislocations often require general anesthesia) or if there are neurovascular complications or associated fractures.

Admission Criteria

Patients with dislocations that have a high potential of neurovascular complication (knee, elbow) should be admitted. *Knee dislocations* often require an angiogram to rule out injury to the popliteal vessels. *Patients with hip dislocations* require admission.

Dislocations are not minor injuries since significant ligamentous disruption is always present, so follow-up is mandatory. The patient should be told to ice intermittently over the first 48 hr; elevate the affected joint; and to immobilize the affected joint by a splint or commercial immobilization device, depending on the joint. Provide analgesia via oral narcotics or nonsteroidal antiinflammatory agents according to the needs of the patient.

Suggested Readings

Rockwood CA Jr., Green DP, Bucholz RW: Rockwood and Green's fractures in adults, 3rd ed. Philadelphia: JB Lippincott, 1991.

Simon RR, Koenigsknecht SJ: Emergency orthopedics: the extremities, 3rd ed. Norwalk, CT: Appleton & Lange, 1995.

16.3. SOFT TISSUE INJURIES

Description

The absence of a fracture does not necessarily mean the absence of a significant injury. A detailed history and physical examination should permit the diagnosis of most injuries (see Table 16.3.1).

The following terms are used to describe soft tissue injuries.

Sprain. Ligamentous injury as a result of an abnormal motion of a joint.

Strain. Injury to the musculotendon unit.

Tendinitis. Painful inflammation of a tendon.

Bursitis. Painful inflammation of a bursa.

Table 16.3.1
Soft Tissue Injuries

Injury	Mechanism	Clinical Findings	Comments
Rotator cuff tear	Fall on shoulder; lifting a heavy object	Shoulder abduction either absent or painful and weak; tender over proximal humerus; passive ROM relatively painless	Surgical treatment in young patient with large tear; conservative management in older patient
Rupture biceps tendon	Repetitive trauma; lifting heavy weights	Palpable defect; asymmetry of muscle belly	Surgical repair
Anterior cruciate ligament tear	Forceful rotation with planted foot	Laxity with anterior drawer test; knee effusion	Patients hear pop; rapid onset of hemarthrosis
Ankle sprain	Abrupt inversion or eversion	Swelling; point tenderness; laxity with grade III injuries	With inversion injury, always palpate base of fifth metatarsal to rule out fracture
Achilles tendon rupture	Violent plantar flexion	Palpable defect in tendon; positive Thompson test	Patient may be able to weakly plantar flex foot with plantaris muscle

Strains and sprains are graded according to extent of injury:

Grade I. Overstretching of ligament or tendon.
Grade II. Partial tear of involved structure.
Grade III. Extensive tear, complete rupture, or avulsion.

History

The following points should be covered in the interview: mechanism of injury, previous injury to the area, increased activity (overuse) including occupational, medications (steroids may predispose to tendon rupture), and underlying disease (renal dialysis, connective tissue diseases).

Physical Examination

Sprain. Check for point tenderness, ecchymosis, swelling, laxity (indicates grade III, although it may be masked by pain and swelling), and decrease or loss of function.

Strain. Check for point tenderness, ecchymosis, swelling, and decrease or loss of function. If grade III, a palpable defect may be present. Active range of motion (ROM) is more painful than passive ROM.

Tendinitis. Check for tenderness. There should be minimal swelling over the site of involvement.

Bursitis. Marked by tenderness, mild swelling, and warmth over the involved bursa. Passive range of motion should be possible with only minimal discomfort; with acute arthritis, passive ROM is extremely painful.

Diagnostic Tests

X-rays. Normal unless associated with fracture, dislocation, or underlying disease.

Arthrocentesis. Aspirate joints or bursae with effusions when infection or gout is suspected. Fluid should be sent for cell count, Gram stain, culture and sensitivity, glucose and protein, and crystal analysis.

Treatment

Conservative management is based on RICE (rest, ice, compression, elevation). Oral analgesics (nonsteroidal antiinflammatory drugs, codeine, hydrocodone) may be given. The injury should be immobilized (Jones dressing or a splint, crutches for lower extremity injuries). Orthopedic follow-up should be arranged. Operative intervention is required for complete tendon and most complete ligament ruptures. Antibiotics should be given if infection is suspected.

Suggested Readings

Browner BD, Jupiter JB, Levine AM, Trafton PG: Skeletal trauma. Philadelphia: WB Saunders, 1992.

Simon RR, Koenigsknecht SJ: Emergency orthopedics: the extremities, 3rd ed. Norwalk, CT: Appleton & Lange, 1995.

16.4. COMPARTMENT SYNDROMES

Description

Most muscle groups are contained within a fascial compartment. A compartment syndrome occurs when intracompartmental pressure is increased to a level at which it compromises the circulation to the structures within the compartment. This condition may occur with or without an associated fracture and must be recognized, as it represents a true orthopedic emergency. Irreversible muscle damage will occur 6 to 12 hr after the onset of symptoms. This injured muscle will be replaced by fibrous tissue, resulting in paralysis and deformity (Volkmann's ischemia).

The etiology of compartment syndrome can be divided into conditions causing a *decrease in compartment space* (constrictive dressing like a cast, military antishock trousers, and prolonged external pressure such as in a comatose patient) and situations that cause an *increase in compartment volume* (hemorrhage, trauma, burns, overuse of muscles, and drug injection).

History

In trauma-related cases, the onset of symptoms is usually 6 to 8 hr after the time of injury, but they may occur up to several days after the insult. Patients taking anticoagulant medications or those with underlying bleeding disorders may develop a compartment syndrome after a seemingly minor trauma. Patients complain of pain out of proportion to the injury, and this pain progresses despite analgesics. Paresthesias are noted in the area supplied by the nerves in the involved compartment.

Physical Examination

Check the extremities. Tenderness and tenseness may be present over the involved compartment. Pain occurs with passive stretching of the affected muscle group. Decreased strength of this muscle group is noted. Similarly, sensation is decreased in the area supplied by the affected nerve. Intact distal pulses and capillary refill do not rule out a compartment syndrome, as these findings may persist after irreversible damage has occurred. **Note:** *Do not depend on a diminished pulse (a late finding) to make the diagnosis of compartment syndrome.* Table 16.4.1 lists clinical findings in the three most common compartment syndromes.

Table 16.4.1
Common Compartment Syndromes

Compartment	Motor Loss	Sensory Loss	Painful Passive Motion
Volar forearm	Finger flexion	Palm	Finger extension
Anterior leg	Dorsiflexion of foot and great toe	Web space between first and second toes	Plantar flexion, foot and great toe
Deep posterior leg	Inversion of foot and flexion of toes	Volar aspect of foot and toes	Toe dorsiflexion

Diagnosis

Usually, the diagnosis can be made from the history and physical examination. Reference is often made to the six P's of compartment syndrome: pain out of proportion, pain on passive stretching, pallor, pulselessness, paraesthesias, and paralysis. Of these six findings, the first two (pain out of proportion and pain on passive stretching) are the most important. *Do not* wait for the other findings to develop in the appropriate clinical setting. Compartment pressure measurements are indicated whenever there is a clinical suspicion but the diagnosis is not clear (see section 21.9).

Several methods are available, including *wick catheter, slit catheter,* and *needle manometer* techniques. Pressures greater than 30 mm Hg suggest compartment syndrome. Some investigators consider the pressure differential between mean arterial pressure and compartment pressure a more accurate indicator of a compartment syndrome; a differential of 40 mm Hg or less is considered diagnostic.

Treatment

Remove any constrictive dressings if present. Perform early surgical decompression (fasciotomy) if compartment syndrome is apparent clinically or compartment pressure is elevated by measurement. Early orthopedic consultation is essential.

Suggested Readings

McGee DL, Dalsey WC: The mangled extremity: compartment syndrome and amputations. Emerg Med Clin North Am 1992;10:783–790.

Moore RE, Friedman RJ: Current concepts in the pathophysiology and diagnosis of compartment syndromes. J Emerg Med 1989;6:657–662.

Chapter 17

Pain Control in the Emergency Department

DESCRIPTION

Acute pain *is the most common presenting symptom* in the ED. Pain is a sensation produced by the noxious (tissue-damaging) stimulation of terminal branches of nerve fibers. The transmission of these signals is influenced by myriad biochemical mediators (prostaglandins, substance P, histamine) and inhibitory and excitatory signals from the brain and spinal column nervous systems. Naturally occurring endorphins play a role in modifying the perception of pain.

Somatic pain (involving the skin, subcutaneous structures, bone) is customarily well localized and described, often equating with the amount of tissue injured. When describing *neurogenic pain* (sciatica, diabetic neuropathy, reflex sympathetic dystrophy), patients employ adjectives such as *shooting, burning, tingling,* or *crushing. Visceral, or referred, pain* arises from organs that share segmental innervation with somatic structures. The specific type of pain depends on the organ affected. Patients writhing in pain frequently suffer from an intraabdominal or vascular disorder. If a hollow organ is obstructed, there will be a periodicity to the pain that corresponds to the contractions of the organ, which is attempting to push against some resistance (e.g., kidney stone in the ureter). *Psychogenic pain* is poorly defined and regularly does not correspond to dermatomal patterns.

Too often, however, the patient's discomfort is discounted, and undue emphasis is placed on diagnostic tests. Explanations for inadequate use of analgesics include exaggerated concerns about drug addiction or respiratory depression from narcotics, inadequate knowledge of appropriate doses and scheduling, and lack of formal and bedside experience in acute pain management.

HISTORY

Perception of pain is quite variable and is affected by co-existing conditions, previous experiences, age, and cultural differences. It is a good rule to *always* give patients the benefit of the doubt when they say they are in pain. Like all symptoms, pain reflects an underlying disturbance. Whenever possible, it is important to explore the attributes of pain. The ED physician ought to make use of the PQRST mnemonic: provocative or palliative factors, quality (sharp, knifelike, burning, dull ache), region (location of pain), severity (ask the patient to relate the pain to common experiences such as toothache, childbirth, and menstrual cramps, or to grade the pain on a scale of 1 to 10), and temporal characteristics (total duration of pain). In addition, determine what pain medications have been used in past (and their efficacy) along with any allergies.

Upon completion of the history, attempt to place the patient in one of five general categories:

1. Acute pain that is severe (MI, ruptured aneurysm, bone fracture, kidney stone);
2. Acute pain that is moderate (ankle sprain, cellulitis);
3. Chronic pain that is severe (metastatic cancer to bone);
4. Chronic pain that is moderate (low back pain, arthritis); and
5. Pain that is suspect (malingerer, substance abuser, psychiatric disturbance).

PHYSICAL EXAMINATION

The physical examination should progress from the history; pain that is acute, traumatic, and well localized is straightforward. The complaint of severe atraumatic abdominal or chest pain necessitates a more thorough physical examination. While certain signs (facial grimacing, posturing, reduced activity, sweating, pallor, dilation of pupils, elevation of blood pressure, tachycardia, and nausea and vomiting) are associated with pain syndromes, their absence *does not* verify the lack of pain.

Very often, one is confronted with uncomfortable or agitated patients who are unable to cooperate because of severe pain. These patients may become more cooperative after using careful increments of appropriate agents. Discuss use of narcotic analgesics for acute abdominal pain with a surgical consultant before use. Also appropriate consent forms for expected treatment should be completed before narcotic analgesia or sedatives are given. Examination before and after the administration of analgesics is advisable. If, however, concern over analgesia interfering with the examination exists, a titratable reversal of analgesia can be accomplished with naloxone.

DIAGNOSTIC TESTS

The need for particular diagnostic studies is governed by the history and clinical findings.

SPECIAL CONSIDERATIONS

Malingerers and Drug Seekers

Malingering is the deliberate act of feigning illness or disability for secondary gain. There is no definitive test for malingering; this is a diagnosis rooted in attentive clinical judgment. Although subsequent benefit is frequently an underlying factor (worker's compensation, disability insurance claims, obtaining controlled substances for resale), the presence of a secondary factor does not mean that the patient is a malingerer. Suspicion of malingering should not preclude a search for an underlying organic disease.

Common complaints of the drug seeker include migraine headaches, renal colic, low back pain, toothache, and even terminal cancer. Many of these patients are quite sophisticated in their medical and pharmacological knowledge (often they use the PDR as a reference). *Narcotics* (especially hydromorphone and oxycodone), *benzodiazepines,* and *amphetamine-like* drugs are the preferred substances of drug seekers. Be wary of patients who are excessively flattering or seductive or who try to control the interview process. Another ploy is to exploit old surgical scars or orthopedic injuries (malunion or nonunion fractures).

It is imprudent to accuse a patient of drug seeking based on a single visit to the ED; in all cases, *grant the patient the benefit of the doubt.* However, if after a careful evaluation, you strongly believe that the patient is a drug seeker (old records reveal multiple ED visits for narcotic analgesics for unclear reasons), advise the patient of your concerns in a professional, nonjudgmental manner. Tell the patient that the reasons for the pain are unclear and that he or she will require a more thorough evaluation in an outpatient setting. Offer the patient a nonnarcotic alternative (NSAID, prochlorperazine for migraine, local anesthetic for toothache). Document all conversations. *Do not* label patients as drug seekers in writing.

Drug Abusers

Drug abusers pose difficult problems with respect to pain management. Contrary to the habit of prescribing normal or lower doses, this group of patients requires *higher* than normal dosing when narcotic medication is necessary. Providing sufficient analgesia in the ED in no way adversely affects the patient's drug dependence. In fact, providing adequate pain relief often betters the physician-patient relationship. Employing inadequate analgesia may provoke the patient to become agitated, uncooperative, or combative.

Elderly Patients

Drug effects tend to be more pronounced in the elderly, and there is an increased incidence of adverse reactions. Therefore, it is advisable to employ lower doses of pain medications and to be aware of the potential for iatrogenic problems (confusion, somnolence, falling).

TREATMENT

The emergency physician is confronted with a wide range of illnesses calling for pain management. However, all too often an improper dose, dosing schedule, and route are chosen. The intravenous route provides the most rapid and consistent drug levels and allows titration so that incremental doses at appropriate intervals can be given to relieve pain. The intramuscular route proves painful, renders variable serum levels (unreliable absorption), and is difficult to titrate. In addition, patients with recurrent pain syndromes (sickle cell disease) are prone to serious complications (such as abscesses, osteomyeliti, and nerve palsies). If the intramuscular route must be used repeatedly, strong oral or intravenous analgesia is a better choice.

Some common misconceptions exist among physicians in the use of analgesics, particularly narcotic analgesics. One in particular is that analgesia will mask the diagnosis. No data exist to support this belief. Another misconception is that the use of narcotics will result in addiction. In fact, the risk of narcotic addiction as a result of treating acute pain is very low and is not an issue in the management of pain in the ED.

Finally, many practitioners believe patients who respond to a placebo (e.g., intramuscular normal saline) are not in pain. This is wrong, and at least one-third of patients with real pain will have a positive response to a placebo. The administration of a placebo has no place in the ED setting.

It is likewise important to extend psychological support to the patient. Tell the patient that supplying relief from the pain is as meaningful to you as uncovering the diagnosis. Let a spouse or friend remain in the room with the patient. Whenever possible, let the patient play a role in the choice of an analgesic; ask the patient what "works" for him or her. Ask the patient to rate the pain on a scale of 1 to 10. Once you have obtained a baseline, check the patient's response at regular intervals.

Nonsteroidal Antiinflammatory Drugs

Unless contraindicated, pharmacologic management of mild to moderate pain should begin with acetaminophen or a NSAID (Table 17.1). NSAIDs decrease levels of inflammatory mediators generated at the site of tissue injury. These agents are rapidly ab-

Table 17.1
Dosing Data for NSAIDs

Drug	Usual Adult Dose
Acetaminophen	650–975 mg q 4 hr
Aspirin	650–975 mg q 4 hr
Choline magnesium trisalicylate	1000–1500 mg BID
Diflunisal	1000 mg initial dose followed by 500 mg q 12 hr
Etodolac	200–400 mg q 6–8 hr
Fenoprofen calcium	200 mg q 4–6 hr
Ibuprofen	400 mg q 4–6 hr
Ketoprofen	25–75 mg q 6–8 hr
Ketorolac	30 or 60 mg IM dose; 10 mg PO q 6–8 hr
Mefenamic acid	250 mg q 6 hr
Naproxen	500 mg initial dose followed by 250 mg q 6–8 hr
Naproxen sodium	550 mg initial dose followed by 275 mg q 6–8 hr
Salsalate	500 mg q 4 hr

sorbed from the gastrointestinal tract, with peak serum levels being obtained within 1 to 2 hr.

NSAIDs offer several advantages, including no respiratory depression or sedation, no addictive qualities, no development of tolerance, and no interference with bowel or bladder function. Caution should be taken when using NSAIDs, as they can inhibit platelet aggregation, cause gastrointestinal irritation, and exacerbate bronchospasm. Careful dosing is important in patients with hepatic or renal disease, because these patients may exhibit toxicity at lower doses.

Opiates and Opioids

Opiates and their synthetic derivatives (opioids) remain the cornerstone of treatment of moderate to severe pain (Table 17.2). They exert their effect primarily on the central nervous system, stimulating specific opiate receptors. Proper use of these potent agents involves selecting an effective drug and route of administration. Equally important is choosing an appropriate starting dose and frequency of administration. Be aware of the incidence and severity of side effects.

Morphine

Morphine remains a standard drug for severe pain. There is substantial experience with this agent, and its effects are easily re-

Table 17.2
Dosing Data for Opiate and Opioid Analgesics[a]

Drug	Oral	Parenteral
Morphine	60 mg q 3–4 hr	10 mg q 3–4 hr
Codeine	200 mg q 3–4 hr	130 mg q 2 hr (IM, SQ)
Hydromorphone	7.5 mg q 3–4 hr	1.5 mg q 3–4 hr
Hydrocodone	10 mg q 3–4 hr	Not available
Levorphanol	4 mg q 6–8 hr	2 mg q 6–8 hr
Meperidine	300 mg q 3 hr	75–100 mg q 2–3 hr
Methadone	20 mg q 6–8 hr	10 mg q 6–8 hr
Oxycodone	30 mg q 3–4 hr	15 mg q 4 hr
Oxymorphone	6 mg q 3–4 hr	1 mg q 3–4 hr
Fentanyl	Not available	0.1 mg IV; additional doses, 0.5–1.0 μg q 3–5 min

[a]Potencies equivalent to 10-mg IM dose of morphine.

versed with naloxone. It is conjugated in the liver, and this pathway is not significantly affected unless total liver failure is present. The elimination half-life is 2 to 3 hr in healthy adults and 4 to 5 hr in older patients. Morphine, like other narcotics, can produce nausea and vomiting, constipation, urinary retention, biliary spasm, sedation, and respiratory depression. Morphine is also associated with the release of histamine, which can cause hypotension and bronchospasm (especially in asthmatics). Respiratory depression generally responds promptly to *naloxone* (0.4 to 0.8 mg IV).

Meperidine

Meperidine is a synthetic derivative of morphine that has one-eighth the potency and a shorter duration of action. Metabolism is significantly affected by liver disease. Complications are similar to other narcotic agents. Meperidine may be favored over morphine for the treatment of biliary and renal colic. Meperidine displays a short duration of action (2 to 3 hr) and should be given in adequate doses (75 to 100 mg q 2 to 3 hr to adults in severe pain). The first metabolite of meperidine, normeperidine, may cause CNS excitation. Although it is common practice, the addition of phenothiazines (promethazine) to the analgesic regimen does not enhance analgesia and may increase the incidence of side effects.

Fentanyl

Fentanyl is a synthetic narcotic well suited for emergency procedures. It is 100 times more potent than morphine, produces analgesia in as little as 1.5 min, and has a brief duration of action (30 min) when administered intravenously. This agent is very safe when dosed correctly. The initial dose in adults is typically 2 to 3 μg/kg IV. Supplemental increments of 0.5 to 1.0 μg/kg q 3 to 5 min may be supplied until adequate sedation and analgesia are obtained. Most adults achieve adequate results after a total dose of 3 to 5 μg/kg. Observe patients closely when titrating the dose, monitoring response, respiratory rate, and oxygen saturation. Use a cardiac monitor and pulse oximeter. Complications other than sedation and respiratory depression are rare.

Miscellaneous Agents

Nitrous oxide is accessible as a self-administered gas (regularly a 50:50 mixture with oxygen) that is employed in both the prehospital setting and the ED. Analgesia generally begins 20 sec after use, peaks in 2 to 3 min, and fades quickly (within minutes) after discontinuation. Contraindications to use include patients with a suspected pneumothorax, decompression illness, drug overdose, altered mental status, abdominal pain with distention, and severe COPD. Interrupt use in any patient too drowsy to handle the mask.

Ketamine gives rise to a dissociative state, leading to analgesia. It can be given intravenously or intramuscularly (0.4 mg/kg). Adverse effects and contraindications to ketamine include increased heart rate and blood pressure (therefore, avoid in patients with severe hypertension), elevation of intracranial pressure (avoid use in head injured patients), increased oral and tracheal secretions, and emergence reactions and dysphoria (do not employ in patients with a history of psychosis; concomitantly use a benzodiazepine to avoid this effect).

Benzodiazepines may be used by the ED physician for sedation and anxiolysis before surgical procedures and for skeletal muscle relaxation. Diazepam (0.1 to 0.3 mg/kg) or midazolam (0.1 to 0.2 mg/kg) is effective. The response to benzodiazepines is individually variable, and it is best to titrate the dose.

Muscle relaxants (orphenadrine, methocarbamol, cyclobenzaprine) may reduce the amount of muscle spasm following an injury. They act mainly by inducing drowsiness. Muscle relaxants possess anticholinergic properties, contraindicating use in patients with narrow angle glaucoma, urinary retention, and prostatic hypertrophy.

Combined Analgesia and Sedation

Often an analgesic is combined with a sedative to reduce the pain and anxiety of ED procedures. Several agents are available for use. Fentanyl and midazolam are a popular combination providing rapid, safe, and short-acting analgesia and amnesia.

Procedure for Combination Analgesia and Sedation
(70-kg Adult)

1. Establish an intravenous line of normal saline. The patient should be in a supine or recumbent position.
2. Pulse, respiratory rate, blood pressure, and level of consciousness should be recorded after each agent is given and every 5 min throughout the procedure.

3. Perform continuous pulse oximeter and cardiac monitoring.
4. Have a resuscitation cart at the bedside.
5. Administer midazolam (1 mg IV over 60 sec); if sedation is not adequate after 3 to 5 min, additional 1-mg IV doses can be given up to a maximum of 0.1 mg/kg.
6. Reassess the patient frequently.
7. Administer fentanyl (0.1 mg, or 100 μg, IV over 60 sec); repeat in 0.5 to 1.0 μg/kg increments every 3 to 5 min until adequate analgesia is obtained (slurred speech and drowsy but responding to pain and verbal stimuli). The maximal total dose is 5 to 6 μg/kg in adults.
8. Administer local anesthesia if needed.
9. Perform the procedure. An additional dose of fentanyl may be given every 3 to 5 min to a total dose of 5 to 6 μg/kg
10. If hypoxemia, slowed respirations, or excessive sedation occurs, assist ventilation with a bag valve mask and administer naloxone (0.4 to 2.0 mg) and flumazenil (0.5 to 1.0 mg) as needed. **Note:** *Flumazenil is contraindicated if the patient is taking benzodiazepines chronically, as it may precipitate a withdrawal reaction.*
11. Continue close observation until the patient is awake and alert. Ensure that the patient can speak and drink before discharge.

Suggested Readings

Aztard AR: Safety of early pain relief for acute abdominal pain. Br Med J 1992;305:554–556.

Acute Pain Management Guideline Panel: Acute pain management: operative or medical procedures and trauma. Clinical practice guideline. AHCPR Pub. 92–0032. Rockville, MD: US Department of Health and Human Services, Feb. 1992.

Coleman N: Check . . . checkmate. Countering the con game of drug abusers. Postgrad Med 1985;77:68–78.

Chapter 18

Environmental Emergencies

18.1 HEAT ILLNESS

Description

Heat-related disorders range from mild cramping to life-threatening. Commonly, symptoms follow excessive exposure to a hot and humid environment, although illness may occur nonseasonally when an underlying disorder, medication, or drug interferes with the body's ability to dissipate heat or illicit drug ingestion provokes excessive muscle activity, thus increasing the amount of body heat generated. When examining a patient with *hyperpyrexia,* the history, physical examination, and laboratory data should focus on eliminating other diagnostic possibilities, particularly *sepsis, meningitis, encephalitis, CVA, SAH, neuroleptic malignant syndrome, malignant hyperthermia, withdrawal states, thyroid storm, malaria,* and *head injury*. However, prompt attention and therapy are essential to prevent significant morbidity and mortality associated with hyperpyrexia regardless of etiology.

History

The patient's level of consciousness determines the line of questioning. Alert patients generally complain of muscular cramping, headache, irritability, fatigue, weakness, or GI disturbances. In obtunded or confused patients, try to obtain a history from bystanders, friends, family, or paramedics. Significant historical clues are the nature and time frame of symptoms, degree of activity before onset of symptoms, and ambient temperature and humidity. Certain conditions increase the susceptibility to heat-related illness (advanced age, Parkinson's disease, chronic skin disorders, hyperthyroidism, spinal cord disorders, CHF, uremia, CVA, malnutrition). Also ask about drugs that may impair sweating or thermoregulation (anticholinergics, antihistamines, phenothiazines, cyclic antidepressants, diuretics, β-blockers, laxatives, alcohol) or cause muscle hyperactivity (PCP, LSD, amphetamines, cocaine).

Physical Examination

Vital signs. Continuously monitor core temperature with a rectal probe. Check for hypotension, tachycardia, tachypnea, and respiratory depression.

HEENT. Look for signs of trauma. Check extraocular movements, pupil response, and fundi.

Neck. Check for stiffness, jugular venous distention, and thyromegaly.

Lungs. Auscultate for bilateral breath sounds, rales, rhonchi, or wheezes.

Heart. Listen for murmurs, gallops, or rubs.

Abdomen. Examine for bowel sounds, distention, guarding, and tenderness.

Rectal. Check stool for blood.

Extremities. Note if they are clammy or cyanotic. Check for presence of muscular rigidity, muscular fasciculations, and track marks.

Skin. Check for presence or absence of sweating, skin turgor, petechiae, and rashes.

Neurologic. Note level of consciousness and focal deficits.

Diagnostic Tests

CBC. The white cell count is frequently elevated (although generally less than 20,000/mm^3). Hemoglobin and hematocrit levels may be higher than normal secondary to hemoconcentration.

SMA. Elevation of liver enzymes is common with heat stroke. The severity of heat stroke correlates with the degree of elevation of the AST. Establish baseline renal function; BUN and creatinine may be elevated due to acute renal failure or dehydration. Hypokalemia can be profound with heat stroke.

PT. Check PT, PTT, and platelets in patients with heat stroke. Both severe heat stroke and sepsis may provoke DIC syndrome.

Cultures. Blood and urine cultures are obligatory when sepsis suspected.

ABG. Helpful to assess oxygenation status and acid-base disruptions.

Urinalysis. Useful in screening for UTI or rhabdomyolysis.

ECG. Hyperthermia may cause ST or T wave changes, premature ventricular contractions, and dysrhythmias.

CXR. May detect pneumonia or pulmonary edema.

CT of head. Indicated in patients with head trauma, focal deficits, or persistent coma despite adequate cooling. However, do not delay therapy for CT.

Toxicology. Specific drug levels may be drawn if indicated.

Lumbar puncture. Necessary when meningitis is suspected.

Special Considerations

Heat Cramps

Heat cramps are painful, involuntary spasms (lasting 1 to 3 min) of major muscle groups (thighs, calves) arising from fluid and/or electrolyte depletion. Typically, heat cramps occur in individuals engaged in vigorous activity and are identified by tenderness and rigidity of the affected muscle groups along with moist skin. The body temperature and mental status should remain normal.

Heat Exhaustion

Heat exhaustion overcomes unacclimatized persons who exercise in hot environments and is characterized by nonspecific, mild CNS disturbances (headache, dizziness, agitation, weakness); GI perturbation (anorexia, nausea, vomiting, diarrhea); and dehydration. The body temperature may be mildly elevated (up to 39°C, 102°F). Presence of serious mental status changes implies progression to frank heat stroke.

Heat Stroke

Heat stroke is the most extreme presentation of heat illness, occurring when the body's ability to dissipate heat is overwhelmed, frequently leading to disturbances of the central nervous system (delirium, disorientation, seizures, coma), cardiovascular system (pulmonary edema, shock), and liver (hepatic necrosis). *Classic heat stroke* occurs primarily in the elderly and patients on medications that interfere with sweating and is characterized by the triad of a temperature ϵ 41°C (106°F), altered mental status, and the absence of sweating. However, younger patients undergoing rigorous exercise or who are agitated due to drugs, agitation, stress, or withdrawal activity may present with hyperthermia and CNS dysfunction, but *with* sweating. This condition is referred to as *exertional heat stroke* and is generally associated with a more acute onset than classic heat stroke.

Treatment

As with all emergencies, the patient's airway, breathing, and circulation must be supported. Perform immediate bedside glucose determination and give 1 amp D_{50} intravenously (if needed) along with *thiamine* (100 mg IV). If lowering of the body temperature is required, ensure adequate circulation. Fluid requirements are highly variable. Exercise caution when replacing fluids in the elderly and patients with heart disease. When significant volume loss is present or anticipated, give isotonic crystalloid (normal saline or lactated Ringer's) in 250- to 500-mL boluses, checking checks of blood pressure, urinary output, and lungs frequently. Patients who remain hypotensive despite fluid support or who develop signs of fluid overload, require invasive monitoring with inotropic support. Continuous monitoring of the core temperature with a *rectal probe* is essential to prevent overshoot and rebound.

For the patient with *heat stroke,* institute immediate *cooling measures.* Methods for removing excess heat include *radiation* (placing the patient in a cool environment and removing clothing), *convection* (fanning the patient), *conduction* (placing ice packs in contact with the body), and *evaporation* (spraying with a cold mist) An exceptionally useful technique is that of *accelerated evaporative heat loss;* in this approach, the patient is disrobed and sprayed with a fine mist of lukewarm water while being exposed to a high-volume fan. Warm water (about 15°C) is advantageous because it both evaporates quickly and does not precipitate shivering. Beds that expose maximal body surface area are best (a hammock is ideal). Stop the cooling measures once the temperature reaches 39°C (102°F) to avoid overshoot.

If severe hyperthermia persists, alternative techniques may be employed, including *ice water immersion* (creates logistic problems as far as monitoring and the initiation of CPR or defibrillation if necessary), *iced gastric lavage,* and *iced peritoneal lavage.* Antipyretics are ineffective for heat stroke. If the patient begins to shiver during the cooling process, administer a *benzodiazepine* (diazepam 5 to 10 mg IV).

Patients with *heat cramps* or *mild heat exhaustion* should be placed in a cool environment and provided rehydration with oral electrolyte solutions or intravenous hydration (1 L NS over 1 to 2 hr).

Admission Criteria

All victims of heat stroke require hospitalization, preferably to an intensive care unit setting. Poor prognostic indicators include patients who are comatose, are hypotensive, have coexisting illness, and have AST levels > 1000 IU. Heat cramps tend to be self-limited, and patients can be safely discharged with instructions encouraging adequate fluid and salt replacement and advice about prevention. Patients with mild to moderate heat exhaustion who respond to ED rehydration and electrolyte replacement after 4 to 6 hr of observation can usually be discharged home. Hospitalization may be necessary for *patients who remain symptomatic, elderly patients, patients with significant underlying illness, when the diagnosis is in doubt, or those with a poor home situation.*

Suggested Readings

Simon HB: Hyperthermia. N Engl J Med 1993;329:483–487.

Tek D, Olshaker JS: Heat illness. Emerg Med Clin North Am 1992;10: 299–310.

18.2 COLD ILLNESS AND INJURY

Description

Hypothermia is defined as a core temperature of < 35°C (95°F). In order not to miss the diagnosis, a special low-reading thermometer must be employed. *Primary hypothermia* results from direct exposure to a cold environment (indoors, outdoors) where the amount of heat loss exceeds the body's ability to generate heat. Routes of heat loss include *radiation* (> 50%), *conduction* (multiplies losses up to 5 times in wet clothing and 25 times in cold water immersion), *convection* (affected by wind velocity), *evaporation,* and *respiration.*

Secondary hypothermia takes place when an underlying illness or disorder (trauma patient, drug overdose, altered mental state) causes the patient to remain exposed to cold conditions, when there is a decrease in heat production (elderly, cachexia, myxedema, hypopituitarism, hypoadrenalism) or an increase in heat loss (burns, skin disorders, poor acclimatization to environment), and when there is impaired thermoregulation (CNS trauma, infection, tumor, spinal cord transection, DKA, uremia). Medications and toxins can predispose patients to hypothermia (impair ability to perceive cold, disturb hypothalamic function, or diminish endogenous heat production).

Peripheral cold injuries are divided into freezing and nonfreezing injuries. *Frostbite* is the most common freezing injury. *Trench foot* and *immersion foot* are nonfreezing injuries following exposure to a wet and cold environment. A nonfreezing injury after exposure to dry cold is referred to as chilblains. Frostbite occurs when the tissue temperature drops below 0°C (32°F), causing extracellular fluid crystallization, dehydration, disruption of cellular structure, and release of cellular breakdown products, which provokes microvascular stasis and sludging. Following tissue thawing, progressive edema intervenes with subsequent thrombosis and tissue necrosis. Predisposing conditions include alcohol and drug use (nicotine), chronic illnesses (peripheral vascular disease), and lack of acclimatization.

History

A history of prolonged exposure to a cold environment readily prompts the diagnosis of hypothermia. However this history is frequently not available, and more subtle presentations are the rule in urban localities. Obtain a thorough past medical history, focusing on underlying systemic disease and medications. Note a history of alcohol or drug abuse. Determine the patient's social supports (if the patient lives in the streets or in an apartment alone).

Physical Examination

Note: *The physical findings of the hypothermic patient are contingent on the core temperature, duration of exposure, and underlying medical condition.* All suspected hypothermic patients should be completely undressed, dried off, insulated with blankets, and examined for signs of trauma or illness. In severely hypothermic patients, limit physical manipulation of the patient to only essential tasks.

General. Shivering is maximum at 35°C (95°F), ceasing when temperature falls to 31°C (87.8°F). When the level of consciousness does not correspond to temperature, think of CNS trauma, infection, or overdose.

Vital signs. The core (rectal) temperature defines the severity of hypothermia; an accurate temperature is crucial and requires a special low-reading probe and continual readings. Decreases in pulse rate, respiratory rate, and blood pressure correspond with core temperature. Palpation of the peripheral pulses may be difficult because of peripheral vasoconstriction combined with extreme bradycardia, leading to the mistaken diagnosis of cardiac arrest in the profoundly hypothermic patient. The finding of tachycardia in the setting of moderate or severe hypothermia suggests a secondary problem (sepsis, hypoglycemia, volume depletion, drug overdose).

Abdomen. May mimic acute abdomen (rectus muscle spasm, ileus) or mask organic pathology.

Diagnostic Tests

CBC. Hematocrit and hemoglobin usually increase secondary to hemoconcentration (Hct rises up to 2% for each 1°C drop in temperature).

SMA. Hypothermia has no predictable effect on sodium, potassium, or chloride levels. Baseline renal function should be established.

Glucose. Hyperglycemia (insulin is inactive when the core temperature drops below 30°C, or 86°F) or hypoglycemia (underlying problem in the elderly, malnourished, or alcoholic) may occur.

Serum amylase and lipase. An elevation in either may be the only clue to cold-induced pancreatitis.

PT, PTT, and fibrinogen. Check for evidence of DIC.

Urinalysis. A dilute urine (< 1.010) typically accompanies hypothermia due to suppression of ADH. Also check for infection.

ABG. In the past, "correcting for cold" was recommended, but it is now generally accepted that decisions are best made on uncorrected gases.

Toxicologies. Drug levels should be sent as indicated.

Blood cultures. Order if sepsis is suspected.

ECG. Required in all patients with significant hypothermia. Temperatures below 32°C (89.6°F) are associated with bradycardia. Atrial arrhythmias with a slow ventricular response emerge once the temperature drops below 30°C (86°F). PR and QT lengthening also occur with decreasing temperatures. The risk of ventricular fibrillation is greatest at temperatures $<$ 30°C. Asystole takes place when the temperature is below 19°C (66.2°F). *Osborne* waves, or elevations of the J point, are considered a distinctive ECG finding of hypothermia, emerging as the temperature approaches 32°C (89.6°F).

Radiology. For the patient with mild hypothermia, order x-rays based on the patient's medical condition and your suspicion of trauma. For moderately and severely hypothermic patients order a CXR (pulmonary edema, pneumonia, pneumothorax). Order *C-spine films* when trauma is suspected, and consider a CT of the head if either mental status does not improve with rewarming or there are indications of head trauma.

Special Considerations

Mild hypothermia is defined as a core temperature of 32.2–35°C (90–95°F). Symptoms include CNS depression (apathy, ataxia, amnesia, dysarthria), tachycardia, pallor, and shivering.

Moderate hypothermia is defined as a core temperature of 27–32°C (80.6–89.6°F). Shivering stops at 31°C (87.8°F). There is a progressive decrease in the level of consciousness and a depression of vital signs (pulse rate decrease 50% at temperatures below 28°C, or 82.9°F). Pupils dilate, and cold diuresis and dysrhythmias may occur.

Severe hypothermia is defined as a core temperature below 27°C (80.0°F). The patient has a loss of reflexes and no response to pain; he or she is comatose (cerebral blood flow is one-third normal). The risk of v-fib is maximal when the temperature is below 30°C(86°F).

Frostbite is the body's attempt to preserve life versus limb; blood is shunted from the periphery to the core to combat systemic hypothermia. Once skin temperature falls below 10°C (50°F), sensory loss (light touch, pain, temperature) follows. Deep frostbite may appear benign. Tissues with severe frostbite have a mottled, violaceous, pale yellow appearance. When the subcutaneous tissue maintains a soft, pliable character, a superficial injury is more likely. In addition, early formation of large clear blebs portends a more favorable prognosis than dark hemorrhagic blisters.

Treatment

The initial management of the *hypothermic* patient starts with the *ABCs*. Contrary to some teachings, there is no evidence that intubation is detrimental to the hypothermic patient. All hypothermic patients require 100% supplemental oxygen (administer heated, humidified oxygen). When asystole or v-fib appears on the cardiac monitor along with an absence of central pulses, institute CPR. CPR is not needed, even in the absence of pulses, if the patient has a viable rhythm. Remove clothing and cover the patient with warm, dry blankets. The cold myocardium may be resistant to defibrillation and pharmacological interventions. Attempt defibrillation once at 2 W·sec/kg, up to 200 W·sec/kg. If defibrillation is unsuccessful, initiate CPR, and delay the next defibrillation attempt until patient's core temperature is above 30°C (86°F). *Bretylium* (5 to 10 mg/kg IV) is possibly an effective antiarrhythmic in the setting of hypothermia and v-fib.

For the hypotensive hypothermic patient, assume fluid depletion; administer normal saline warmed to 40 to 42°C (104 to 108°F) in the microwave. Give intravenous $D_{50}W$ (50 mL), thiamine (100 mg), and naloxone (2 mg) as indicated. Limit the amount of movement and stimulation of the moderately or severely hypothermic patient. Intubation and cardiac monitoring are relatively harmless if done cautiously. If a central venous catheter is essential, avoid contact with heart. Foley catheters and nasogastric tubes are generally considered safe.

For patients who are hypothermic but hemodynamically stable with temperatures above >32°C (90.5°F), *passive external rewarming* is sufficient. Remove wet clothing, and insulate the patient with blankets. *Active external rewarming* (AER) entails the external application of heat to the patient via radiant heating lights, heating blankets, warm water immersion, etc. For patients with severe hypothermia (temperature < 27°C, or 0.6°F) or those with cardiovascular instability, it is generally recommended that *active core rewarming* (ACR) techniques be used. ACR includes inhalation of heated humidified oxygen; use of warmed intravenous fluids; heated irrigation of the peritoneum (peritoneal lavage with 2 L of dialysate heated to 40 to 42°C), thorax (thoracostomy tube irrigation with warm sterile saline), and GI tract; and extracorporeal warming. Extracorporeal warming with cardiopulmonary bypass provides the most efficient core rewarming (can increase core temperate by 1 to 2°C every 5 min) and is the procedure of choice, when accessible, for patients in cardiac arrest or those with temperatures < 27°C in extremis. Failure of a patient to rewarm quickly (at least 1°F/hr) suggests underlying illness or disease. Standard criteria of death do not apply to the hypothermic patient unless the temperature is above 32°C (90°F). Resuscitative efforts must be aggressive until the temperature is ≥ 32°C (90°F). Early work suggests that an elevated serum potassium (K > 10 meq/L) implies irreversible cell death and a poor prognosis.

Once hypothermia is corrected, attention can be directed to treating any *frostbite injuries.* Rapid rewarming of the frozen extremity in a circulating warm (40 to 42°C) water bath is ideal. *It is essential to avoid partial thawing and refreezing of extremity.* A common error is to prematurely terminate rewarming. Reestablishment of perfusion to the affected extremity is frequently accompanied by severe pain, necessitating parenteral analgesia. Tetanus prophylaxis should be provided if necessary. Tissues must be handled gently, avoiding compressive dressings. Further therapy should be discussed with the consultant.

Admission Criteria

Patients with *moderate to severe hypothermia* (< 30°C) obligate admission, usually to a monitored bed (especially if there is cardiovascular instability, metabolic derangement, or a complicating illness). Hospitalization is indicated for *all but the most mild cases of frostbite.* Patients with mild primary hypothermia (30 to 32°C) who promptly respond to rewarming measures, are free of underlying disease and complications, have been properly observed, and possess adequate social support may be discharged with appropriate cautions.

Suggested Readings

Danzl DF, Pozos RS: Accidental hypothermia. N Engl J Med 1994;331: 1756–1760.

Delaney KA, Howland MA, Vassallo S, et al.: Assessment of acid-base disturbances and their physiologic consequences. Ann Emerg Med 1989;18:72–82.

18.3 NEAR DROWNING

Description

Drowning victims die from suffocation subsequent to submersion in a liquid medium; if the victim survives the initial insult then a *near drowning* is said to have occurred. *Secondary* drowning depicts mortality taking place minutes to days following the initial recovery from the original event. Hypoxia associated with drowning or near drowning is usually due to aspiration of fluids (*wet* drowning) in 80% of cases; however, 20% of victims develop laryngospasm and never aspirate water (*dry* drowning). The resultant hypoxia following both fresh water and saltwater submersion leads to intrapulmonary shunting, decreased lung compliance, and $\dot{V}/\dot{Q}$ mismatches. Hypothermia may accompany submersion episodes and influences treatment and outcome. Case reports recount situations in which neurologically intact survival has followed prolonged submersion in cold water.

History

Presentation is highly variable; from the asymptomatic patient, to the restless patient complaining of dyspnea and chest pain, to the patient with frank cardiopulmonary arrest. Significant facts include the length of time submerged, water temperature, and type of water. Additional information should include any trauma (diving accident), use of drugs or alcohol, and underlying medical problems (seizure disorder, cardiac disease). Consider possible suicide attempt. Inquire about initial assessment and treatment at the scene (EMT, bystanders).

Physical Examination

Vital signs. Spontaneous respirations after resuscitation are a reliable predictor for neurologically intact survival from near drowning. A core temperature is imperative in all near drowning victims, as prolonged resuscitation efforts may be obligatory. Remember that the initial appearance of near-drowning patients can be deceptively benign.

HEENT. Look for signs of trauma.

Neck. Maintain cervical spine immobilization until radiography is available if trauma is suspected.

Lungs. Note presence, extent, and quality of breath sounds.

Extremities. Look for obvious deformities or needle tracks.

Neurologic. Classification scales for both assessment and prognosis have been developed for the near-drowning victim (Table 18.3.1)

Diagnostic Tests

Radiology. A baseline CXR is required in all near-drowning victims. In any patient with a history of trauma or altered mental status, C-spine injury should be suspected. Additional films should be guided by the history and physical exam.

ABG. Generally required on all near-drowning victims to ascertain oxygenation and acid-base status.

Pulse oximetry. Provides continuous monitoring of oxygenation.

ECG. Indicated in all class B and C patients and any class A patient with findings that suggest cardiac disease.

Blood counts and chemistries. While there are no abnormalities specific for near drowning, *a lab stick for glucose, CBC, serum chemistries, coagulation profile, urinalysis,* and *toxicological studies* (including alcohol level) are warranted in all class B and C patients.

Table 18.3.1
ABC Classification of Near-Drowning Victims

Class	Glasgow Coma Scale	Description	Prognosis
A (alert)	15	Alert, fully conscious	Near 100% survival
B (blunted)	9–13	Stuporous, but responds to painful stimulation; respirations normal	90% neurologically intact survival
C (comatose)	6–8	Comatose, not rousable to pain; respirations usually abnormal	Approximately 70% survival
C-1	5	Decorticate posturing	Approximately 50% chance of neurologically intact survival
C-2	4	Decerebrate, extensor response with hyperventilation and dilated pupils	< 50% chance of neurologically intact survival
C-3	3	No response to pain, flaccid; respirations absent	< 5%

Special Considerations

Although there are no absolute prognostic indicators for survival from near drowning, factors predicting an unfavorable outcome include submersion time > 5 min, no resuscitation efforts for > 10 min, CPR required in ED, Glasgow coma score < 3, and arterial pH < 7.1.

Treatment

Aggressive treatment of hypoxia is the key to management of near-drowning victims. Early use of endotracheal intubation (with C-spine precautions) allows both protection of the airway from aspiration and the ability to deliver high oxygen concentrations. In addition, positive end expiratory pressure (PEEP) may be necessary to achieve a PaO_2 > 60 mm Hg. For awake patients, oxygen can be supplemented with a face mask and continuous positive airway pressure (CPAP) if necessary. For patients without a pulse and respiration, CPR should be initiated.

Hypothermia should be treated as outlined in section 18.2.

Prophylactic steroids or antibiotics have not been found to be beneficial. Bronchodilators (albuterol) may be advantageous in treating bronchospasm. Severe metabolic acidosis (pH < 7.1) may obligate the use of sodium bicarbonate. If aspiration of large particulate matter is suspected, bronchoscopy may be required.

Invasive monitoring may be necessary to determine fluid balance. An indwelling Foley catheter and nasogastric tube are helpful in managing symptomatic patients.

Admission Criteria

All symptomatic patients require admission and at least 24 hr of supplemental oxygenation and observation. Asymptomatic patients may be discharged if they remain symptom-free after 6 to 8 hr of observation, the repeat CXR and ABGs are acceptable, they are reliable, and close follow-up is available.

Suggested Readings

Modell JH: Drownings. N Engl J Med 1993;328:253–256.
Olshaker JS: Near drowning. Emerg Med Clin 1992;10:339–350.

Chapter 19

Psychiatry

19.1 MEDICAL EVALUATION OF PSYCHIATRIC PATIENTS

Description

The emergency medical evaluation of an acutely disturbed patient is one of the most demanding assignments. The emergency physician must have an unusual amount of skill, patience, and concern for these patients. All too often, "medical clearances" are perfunctory and superficial because of the aversion that many doctors have toward people who act "crazy." Up to 80% of patients who are deemed to be medically clear from the ED are later found to have organic factors that should have been detected on the initial assessment.

The psychiatric patient is no different from any other ED patient; the history and physical examination are especially meaningful in determining a working diagnosis and developing a plan of action. In the absence of a life-threatening problem, ruling out organic disease is the first task in assessing the patient, not only because the medical problem may be the cause of the behavioral disturbance but also because the medical disease may go undetected and untreated if the patient is confined in a psychiatric facility. The most commonly encountered problems include infection; pulmonary, gastrointestinal, or neurologic disease; malignancy; drug toxicity or reaction; drug or alcohol withdrawal; and trauma.

History

Ask the patient to describe the current problem; inquire about hallucinations and suicidal or homicidal thoughts. Comments from family members, friends, paramedics, and police who have had contact with the patient are helpful, especially in patients who are acting violent or bizarre. The history should include a description of the current episode and its duration, past psychiatric history, past medical history (including any hospitalizations or ongoing medical problems), current medications (if possible check medication containers), history of drug or alcohol abuse, allergies, and a brief review of systems.

Physical Examination

General. Note if the patient is agitated, confused, depressed, or lethargic. Examine the patient's posture and grooming. Inform the patient about what you are going to do and then proceed confidently. Advance through the exam, starting with the most nonthreatening evaluations first, deferring potentially embarrassing or painful parts of the exam to the end.

Vital signs. Pay particular attention; any abnormality must be addressed.

Skin. Examine for warmth, moisture, rashes, bruising, texture, and turgor.

HEENT. Search for signs of head trauma. Examine EOMs, pupillary responses, and the presence of nystagmus (vertical nystagmus is seen with certain drug ingestions and cerebellar problems). Perform a careful fundiscopic examination. Tongue lacerations may imply seizure. Note any abnormal breath odors. Check for dry mucous membranes (suggest dehydration), jaw spasm (associated with extrapyramidal side effects of neuroleptics and related medications), and lingual and facial grimacing (may also be a late complication of neuroleptic therapy).

Neck. Note presence of rigidity or *torticollis* (twisting motions of the neck that suggest dystonic reactions). Evaluate for thyroid enlargement.

Chest. Barrel-shaped appearance may indicate underlying COPD. Carefully auscultate for signs of pneumonia or pulmonary edema.

Heart. Identify presence of abnormal and irregular sounds.

Abdomen. Palpate and inspect for tenderness, hepatosplenomegaly, masses, scars, or self-inflicted wounds.

Rectal. Check stool for occult blood and evaluate the prostate gland (hypertrophy, nodules).

Extremities. Look for any signs of trauma (including self-inflicted wounds), track marks, skin ulcers, and rashes.

Neurologic. Perform a thorough examination, including assessment of cranial nerves, sensory, motor, cerebellar function, and gait. Check for deep tendon reflexes. Search for characteristic findings (resting tremor, shuffling gait, cogwheel rigidity of extremities) that tend to support an adverse drug effect. In addition, test for abnormal reflexes (snout and grasp) and asterixis. *Any abnormal or focal finding must be presumed due to an organic problem.*

Mental status. In addition to orientation to person, place, and time, a basic mental status examination consists of five customary areas: (1) general appearance and behavior of the patient, (2) stream of conversation (both structure and content), (3) intellectual function (short- and long-term memory, judgment capacity), (4) patient's mood (depressed, manic), and (5) mental content (Table 19.1.1). The *Folstein Mini-Mental Status Examination* is a good screening test of sensorium, incorporating tests of attention, memory, cognition, and constructional ability as well as language.

Diagnostic Tests

The use of ancillary tests can be helpful in confirming an organic disorder underlying a behavioral disturbance.

CBC. Presence of anemia implies possible impairment of oxygen delivery and suggests potential underlying organic problems (vitamin B_{12} or folate deficiency). Leucocytosis may be associated with infection or leukoplastic disease.

SMA. Look for alterations in blood glucose, serum sodium, calcium, renal failure, and liver function.

ABG. Check for *hypoxia, CO_2 retention,* and acidosis.

Toxicology. Order on an as-needed basis (alcohol, lithium, digoxin, aspirin, acetaminophen, antiepileptic drugs).

ECG. Useful in older patients (where MI can present as altered mental status) and patients suspected of electrolyte disorders or ingestion of tricyclic antidepressants.

Urinalysis. Look for evidence of UTI.

Lumbar puncture. Indicated when meningitis or subarachnoid hemorrhage (first ensure that there is no evidence of focal deficits or increased intracranial pressure) is suspected.

CXR. Often useful to screen for both cardiac (cardiomegaly) and respiratory diseases (pneumonia, TB).

Table 19.1.1
Mental Status Examination

Condition	Comments
	MENTATION
Delirium	The most common; note clouding consciousness, perceptual disturbances (illusion, hallucinations), incoherent speech, increased or decreased psychomotor activity, disorientation, and memory impairment; usually acute and has a waxing and waning course
Dementia	Includes progressive loss of intellectual abilities, impaired judgment, and other disturbances of cortical functioning (e.g., aphasia, apraxia, agnosia, constructional difficulty, personality change); the state of consciousness is not clouded; usually chronic; mental status is static (does not wax and wane); memory deficit and a loss of cognitive ability are prominent
Organic personality disorder	Seen with psychomotor epilepsy, frontal lobe lesions, and metabolic disturbances (uremia, hypercalcemia, and hypoxia); a marked change in behavior associated with emotional lability, impairment of impulse control, marked apathy or indifference, suspiciousness, or paranoid ideation
Hallucination and delusions	Note the presence or absence of auditory, visual, tactile, or other types of hallucinations and paranoid or grandiose delusions.
	MEMORY
Short-term memory	Test with five unrelated objects; go over them with the patient until he or she can repeat them; ask for recall 5 min later
Long-term memory	Test by asking about famous people or events compatible with the patient's education and cultural background
	OTHER
Attention	Ask the patient to repeat progressively increasing consecutive digits
Affect	Note any evidence of alteration of mood, inability to control emotions, or inappropriate affect
Cognitive ability	Ask patients to do serial subtraction of 7 from 100; try to tailor the intellectual task to the patient's educational level
Orientation	Test orientation to time (year, month, day of the week, date), place, and person
Construction and naming	Test the patient's ability to copy a star, triangle, and cross (nondominant hemisphere) and to name simple objects (dominant hemisphere)

Abdominal films. Request if you suspect foreign body ingestion, obstruction, or perforation.

CT of head. May be indicated when head trauma or intracranial mass is suspected and with focal neurologic findings.

Additional laboratory tests. The following tests may be germane in the appropriate clinical setting: blood cultures, serum ammonia, ESR, osmolality, serum ketones, VDRL, and endocrine studies (especially thyroid fucntion tests).

Special Considerations

The first step in the differential diagnosis is determining if the problem is *organic* or *functional.* Any potentially *life-threatening disorder* (meningitis, encephalitis, hypoglycemia, hypertensive encephalopathy, hypoxia, poisonings, cardiac, pulmonary disease, intracranial hemorrhage, Wernicke's encephalopathy) needs to be promptly identified and addressed. It is the task of the emergency physician to exclude organic disorders before labeling a patient with a functional diagnosis.

Characteristics supporting an organic etiology include abrupt onset, onset after age 40, visual or tactile hallucinations, underlying medical disorder, substance abuse, abnormal vital signs, and impaired cognitive ability or loss of recent memory. *Characteristics supporting a functional disorder* include gradual onset, onset before age 40, auditory hallucinations, previous psychiatric history, normal vital signs, alteration in mood, and delusions or bizarre thinking with intact cognition.

Treatment

As for any patient, the initial focus is on stabilization and treatment of underlying condition. For behavioral control, see section 19.2.

Admission Criteria

Disposition of the patient with a behavioral disturbance is predicated on the nature and duration of the underlying illness, i.e., *patients with an organic cause for their disturbance of mental status* obligate admission to the appropriate service. *Certain functional disturbances* may also call for admission (acute psychosis, mania, suicidal or homicidal ideation, demented patients unable to care for themselves, catatonia, and severe depression). *If the etiology re-*

mains unclear, the patient should be admitted (general medicine or neurology) for further evaluation.

Many patients with a psychobehavioral disturbance will not be amenable to treatment or admission. In most cases, physicians must obtain an informed and voluntary consent for medical treatment. Most patients have the right to refuse treatment, unless they are suicidal or their judgment is impaired. There are several exceptions (see section 20.4). In a true emergency, where time is of the essence, the emergency physician may obtain either *substituted consent* (next of kin, designated person) or may act under the principal of *presumed consent.* Other exceptions are patients who are judged incompetent or incapable to accept or refuse treatment. Psychiatric consultation should be sought, and the need for involuntary commitment must be discussed.

Suggested Readings

Bauer J, Roberts MR, Reisdorff EJ: Evaluation of behavioral and cognitive changes: the mental status examination. Emerg Med Clin North Am 1991;9:1–12.

Riba M, Hale M: Medical clearance: fact or fiction in the hospital emergency room? Psychosomatics 1990;31:400–404.

Tintanelli JE, Peacock FW, Wright MA: Emergency medical evaluation of psychiatric patients. Ann Emerg Med 1994;23:859–862.

19.2 THE VIOLENT PATIENT

Description

Violent patients are encountered with regularity in the ED. Some are brought in by family or police because of acts or threats of violence outside the hospital, and others may become violent during their course of stay in the ED. Medical staff must be prepared to deal with violent patients quickly and effectively to prevent physical harm to the patient, staff, and other patients. Once the patient is under control, the task is to recognize any possible underlying cause of the disturbance.

Contrary to popular belief, acute psychosis is not the cause of most episodes of violent behavior. Specific causes of violent behavior include *drug intoxication* or *withdrawal, metabolic disturbances* (especially hypoglycemia), *infection* (sepsis, meningitis, encephalitis), *organ failure* (hypoxia, hepatic, renal failure), *environmental emergencies* (heat stroke), *seizures, CNS trauma, tumor, acute psychosis* (paranoid schizophrenia, bipolar disorders), *be-*

havioral disorders (manipulative, antisocial, borderline personalities), and *acute situational crises* (domestic dispute, unemployment, gang-related activity).

History

Every effort must be made to ensure that a serious or life-threatening disorder is not responsible for the violent behavior. There is no substitute for an adequate history, physical examination, and mental status examination (see section 19.1). The history should focus on the acuity of the violent behavior, including its onset and duration. Ask about associated symptoms (disorientation, hallucinations, delusions, memory or thought problems). The single most important predictor of future violence is the patient's history of violent behavior (check patient's old records). High-risk patients tend to be young adult males 15 to 40 years old.

Physical Examination

General. Behavioral clues to a potentially violent patient include posture for tension (poised for flight or fight), speech (loud, profane, pressured speech), and excessive motor activity (angry gestures, restlessness, or pacing).

Vital signs. A good rule of thumb is that *if the patient is not calm enough to obtain accurate vital signs, further measures will be necessary to control the situation.*

Diagnostic Tests

See section 19.1.

Treatment

The number one priority of the emergency physician is to ensure the safety of the staff and patient. Only after the situation is controlled will the emergency caretaker be able to attempt to identify the presumptive etiology and initiate any treatment that may be required.

It may be possible to defuse a potentially violent situation without resorting to chemical or physical restraints. Verbal techniques can be helpful. Refer to patients respectfully. Allow the patient to vent their anger and frustration. Strive to form an alliance with the patient; act as the patient's advocate, empathize with realistic problems. Offer the patient food or drink but avoid hot liquids (coffee) because they can be used as weapon against you. Avoid escalating the situation by getting into a shouting match or threatening the patient. Speak in a confident, nonjudgmental, controlled manner. Reduce environmental stimuli. Enlist the aid of family, friends, or patient representatives.

Certain basic rules should guide all encounters with potentially violent patients: (1) define acceptable and nonacceptable behavior; (2) leave the door open; (3) never turn your back on the patient; (4) never place a patient between you and the door, provide a means of escape for yourself; and (5) ensure that adequate assistance is available (notify security personnel) and that the staff is aware of the potential for violence. Ask the patient if he or she is carrying a weapon. If the patient is armed, do not try to take any weapon directly from him or her; notify hospital police or security and attempt to have patient voluntarily surrender arms. Often the best way to deal with potential violence is to prevent any such situation from occurring. Many hospitals in urban areas have adopted the use of permanent and hand-held metal detectors. When weapons are found they are confiscated by security personnel.

Although communicating with the patient should always be tried initially, a significant subset of violent patients may be beyond the reach of verbal control. While competent patients have the right to refuse treatment, case law has reinforced the right and duty of emergency personnel to detain and restrain individuals who may pose a danger to themselves or others. Never attempt to subdue a patient alone. If you feel yourself being threatened or your personal discomfort increases, stop the interview process immediately. If the patient continues to threaten staff, mobilize a security team. Ideally, the team will have five members: one member is assigned to each limb and a team leader takes the head (if the patient is female, one member of the team ought to be a female).The team leader should make one request to the patient to cooperate with the placement of restraints. If the patient refuses, the patient is approached from two sides. Each limb (grab arms at elbows and legs at knees) and the head are restrained, with the patient being secured to the stretcher. It is best to use padded restraints and place the patient in a lateral decubitus position to help prevent aspiration. Do not forget to document both the orders for restraints and the indications for them. Check the patient immediately after he or she is restrained for injuries and periodically reexamine the patient, verifying the neurovascular status of the extremities and the overall state of the patient. Document fully the reasons for the restraints and the specific orders in the chart.

In general, patients who remain combative will require chemical restraint. Rapid tranquilization can be accomplished with benzodiazepines and/or neuroleptics. Oral medications can be offered to the patient. However, if the patient refuses oral medication, be prepared to administer injectable agents. *Haloperidol* is the most commonly used agent for rapid tranquilization of the violent patient. It can be given orally, intramuscularly, or intravenously (not FDA approved for intravenous use). The dosage of haloperidol is titrated to patient response; an initial dose of 5 to 10 mg is acceptable in previously healthy, young adults, while elderly patients should receive 1 to 2 mg boluses. The dose can be repeated every 30 to 60 min, up to three times. The most frequent undesirable side effect of haloperidol is acute dystonia (see section 19.5). *Lorazepam,* a benzodiazepine, has been used alone and in combination with haloperidol. It is the preferred agent when the cause of violence is thought to be drug withdrawal or intoxication. The usual initial dose is 2 mg (IV or IM) in adults, repeated every 30 to 60 min, up to a 5- to 6-mg total dose. *Alprazolam* (1 mg PO q 2 hr, up to 4 mg) is an alternative benzodiazepine that may be effective in the management of psychiatric emergencies. *Droperidol* (1 to 2 mg IV q 20 to 30 min) may also be employed to sedate the violent patient.

Admission Criteria

In general, *patients who specifically threaten harm to themselves or someone else, are floridly psychotic, or are suspected of having an organic basis to violence* necessitate hospitalization. If the patient is considered dangerous and refuses admission, he or she ought to be held involuntarily (all states allow a mental health hold) for evaluation by psychiatry. In addition, emergency physicians have a duty to warn potential victims of violence. If a patient escapes or cannot be held, the police should be notified.

Suggested Readings

Dubin WR, Feld JA: Rapid tranquilization of the violent patient. Am J Emerg Med 1989;7:313–320.

MacPherson DS, Lofgren RP, Granieri R, et al.: Deciding to restrain medical patients. J Am Geriatr Soc 1990;38:516–620.

19.3 THE SUICIDAL PATIENT

Description

Suicide is the tenth leading cause of death in the United States. Males complete suicide attempts 4 times more often than females, although females attempt suicide (gesture) 10 times more frequently than males. There is also an increased risk of suicide in the elderly. Besides age and sex, other factors relating to likelihood of suicide include history of mental illness or symptoms of major depression, use of alcohol or drugs, chronic illness or disability, tenuous economic status, family history of suicide or suicide attempt, and lack of social supports (separated, widowed, divorced, no close family or friends).

History

It is the task of the emergency physician to assess both the possibility and the level of risk for suicide. The threat of suicide should always be considered an emergent problem and not dismissed. Subtle clues to suicide potential include single vehicle, single driver accidents; high-risk behavior; unclear reasons for seeking medical care; family or friends noting marked change in personality; and victims of violence. In assessing the patient's risk, the interviewer needs to ask frank questions, from assessing feelings of depression to specifically asking the patient if he or she is having suicidal thoughts. It is much more dangerous not to ask and to overlook suicidal depression.

Determine the seriousness of the suicide attempt. Violent acts (self-inflicted gunshots, stabbing) indicate a serious suicidal attempt. Assess the three P's: premeditation, plan, and probability of rescue. Corroborating history from family, friends, and private physicians will be helpful in judging risk.

Physical Examination

See section 19.1.

Diagnostic Tests

See section 19.1.

Treatment

Stabilize the patient's condition. Never leave the patient alone. The suicidal patient must be observed closely at all times while in the ED, not only to prevent self-injury but also to prevent elopement from the hospital. Ensure that no potentially dangerous objects (including matches) are on the person or left in the room. The patient should be accompanied when using the bathroom.

Be nonjudgmental and concerned. Do not reprimand the patient. Emphasize the fact that family and friends and the medical staff are supportive. Allow family and friends to speak to patient. Permit the patient to vent feelings of unhappiness, as this may defuse suicidal energy.

Notify the primary therapist. If the patient is in therapy, the primary therapist should be contacted as soon as possible and is often able to offer valuable insight into acute management.

Avoid sedation. Generally, sedatives should not be given to patients with drug overdoses or intoxications (exceptions include severe sympathomimetic, PCP, hallucinogenic overdoses). Patients who are violent or combative may require rapid tranquilization (see section 19.2).

Consult a psychiatrist as soon as possible. No potentially suicidal patient should leave the ED without a psychiatric consult. All attempts and gestures must be taken seriously. Patients with an altered mental status and those with homicidal or suicidal tendencies should be held, against their will if necessary, until they are evaluated by a psychiatrist.

Admission Criteria

The decision to admit a suicidal patient is usually made by a psychiatrist. However, on occasion, a suicidal patient obligates admission to a medical or surgical service because of *complications of the suicide attempt.* These patients should be carefully evaluated for suicidal potential before leaving the ED. Patients who are judged to be seriously suicidal or whose suicidal risk cannot be judged with certainty (comatose patients) should have arrangements made for continuous observation at all times while hospitalized.

Suggested Readings

Hockberger RS, Rothstein RJ: Assessment of suicide potential by nonpsychiatrists using the SAD PERSON'S score. J Emerg Med 1988;6: 99–107.

Hoffman DP, Dubovsky SL: Depression and suicide assessment. Emerg Med Clin North Am 1991;9:107–122.

19.4 ORGANIC BRAIN SYNDROMES

Description

Delirium and *dementia* are both classified as organic brain syndromes, arising from a primary brain disturbance or as a secondary manifestation of an underlying disorder. *Delirium* is characterized as an acute, transient confusional state, and *dementia* is considered an acquired loss of cognitive function. The emergency physician is frequently called on to differentiate between patients with chronic, irreversible causes of impaired intellectual function (Alzheimer's) from those with a treatable, reversible etiology. Failure to recognize potentially correctable states of confusion can result in irrevocable brain damage and even death. Delirium is a symptom, not a disease, and may arise from multiple causes (see Table 19.4.1).

The prevalence of dementia increases after age 65 years (affecting 5 to 10% of patients), reaching a peak of 30 to 40% in per-

Table 19.4.1
Causes of Delirium

Metabolic (hypoglycemia, diabetic ketoacidosis, nonketotic hyperosmolarity)
Hypoxia (MI, pneumonia, pulmonary embolus, COPD)
Infection (meningitis, encephalitis, pneumonia, sepsis)
Low cardiac output states (MI, arrhythmia, CHF)
Seizure disorders (postictal, temporal lobe states)
Intracranial hemorrhage or ischemia (subdural hematoma, SAH, CVA, TIA)
Uremia and dialysis syndromes
Hypertensive and hepatic encephalopathy
Acute intoxication
- Alcohol
- Illicit drugs (cocaine, amphetamines, LSD)
- Prescribed medications (digitalis, antihypertensives anticholinergics, antidepressants, anticonvulsants, corticosteroids, cimetidine)
- Poisons (carbon monoxide, organophosphates, heavy metals)
- Over-the-counter medications (antihistamines, decongestants, diet or weight loss drugs)[a]

Acute withdrawal (alcohol, sedative-hypnotics)
Miscellaneous
- Hypothermia or hyperthermia
- Autoimmune disorders (SLE, polyarteritis nodosa)
- Endocrine disorders (Addison's, hypothyroidism or hyperthyroidism, hypocalcemia or hypercalcemia, porphyria).

[a]Polypharmacy is especially a problem in the elderly.

sons older than 80 years. Primary degenerative (Alzheimer's) and atherosclerotic (multiinfarct) dementia are the most common chronic causes. Reversible causes of dementia are listed in Table 19.4.2. In addition, delirium may be superimposed on dementia.

History

The chief complaint usually involves some disturbance in cognition, behavior, memory, or intellectual function. Employ all available sources when obtaining a history (family, caretakers, old records). The bedside evaluation includes a careful review of previous medical and psychiatric evaluations (baseline), prior trauma (head injuries, elder abuse), underlying illness, medications, and social history (alcohol, drug abuse, living situation).

Symptoms that suggest *delirium* include a rapid evolution of symptoms (hours to days), fluctuating mental state (lucid intervals), impairment of short-term memory, hallucinations (especially visual or tactile hallucinations), presence of a significant underlying illness (AIDS, hypertension, diabetes mellitus, cancer), age < 65 years, and no previous psychiatric history. *Dementia* is more likely in elderly patients and is associated with a more protracted onset of symptoms (months), impairment of long-term memory, auditory hallucinations, and previous history of altered mental status.

Table 19.4.2
Reversible Causes of Dementia

A useful mnemonic for recalling the reversible basis of dementia is the term DEMENTIA.

- D Drug toxicity (psychoactive drugs, sedatives, hypnotics, anti-Parkinson drugs)
- E Emotional disorders (so-called pseudo-dementia, i.e., major depression)
- M Metabolic and endocrine disturbances (hypoglycemia, myxedema, hyperosmolar states, electrolyte imbalances, hepatic encephalopathy)
- E Eyes and ears (visual and hearing disorders)
- N Nutritional disorders (B12, folate, thiamine) and normal pressure hydrocephalus
- T Tumors (primary or metastatic neoplasms) and trauma (subdural)
- I Infection (meningitis, encephalitis, pneumonia, tertiary syphilis)
- A Atherosclerotic complications (strokes, TIAs, MI, CHF)

Physical Examination

Note: *Physical findings are highly variable and reflect the cause.* Particular emphasis is placed on the general appearance, vital signs, neurologic examination, and mental status.

General. Observe overall appearance (sick, cachectic) and behavior (agitation, somnolent), and look for signs of autonomic dysfunction (diaphoresis, dilated pupils).

Vital signs. Any abnormality (fever, tachycardia, hypertension) should prompt an attentive search for underling illness.

Neurologic. Note gross abnormalities (tremors, ataxia, myoclonic jerking, asterixis), and conduct careful motor, sensory, reflex, cerebellar, and gait examinations.

Mental status. In differentiating delirium from dementia a key clinical finding is the patient's state of arousal. The demented person generally has a consistent pattern of response to attention, while the patient with delirium has a variable level of response.

Diagnostic Tests

Use a tiered approach; first screening for major physiologic derangement (lab stick for glucose, pulse oximetry, CBC, serum electrolytes, glucose, BUN, creatinine, calcium, ECG, CXR, ABG). Further testing (CT scan of head, lumbar puncture, liver function tests, toxicological screens, VDRL, thyroid studies) is guided by subsequent findings on the clinical examination and initial laboratory studies.

Treatment

Initial assessment and management should proceed as any other medical emergency, with foremost attention and support to the ABCs in urgent and emergent cases. Hypoglycemia must always be considered, with either a bedside test being performed or the empirical administration of glucose being provided. Thiamine should be given if the etiology is unclear or there is a history of alcoholism. Give antibiotics whenever meningitis is considered. Treat the underlying cause if possible.

In cases of extreme agitation and disturbances in behavior, the patient may need to be restrained to avoid harming himself or herself or others. Be cautious when deciding whether or not to medicate a patient, as this may further confuse the clinical picture.

Admission Criteria

The majority of patients with delirium have an acute medical disorder that will require hospitalization. Exceptions to this rule include the following:

- Postictal states in patients with known seizure disorders;
- Acute intoxication with alcohol or drugs; and
- Hypoglycemia in a diabetic with a clear etiology that is self-limited and not likely to recur (e.g., forgot to eat).

Patients with chronic dementia will require admission for the following:

- Dementia not worked up in past and outpatient work-up not possible;
- Acute medical illness that is causing deterioration of mental status; and
- Lack of necessary social supports (cannot continue to live alone, homeless).

Management of the chronically demented patient is generally a multidisciplinary endeavor, involving the medical doctor, psychiatrist, and social worker.

Suggested Readings

Eisdorfer C: Evaluation of the demented patient. Med Clin North Am 1994;78:773–784.

Tueth MJ: Diagnosing psychiatric emergencies in the elderly. Am J Emerg Med 1994;12:364–369.

19.5 EXTRAPYRAMIDAL REACTIONS

Description

Extrapyramidal reactions proceed from a disturbance in the balance between the dopaminergic and the cholinergic neurotransmitters, frequently leading to movement disorders. Adverse side effects due to neuroleptic agents are often related to drug dose and potency, occur more commonly in the elderly, and may present after a single dose or subsequent to chronic use.

Akathisia, or motor restlessness, is the most common extrapyramidal disorder due to psychotropic agents. Additional extrapyramidal disturbances include *akinesia* (a drug-induced Parkinson's disease), *tardive dysknesia* (involuntary, stereotyped movements, most often involving the mouth, tongue, and lips), *perioral tremor* (rabbit syndrome), and *acute dystonic reactions* (dyskinetic, involuntary, stereotyped, rhythmic, or bizarre muscle activity that occurs 48 to 72 hr after the initial dose of a neuroleptic-type drug) (Table 19.5.1).

Neuroleptic malignant syndrome (NMS) is the most serious complication resulting from use of antipsychotic-type drugs. It is characterized by an altered mental status, muscular rigidity, hyperthermia, and autonomic instability. NMS reactions are idiopathic and may occur anytime during neuroleptic treatment (even after the drug has been discontinued).

The differential diagnosis for extrapyramidal reactions includes conversion reaction, seizures, tetanus, black widow spider bites, cerebrovascular accidents, and idiopathic Parkinsonism.

History

Patients prescribed neuroleptic and related medications (primarily phenothiazine antiemetics) may present to the ED with a variety of short- and long-term side effects. Extrapyramidal symptoms include restlessness, tics, stiffness, tremor, postural instability, shuffling gait, disrupted speech, and difficulty swallowing (drooling) or chewing. Symptoms may become oppressive enough to be disabling. Acute dystonia can be quite frightening and uncomfortable for the patient. Patients may also complain of anticholinergic side effects (dry mouth, blurring of vision, sedation, urinary retention, menstrual cycle irregularities, gynecomastia, orthostatic hypotension, cognitive disturbances).

Physical Examination

Vital signs. Consider NMS when the temperature is elevated. (In an uncoopertaive patient, use a rectal probe.) Elevated heart

Table 19.5.1
Commonly Used Drugs and Toxins Capable of Causing Dystonic-Type Reactions[a]

Haloperidol and butyrophenones
Metoclopramide
Phenothiazines (chlorpromazine, prochlorperazine, fluphenazine)
Miscellaneous: PCP, strychnine, phenytoin, cocaine, lithium, MPTP

[a]Patients may come to the ED with a dystonic reaction attributed to street Valium; this usually turns out to be haloperidol or a phenothiazine. There appears to be a higher incidence of dystonic reactions in parenteral drug abusers.

rate, an alteration in blood pressure (hypotension or hypertension), or signs of autonomic instability (diaphoresis) exist. Ensure that respirations are adequate; a rare, but potentially fatal form of dystonic reaction is *acute laryngeal spasm,* in which spasms of the larynx and pharynx cause gagging, cyanosis, respiratory distress, and eventually asphyxia if not rapidly treated

Neurologic. The spectrum of dystonia includes oculogyric crisis; spasms of the jaw, tongue, and throat; torticollis (neck twisting); retrocollis; opisthotonos (extreme hyperextension of the spine); lingual and facial grimacing; and tortipelvis (abdominal wall spasm). Drug-induced Parkinsonism may present with bradykinesia, cogwheel rigidity, shuffling gait, tongue tremors, mask-like facies, and a resting tremor that may be unilateral.

Diagnostic Tests

Laboratory abnormalities associated with NMS include leukocytosis; hyperkalemia; myoglobinuria; and elevations in creatine kinase (CK), serum transaminases, lactic dehydrogenases, and alkaline phosphatases. Use of antipsychotic agents can lead to *agranulocytosis* (especially clozapine) and *hepatic dysfunction.*

Treatment

Initial management is focused on maintaining the airway and circulation, providing supplemental oxygen, and monitoring as needed. If a vasopressor is required to manage refractory phenothiazine-mediated hypotension, give fluids. Avoid epinephrine and dopamine (phenothiazines are potent α-adrenergic antagonists); instead employ *levarterenol* or phenylephrine. Consider decontamination measures when overdose is suspected.

Acute dystonic reactions respond rapidly to treatment with *diphenhydramine* (50 mg IV or IM) or *benztropine* (1 to 2 mg IV or IM). Benzodiazepines (diazepam, 0.1 mg/kg) are effective when anticholinergic agents have failed or in febrile patients who display impaired thermoregulatory control. If a patient fails to respond or exhibits only a partial response, the dose may be repeated in 15 to 30 min. Failure to respond to a second dose should make the ED physician highly suspicious of another disease process. Patients will need three days of oral therapy upon discharge, either *diphenhydramine* (50 mg PO QID), *benztropine* (1 to 2 mg PO BID), or *trihexyphenidyl* (5 mg PO BID). If the patient requires long-term therapy on neuroleptics, concomitant use of benztropine should be discussed with the primary physician.

Akathisia and *akinesia* may or may not respond to the addition of an anti-Parkinson agent. Options include administering a benzodiazepine, decreasing the dose of the neuroleptic agent, or changing to a different neuroleptic.

Currently, there is no definite effective therapy for *tardive dyskinesia.* Anticholinergic agents not only are useless but may worsen the patient's condition. Various drugs being studied include baclofen, benzodiazepines, levodopa, bromocriptine, and lithium.

Treatment for *NMS* must be prompt. After excluding other possible life-threatening etiologies, the management of NMS consists of supportive actions (protect the airway, maintain circulatory support, monitor for arrhythmias, check for hypoglycemia, etc.), rapid cooling measures (see section 18.1), arresting muscle hyperactivity (intravenous benzodiazepines), and discontinuing the neuroleptic agent. Two medications often used to relieve the symptoms of NMS are dantrolene and bromocriptine. However, neither of these agents has been shown to definitively alter either the severity or the duration of NMS. Do not use anticholinergics, as they may interfere with sweating and worsen hyperthermia.

Admission Criteria

Neuroleptic malignant syndrome is a life-threatening emergency (death is usually due to respiratory, renal, or cardiovascular complications), and NMS necessitates intensive-level care. In general, most other extrapyramidal reactions are readily managed in the ED and do not require admission. Before prescribing additional antipsychotic therapy or discontinuing any prescribed neuroleptic, discuss the case with the patient's personal physician or the consultant on call to the ED.

Suggested Readings

Lewin NA, Wang RY: Neuroleptic agents. In Goldfrank LR, Flomenbaum NE, Lewin NA, et al., eds. Goldfrank's toxicology, 5th ed. Norwalk, CT: Appleton & Lange, 1994;739–747.

Tueth MJ. Emergencies caused by side effects of psychiatric medications. Am J Emerg Med 1994;12:212–216.

Chapter 20

Social, Legal, and Ethical Issues

20.1 DOMESTIC VIOLENCE

Description

Domestic violence, a major public health disorder that has reached epidemic proportions, is characterized by coercive behavior that allows one person to dominate another to gain power and control over that other person's life. Physicians play a significant role in recognizing domestic violence and failure to do so results in the physician perpetuating the problem. Unfortunately, many of these relationships develop into the "battering syndrome." The battering syndrome includes repeated battering and injury; general medical complaints; psychological abuse; sexual assault; and progressive social isolation, deprivation, and intimidation.

The characteristic of power over and victimization of a less physically powerful individual by a physically more powerful person may explain why men more frequently batter women. It is known that men may be assaulted by women but this rarely, if ever, provokes a battered syndrome as seen in women. Although the gender-neutral term *spouse abuse* is often used, men commit 95% of all abuse. Women in the United States are more likely to be victimized through assault, battery, rape, or homicide by a current or former male partner than by all other assaults combined. Battering is the most common cause of injury to women, more common than auto accidents, muggings, and rape combined. It is estimated that every 7.4 sec a woman is beaten by her husband. It appears that women who try to escape their perpetrators by divorce or separation may heighten their risk for violence and homicide. Domestic violence is a global problem of both genders, involving all racial, ethnic, and socioeconomic backgrounds.

The battering syndrome as defined involves a history of abuse and injury with unsuccessful help seeking, along with sexual assault, general medical illnesses, and serious psychosocial problems. The extent of injury is often minor and only 4% of domestic violence injuries require hospitalization. It is the accumulation of repetitive ED visits that is the usual hallmark of domestic violence. The injury pattern is to the central areas of the body. Although injury is common in most cases, it may actually be only a small part of the pathological profile. Between 20 and 45% of all injured women who present to the ED are physically abused. These repeated episodes of injury and other abuses (e.g., psychological, emotional) lead to a posttraumatic syndrome, which presents itself clinically with a host of somatic complaints.

History

A battered woman coming to the ED has just been severely traumatized and is in physical and emotional pain. She often feels shame and fears ridicule and humiliation if she admits being beaten by her husband or boyfriend. She may feel guilty, believing that she was responsible for the beating (e.g., dinner wasn't ready, the kids were crying). She may have been threatened with further violence if she tells the truth. ED staff not only must maintain a high index of suspicion but must also question the patient gently. Patterns of injury or behavior that suggest battering include the following.

Multiple trauma to the trunk. Most accidental trauma involves the extremities. In addition, there are very few ways other than assault to sustain injuries to multiple sites, particularly bilateral injuries.

History that does not explain the injury. An explanation that does not adequately explain an injury should be considered suspicious for battering (e.g., a black eye from falling down stairs).

Frequent ED visits. Battered women often have a record of repeated visits for minor injuries or seemingly insignificant medical complaints.

Late presentation of injuries. Battered women are often prevented from seeking medical care after a beating and may present later than might reasonably have been expected.

Pregnancy. Battering often begins or escalates during pregnancy, and a pregnant woman who is injured or complains of abdominal pain or bleeding may have been beaten. Battered women have a higher frequency of spontaneous abortion than other women.

Aggressive male companion. A battered woman is often brought to the ED by her batterer, who is frightened both that he may have seriously injured her and that she may implicate him. An aggressive, "overprotective" male companion who insists on giving the history or refuses to leave the room should be viewed with suspicion.

Attempted suicide. A battered woman may be extremely depressed and see no other solution.

Depression and drug abuse. Repeated abuse will lead to depression and loss of self-respect, and the battered woman may seek escape through drug or alcohol abuse.

Somatic complaints. Such complaints as insomnia, vague stomach or chest pain, dysphagia, or hyperventilation may reflect a constant state of fear and anxiety.

Physical Examination

General. The woman may be agitated, hysterical, or fearful.

Vital signs. Note hyperventilation or tachycardia.

Skin. Note location and size of traumatic lesions.

HEENT. Examine skull for evidence of trauma, raccoon eyes, and Battle's sign.

Abdomen. Examine abdomen carefully for tenderness. Examine for tenderness over the spleen gently (splenic trauma).

Pelvic. Should be done in all women complaining of vaginal bleeding or sexual assault.

Extremities. Check for sprains, dislocations, burns, and fractures.

Diagnostic Tests

Dictated by clinical findings; be alert for concealed injuries. Photographs are very helpful to document the extent of injuries.

Treatment

The interview process is an extremely important component of the ED visit. The patient must be interviewed alone, without her partner present. Questioning should be supportive and generalized, as if part of your routine. Some examples of recommended questions are the following:

"I noticed that you have a number of bruises. We see bruises like this in cases of personal injury. Could someone be doing this to you?"

"Are you in a relationship in which you have been physically hurt or threatened by your partner?"

"Many patients tell me they have been hurt by someone close to them. Has this happened to you?"

"Has any household member hurt you or threatened you?"

Establishing a multidisciplinary team in the ED provides for a systematic and thorough approach. Nurses, social workers, crisis intervention teams, psychiatric staff members, hospital security, clergy, and volunteers are all essential components. The team's primary goal is to provide support, safety, and privacy while the physician does a complete assessment. There are seven roles and responsibilities for the physician and the ED staff:

1. Establish a positive environment.
2. Examine and identify possible abuse.
3. Provide emotional and social assessment.
4. Treat injuries appropriately.
5. Document and report.
6. Establish prehospital emergency medical services programs and educational protocols for victims of domestic violence.
7. Provide referrals and shelters.

The patient's story in her own words, including the name of the batterer, should be written in the ED chart, along with a careful description of her injuries. Photographs can be taken after the woman signs a consent; it is advisable to have a Polaroid camera available for this purpose. Other evidence of the beating, such as bloody or torn clothing, should be collected and labeled. The battered woman will need all of this as evidence when she goes to court. The staff member seeing the patient should inform the social worker assigned to the ED. The social worker should assume responsibility for crisis intervention, act as a patient advocate, and arrange for future counseling. When no social worker is available, it is the ED staff's responsibility to see that a safe disposition is arranged. Remember, most female homicide victims are killed by their husbands or lovers. You may be saving a life.

If the woman feels that she can return home, she should be given literature about facilities available to assist battered women and any phone numbers that might be of assistance in the future. She should be informed of her legal options for protection of herself and her children (with a court order of protection) and her right to request a copy of her chart and any photographs. If she cannot go home, she should be assisted in finding shelter or in locating a friend or relative with whom she and her children can stay temporarily. She should be advised not to leave any children behind (a neglect charge may be brought against her and she may lose custody) and not to stay with a nonrelated male (construed as adultery). If she has no place to go, she should be held in the ED until a social worker is available.

The police are required by law to take down her complaint if she wishes to press criminal charges. If she has an order of protection from family or criminal court, they must make an arrest upon her request. She has a right to police escort to her house to pick up children, clothes, etc. Find out what precinct she lives in before calling the police. Hospital police can be helpful in this regard. Patients should not be sent home with tranquilizers or sedating pain medication. A battered woman's survival may depend on her ability to think and react quickly. If a battered woman is admitted to the hospital, the medical and nursing staff should be informed that she is a battered woman. This is essential so that her personal safety in the hospital can be ensured and adequate discharge planning done.

Follow-Up

One of the most frustrating aspects of caring for battered women is that many of them will return to their batterers after leaving the ED. The problems these women face are complex and often involve emotional or financial ties to the batterer, fear of retaliation, or feelings of guilt. Many women will return to the home in the hope that improved behavior on their part or on the part of the batterer will help them avoid future episodes of violence. Medical personnel must maintain a sense of perspective when confronted with this situation and must avoid blaming the battered woman for her victimization. Providing an atmosphere that preserves a woman's dignity and respects her capacity for self-determination is the main goal.

Suggested Readings

Berrios DC, Grady D: Domestic violence—risk factors and outcomes. West J Med 1991;155:133–135.

Council on Scientific Affairs, American Medical Association: Violence against women: relevance for medical practitioners. JAMA 1992;267: 3184–3189,

McLeer S, Anway R: The role of the emergency physician in the prevention of domestic violence. Ann Emerg Med 1987;16:1155–1161.

20.2 THE HOMELESS PATIENT

Description

As a group, homeless people suffer a greater burden of disease, are more vulnerable to illness, and frequently present for medical care in a more advanced stage of disease. The homeless constantly confront exposure to the elements, overcrowding, lack of food and shelter, street violence, alcoholism, and drug abuse; all conspiring to make the homeless predisposed to a host of diseases (malnutrition, hypothermia, frostbite, infestations, tuberculosis, trauma). In addition, recent studies of the homeless estimate the prevalence of serious mental disorders to be approximately 30%. The consequence is that the homeless person is placed in double-jeopardy; they are not only more likely to have a health problem but they are also less likely to be able to care for themselves when ill. The ED is often the final recourse for this neglected group.

History

Be sensitive to the possibility that the person may be chronically confused, intimidated, or angered by the medical bureaucracy or reluctant or ashamed to reveal details. Be gentle and nonjudgmental. Previous medical history should focus on major disease, such as heart, lung, or kidney disease. A history of drug or alcohol abuse should be quantified.

Physical Examination

General. Note cachexia, bloating, or disorders of affect.

Vital signs. Always verify temperature in addition to pressure, pulse, and respirations.

HEENT. Inspect for signs of trauma. Look for nits or scalp lesions that suggest lice. Examine extraocular movements, pupillary responses, and fundi. Check dentition.

Neck. Check for stiffness. Palpate the thyroid for size and consistency.

Lungs. Listen for rales or wheezes.

Heart. Listen for murmurs, gallops, or rubs.

Abdomen. Observe for distention. Palpate for ascites. Assess for hepatosplenomegaly. Note any masses.

Rectal. Check stool for blood.

Extremities. Look carefully for skin ulcers, pedal edema, track marks, and the burrows of scabies. Do not neglect the palms and soles (secondary syphilis).

Neurologic. Do a thorough neurologic examination with particular attention to mental status. Examine for abnormal reflexes, cerebellar signs, tremor, and asterixis. Assess gait (ataxia).

Diagnostic Tests

The rational ordering of tests ought to be guided by the history and clinical findings.

Special Considerations

Immersion Foot and Frostbite

Considering the relative lack of shelter from the elements (cold, rain, snow), poor hygiene, malnutrition, and history of repetitive trauma, the homeless are at greater risk for both *trench foot* and *frostbite* (see section 18.2). Dampness and wind hasten the process of cold injuries to the extremities. Compounding the problem is that many homeless patients demonstrate an impaired mentation (psychiatric, drugs, alcohol, systemic disease), and many smoke nicotine, which is a vasoconstrictor.

Homeless people also do not have the opportunity to "prop their feet up at night" (continuous leg dependency), leading to gravitational and mechanical outflow obstruction of the deep venous system, which can advance to *chronic stasis ulcers.* The incidences of arteriosclerosis and diabetes are also higher in this group, further predisposing them to peripheral vascular disease. Also, because the homeless frequently wear the same cold, damp socks and shoes for days, bacteria rapidly proliferate on their feet.

Eventually, all these factors (vasoconstriction, tissue destruction, myonecrosis) contribute to immersion foot syndrome.

Ectoparasitic Infestations

Lice and *scabies* infestations are especially widespread in the homeless, because these people seldom change their garments or bedding, borrow clothing or bunks and bed sheets, and often sleep huddled together. The infested patient may come in complaining specifically of itching (often worse at night) or infestation may be noticed while evaluating the patient for another problem.

Lice can be found on the head, body, or in pubic area. Head lice deposit white eggs called nits, which are attached closely to the base of the hair. The sensitivity to bite marks varies among individuals, ranging from a stinging sensation to intense itching that soon leads to scratching causing erythema, irritation, and inflammation and ultimately an oozing dermatitis with a secondary bacterial infection. When a large number of lice have beset the patient in a short time, systemic complaints (muscle aches, fever, malaise, lymphadenopathy) may evolve. Employ a Wood's lamp (ultraviolet light) when screening for head lice (will fluoresce). Head lice typically bite behind the ears and nape of the neck, while body lice prefer the chest and abdomen. The favorite "haunt" of the pubic, or crab, louse is the pubic hair, but the thighs, lower abdomen, and axilla may also be affected.

The mite *Sarcoptes scabiei* is the responsible organism for scabies. Scabies is notorious for provoking an intense pruritus, often worse at night when the patient wants to sleep. Most patients with scabies display a papulosquamous rash along with tiny blisters; excoriations; and small, linear, gray-white marks, which are burrows in which the females lay their eggs. Lesions are found in greatest concentrations along the finger webs, ventral wrists, axilla, breasts (intermammary folds), intergluteal crease, and genitalia (the head and neck are characteristically spared in adults). Consider the diagnosis of scabies anytime a patient (especially someone subjected to poor living conditions) presents with a pruritic dermatitis. Definite diagnosis depends on identification of the mite: This can be attempted by scraping a fresh papule or burrow with a #15 scalpel, placing the sample on a slide, immersing it with mineral oil, and observing it under low power. It may be difficult to find a virgin burrow from which to obtain a fresh sample.

Norwegian scabies occurs in immunosuppressed patients (AIDS) and may not itch. Infestations manifest as thick, yellow, scaly skin, that can be easily mistaken for eczema or contact dermatitis. Patients may be overwhelmed by a tremendous number of mites (> 10,000).

Tuberculosis

An association of homelessness and TB has been known for some time. Not only does living in close quarters (shelters) predispose patients to infection but alcoholism increases the risk. In addition, there has been a surge in the number of cases of TB among younger homeless patients, especially intravenous drug users and victims of AIDS. Along with this increased prevalence, emergence of a multidrug-resistant form of TB has appeared (see section 9.2).

A major problem in treating homeless persons with TB is noncompliance. Because of the need for long-term therapy, cities like New York have established direct observation programs to ensure proper treatment of infected persons.

Trauma

Trauma is the leading cause of death and disability among the homeless. Many homeless people who are victims of beatings, stabbing, falls, burns, motor vehicle accidents are either ignored while they lie on the street, end up in areas out of sight, or purposely chose not to seek medical attention because of past experiences with the health care bureaucracy.

Treatment

The treatment of many of the medical problems listed above is discussed elsewhere in this text. However, several disorders warrant brief mention here.

Therapy for immersion foot is mainly supportive. Focus on ensuring good local hygiene (adequate warming, drying, cleaning), provide a change of clothes, update tetanus prophylaxis, limit weight bearing (including admission if necessary), and prescribe appropriate antibiotics and analgesics.

Individualize treatment regimens for lice infestations. Partners and close contacts will also require examination and treatment to prevent reinfection. All clothing and bedding must be laundered in hot water (> 51.5°C, or 125°F) to effectively kill the adult lice, nymphs, and nits.

Pyrethrins with *piperonyl butoxide* (RID) is an efficient nonprescription product for eradicating body lice: Apply the lotion to entire body, leave on for 10 min, then bathe. Retreatment may be required in 7 to 10 days. *Permethrin* (1% liquid, available over the counter) is employed for head lice: Wash hair, apply lotion, leave on for 10 min, rinse hair, then comb with a fine-toothed comb. An alternative prescription medication for the treatment of lice is *lindane,* available as a lotion, cream, or shampoo. Because lindane is potentially toxic and is able to be absorbed percutaneously, avoid use in small children, older patients, pregnant women, patients with multiple excoriations or many lesions (especially over the scrotum), and those being treated repeatedly. For body lice, it is recommended that two 8-hr applications of lindane be used, preceded and followed by showering. For head lice, follow rinsing again by combing with a fine-toothed comb to remove nits. When lice are found attached to eyelids or eyelashes, apply petroleum jelly BID; *do not* use insecticides near the eyes.

Treatment options for scabies include permethrin, crotamiton, and lindane. For *permethrin* (5% cream), apply 30 g, massaging from head to sole of feet; leave on for 8 to 14 hr before washing it off. Side effects include a transient burning, associated with severity of infestation. For *crotamiton* (10% cream), massage the cream into the skin from the neck down (especially into skin folds and creases), repeat the treatment in 24 hr, then bathe at 48 hr. The main side effects occurring with crotamiton are allergic skin reactions.

Lindane is a prescription medication that can be applied as a 1-oz lotion or 30-g tube of cream. Spread on a thin layer, from the neck to the toes (including the soles of the feet), with special attention to the areas most involved. Wash off in 8 to 12 hr. The treatment can be repeated in 1 week if no improvement is noticed. Precautions mentioned for lice treatment with lindane apply here, too: There is a risk of CNS toxicity (seizures) as well as bone marrow suppression.

Note that mites tend to persist in subungual areas; thus the fingernails should be trimmed, the fingers scrubbed, and a scabicide applied.

Inform the patient, that no matter what medication is chosen for treatment of scabies, he or she may continue to experience itching for up to 4 weeks subsequent to therapy. Supplemental relief for troublesome symptoms may be provided with topical steroids and antihistamines.

Admission Criteria

Any homeless patient with acute disease or an acute exacerbation of chronic disease will probably require inpatient hospitalization. *Homeless patients with complex outpatient regimens* generally should be admitted. ED staff must not be afraid to admit patients for social reasons because a large number have significant medical illness. Hospitalization may offer the homeless person not only the opportunity to regain his or her health but also the chance to make contact with the necessary social services.

Unfortunately, some refuse hospitalization. Unless such patients have been judged incompetent in a court of law or constitute an immediate threat to themselves or others, they have the right to refuse medical treatment or hospital admission. If a serious medical problem exists, however, and the patient is refusing treatment, immediate psychiatric consultation should be obtained.

Suggested Readings

Breakey WR, Fischer PJ, Kramer M, et al.: Health and mental health problems of homeless men and women in Baltimore. JAMA 1989;262: 1352–1357.

Concato J, Rom WN: Endemic tuberculosis among homeless men in New York City. Arch Intern Med 1994;154:2069–2073.

Fischer PJ, Breakey WR: The epidemiology of alcohol, drug, and mental disorders among homeless persons. Am Pscyhol 1991;46:1118–1125.

20.3 INFORMED CONSENT

Patients have the right to determine what is and is not done to them during a medical evaluation or treatment. Patients also have the right to accept some but not all parts of a recommended evaluation or treatment. Consent for the intended evaluation or treatment should be obtained from the patient or the responsible guardian. *Expressed consent* is the process by which the patient overtly, by either a written or an oral statement, agrees to a procedure or treatment. Implied consent refers to the condition where the patient acts in such a way as to indicate agreement with a plan or regimen (when a patient extends an arm to allow blood to be drawn). To be valid, consent should be informed. This requires that the patient have enough information to understand what is being consented to. The patient should understand (1) the nature of the illness or injury, (2) the recommended treatment, (3) possible risks from the treatment, (4) alternative treatment possibilities, and (5) the risks of refusing treatment.

To give consent, the patient must have the legal capacity to do so. Minors cannot consent to or refuse treatment except in special circumstances such as an emancipated minor. Emancipated minors are able to give consent with no parental or court involvement. An emancipated minor may be a person who:

Lives apart from and is financially independent from his or her parents;
Is married currently or was so in the past;
Is pregnant now or was so in the past; and/or
Is a minor removed by court order.

Most states also allow minors to present for treatment without parental consent for the following conditions:

Sexually transmitted diseases;
Suspected pregnancy; and
Alleged child abuse.

When minors present without parental consent for treatment of true emergencies, evaluation and treatment should be initiated while the parents are located or a court order is obtained.

Suggested Reading

Siegel DM: Consent and refusal of treatment. Emerg Med Clin North Am 1993;11:833–840.

20.4 REFUSAL OF TREATMENT

Patients may refuse part or all of their recommended evaluation and treatment. Refusal (nonconsent) may be implied, verbal, or written. This situation represents one of the most frustrating professional encounters. When a patient refuses treatment, the ED physician must first establish that the patient is mentally capable to do so. The patient must have the capacity to understand the illness, the treatment recommended, the alternative treatments, and most important, the possible deleterious consequences associated with refusal of treatment. Incapacitated patients are unable to consent or refuse their own treatment. Such patients include those with (1) drug or alcohol intoxication, (2) severe depression, (3) altered mental status, (4) psychosis, (5) injury-induced shock, (6) suicidal ideation, and/or head injury. Patients who are determined to be lacking the capacity to refuse treatment must be restrained or sedated and held in the hospital for further evaluation and treatment. If possible, have the patient deemed incapacitated to make decisions by another qualified physician (other than the treating doctor) or obtain a court order of incompetence.

When patients refuse treatment and their mental competence is established, all options should be discussed with them, and they should sign an informed refusal document, which becomes part of the permanent medical record. The form should include the following:

Documentation that the patient was given an initial screening examination and its results;
Description of evaluation and treatment recommendations and options;
List of which specific parts of the evaluation or treatment were refused;
Description of the risks and benefits related to refusal and that the patient was informed of these; and
Patient signature acknowledging refusal of treatment and the signature of a witness.

If the patient refuses a specific treatment or evaluation, attempt to provide the next best option. All too often practitioners become angry with the patient and present "all or none" options. An example is the patient who refuses sutures for a laceration; rather than giving the patient a bandage and discharging him or her, the physician can cleanse, explore, and débride the wound; close with Steri-Strips; and provide antibiotics.

Suggested Reading

Hamilton FN, Lyndon DR: Significant legal developments affecting the practice of emergency medicine in the last year. Emerg Leg Briefings 1993;4:25–32.

20.5 ADVANCE DIRECTIVES

Advance directives include living wills, durable powers of attorney for health care, the medical directive, and do not resuscitate (DNR) orders. All are designed to preserve an individual's autonomy in determining the course of his or her medical care.

Living wills allow competent adults to prospectively refuse certain types of life-saving treatment. They are legal documents in which an individual may outline medical procedures (e.g., intubation) or treatments (e.g., vasopressors) that are not to be initiated. Living wills have limitations. Patients are restricted to simple refusal of specific treatments, which is unlikely to address all possible medical options. Many states allow a physician to refuse a living will, as emergency situations do not logistically permit one's will to be scrutinized before treatment decisions. Living wills are not yet accepted in all states, and often their use is restricted to the vaguely defined terminally ill.

Durable powers of attorney and court orders appoint a proxy (family member or friend) to make specific medical decisions for a person who is suddenly unable to do so. This practice is not accepted in every state and many problems arise from family and friend disagreements. In addition, the presumption that family and friends are more likely than hospital staff to act in a patient's best interest does not always hold true.

Medical directives are more structured living wills that specify certain protocols to follow if certain general clinical situations arise. These may include a checklist of both general and specific initiatives that should or should not be taken if a patient is in a particular clinical predicament (e.g., coma). Obvious problems arise with semantics and divergent medical management opinions.

Do not resuscitate, or no code, orders have been simply defined by the President's Commission for the Study of Ethical Problems in Medicine in 1983: "In the event of an acute cardiac or respiratory event, no CPR efforts will be initiated." Current medical practice is far more complex and complicated than this simple statement indicates. The ED physician needs to be quite clear as to precisely what orders for DNR, no code, and no extraordinary measures mean at each hospital. Documentation of the patient's desires in the medical record (including specific interventions like intubation, transfusion by name) is of paramount importance so that other caregivers need not interpret the record.

Determinations of death, patient autonomy, and when to resuscitate are all interrelated concepts physicians must consider when life-saving medical interventions are required. The Uniform Determination of Death Act (adopted in 1981 by the American Medical Association and American Bar Association) defined death as (1) irreversible cessation of circulatory and respiratory functions or (2) irreversible cessation of all functions of the entire brain, including the brainstem. The first criterion is proven if a patient fails to respond to medical treatments established by the advanced cardiac life support (ACLS) protocols. The second criterion (brain death) requires specialized equipment and physicians (often neurologists or neurosurgeons) and is often not performed in the ED.

Patient autonomy refers to the patient's right of self-determination. As a general rule, the competent adult patient should be directly approached with questions pertaining to the use of resuscitative measures and equipment before the actual need. Most people have thoughts about use of life support measures. Their specific requests should be documented in the medical record. Hospital policies often require an attending physician's signature on DNR orders. In situations where the patient is not capable of making decisions (e.g., severe hypoxia), there is an established hierarchy within the family as to who serves as the patient's proxy (see Table 20.5.1). After addressing resuscitative issues with the patient or proxy, be sure to inform other family members regarding the decision and address family concerns.

When to resuscitate: The move toward advance directives in recent years has been fueled by a desire to protect patients from the additional physical pain, suffering, and financial costs incurred in futile resuscitative efforts. The decision of when to resuscitate

Table 20.5.1
Medical Proxy Hierarchy

1. Spouse
2. Parent
3. Adult child
4. Adult brother or sister
5. Adult aunt or uncle
6. Grandparent
7. Any person with obvious responsibility or authority to grant consent

is not an easy one, and often in the ED setting there is not enough information to guide the clinician. Resuscitation of all those in cardiac arrest, regardless of the circumstances, is an alternative but may not always be appropriate. The absence of DNR orders or an advance directive does *not* obligate emergency medicine personnel to resuscitate. The best approach is to consider all the variables (e.g., underlying disease state, possibility of recovery, family desires) before making a decision. If the decision is equivocal, there should be a presumption in favor of resuscitation. If resuscitation would be futile, then it should not be initiated.

Suggested Readings

Adams JE, Derse AR, Gotthold WE et al.: Ethical aspects of resuscitation. Ann Emerg Med 1992; 21:1273–1276.

Iversor KV: Getting advance directives to the public: a role for emergency medicine. Ann Emerg Med 1991;20:692–696.

20.6 ORGAN DONATION

Organ transplantation is becoming increasingly common. Unfortunately, suitable donors are becoming increasingly difficult to find. It is estimated that from one-third to one-half of patients waiting for organ transplants will die before a suitable donor is found. The majority of organ donors are between the ages of 18 and 45 years and have been previously healthy. Organ procurement starts with potential organ donors; the 12 R's of procurement (see Table 20.6.1) are the widely accepted guidelines that must be followed in each case. Local organ procurement agencies (OPA) provide both state and local services through transplant teams, which in turn work through individual hospitals. Referring physicians, transplant teams, and patients' families must collectively determine when potential donors are suitable with respect to medical and ethical (especially religious) criteria.

Clinical brain death criteria were established in 1981 and have now been accepted by all but a few states. Once a person is declared brain dead by a physician (usually a neurologist), the family may be approached by a physician and the decision to donate (or not) can be made. If the decision is made to donate, the organ procurement team is then involved. Specifics pertaining to which organs the family wishes to donate and which are suitable for donation (each organ has its own criteria) are then explored.

Table 20.6.1
Potential Organ Donors—The 12 R's

Resuscitation	ABCs of resuscitation of all prospective organ tissue donor patients with catastrophic brain injury from trauma or medical disease
Recognition and referral	Initial assessment and evaluation of a prospective donor
Regard and request	Clergy involvement; family and religious orientation
Requirements	Neurology or neurosurgery; consent
Remember	Medical examiner; hospital administrator; legal advice
Record	Accurate record keeping; time of brain death
Regulate	Maintenance of optimal organ-tissue donor homeostasis for optimal retrieval and function
Resource	Involve procurement and transplantation team
Recovery	Organ-tissue retrieval
Reverence	For family and patient after donation or if donation is denied

Approaching grieving family members with questions regarding organ donation may make some health care professionals uncomfortable. It is helpful to view this as part of the continuum of care for both the patient and the family. Follow-up studies with donor families have found that most have positive feelings about donation and that donations in many instances actually lessened the grief.

Suggested Readings

Adams JE, Derse AR, Gotthold WE, et al.: Ethical aspects of resuscitation. Ann Emerg Med 1992;21:1273–1276.

Buse S, Bivins B, Horst H, Rivers E: Organ and tissue procurement in the acute care setting: principles and practice. Parts 1 and 2. Ann Emerg Med 1990;19:78–85, 193–200.

Chapter 21

Emergency Procedures

21.1 VENOUS ACCESS

Peripheral Vein Cannulation (Needle within Catheter Type)

1. Apply a tourniquet.
2. Prep the skin.
3. Hold the skin taut.
4. Puncture at a 30° angle to the skin and bevel the needle upward.
5. Easy blood return indicates good position.
6. Gently advance the catheter while withdrawing the needle.
7. Attach and regulate the intravenous fluid tubing or saline lock device.
8. Tape the catheter securely to the skin.

Brachial Vein Cannulation (Needle within Catheter Type)

The brachial vein lies just medial to the brachial artery in the groove between the biceps and triceps muscles, two finger breadths above the antecubital crease.

1. Apply a tourniquet and prep the skin.
2. Palpate the pulsating brachial artery and pull the skin taut with two fingers.
3. Puncture just medial to the artery, at a 30° angle to the skin, with the bevel facing superficially.
4. Easy blood return indicates good position.
5. Advance the catheter while withdrawing the needle.

Note: *The brachial vein lies close to the median nerve so it is best to attempt this procedure in an awake patient.* This is an excellent intravenous site in patients with no apparent access, such as intravenous drug abusers.

External Jugular Vein Cannulation (Needle within Catheter Type)

Refer to Figure 21.1.1.

1. Place the patient supine with legs elevated and perform the Valsalva maneuver to engorge the neck veins.
2. Prep the skin.
3. Press your finger over the vein just above the clavicle.
4. Puncture the skin as high on the neck as the vein is visible, guiding the catheter into the lumen of the vein. Be sure to pull the skin taut, as the vein rolls very easily.
5. Blood return indicates good position; advance the catheter while withdrawing the needle.
6. Attach intravenous tubing and tape in place securely.

Caution: *The tortuousity and valves present in this vessel make cannulation difficult.* The Seldinger technique (see below) may increase the frequency of vessel cannulation.

Internal Jugular Vein Cannulation (Anterior Approach)

This method uses the Seldinger technique. Refer to Figure 21.1.2.

1. Place the patient supine, with legs or foot of stretcher elevated and head turned 15 to 20° to the side opposite the puncture. The right side is preferred for puncture.

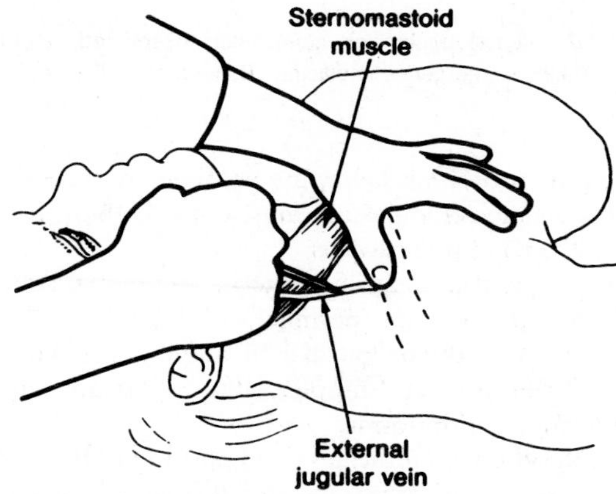

Figure 21.1.1. External jugular vein cannulation. (Reprinted by permission from RR Simon and BE Brenner: Emergency procedures and techniques. Baltimore: Williams & Wilkins, 1994:386.)

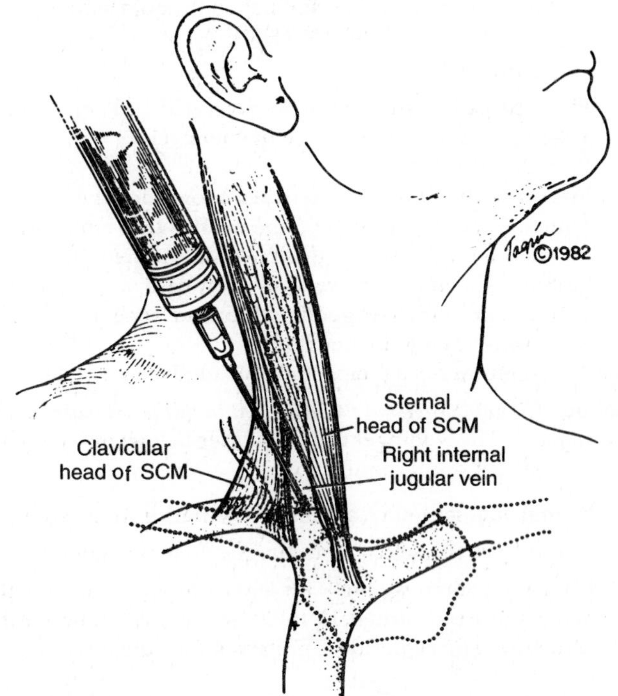

Figure 21.1.2. Internal jugular vein cannulation. (Reprinted by permission from EW Wilkins: Emergency medicine. Baltimore: Williams & Wilkins, 1989:1005.)

2. The puncture site is below the point where the two bodies of the sternocleidomastoid muscle meet, about two finger breadths above the clavicle.
3. Prep skin and drape using a sterile technique. Administer local anesthetic if time permits.
4. Puncture with the needle at a 30° angle to the skin, aiming toward the ipsilateral nipple, withdrawing the plunger of the syringe continuously.
5. Easy blood return indicates good position of the needle.
6. A curved-tip guidewire is inserted through the needle a few centimeters past the bevel.
7. Remove the needle from the skin while grasping the guidewire and then slide the needle off the wire.

8. Incise the skin with a #11 blade approximately 0.5 cm.
9. Slide the dilator over the guidewire making sure that the wire extends beyond the dilator at all times.
10. While holding the guidewire at the free end, slide the dilator into the puncture site with a corkscrew motion.
11. Use the same sequence for the catheter after the dilator has been removed from the wire.
12. Remove the wire after the catheter is in place. Check for good blood return and secure the catheter with sutures.

Note: *These steps can also be used for subclavian vein and femoral vein cannulation after the needle is in place. Do not expose the free end of the catheter to air but cover at all times with a gloved finger when it is not connected.* This avoids possible air embolism. If blood return is pulsating and bright red, this indicates inadvertent carotid artery puncture. Immediately withdraw the needle and compress for 5 min. Always have control of the guidewire.

Subclavian Vein Cannulation

Refer to Figure 21.1.3.

1. Place the patient supine with legs or foot of stretcher elevated, face turned to the side opposite the puncture, and ipsilateral arm abducted 10 to 20°. Traction on the ipsilateral arm inferiorly may be of benefit.
2. The puncture site should be just inferior to the clavicle at the junction of the medial and middle third of the clavicle.

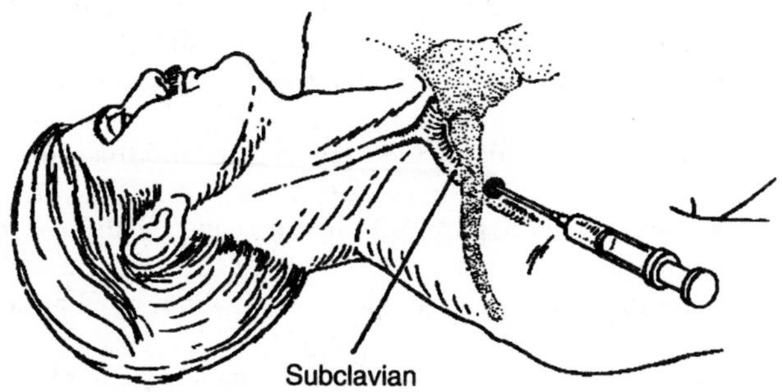

Figure 21.1.3. Subclavian vein cannulation. (Reprinted by permission from P Rosen and GL Sternbach: Atlas of emergency medicine, 2nd ed. Baltimore: Williams & Wilkins, 1983.)

3. Prep the skin; give local anesthetic if time permits.
4. Keeping the needle and syringe flat against the patient's body with the bevel caudal, insert the needle, aiming toward the suprasternal notch while maintaining slight traction on the plunger of the syringe.
5. Easy blood return indicates good position of the needle. If blood return is pulsating and red, this indicates inadvertent subclavian artery puncture. Immediately withdraw needle and compress for 5 min.

Note: *The Seldinger technique (see above) can be used for catheter placement after the needle is in the vessel. All central venous cannulations should be followed by immediate chest x-ray to check catheter position and to rule out pneumothorax.*

Cutdowns

Refer to Figure 21.1.4.

1. Choose the incision site.
   a. *Saphenous vein at groin.* Make a 5-cm incision just distal and parallel to the crural fold below the pubic tubercle; feel for the pubic tubercle and make an incision two finger breadths lateral and one finger breadth inferior to it.
   b. *Saphenous vein at ankle.* A 3-cm incision is made in a posteroanterior direction, just proximal to the medial malleolus, centered above the anterior border of the medial malleolus. A tourniquet may be placed in the midleg to facilitate vein cannulation.
2. Prep and drape the area to be used, using a sterile technique. Administer local anesthetic if possible.
3. Incise the skin and superficial subcutaneous tissue with scalpel.
4. Bluntly dissect with curved hemostat around the vein, freeing it.
5. Pass two 3-0 silk ties around the vein, tying the distal one securely.
6. Incise the vein at a 45° angle through about one-half its diameter.
7. Insert a sterile intravenous catheter, small feeding tube, or intravenous tubing into the vein, and advance 3 to 4 cm. Secure by tying the proximal ligature snugly. An alternative method is to use the Seldinger technique (see above) after

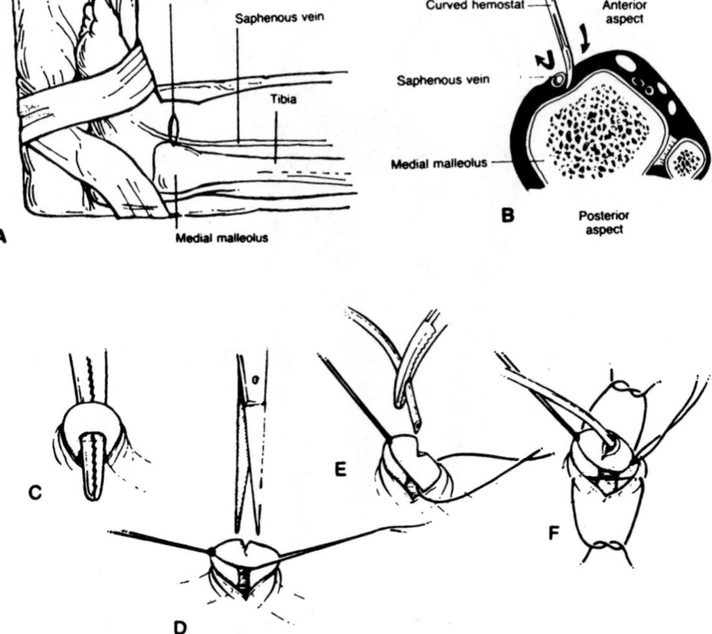

Figure 21.1.4. Cutdowns. (Reprinted by permission from PM Suratt, RS Gibon: Manual of medical procedures. St. Louis: Mosby, 1982.)

the vein is incised and insert an 8.5-French or 10-gauge catheter into the vein.

8. Place the catheter in the corner of the incision and close the skin with interrupted sutures. The skin suture nearest the catheter can be placed around it, securing the catheter in place.

Intraosseous Infusion

Equipment needed includes an intraosseous needle or sternal bone marrow needle. *Absolute contraindications* include infection at the puncture site and fractures of the bone intended for insertion. Refer to Figure 21.1.5.

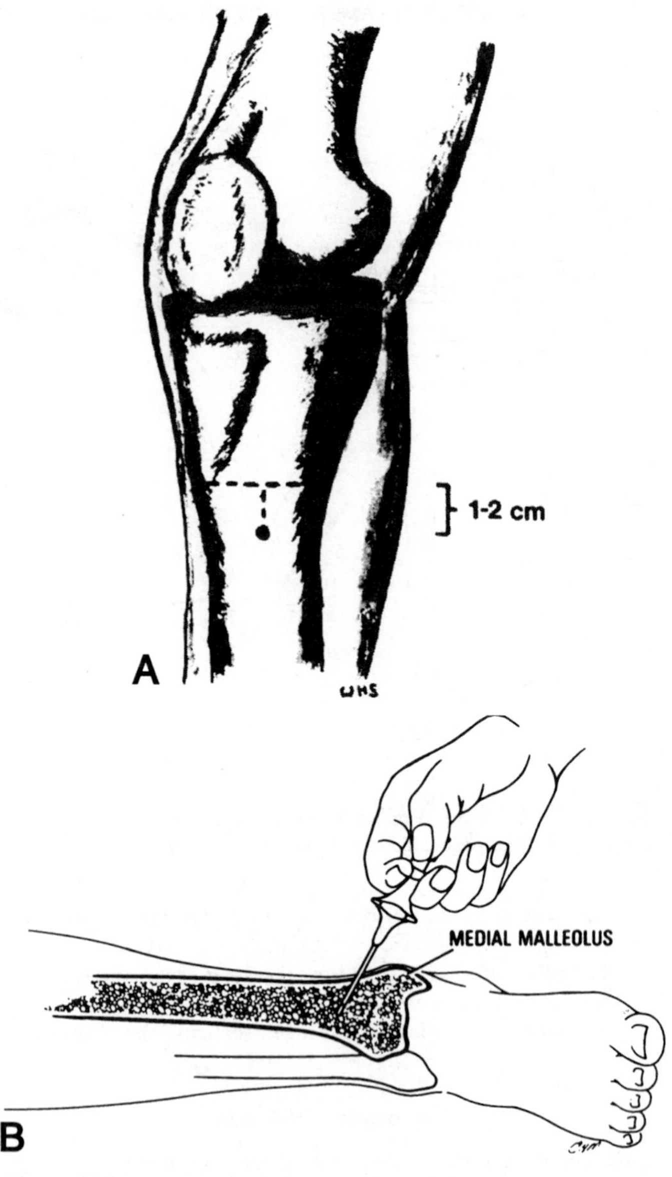

Figure 21.1.5. Intraosseous infusions. (Reprinted by permission from J Roberts and J Hedges: Clinical procedures in emergency medicine. Philadelphia: WB Saunders, 1991:366.)

1. Choose the site.
    a. *Proximal tibia.* An imaginary mark is drawn one-half the distance between the tibial tuberosity and the most medial portion of the tibia. The puncture site is 2 cm distal to this mark.
    b. *Distal tibia.* The puncture site preferred in an adult is the medial surface of the tibia one to two finger breadths superior to the medial malleolus.
2. Prep and drape. Anesthetize the area if time permits.
3. Grasp the needle firmly in the palm of your hand with the bevel pointed away from the joint surface. Stabilize the needle shaft with your index finger and with a twisting-type motion cut through the cortex of the bone.
4. Decreased resistance signals intermedullary placement of needle. Be sure not to go through the opposite cortex.
5. Remove the stylet and aspirate the contents—bone and marrow—to confirm placement.
6. Attach intravenous tubing and secure.

21.2 THORACIC PROCEDURES

Intercostal Nerve Block

Refer to Figure 21.2.1.

1. Locate the painful rib by palpation. Correlate to the x-ray when possible.
2. Follow the rib posteriorly to the posterior axillary line, the site of infiltration. One or two ribs above and below the affected one should also be blocked.
3. Prep and drape the area. Place gentle cephalad skin traction over the rib to be blocked. Place a wheal of rapid-acting anesthetic, such as lidocaine, over the inferior border of the rib.
4. Using a 1.5-inch, 22- to 23-guage needle on a syringe filled with long-acting anesthetic such as bupivacaine (Marcaine), insert the needle through the wheal at an 90° angle with the needle pointing cephalad; advance the needle to the inferior border of the rib.
5. Release traction on the skin and insert the needle 3 mm deeper, being careful not to go too deeply (in order not to penetrate the thoracic cavity).
6. Withdraw the plunger of the syringe to ensure that the nee-

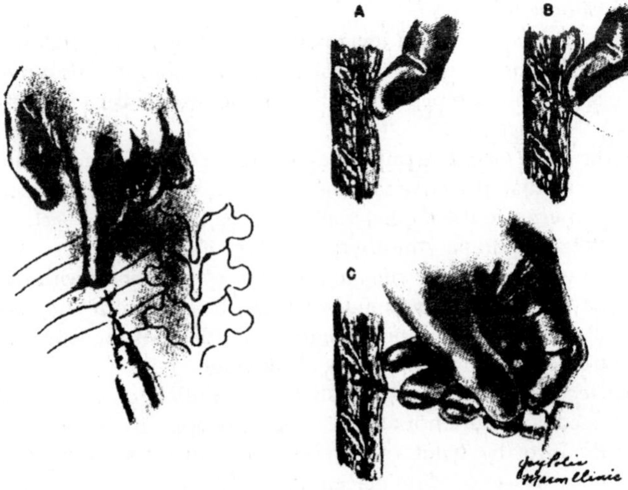

Figure 21.2.1. Intercostal nerve block. (Reprinted by permission from DC Moore: Regional block: a handbook for use in clinical practice of medicine and surgery. Springfield, IL: Charles C Thomas, 1971:153.)

dle is not in the blood vessel or the pleural space. Inject 4 to 5 mL of anesthetic.

7. Cover the area with a sterile dressing.

Pericardiocentesis

Refer to Figure 21.2.2.

1. Prep, drape, and anesthetize the anterior chest over the left costosternal angle. The patient should be supine.
2. Using a 5-inch, 18-gauge cardiac or spinal needle with a 20-mL syringe, attach the precordial lead of an ECG machine to the hub end of the needle, using a wire with two alligator clips.
3. Insert the needle at a 30° angle to the skin, between the xiphoid process and the left costal margin, aiming toward the left shoulder.
4. While inserting the needle, maintain aspiration traction on the syringe. A current of injury on a precordial lead means the needle is in contact with the epicardium; withdraw slightly until the ECG pattern returns to normal.
5. Aspirate—a collection of nonclotting blood indicates a probable hemopericardium.

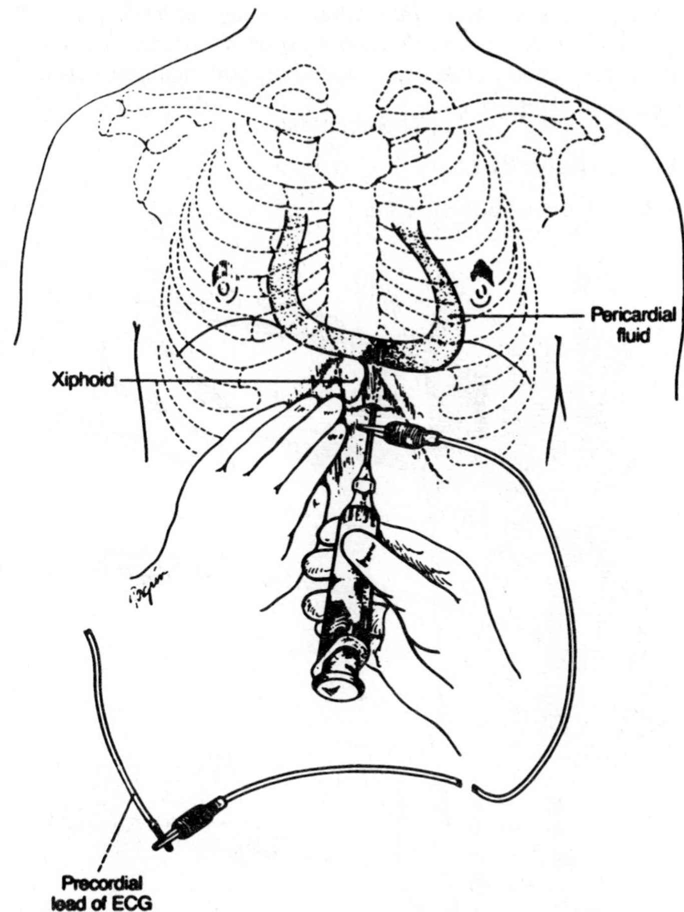

Figure 21.2.2. Pericardiocentesis. (Reprinted by permission from EW Wilkins: Emergency medicine. Baltimore: Williams & Wilkins, 1989:1017.)

Remember: *A negative pericardiocentesis does not rule out tamponade.* Also, clotted blood may be obtained from a very recent hemopericardium.

6. If a large amount of fluid or blood is evacuated, evacuation can continue with the needle left in place by attaching a three-way stopcock.

Note: *If the patient is in cardiac arrest or an agonal rhythm, the ECG leads attached to the needle should be disregarded.* Echocardiographic guidance should be used in the nonarrest patient if time permits.

Thoracentesis

Refer to Figure 21.2.3.

1. Choose the puncture site.

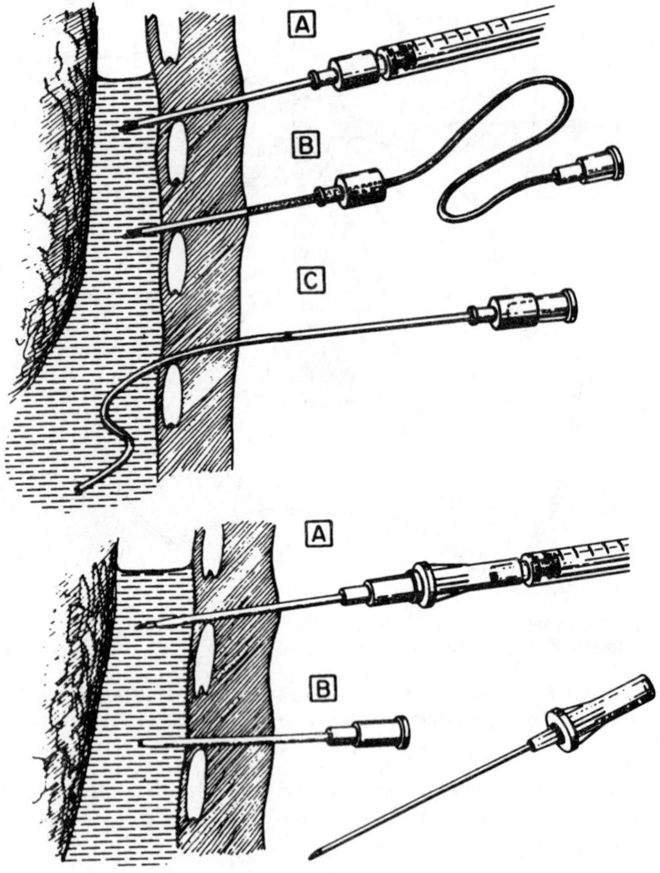

Figure 21.2.3. Thoracentesis. (Reprinted by permission from NH Fishman: Thoracic drainage: a manual of procedures. St. Louis: Mosby, 1983:30.)

a. *For evacuation of air.* The second intercostal space at the midclavicular line (anterior chest), with the patient placed supine.
b. *For evacuation of fluid.* The seventh intercostal space at the point of the scapula, with the patient sitting erect.

2. Prep the skin; anesthetize locally down to the periosteum of the inferior rib.
3. Attach a three-way stopcock and 50-mL syringe to a through-the-needle catheter. The tubing to the third port of stopcock may be attached to a water seal, 500-mL evacuated bottle, etc. A 15- to 18-gauge over-the-needle catheter may also be used.
4. Puncture the skin over the rib just inferior to the landmarked space. Walk the needle over the superior edge of rib, puncturing through to the pleural space just above the rib, while aspirating constantly with the syringe. Stop advancing as soon as any air or fluid return is felt.
5. The catheter may be advanced to 6 to 8 cm, the needle withdrawn, and the catheter secured in place if continued drainage is desired. Alternatively, an over-the-needle catheter may be used.
6. Check a chest x-ray after the procedure is completed.

Note: *The Seldinger technique (section 21.1) can also be used for the placement of the catheter.*

Tube Thoracostomy

Refer to Figure 21.2.4.

1. Place the patient supine. The incision site is the fifth intercostal space in the midaxillary line.
2. Prep and drape the skin. Infiltrate the skin, subcutaneous tissue, periosteum of the rib inferior to the fifth intercostal space, and parietal pleura with local anesthetic.
3. Make a 3-cm incision parallel to and over the sixth rib, nearly to the depth of the rib. Now tunnel up and over the rib. Tunneling may be contraindicated in obese patients; an incision directly over the intercostal space at which the pleura is punctured is advisable.
4. Use a blunt curved clamp to dissect into the pleural space with firm, controlled motions. Widen the track with spreading motions, staying below the neurovascular bundle that lies inferior to each rib.

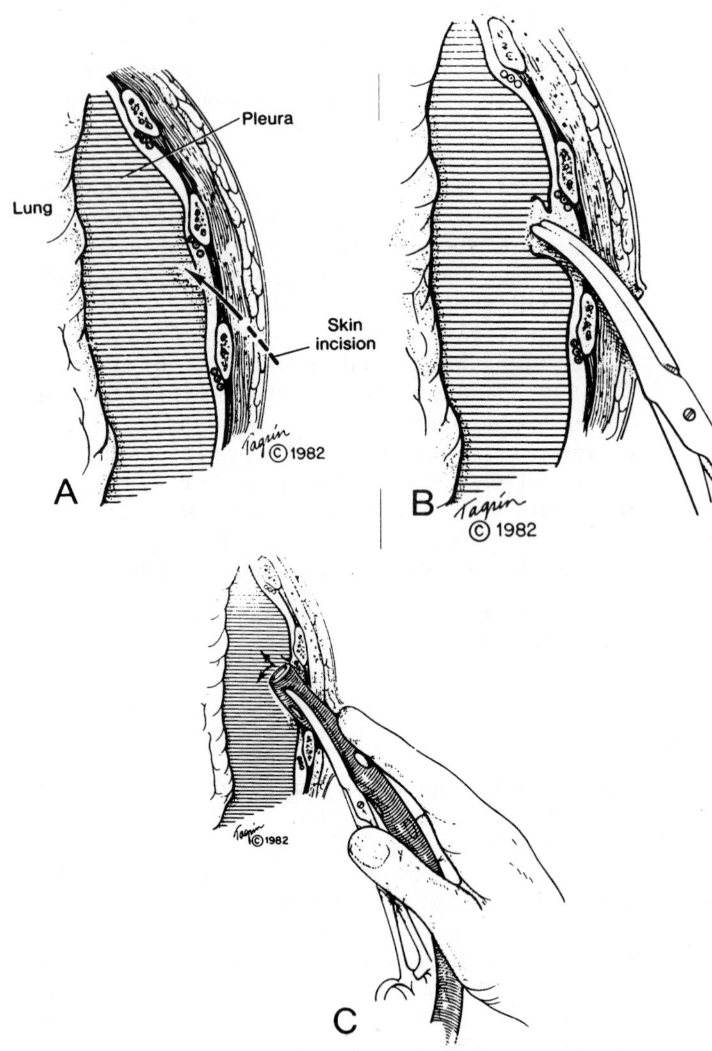

Figure 21.2.4. Tube thoracostomy. (Reprinted by permission from EW Wilkins: Emergency medicine. Baltimore: Williams & Wilkins, 1989: 1024–1025.)

5. Insert a gloved finger into the pleural space to check for pleural adhesions.
6. Insert a chest tube by grasping with a clamp as shown in Figure 21.2.4*C* and inserting superiorly, medially, and posteriorly. Be sure all the holes in the chest tube are in the pleural space.
7. Connect the tube to a water seal.
8. Place a simple suture across the incision next to the tube, leaving the ends long. Wrap the ends of the suture numerous times around the tube, securing it in place. Now place a single horizontal mattress suture across the incision and around the tube.
9. A dressing of petrolatum gauze completes the seal, and the tube is double taped for security.
10. Check a chest x-ray for tube placement.

Thoracotomy

Refer to Figure 21.2.5.

1. The patient should be prepared with endotracheal intubation, adequate venous access, sedation, and muscle relaxation, if necessary. Prep of the hemithorax (most often the left side). A thoracic surgery team should be on the way for immediate definitive management.
2. Using a large scalpel blade, incise from the sternum to the posterior axillary line following the curve of the fourth or fifth intercostal space. In one brisk motion, incise the skin, subcutaneous, and wall-muscle layers. Intercostal muscles should then be separated quickly but gently with blunt dissection using scissors to protect the subjacent lung. The pleura should now be lifted up with forceps and then incised.
3. Insert the rib spreader and separate the ribs.
4. Evacuation of the pericardium, temporizing repair of cardiac or major vessel wounds, control of the aorta, and internal cardiac massage may now be accomplished.

Note: *Care must be taken to identify the phrenic nerve before incising the pericardium.* The pericardium should then be incised vertically anterior to the nerve. To gain access to both hemithoraces simultaneously, a median sternotomy should be performed with a Lesky knife or a sternal saw.

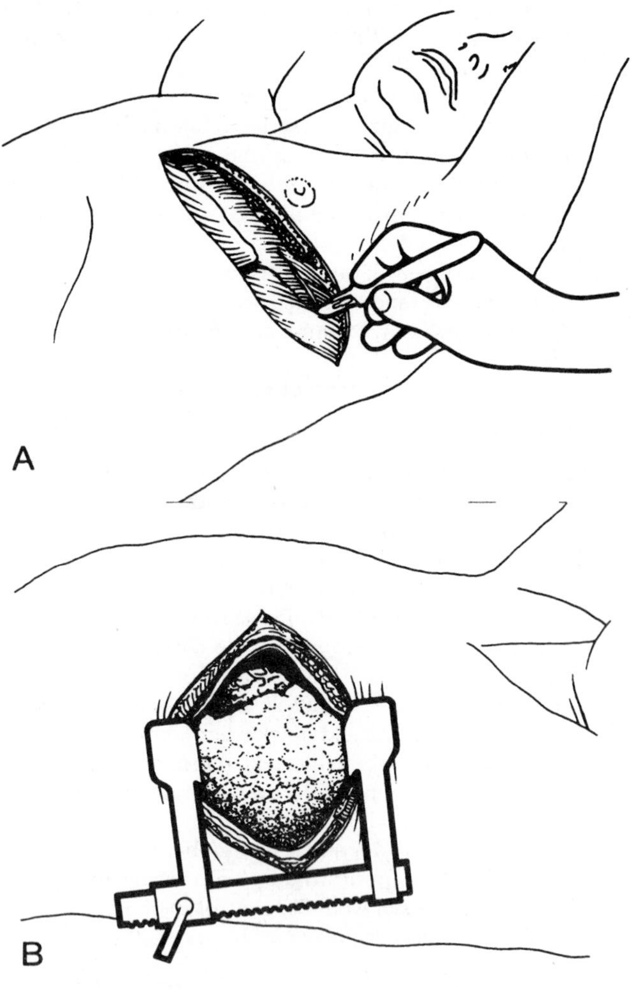

Figure 21.2.5. Thoracotomy. (Reprinted by permission from RR Simon and BE Brenner: Emergency procedures and techniques. Baltimore: Williams & Wilkins, 1994:135.)

21.3 SURGICAL AIRWAY MANAGEMENT

Needle Cricothyrotomy

Refer to Figure 21.3.1.

1. The patient is supine. Prep and drape the anterior neck, if possible.
2. Identify the thyroid and cricoid cartilages, as shown in Fig-

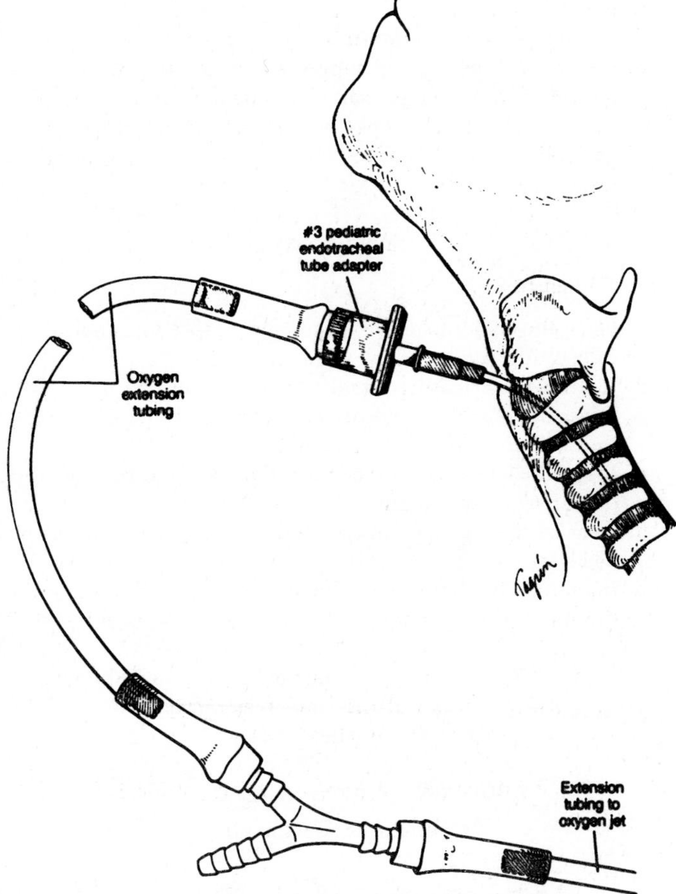

Figure 21.3.1. Needle cricothyrotomy. (Reprinted by permission from EW Wilkins: Emergency medicine. Baltimore: Williams & Wilkins, 1989:1001.)

ure 21.3.1. The narrow space between the cartilages is the cricothyroid membrane, the midline of which will be the puncture site. Infiltrate the skin with local anesthetic, if possible.

3. Using a 10- to 12-gauge catheter over the needle, puncture at a 45° angle, as shown, inserting the needle only 1.5 to 2 cm while constantly aspirating until air returns easily.
4. Gently advance the plastic catheter while withdrawing the needle.
5. Recheck catheter position by aspirating air again.
6. Ideally, a 50 psi oxygen supply is attached to pressure tubing with a Y connector, and this in turn is connected to the catheter. Ventilation is performed using a 1-sec burst of oxygen followed by a 2-sec expiratory phase. A bag-valve apparatus may be used but is not as efficient.

Cricothyrotomy

Refer to Figure 21.3.2.

1. Place the patient supine, prep, and drape. Anesthetize locally if time allows.
2. Identify the cricothyroid membrane (see Fig. 21.3.1).
3. Incise the skin above the membrane with a #10 scalpel blade with a vertical incision.
4. Incise the subcutaneous tissue and platysma to visualize the cricothyroid membrane.
5. Visualize the cricothyroid membrane and incise it horizontally, taking care not to cut too deeply, avoiding complications.
6. Immediately insert the scalpel handle and turn 90° to hold the incision open widely. The incision may be widened if necessary.
7. A cuffed #5 to 6 tracheostomy tube or a #4 to 6 Shiley tube may now be inserted. Insertion may be facilitated with a Trousseau dilator and tracheal hooks.

21.4 ABDOMINAL AND PELVIC PROCEDURES

Open Peritoneal Lavage

Refer to Figure 21.4.1.

1. The patient is supine. Prep and drape the infraumbilical area after emptying the bladder.

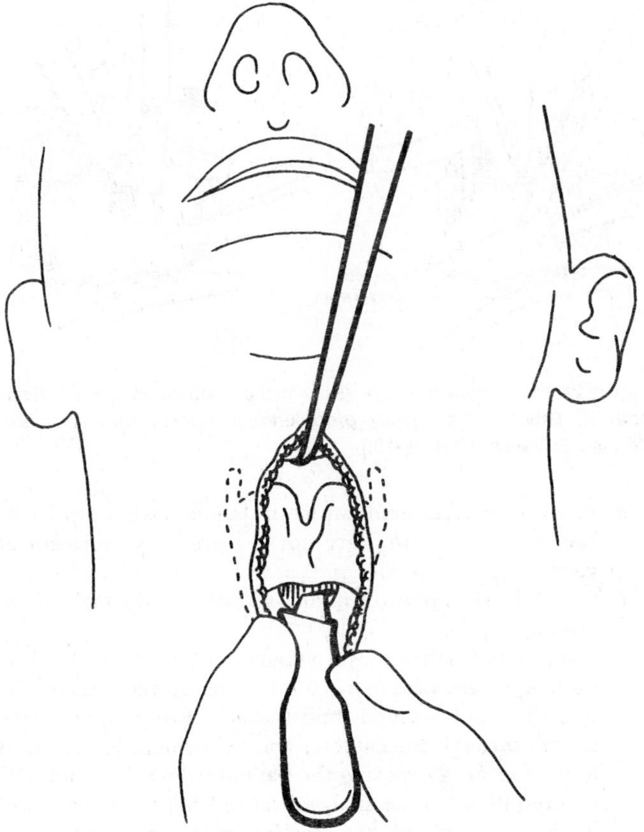

Figure 21.3.2. Cricothyrotomy.

2. Infiltrate the skin with local anesthetic containing epinephrine in the midline, 2 to 3 cm below the umbilicus. For patients with pelvic fractures or pregnancy incise above the umbilicus.
3. Make a 2- to 3-cm vertical incision of skin and subcutaneous tissue, down to the fascia (linea alba). Good hemostasis is essential at each layer. Gently cut through the fascia to expose the peritoneum.

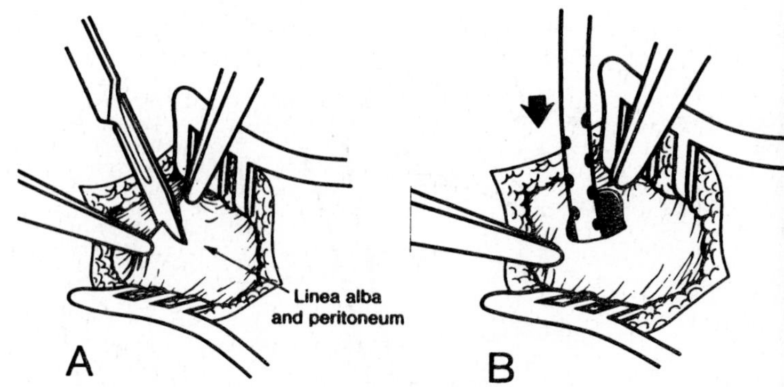

Figure 21.4.1. Peritoneal lavage. (Reprinted by permission from RR Simon and BE Brenner: Emergency procedures and techniques. Baltimore: Williams & Wilkins, 1994:14–15.)

4. Pick up the peritoneum with two clamps and gently nick between clamps, taking care not to pierce any subjacent organs.
5. Gently insert a peritoneal dialysis catheter through the incision.
6. Aspirate the catheter. More than 10 mL of frank blood is a positive result. Less than 10 mL of blood requires instillation of 1 L of warmed fluid (lactated Ringer's or normal saline) through the catheter and subsequent aspiration of fluid after gently rocking the patient from side to side. Recovered fluid may be analyzed for red cell count, white cell count, particulate matter, amylase, and Gram stain/culture. See section 4.5 for interpretation of lavage fluid.
7. Layer-by-layer closure should be done and a sterile dressing should be applied. The catheter may be left indwelling for repeat lavage later, if properly secured.

Note: *A supraumbilical approach may be used in patients with pelvic fractures, pregnancy, and obesity.* Some physicians prefer the use of a Seldinger wire kit (closed technique) to perform peritoneal lavage.

Culdocentesis

Refer to Figure 21.4.2.

1. Have the patient void before the procedure if at all possible.

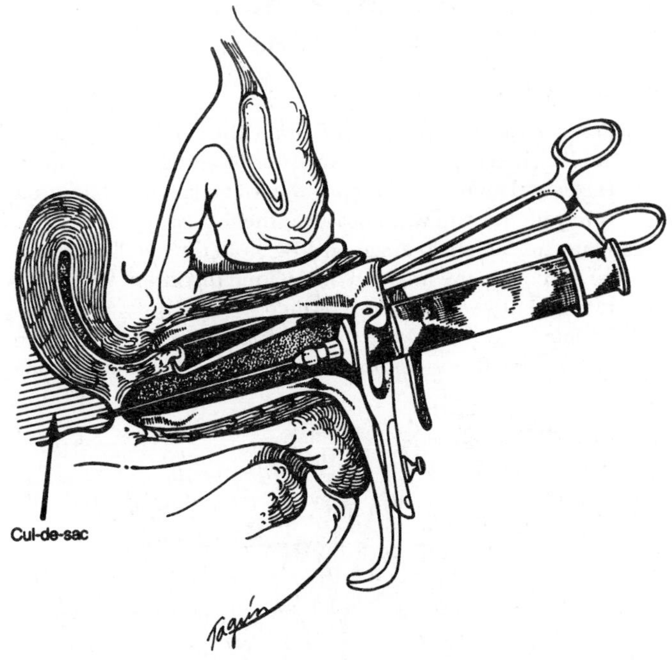

Figure 21.4.2. Culdocentesis. (Reprinted by permission from EW Wilkins: Emergency medicine. Baltimore: Williams & Wilkins, 1989:1035.)

2. Place the patient in the lithotomy position, with a speculum in the vagina.
3. The posterior lip of the cervix is grasped with a tenaculum and drawn anteriorly. Local anesthesia may be used as needed.
4. The vaginal mucosa of the posterior cul-de-sac is punctured with a long #18-gauge needle on a 10- or 20-mL syringe and aspirated as shown in Figure 21.4.2. A total of 5 mL of air may be injected before aspiration to expel any epithelial plugs.
5. More than 2 mL of nonclotting blood is usually considered a positive result for ruptured ectopic pregnancy. A purulent aspirate indicates pelvic infection. Serosanguinous fluid suggests a ruptured ovarian cyst. Aspiration of clear fluid or no fluid indicates a negative examination. These results need to be interpreted with caution.

21.5 ARTHROCENTESIS

Ankle Arthrocentesis

Refer to Figure 21.5.1.

1. For lateral swelling, prep and drape the lateral aspect of the ankle. The landmark is 1 cm anterior and 1 cm inferior to the lateral malleolus, keeping the foot in a neutral position. Infiltrate the skin with local anesthetic.
2. Using a 1.5-inch 20-guage needle, hold the needle horizontal and enter the ankle in an oblique direction, while aspirating gently with a 20-mL syringe.
3. For medial swelling, keep the foot in a neutral position and insert the needle just anterior to the medial malleolus and me-

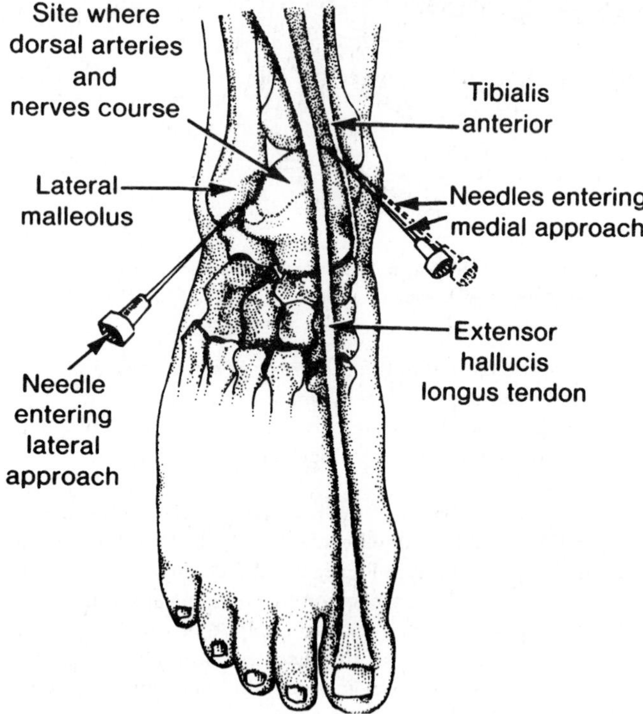

Figure 21.5.1. Ankle arthrocentesis. (Reprinted by permission from RR Simon and BE Brenner: Emergency procedures and techniques. Baltimore: Williams & Wilkins, 1994:210.)

dial to the tibialis anterior tendon, avoiding the dorsalis pedis artery. The needle is held horizontally and at an oblique angle. Advance the needle 2 to 3 cm into the joint space.

4. Apply a sterile dressing with slight pressure.

Knee Arthrocentesis

Refer to Figure 21.5.2.

1. The patient is supine. Prep, drape, and infiltrate the skin with local anesthetic while the knee is slightly flexed. The landmark is the medial surface of the patella near the inferior pole.
2. Insert an 18-gauge needle just posterior to the patella medially, aiming for the intercondylar notch. As the flow of fluid stops, milk the suprapatellar bursa to facilitate drainage.

21.6 LUMBAR PUNCTURE

Contraindications include signs of increased intracranial pressure (e.g., papilledema, focal neurological signs, history of slowly worsening headache). A CT scan should be obtained in these pa-

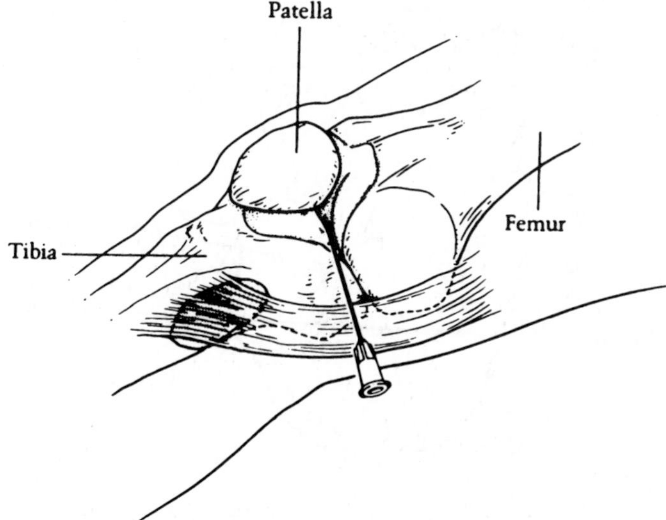

Figure 21.5.2. Knee arthrocentesis. (Reprinted by permission from TJV Vandersalm: Atlas of bedside procedures. Boston: Little, Brown & Co., 1979.)

tients before lumbar puncture because of the risk of herniation. Anticoagulation therapy or a history of bleeding diathesis is a relative contraindication.

Midline Approach

Refer to Figure 21.6.1.

1. The patient is placed on the examining table in the lateral decubitus position with the spinal column in as much flexion as possible, while the back is kept perfectly perpendicular to the tabletop.
2. The landmark is the L3–4 intervertebral space (L-4 is at the level of the iliac crests). Prep and drape the area, and infiltrate with local anesthetic.

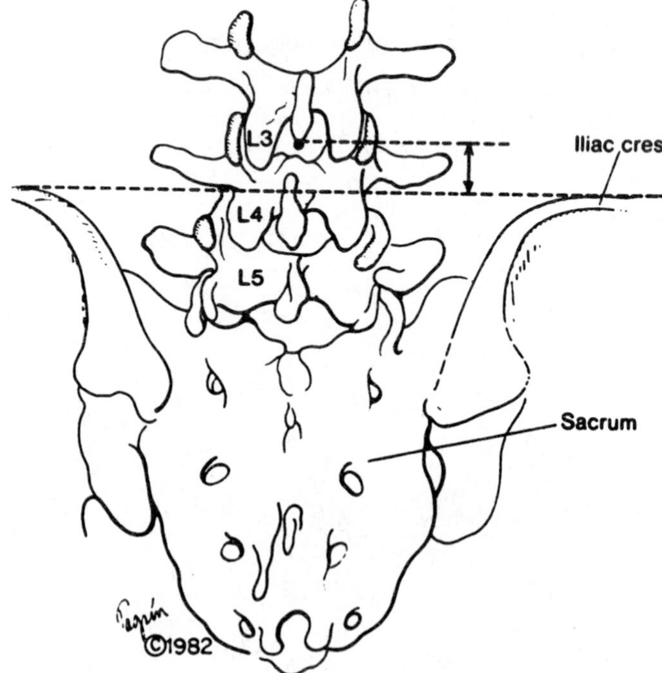

Figure 21.6.1. Lumbar puncture: midline approach. (Reprinted by permission from EW Wilkins: Emergency medicine. Baltimore: Williams & Wilkins, 1989:1027.)

3. Using a long 20- or 22-gauge spinal needle with a trocar, enter the intervertebral space with the needle angled cephalad (80° from the skin), aiming for the umbilicus. Keep the needle horizontal to the table and advance gently.
4. Three small pops are felt as the bevel of the needle pierces the skin, ligamentum flavum, and dura. Cease advancing immediately.
5. Removing the trocar with one hand while stabilizing the needle with the other will allow the cerebrospinal fluid to begin dripping out of the barrel of the needle.
6. An opening pressure may be obtained with the leg extended and 1 mL of fluid collected in each of four sterile tubes.
7. Gram stain, red cell count, white cell count with differential, glucose, protein, culture, and specialized laboratory examinations (VDRL, cryptococcal antigen, CIE, etc.) may be performed on the fluid. Fluid that is initially streaked with blood but clears progressively with each sample tube suggests a traumatic tap, whereas consistently bloody fluid in all tubes is more likely due to subarachnoid bleeding. If the fluid is not crystal clear, spin it down to check for xanthochromia.

Paramedian Approach

The Paramedian approach may be used in older patients who have calcified supraspinal and intraspinal ligaments. Not as much flexion is needed as with the midline approach.

1. The patient is in the lateral decubitus, slightly flexed position, while the back is perpendicular to the table.
2. The landmark is the L-4 vertebral body spinous process. Prep and drape, and infiltrate 1.5 cm lateral to the spinous process with local anesthetic.
3. Using a 3.5-inch, 20- to 22-gauge needle, puncture the skin 1.5 cm lateral to the spinous process. Direct the bevel of the needle toward the midline of the L3–4 interspace. The cranial angle of the needle should be approximately 120 to 135° to the plane of the back.
4. Three pops signal penetration of the skin, ligamentum flavum, and dura. Stop advancing immediately.
5. The remaining steps are the same as in the midline approach (see above).

Note: *Extreme flexion of the neck is not required with either approach.* This is uncomfortable and may decrease patient cooperation. The smaller-gauge needles and restraint in the volume of CSF sampled may lessen the risk of spinal headache postprocedure.

21.7 EMERGENCY CARDIAC PACING

Transvenous Cardiac Pacing

Refer to Figure 21.7.1.

1. Choose the site. The right internal jugular followed by the left subclavian vein is preferred for the most direct approach.
2. Place the introducer sheath as previously described under sterile technique (6.5- to 8.0-French introducers are ideal).

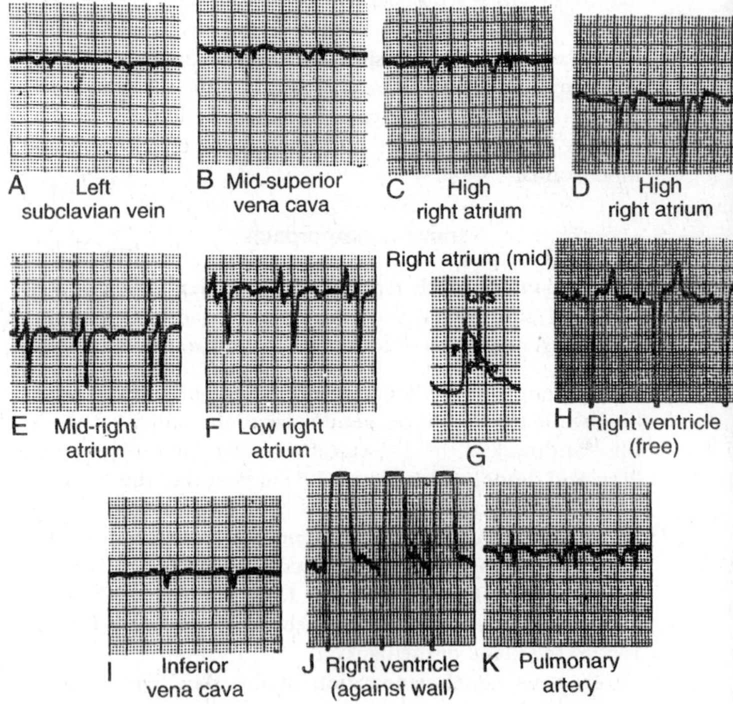

Figure 21.7.1. Transvenous cardiac pacing. (Reprinted by permission from OH Bing et al.: N Engl J Med 1972;287:651.)

3. A bipolar balloon-tipped pacing catheter is placed 10 to 12 cm into the introducer, and the balloon is inflated.
4. The patient is connected to a monitor and the limb leads of an ECG machine, with the distant terminal of the pacer being connected to the V lead of the ECG.
5. The pacer should be advanced quickly and smoothly while one monitors the V lead.
6. The pacer should be advanced into the right ventricle until contact is made with the endocardial wall. This is signaled by ST segment elevations of the monitoring ECG.
7. The pacer is now disconnected from the ECG, and the leads are connected to their respective terminals in the pacer generator. Set the generator to demand mode at 80 bpm or 10 bpm above the patient's intrinsic rate. The output is placed at 5 mA and the pacer is turned on.
8. If full capture is noted, slowly decrease the output until the capture is lost; this is called the threshold (usually 0.3 to 0.8 mA). Repeat this three times to get an average and set the output to 2.5 times the threshold level.
9. If complete capture does not occur, the pacer should be repositioned.
10. Gentle clockwise and counterclockwise rotations of the pacing catheter can be used if repositioning is needed.
11. Sensing can be tested by placing the generator in the demand mode with full capture. Slowly turn down the rate until the pacer is sensing and not pacing. Return the pacer to the desired rate.
12. Placement is confirmed with a chest x-ray (PA and lateral views), 12-lead ECG, and physical examination.

Blind Transvenous Pacer Placement

1. The pacer is attached to the pacer generator in the demand mode with the rate set at two times the intrinsic patient rate and the output below the patient's threshold.
2. The pacer is turned on and advanced with balloon up, while sensing (not pacing). As the catheter enters the ventricle, the pacer senses on every other beat if it is set at two times the intrinsic rate.
3. Increase the output to 5 mA and advance to capture the ventricle.

4. Reduce the rate to the desired level. Adjust the output and check sensing as above.

Note: *In cardiac arrest or critically low flow states, the pacer generator can be set to asynchronous mode and maximal output with a rate of 80 to 100. Blind advancement is undertaken until ventricle is captured.*

Transcutaneous Cardiac Pacing

Transcutaneous cardiac pacing is indicated for bradydysrhythmias that have not responded to atropine treatment and are associated with hypotension, chest pain, pulmonary edema, or decreased cerebral perfusion.

1. Place the anterior electrode over the left anterior chest wall at the point of maximal impulse (usually just inferior to the nipple in the midclavicular line). The electrodes are marked *front* and *back*. The front electrode is round, and the posterior electrode is rectangular.
2. The posterior electrode is placed directly opposite the anterior electrode on the patient's back near the scapula.
3. The electrodes are attached to the pacing unit, and the patient is attached to an appropriate ECG monitor that accompanies the pacing unit. The special ECG monitor is needed to monitor the patient's rhythm as the pacer is firing.
4. If the patient is bradycardic, place the unit in the demand mode at a rate of 80 to 90.
5. Now slowly increase the output (mA) until capture occurs. Check for improvement in blood pressure and symptoms. Barrel-chested patients, patients with pneumothoraces, and patients with pericardial tamponade or effusions will require a much higher output for capture.
6. Sedation and analgesia may be required for patient comfort. Be careful not to compromise the patient's blood pressure or respiratory status.
7. The asynchronous or fixed mode may be used if the patient has progressed to an asystolic arrest. Transcutaneous cardiac pacing should only be used early in an arrest situation (the first 5 min) and is usually unsuccessful.

Note: *Repositioning of the pacer electrodes may facilitate capture. The major complication of this type of pacing is failure to recognize treatable* *ventricular fibrillation. If used prophylactically, always test first to make sure it captures before placing it in demand mode.*

21.8 RAPID-SEQUENCE INDUCTION

Rapid sequence induction of anesthesia is used to facilitate intubation. *Indications* include obtaining an airway in a nonfasting patient, avoiding an increase in intracranial pressure during intubation (important for head trauma and stroke patients), controlling the airway and patient for certain procedures (e.g., CT scan or MRI), and improving mechanical ventilation (Table 21.8.1).

1. Preoxygenate the patient. Establish intravenous access and set up monitoring equipment. Avoid manual ventilation with a bag-valve mask, as this may cause gastric distention, increasing aspiration risk.
2. Administer lidocaine (1.5 mg/kg IV). In the presence of head injury this might help to attenuate the increase in intracranial pressure secondary to intubation.
3. Administer pancuronium (0.01 mg/kg IV; in preparalyzing dose) to decrease the intensity of fasciculation due to succinylcholine. A preparalyzing dose is not necessary if a nondepolarizing agent is substituted for succinylcholine.
4. Administer atropine 0.01 mg/kg IV to prevent bradycardia.
5. Administer thiopental (4 mg/kg IV) to induce unconsciousness. Alternative agents are midazolam (0.1 mg/kg), ketamine (1 to 2 mg/kg), and diazepam (0.1 to 0.5 mg/kg). The agent should be chosen with consideration of side effects. Thiopental is a myocardial depressant and can decrease blood pressure. Ketamine raises intracranial pressure but is a bronchodilator and may be useful in asthmatic patients.
6. Sellick's maneuver increases cricoid pressure to prevent aspiration. Pressure should not be released until the endotracheal tube balloon is inflated.
7. Succinylcholine (a depolarizing neuromuscular blocking agent) is given at a dose of 1.5 mg/kg IV to cause paralysis. Contraindications include penetrating eye injuries (due to rise in intraocular pressure), burns older than 8 hr, crush injuries, hyperkalemia, and history of plasma pseudocholinesterase deficiency.
8. Following oral intubation, inflate the endotracheal tube

Table 21.8.1
Neuromuscular Paralyzing Agents

Agent	Dose (mg/kg)	Onset	Duration	Advantages	Disadvantages
Succinylcholine	1.0–1.5	30–60 sec	3–10 min	Fast onset and short duration	Increased intragastric and intraocular pressure; fasciculation; release of potassium
Vecuronium	0.1–0.25	2–4 min	25–60 min	No fasciculation; no increase in intraocular and intragastric pressures	Long recovery time at higher dose and with hepatic-renal dysfunction
Pancuronium	0.1	1–5 min	30–90 min		Can cause tachycardia
Atracurium	0.3–0.5	2–5 min	30 min	No renal excretion (better in patients with chronic renal failure)	Histamine release; hypotension; tachycardia

balloon, release the cricoid pressure, and confirm the positioning of the endotracheal tube.

Note: *These steps are only an outline. Any practitioner who plans to use rapid-sequence induction should be familiar with all the medications and techniques involved. Equipment must be prepared to perform a surgical airway in the event that intubation is not possible.*

The mnemonic for rapid-sequence induction is PLATS:

Prepare the patient, preoxygenate, and partial paralysis (defasciculating agent);
Lidocaine;
Atropine;
Tranquilization (thiopental); and
Succinylcholine and Sellick's maneuver.

21.9 COMPARTMENT PRESSURES

The diagnosis of a compartment syndrome must be made early to prevent permanent neuronal, muscular, and vascular injury. The following compartments can be monitored for increased pressure: forearm (dorsal and volar), hand, leg (anterior, lateral, superficial posterior, and deep posterior), and gluteal. Indications include clinical suspicion of a compartment syndrome, fractures, crush injuries, burns, hematomas, and venous obstruction. Refer to Figures 21.9.1 and 21.9.2.

1. Assemble the following:
   A 20-mL syringe;
   Three-way stopcock;
   Two pieces of intravenous tubing;
   Two 18-gauge needles;
   A column mercury manometer; and
   Sterile normal saline.
2. Draw up 10 to 15 mL of normal saline from the vented container. An air-fluid meniscus should be created by introducing air from the syringe into the proximal intravenous tubing.
3. Prep and drape the skin overlying the compartment to be monitored, using an antiseptic technique.
4. Apply local antiseptic to the superficial skin layer.
5. Carefully insert the needle into the compartment. **Note:** *Most compartments are relatively superficial.* The deep posterior leg

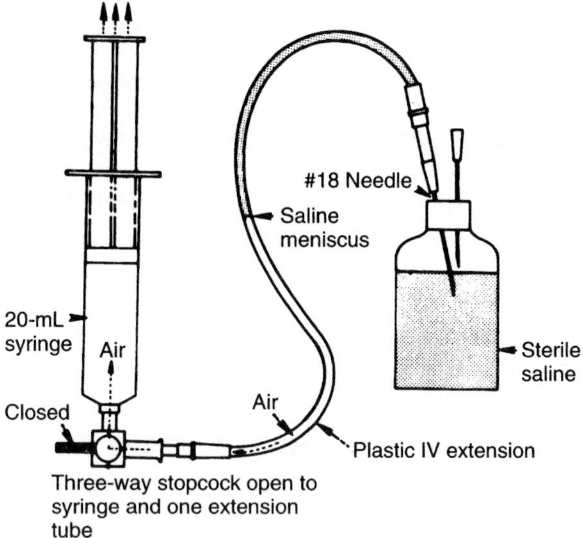

Figure 21.9.1. Equipment for measuring compartment pressure.

compartment and the gluteal compartment require deeper placement.

6. Connect the second intravenous tubing to the manometer and turn the stopcock so that all three ports are open.
7. Slowly depress the plunger of the syringe until the air-fluid meniscus moves toward the patient.
8. Read the manometer.
9. Obtain two additional readings of the compartment pressure to ensure accuracy.
10. Repeat the procedure on the nonaffected side for a comparison pressure reading if necessary. The normal compartment pressure is 8 to 15 mm Hg (10 to 20 cm H_2O).

21.10 EMERGENCY INTUBATION

Indications for emergency intubation include the following:

Multiple trauma and hypovolemic shock without response to supplemental oxygen;
Head trauma, coma, or stupor with risk of aspiration;

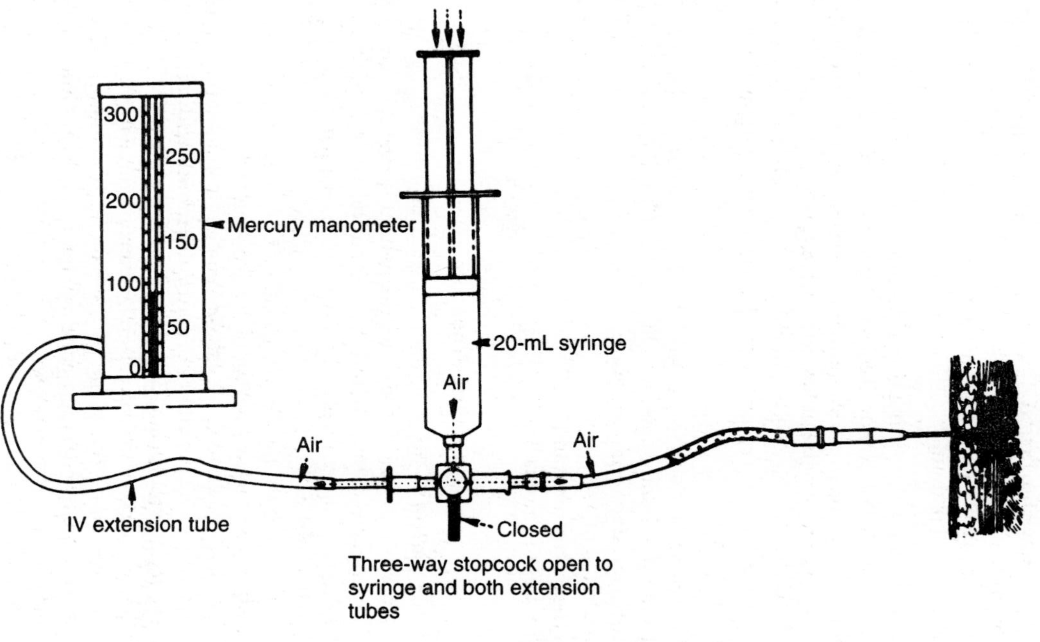

Figure 21.9.2. Compartment pressure measurement.

Inability to clear secretions, or an unconscious patient without a gag reflex 7;
Upper airway obstruction;
Poor or deteriorating blood gases; and
Acute respiratory failure or inadequate respiratory status in the critically ill patient.

Intubate immediately if necessary. Intubation should be performed by the most experienced physician in attendance. Administer positive pressure ventilation via bag valve mask with 100% oxygen. Hyperventilate to hyperoxygenate.

Assess the patient for difficulty in orotracheal intubation. These patients may require surgical airways. Patients in this group include those with:

Anatomic variation or short necks (less than three finger breadths from hyoid bone to mentum of chin when head is extended);
Massive facial trauma with distorted anatomy;
Intraoral hemorrhage;
Laryngeal fracture; and
Edema of the glottis or epiglottis.

The Procedure

1. The patient is hyperoxygenated via a bag valve mask; the hands should be restrained if the patient is awake.
2. The neck is extended and the occiput raised (sniffing position) to facilitate direct alignment of the oropharynx, larynx, and intubator's field of vision.
3. The mouth is opened with jaw thrust or finger scissor technique. Dentures or partial plates are removed.
4. The laryngoscope blade (#3 or 4 curved or straight blade) is introduced at the right corner of the mouth and displaces the tongue to the left.
5. The vocal cords are visualized by exerting force to the laryngoscope along the plane of the handle. It is important to avoid using the laryngoscope as a lever or coming into contact with the patient's teeth.
6. The Sellick's maneuver of cricoid pressure must be used to prevent passive regurgitation and augment visualization of cords. Suctioning is done at this point if needed.
7. The endotracheal tube is passed through the vocal cords to

the 19- to 21-cm mark on the tube as measured to the right corner of the mouth.

8. The balloon is inflated with air and the endotracheal tube is connected to the ball valve mask Ambu bag with 100% oxygen.
9. Auscultate the stomach. If an air rush is heard, the endotracheal tube is in the esophagus and must be removed immediately. Hyperoxygenate the patient via bag valve mask and begin endotracheal intubation again. Following endotracheal tube placement, auscultate the stomach again. If no air is heard, check both lung fields (anteriorly and laterally) to determine the presence of equal breath sounds. If breath sounds are decreased on the right, the endotracheal tube should be pulled back while the balloon is deflated. Recheck the new position with auscultation, secure the endotracheal tube, and reauscultate.
10. Confirm the placement of the endotracheal tube and check for pneumothorax immediately with a portable chest x-ray.
11. Empirically set the ventilator at FIO_2 100%, tidal volume 10 to 15 mL/kg, and respiratory rate of 12 to 16/min. Check an ABG in 15 min.
12. Attempt to decrease the FIO_2 to $< 60\%$, as alveolar-capillary membrane damage can occur in 12 to 24 hr at higher percentages. Begin treatment of the underlying pathology (e.g., bronchodilators for asthma or COPD, antibiotics and pulmonary toilet for pneumonia).
13. Always sedate an intubated or paralyzed patient. Analgesia must be remembered, as intubated patients cannot verbalize their pain.

Suggested Readings

Roberts J, Hedges J: Clinical procedures in emergency medicine. Philadelphia:, WB Saunders, 1991.

Rosen P, Barkin R: Emergency medicine: concepts and clinical practice. St. Louis: Mosby, 1992.

Rosen P, Sternbach GL: Atlas of emergency medicine. Baltimore: Williams & Wilkins, 1980.

Simon RR, Brenner BE: Procedures and techniques in emergency medicine. Baltimore: Williams & Wilkins, 1982.

Wilkens EW et al.: Emergency medicine. Baltimore: Williams & Wilkins, 1989.

Chapter 22

Formulas and Emergency Drugs

22.1 ACID-BASE CALCULATIONS

1. **Respiratory acidosis-alkalosis.** A change in P_{CO_2} of 10 mm Hg (10 torr) results in a reciprocal change in pH of 0.08 units.
2. **Metabolic acidosis.** In metabolic acidosis, the compensation of P_{CO_2} is calculated as 1.5 (HCO_3) + 8 (± 2).
3. **Metabolic alkalosis.** In metabolic alkalosis, the compensation of P_{CO_2} is calculated as 0.9 (HCO_3) + 9 (± 2).
4. **Differential diagnosis of anion gap metabolic acidosis.** Use the mnemonic MUD PILES:
   Methanol;
   Uremia;
   Diabetic ketoacidosis;
   Paraldehyde, phenformin, propylene glycol;
   Iron, isoniazid, inhalants (CO, CN, H_2S);
   Lactic acidosis;
   Ethanol ketoacidosis, ethylene glycol; and
   Salicylates, solvents (e.g., toluene), severe starvation.
5. **Differential diagnosis of nonanion gap acidosis.** Use the mnemonic HARD UP:

   Hypocapnia, hyperaldosteronism, hyperalimentation, hypoparathyroidism;
   Acetazolamide, ammonium chloride, arginine administration, aldactone;
   Renal (renal tubular acidosis, chronic pyelonephritis, interstitial nephritis);
   Diarrhea, dilution acidosis;

Uropathy (obstructive), ureteroenteric fistula; and Pancreatic fistula.

22.2 ALVEOLAR-ARTERIAL GRADIENT

Calculate alveolar oxygen tension (PAO_2):

$$PAO_2 = FIO_2\,(PATM - PWATER\ VAPOR) - \left(\frac{PCO_2}{0.8}\right)$$
$$= FIO_2\,(760 - 47) - \left(\frac{PCO_2}{0.8}\right)$$

Note: *If the patient is breathing room air (21% oxygen), then:*

$$PAO_2 = (0.21)(713) - \left(\frac{PCO_2}{0.8}\right)$$
$$\approx 150 - (1.2)\,PCO_2$$

Alveolar-arterial (A-a) gradient: $PAO_2 - PaO_2$ (PaO_2 taken from ABG). Normal A-a gradient = 3 to 20 mm Hg, with an age correction of 2.5 + age/4.

Causes of increased A/a gradient: Diffusion defect, right to left shunt (does not correct with 100% oxygen), and $\dot{V}/\dot{Q}$mismatch.

22.3 ANION GAP

Anion gap (AG): (Na + K) − (Cl + HCO_3); normal anion gap = 8 to 16 mEq/L. **Note:** *Normal AG is 8 to 12 mEq/L if potassium is not included.* Also, since chloride determinations may vary based on the laboratory method used, the normal anion gap should be adjusted for each institution.

Causes of an elevated anion gap: Metabolic acidosis, dehydration, sodium salts of strong acids (citrate, lactate, acetate), sodium penicillin in high doses, and metabolic and respiratory alkalosis.

Causes of a depressed anion gap: Decreased unmeasured anions; dilution (hypoalbuminemia); increased unmeasured cations; increased calcium, magnesium, lithium, paraproteinemia (multiple myeloma), and polymyxin B); underestimation of serum sodium, severe hypernatremia, and hyperviscosity; overestimation of serum chloride; and iodide or bromide ingestion.

22.4 ARTERIAL OXYGEN SATURATION (FIG. 22.4.1)

Causes of shift to the right (decreased affinity): Acidosis; hyperthermia; increased concentration of 2,3-DPG; sulfhemoglobin; and high altitude acclimatization.

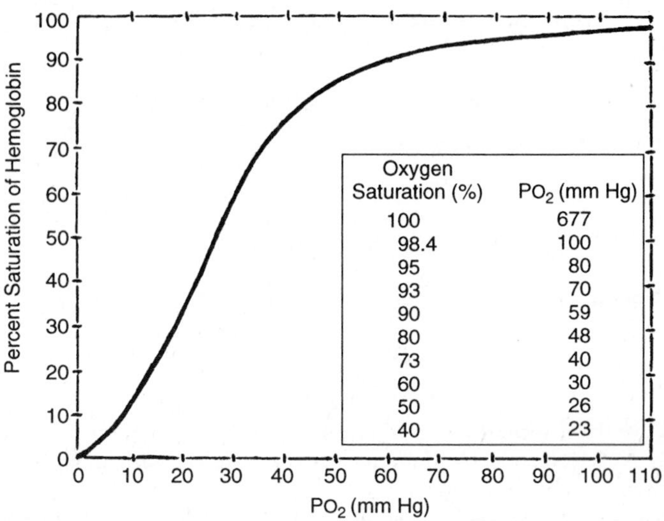

Oxygen Saturation (%)	PO_2 (mm Hg)
100	677
98.4	100
95	80
93	70
90	59
80	48
73	40
60	30
50	26
40	23

Figure 22.4.1. Oxyhemoglobin dissociation curve (pH 7.40; temperature 37°C).

Causes of shift to the left (increased affinity): Alkalosis; hypothermia; decreased concentration of 2,3-DPG (banked blood, low phosphate); fetal hemoglobin; methemoglobin; and carbon monoxide.

22.5 ARTERIAL OXYGEN CONTENT

Arterial oxygen content: $CaO_2 = 1.36$ (Hgb) (SaO_2) + 0.003 (PaO_2); normal $CaO_2 = 20$ vol %, or 20 mL/100 mL blood.

Mixed venous oxygen content: $CvO_2 = 1.36$ (Hgb) (SvO_2) + 0.003 (PvO_2); should be drawn from the pulmonary artery.

Arterial-venous oxygen difference: Normal $CaO_2 - CvO_2 = 2$ to 5 vol %. Values greater than 5 vol % imply inadequate tissue perfusion (e.g., shock).

22.6 CREATININE CLEARANCE

$$Cl_{cr} = \frac{U_{cr} \times U_{vol}}{S_{cr} \times 1440}$$

where U_{vol} is expressed in mL/24 hr.

$$= \frac{(140 - \text{Age})\ (\text{Weight})}{72 \times S_{cr}}$$

where weight is given in kilograms.

Normal creatinine clearance = 100 to 125 mL/min.

22.7 FRACTIONAL EXCRETION OF SODIUM

Fractional excretion of sodium (FENa) is described by the following equation:

$$\text{FENa} = \left[\left(\frac{U_{Na} \times U_{vol}}{S_{Na}}\right) \div \left(\frac{U_{cr} \times U_{vol}}{S_{cr}}\right)\right] \times 100$$

$$= \left(\frac{U_{Na}}{S_{Na}}\right) \times \left(\frac{S_{cr}}{U_{cr}}\right) \times 100\%$$

Note: *An FENa > 1% is often associated with oliguric renal insufficiency (acute tubular necrosis) and an FENa < 1% with prerenal azotemia.*

22.8 OSMOLAL GAP

Estimated serum osmolality: $2\text{Na} + \frac{\text{Glu}}{18} + \frac{\text{BUN}}{2.8}$; normal serum osmolality = 285 to 295 mOsm/kg · H_2O.

Osmol gap: Osm (measured) − Osm (calculated); normal osmolal gap is < 10 mOsm/kg · H_2O.

Causes of increased osmolal gap: Decreased serum water content, hyperproteinemia, hyperlipidemia, and additional substances in serum (sorbitol, glycerol, mannitol, ethanol, isopropyl alcohol, methanol, acetone, ethylene glycol, propylene glycol).

22.9 CARDIOVASCULAR CALCULATIONS—PRESSURES

Right atrium: 1 to 10 mm Hg (equivalent to CvP).

Right ventricle: 15 to 30 mm Hg systolic; 0 to 8 mm Hg diastolic (mean 10 to 15 mm Hg).

Pulmonary artery: 15 to 30 mm Hg systolic; 5 to 25 mm Hg diastolic (mean 10 to 22 mm Hg).

Pulmonary capillary wedge (PCWP): 8 to 10 mm Hg.

Mean arterial pressure (MAP):

$$\text{Diastolic} + \frac{\text{Systolic pressure} - \text{Diastolic pressure}}{3}$$

Systemic vascular resistance (SVR): $\text{SVR} = \frac{\text{MAP} - \text{RAP}}{\text{CO}} \times 80$; normal is 800 to 1400 dynes/sec/cm^3.

Emergency medications: See Table 22.9.1.

Table 22.9.1
Emergency Medications

Generic	Brand Name	Indication	Preparation	Dosage	Comments
Atropine	—	Asystole, bradycardia, heart block	1 mg (5 mL) = 0.5 mg	Give 1 mg IVp for asystole; 0.5 mg q 5 min IVp (0.04 mg/kg total)	May be given via ET tube
Adenosine	Adenocard	Drug of choice for paroxysmal supraventricular tachycardia	1 vial (2 mL) = 6 mg	Give 6 mg rapid IVp; follow with 20 mL NS flush; may repeat 12 mg IVp	Bradycardia, flushing dyspnea, chest pain; Theophylline is an antagonist
Amrinone	Inocor	Congestive heart failure	Place 11 amp (20 mL) = 100 mg in 100 mL NS (1 mg/mL)	Give 0.75 mg/kg IVp over 5 min; follow with 5–10 μg/kg/min infusion via pump	Can see nausea and vomiting and hypotension
Bretylium	Bretylol	Ventricular instability, ventricular fibrillation, and tachycardia	1 mg (10 mL) = 500 mg 2 g in 500 mL = 4 mg/mL	Give 5 mg/kg slow IVp (may give 5–10 mg/kg to 35 mg/kg total)	Nausea and hypotension may occur if injected too rapidly
Clonidine	Catapres	Hypertensive urgency or opiate withdrawal	0.1 mg tablets	Give 2 tabs PO stat followed by 0.1 mg PO q 1 hr	Not for hypertensive crisis or vomiting patient

Diazoxide	Hyperstat	Hypertensive crisis	1 amp = 300 mg (20 mL)	Give 100 mg slow IVp over 5 min three times, or 5 mg/kg at 15 mg/min IV via infusion pump	Give slowly and do not overshoot
Digoxin	Lanoxin	CHF, rapid atrial fibrillation	1 amp (2 mL) = 0.5 mg	Give 0.25–0.50 mg IVp slowly, followed by 0.2 mg q 3–5 hr to a total of 1.0–1.5 mg	Always check potassium and renal function
Diltiazem	Cardizem	Supraventricular tachycardia, atrial fibrillation or flutter	1 vial (5 mL) = 25 mg	Give 0.25 mg/kg IV over 2 min; repeat 0.35 mg/kg over 2 min and as needed	Caution with AV block
Dobutamine	Dobutrex	Refractory CHF	1 amp (20 mL) = 250 mg 250 mg in 500 mL = 500 μg/mL	Give 2–20 μg/kg/min IV via infusion pump	May see increase in heart rate
Dopamine	Intropin	Shock states	1 amp (5 mL) = 200 mg	Give 2–10 μg/kg/min IV via infusion pump; for easy dosing, multiply body weight (kg) by 30, and place that amount of dopamine (mg) in 500 mL D_5W, so 1 mL/hr = 1 μg/kg/min	May see nausea or tachycardia at doses > 10 μg/kg/min; essentially an α-agonist at high doses

Table 22.9.1—*Continued*

Generic	Brand Name	Indication	Preparation	Dosage	Comments
Edrophonium	Tensilon	Supraventricular tachycardia; also used as a test for myasthenia	1 amp (1 mL) = 10 mg	Give 1 mg slow IVp for a test dose; up to 10 mg total	Possible SLUD reaction; caution in asthmatics
Enalapril	Vasotec	Hypertensive urgency	1 vial (1 mL) = 1.25 mg	Give 1.25–2.50 mg IVp over 5 min	Angioedema, headache, nausea, and vomiting
Epinephrine	Adrenalin	Anaphylaxis and cardiac arrest (asystole or ventricular fibrillation)	1 amp (10 mL) of 1:10,000 = 1 mg	Give 5–10 mL IVp	Can give via ET tube; high doses (10 mg) have been used with equivocal results
Esmolol	Brevibloc	A-fib, A-flutter, hypertensive episodes	1 amp (2.5 g); add 2 amps to 500 mL D_5W = 10 mg/mL	Give 50–200 μg/kg/min	Can cause bradycardia or precipitate CHF
Glucagon	—	Hypoglycemia	1 vial (10 mL) = 10 mg	Give 1–3 mg IM or slow IVp; may repeat once	Nausea and vomiting
Hydralazine	Apresoline	Hypertensive crisis	1 amp (1 mL) = 20 mg	Give 10–20 mg IM; may repeat with increased dose after 45–60 min	May cause tachycardia and worsen angina; do not use in ASHD

Isoproterenol	Isuprel	Asystole, bradycardia, heart block, shock states	1 amp (5 mL) = 1 mg; 4 mg in 500 mL = 8 μg/mL	Give 2–10 μg/min IV via infusion pump	Can cause ventricular arrhythmias and exacerbate ischemia
Labetalol	Normodyne, Trandate	Hypertensive urgencies	1 vial (20 mL) = 100 mg	Give 0.25 mg/kg IVp over 2 min; can give 0.125–0.250 mg/kg q 10 min to total 300 mg; may give 2 mg/min infusion via pump	Dizziness, nausea, vomiting, and wheezing
Lidocaine	Xylocaine	Ventricular arrhythmias, prophylaxis in acute MI	1 amp (5 mL) = 100 mg 2 g/500 mL = 4 mg/mL	Give 1–1.5 mg/kg IVp (may repeat boluses of 0.5–1.5 mg/kg q 5–10 min to total of 3 mg/kg	May be given IM or via ET tube; give regular bolus and half-infusion in elderly and patients with HTN, CHF, and/or liver disease
Magnesium	—	Torsades de pointes, MI prophylaxis, eclampsia, magnesium deficiency	20 or 50% solution; mix 1–2 g in 50 mL D_5W	Give 1–2 g (8–16 mEq) over 5 min; can give 0.5–1 g q 1 hr; give 12 g/24 hr for MI	Flushing, hypotension, and depressed reflexes
Metaraminol	Aramine	Hypotension, supraventricular tachycardia	1 amp (10 mL) = 100 mg; 100 mg in 250 mL = 0.4 mg/mL	Give 0.2–1.0 mg/min IV via infusion pump	Possible ventricular arrhythmias; tissue sloughs if extravasates
Nifedipine	Procardia	Hypertensive urgency	1 capsule = 10 mg	Break sublingually, then chew and swallow	Not to be used for hypertensive crisis

Table 22.9.1—*Continued*

Generic	Brand Name	Indication	Preparation	Dosage	Comments
Nitroglycerin	Nitrol	Refractory angina	1 amp (10 mL) = 8 mg	Start with 5–10 μg/min IV; increase by 5 μg/min to a total of 100 μg/min via infusion pump; for easy dosing, put 50 mg in 500 mL D_5W; now each 3 mL/hr = 5 μg/min	Monitor BP; use special tubing
Nitroprusside	Nipride	Hypertensive crisis	1 amp (5 mL) = 50 mg; 50 mg/500 mL = 100 mg/mL	Give 0.5–10 μg/kg/min IV via infusion pump	Use tin foil; cyanide toxicity with high doses
Norepinephrine	Levophed	Shock states	1 amp (4 mL) = 4 mg; mix 8 mg in 500 mL D_5W = 16 μg/mL	Give 8–12 μg/min infusion via pump; must use central line	Extravasation may cause tissue sloughing
Phenylephrine	Neosynephrine	Hypotension	1 amp (1 mL) = 10 mg; dilute 10 mg in 9 mL D_5W or mix 10 mg in 500 mL D_5W (20 μg/mL)	Give 0.1–0.5 mg slow IVp; give 100–200 μg/min infusion via pump	Headache, arrhythmias, reflex bradycardia

Procainamide	Pronestyl	Ventricular arrhythmia, paroxysmal atrial fibrillation	1 amp (10 mL) = 100 mg	Give 20 mg/min slow IVp to total 17 mg/kg or until arrhythmia is suppressed, hypotension ensues, or QRS is widened 50%; follow with 1–4 mg/min IV infusion via pump	Monitor BP and ECG; may see hypotension and widening of QRS
Propranolol	Inderal	Ventricular arrhythmias, atrial fibrillation, SVT, refractory angina	1 amp (1 mL) = 1 mg	Give 0.5–1 mg slow IVp to total 0.1 mg/kg (can also use atenolol or metoprolol 5–10 mg IV over 5 min)	May cause acute bronchospasm; negative inotrope
Trimethaphan	Arfonad	Hypertensive crisis, especially aortic dissection	1 amp (10 mL) = 500 mg; 500 mg/500 mL = 1 mg/mL	Give 0.5–10 mg/min IV via infusion pump	Can see tachycardia and ileus
Vasopressin	Pitressin	Gastrointestinal bleeding due to varices	1 amp (10 mL) = 5 units; 100 units in 250 mL = 0.4 units/mL	Give 20 units slow IVp then 0.4 units/min infusion via pump	May see acute water retention; coronary or mesenteric ischemia
Verapamil	Isoptin, Calan	Atrial fibrillation, supraventricular tachycardia	1 amp (2 mL) = 5 mg	Give 2.5–5 mg slow IVp; may repeat in 15–30 min to total 20 mg.	Not with second- or third-degree block, sick sinus, preexcitation syndromes, or severe CHF

Index

Page numbers in *italics* indicate figures; page numbers followed by "t" indicate tabular material.

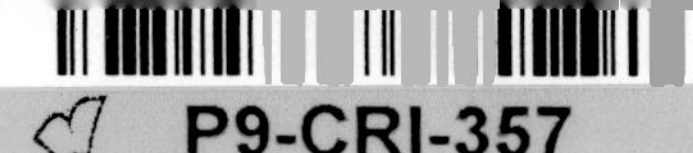

Praise for *Total Power*

"Mills's suspenseful, strikingly original sixth Mitch Rapp novel . . . is as riveting as anything penned by Mitch's creator, Vince Flynn (1966–2013). Mills has really hit his stride with this franchise entry."

—*Publishers Weekly* (starred review)

"A tour de force."

—*The Providence Journal*

"One of the best thriller writers on the planet."

—The Real Book Spy

Praise for *Lethal Agent*

"The writing is stellar, and the action is nonstop, as always, continuing the legacy that makes the Rapp series the best of the best when it comes to the world of special ops."

—*Booklist* (starred review)

"Mitch Rapp is the hero we need, maybe now more than ever."

—The Real Book Spy

"*Lethal Agent* is a gut punch of a tale that exploits our greatest fears, and it's as brilliantly conceived as it is wondrously crafted."

—*The Providence Journal*

Praise for *Red War*

"Heart-pounding, page-turning, riveting right from the start."

—*The Washington Times*

"Outstanding . . . Mills is writing at the top of his game in this nail-biter."

—*Publishers Weekly* (starred review)

"In the world of black-ops thrillers, Mitch Rapp remains the gold standard. Mills has embraced the high-concept-thriller style and continues to exceed expectations."

—*Booklist* (starred review)

PRAISE FOR *ENEMY OF THE STATE*

"In the world of black-ops thrillers, Mitch Rapp continues to be among the best of the best."

—*Booklist* (starred review)

"This novel perfectly combines geo-politics, covert operations, and the backstory of the characters. Readers can close their eyes and remember past books written by Vince Flynn and will not skip a beat with Kyle Mills at the helm."

—*Crimespree Magazine*

PRAISE FOR *ORDER TO KILL*

"This series continues to be the best of the best in the high adventure, action-heavy thriller field . . . . Flynn's name, Flynn's characters, and Mills's skill will take this one to the top of the charts, territory already familiar to Mitch Rapp."

—*Booklist* (starred review)

"What thriller readers live for: tense and dramatic with a nice twist."

—*Kirkus Reviews*

PRAISE FOR *THE SURVIVOR*

"The biggest compliment one can give Mills is that it's totally unclear where Flynn's work ends and his begins in *The Survivor*."

—*San Jose Mercury News*

"Mills has created a wonderful tribute to Flynn while also writing a great novel. While thriller readers and fans miss Flynn, Mills was the perfect choice, and Rapp will continue in good hands."

—Associated Press

PRAISE FOR

• *THE LAST MAN* • *KILL SHOT* • *AMERICAN ASSASSIN* •

• *PURSUIT OF HONOR* • *EXTREME MEASURES* •

• *PROTECT AND DEFEND* • *ACT OF TREASON* •

• Consent to Kill • Memorial Day •
• Executive Power • Separation of Power •
• The Third Option • Transfer of Power •
• Term Limits •

"Complex, chilling, and satisfying."

—*The Cleveland Plain Dealer*

"Just fabulous."

—Rush Limbaugh

"A Rambo perfectly suited for the war on terror."

—*The Washington Times*

"Pure high-powered exhilaration."

—*Lansing State Journal*

"Suspenseful . . . satisfying and totally unexpected."

—*The Roanoke Times*

"[A] thriller with deadly aim. . . . Moves at the speed of a Stinger missile."

—*People*

"Flynn has done his homework on military and security matters."

—*The Washington Post*

"Every American should read this book."

—Bill O'Reilly

"A page-turning read."

—Larry King, *USA Today*

"A roller-coaster, edge-of-your-seat thriller."

—*Minneapolis Star Tribune*

"Truly entertaining—even for those not particularly politically inclined."

—*The Cedar Rapids Gazette*

Novels by Vince Flynn

The Last Man
Kill Shot
American Assassin
Pursuit of Honor
Extreme Measures
Protect and Defend
Act of Treason
Consent to Kill
Memorial Day
Executive Power
Separation of Power
The Third Option
Transfer of Power
Term Limits

And by Kyle Mills

Enemy at the Gates
Total Power
Lethal Agent
Red War
Enemy of the State
Order to Kill
The Survivor

VINCE FLYNN

LETHAL AGENT

A MITCH RAPP NOVEL
BY KYLE MILLS

EMILY BESTLER BOOKS

ATRIA

New York London Toronto Sydney New Delhi

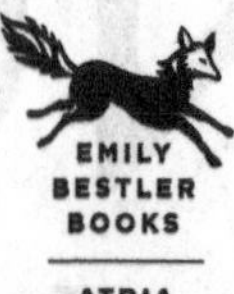

ATRIA
An Imprint of Simon & Schuster, Inc.
1230 Avenue of the Americas
New York, NY 10020

This Emily Bestler Books/Atria Paperback edition September 2021

EMILY BESTLER BOOKS / ATRIA PAPERBACKS
and colophon are trademarks of Simon & Schuster, Inc.

Manufactured in the United States of America

3 5 7 9 10 8 6 4 2

ISBN 978-1-5011-9062-9
ISBN 978-1-9821-4754-9 (pbk)
ISBN 978-1-5011-9064-3 (ebook)

Acknowledgments

Sitting alone in your basement all year can make producing a book seem like a solo effort. Nothing could be further from the truth. Thankfully, I've managed to fall in with a good crowd.

Emily Bestler and Sloan Harris were always there for Vince and they've been every bit as supportive of me. Lara Jones keeps me on track. Simon Lipskar and Celia Taylor Mobley keep me from getting tangled in the complex web I've created over the last twenty years. David Brown leaves no marketing stone unturned. Ryan Steck props me up with his enthusiasm and unparalleled knowledge of the Rappverse. My mother and wife are my first editorial stop, providing early criticism and ideas. Rod Gregg has become a recurring character—making sure I don't make any fatal firearms errors.

Without all of you, I'd just be staring at a blank computer screen . . .

AUTHOR'S NOTE

In *Transfer of Power*, Vince wrote that he intentionally omitted details relating to the White House and Secret Service. I find myself in a similar position with *Lethal Agent*.

Because of the sensitivity of border security at the time of writing, I've kept the details of crossings vague. Further, I either omitted or obscured the details of anthrax production.

PRELUDE

NORTHERN IRAQ

THE cave was more than ten meters square, illuminated with a handful of battery-powered work lights. The glare and heat from them was centered on two rows of men kneeling on colorful cushions. Armed guards lurked near the jagged walls, barely visible in the shadows.

Mullah Sayid Halabi sat cross-legged, gazing down from a natural stone platform. Most of the men lined up in front of him were in their middle years—former junior officers from Saddam Hussein's disbanded army. Their commanders had been either captured or killed over the years, but these simpler soldiers were in many ways more useful. Their superiors had left the details of war to them while they focused on the much more critical activity of currying favor with Hussein.

The prior leader of ISIS had recruited these men in an effort to turn his motivated but undisciplined forces into an army capable of holding and administering territory. After his death in a drone strike, Halabi had taken over the organization with a much more ambitious goal: building a military capacity that could stand against even the Americans. Unfortunately, it was proving to be an infuriating, slow, and expensive process.

His men, generally prone to bickering and loud displays of fealty, had fallen silent in order to contemplate the rhythm of approaching footsteps. Halabi did the same, turning his attention to an inky black tunnel in the wall facing him. A few moments later, Aali Nassar appeared.

His expensive clothing was torn and covered in the dust that made up this part of Iraq. His physical suffering was admirably absent from his expression but evident in both his posture and the broken section of collarbone pressing against the luxurious cotton of his shirt.

Only hours ago, he had been the highly respected and greatly feared director of Saudi intelligence. A man who had never failed to prove himself—first in the Saudi Special Forces and then during his meteoric rise through the ranks of his country's intelligence apparatus. He had the ear of the king, a devoted family, and a lifestyle marked by privilege and power.

But now all that was gone. His plot to overthrow the Saudi royalty had been discovered and he'd been forced to flee the country. The great Aali Nassar was now alone, injured, and standing in a cave with nothing more than the clothes on his back and the contents of his pockets. It was the latter that he hoped to exchange for protection and a position in the ISIS hierarchy.

"Welcome, Aali," Halabi said finally. "I trust your journey wasn't too uncomfortable."

"Not at all," he said, revealing only a hint of the pain that speaking caused him.

"I understand that you have something for me?"

The thumb drive Nassar was carrying had been discovered when he'd been searched for tracking devices in Mecca. He'd been allowed to keep it and now retrieved it from his pocket. When he stepped forward to hand it to Halabi, the men at the edges of the cave stirred.

"Don't give it to me." The ISIS leader pointed at a man to Nassar's right. "Give it to him."

He did as he was told and the man slipped the drive into a laptop.

"It's asking for a password."

"Of course it is," Halabi said. "But I suspect that Director Nassar will be reluctant to give us that password."

Prior to his escape from Saudi Arabia, Nassar had downloaded an enormous amount of information on that country's security operations, government officials, and clandestine financial dealings.

"The intelligence and bank account information on that drive are yours," Nassar said.

Halabi smiled. "A meaningless response. Perhaps politics was your true calling."

"Perhaps."

"Can we break his encryption?" Halabi asked.

His very capable technological advisor shook his head. "Unlikely. Torturing him for it would have a higher probability of success."

"I wonder," Halabi said thoughtfully. "It seems likely that there's a password that would put the information forever out of our reach. Isn't that so, Aali?"

"It is."

Halabi rubbed his palms together in front of his face. "The money that drive gives us access to will quickly slip through our fingers and the intelligence will just as quickly become dated. Is it the information it contains that's valuable or is it the cunning and experience of the man who brought it here?"

The question was clearly rhetorical, but one Halabi's people answered anyway. "Do those qualities make him valuable or do they make him dangerous? He's betrayed his king and country. Why? For the cause? For Allah? Or is it for personal gain? Can he be trusted, Mullah Halabi? Is he here to assist you or is he here to replace you?"

"I had power," Nassar responded. "I had wealth. I had the respect of the king and the Americans. But I jeopardized it all. I—"

"The king is old and weak," the man interrupted. "You feared the collapse of the kingdom and were playing both sides. The Americans discovered your treachery and now you've had to run."

Nassar fell silent for a moment before speaking again.

"They discovered my allegiance to Mullah Halabi, yes. Regrettable, because while I can be of great assistance to you from here, I would have been much more effective at the king's side. The effort that went into gaining his confidence isn't something that I'd expect a simple soldier to understand."

The man stiffened at the insult, but Nassar continued. "I've worked closely with the Americans on their homeland security protocols and preventing terrorist attacks on their soil. It's given me an intimate knowledge of their borders and immigration policy, their power grid and nuclear plants. Even their water supply. If we strike surgically, we can turn the tide of the war. We can make the Americans lash out against all Muslims and turn your thirty thousand soldiers into a billion."

Halabi stared down at Nassar, who averted his eyes in an obviously insincere gesture of fealty.

Then his forehead exploded outward.

In the split second of stillness that followed, Halabi saw a bearded face flicker into view at the tunnel entrance. It was the face of the devil that had been burned so indelibly onto his mind and soul. The face of Mitch Rapp.

And then everything was in motion. Members of Halabi's guard charged toward him while others fired into the tunnel. Three of his men began dragging him toward a small opening at the back of the cavern as the roar of gunfire and acrid stench of gunpowder became overwhelming.

A blinding flash preceded the sensation of shrapnel tearing through his lower leg. The man behind him took the brunt of the blast, slamming into Halabi from behind and driving him to the ground. The lights were immediately extinguished and debris began cascading from the ceiling. The men with him were either dead or unconscious, and Halabi struggled to get out from beneath the weight of the one sprawled across his back.

As he did so, the extent of his injuries became clear. His right arm was useless and completely numb. His left leg felt as though it was on fire and a dagger-like pain in his side made it difficult to breathe. The warm, wet sensation of flowing blood seemed to cover nearly his entire body, but it was impossible to know if it was his or that of his men.

A few muffled shouts became audible but were quickly drowned out by a collapse somewhere not far from him. A rush of air washed over him, filling the cavern with a choking cloud of dust and pulverized rock. He buried his face in his blood-soaked tunic and fought to stay conscious.

It couldn't end this way. God wouldn't allow it. He wouldn't allow his faithful disciple to die at the hands of Satan's representative on earth. Not before His work was done.

A test. That had to be the explanation. It was a test of his strength. His worthiness. His devotion.

Bolstered by that realization, Halabi managed to drag himself from beneath his man. The darkness was now absolute, but he was able to find the back wall of the cave and feel along it as the last weak shouts around him fell silent. Finally, he located the narrow opening he was looking for and, by the grace of God, it was still passable.

Reports were that it was six hundred meters long and varied from three meters in diameter to barely wide enough for a full-grown man. He dragged himself through the broken rock, feeling his way forward. In places the passage seemed blocked, but after a few moments of blind exploration, he always managed to progress a few more meters.

Finally the walls narrowed to the point that it was impossible to continue. He tried to retreat but found himself trapped.

The world seemed to disappear, adding to his confusion and amplifying the pain that racked his body. For a time, there was little else. No sound that wasn't produced by him. No light that his eyes could process. Only the pain, the taste of earth, and the swirl of his own thoughts.

The elation he'd felt when he'd concluded this was a test became lost in the realization that what he was experiencing felt more like a punishment. What had he done to deserve Allah's wrath?

He slipped in and out of consciousness, though in the darkness it was difficult to differentiate the two. He saw America. The gleaming buildings. The mass of humanity pursuing pleasure and comfort as a replacement for God. He saw the glorious collapse of the World Trade Center and the horror and vulnerability that attack had instilled in the American people. An incredible victory wasted by Osama bin Laden, who had turned to blithering endlessly about Islam on hazy video.

He saw the rise of ISIS fueled by its grasp of social media and intimate understanding of what motivated young men throughout the world. And, finally, he saw its battlefield victories and ability to terrify the Americans in a way that even September 11 hadn't.

He tried to pull himself forward again and again collapsed into the bed of shattered rock beneath him. The darkness and silence was deeper than anything he'd ever experienced. It blurred not only the lines between consciousness and lucidity but between life and death. Only the pain and sound of his own breathing assured him that he hadn't crossed over.

He didn't know how long he lay there but finally the darkness began to recede. He opened his eyes but didn't see the earthen tunnel around him. Only the blinding white light of God. It was then that he understood. It was his own arrogance that had brought him to this place. He had allowed his own hate and thirst for victory to deflect him from the work God had charged him with. He had become seduced by the power he wielded over his followers and the fear he commanded from his enemies. By visions of a new caliphate with him at its head, locked in righteous battle with the forces of the West.

He felt the panic rising in him, growing to a level that was nearly unbearable. The life he'd lived was a lie and God had finally shown him that fact. He had served only himself. Only his own vanity and hate.

Halabi clawed at the walls around him, unwilling to die in this graceless state. He felt something in his shoulder tear, but ignored it and was finally rewarded with a cascade of rock that created a path forward.

He was free.

CHAPTER 1

SOUTHWEST OF THAMUD
YEMEN

MITCH Rapp started to move again, weaving through an expansive boulder field before dropping to his stomach at its edge. A quick scan of the terrain through his binoculars provided the same result it had every time before: reddish dirt covering an endless series of pronounced ridges. No water. No plant life. A burned-out sky starting to turn orange in the west. If it were ninety-five below zero instead of ninety-five above, he could have been on Mars.

Rapp shifted his gaze to the right, concentrating for a good fifteen seconds before spotting a flash of movement that was either Scott Coleman or one of his men. All were wearing camo made from cloth specifically selected and dyed for this op by Charlie Wicker's girlfriend. She was a professional textile designer and a flat-out genius at matching colors and textures. If you gave her a few decent photos of your operating theater, she'd make you disappear.

A couple of contrails appeared above and he followed them with his eyes. Saudi jets on their way to bomb urban targets to the west. This sparsely populated part of Yemen had become the exclusive territory of ISIS and al Qaeda, but the Saudis largely ignored it. Viable targets were hard to engage from the air and the Kingdom didn't have the stomach to get bloody on the ground. That job had once again landed in his lap.

Satisfied they weren't being watched, Rapp started forward in a crouch. Coleman and his team would follow, watching his back at perfect intervals like they had in Iraq. And Afghanistan. And Syria. And just about every other shithole the planet had to offer.

The Yemeni civil war had broken out in 2015 between Houthi rebels and government forces. Predictably, other regional powers had been drawn in, most notably Iran backing the rebels and Saudi Arabia getting behind the government. The involvement of those countries had intensified the conflict, creating a humanitarian disaster impressive even by Middle Eastern standards.

In many ways, it was a forgotten war. The world's dirty little secret. Even among U.S. government officials and military commanders, it would be hard to find anyone aware that two-thirds of Yemen's population was surviving on foreign aid and another eight million were slowly starving. They also wouldn't be able to tell you that hunger and the loss of basic services were causing disease to run rampant through the country. Cholera, antibiotic-resistant bacteria, and even diphtheria were surging to levels unheard-of in the modern era.

And anyplace that could be described using words like "forgotten," "rampant," and "war" eventually became a magnet for terrorists. They were yet another disease that infected the weakened and wounded.

An unusually high ridge became visible to the northwest, and Rapp dropped to the ground again, studying it through his lenses. He could make out a gap just large enough for a human about three hundred yards away.

"Whatcha got?" Coleman said over his earpiece.

"The cave entrance. Right where they said it would be."

"Are we moving?"

"No, it's backlit. We'll let the sun drop over the horizon."

"Roger that. Everybody copy?"

Bruno McGraw, Joe Maslick, and Charlie Wicker all acknowledged. The four men made up about half the people in the world Rapp trusted. Probably a sad state of affairs, but one that had kept him alive for a lot longer than anyone would have predicted.

He fine-tuned the focus on his binoculars, refining his view of the dark hole in the cliff face. It was hard to believe that Sayid Halabi was still alive. If Rapp had been any closer with that grenade, it would have gotten jammed in the ISIS leader's throat. But even if his aim had been way off, it shouldn't have mattered. The blast had brought down a significant portion of the cavern he'd been hiding out in.

The collapse had been extensive enough that Rapp himself had been trapped in it. In fact, he'd have died slowly in the darkness if Joe Maslick wasn't a human wrecking ball who had spent much of his youth digging ditches on a landscaping crew. Oxygen had been getting pretty scarce when Mas finally broke through and dragged him from the grave he'd made for himself.

Despite all that, the intel on Halabi seemed reasonably solid. A while back, someone at NSA had decrypted a scrambled Internet video showing the man standing in the background at an al Qaeda meeting. The initial take had been that it was archival footage dredged up to keep the troops motivated. Deeper analysis, though, suggested that the images may have been taken six months *after* the night Rapp thought he'd finally ground his boot into that ISIS cockroach.

The video had led to the capture of one of the people at that meeting, and his interrogation led Rapp to this burned-out plain. The story was that Halabi had been severely injured by that grenade and was hiding out here convalescing. The sixty-four-thousand-dollar question was whether it was true. And if it was true, was he *still* here. Clearly, he was healthy enough to be going to meetings and starting the process of rebuilding ISIS after the beating it had taken in his absence.

The sun finally hit the horizon, causing an immediate drop in temperature and improvement in visibility. Waiting for full darkness was an option, but it seemed unnecessary. He hadn't seen any sign of exterior guards and night versus day would have little meaning once he passed into that cave.

"We're on," he said into his throat mike.

"Copy that," came Coleman's response.

Rapp angled left, moving silently across the rocky terrain until he reached a stone wall about twenty yards from the cavern entrance. Staying low, he crept along the wall's base until he reached its edge. Still no sign of ISIS enforcers. Behind him, the terrain was similarly empty, but that was to be expected. Coleman and his team would remain invisible until they were needed. It was impossible to anticipate the environment inside the cave, and Rapp was concerned that it could get tight enough to make a force of more than one man counterproductive.

When he finally slipped inside, the only evidence that it was inhabited was the churned dirt beneath his feet. He held his weapon in front of him as he eased along a passage about three feet wide and ten feet high. The familiar weight of his Glock had been replaced with that of an early-model Mission crossbow. His weapons tech had modified it for stealth, pushing the decibel level below eighty-five at the bow. Even better, the pitch had been lowered to the point that it sounded nothing like a weapon. Even to Rapp's practiced ear, it came off more like a bag of sand dropping onto a sidewalk.

Crossbows weren't the fastest things to reload and there hadn't been much time to train with it, but he still figured it was the best tool for the job. The quietest pistol he owned—a Volquartsen .22 with a Gemtech suppressor—was strapped to his thigh, but it would be held in reserve. While it was impressively stealthy, the sharp crack it made was too loud and recognizable for this operating environment.

The darkness deepened the farther he penetrated, forcing him to move slowly enough for his eyes to keep pace. Based on what had happened last time he'd chased Sayid Halabi into a hole, it made sense to prioritize caution over speed. Mas might have forgotten his shovel.

A faint glow became visible at the end of the passage and Rapp inched toward it, avoiding the rocks beneath his feet and staying on the soft earth. As he got closer, he could see that the corridor came to a T. The branch going right dead-ended after a few feet but the one to the left continued. A series of tiny bulbs wired to a car battery was the source of the glow.

One of the downsides of LED technology was that it made hiding out in caves a lot easier. A single battery could provide light for days. But it also created a vulnerability. Power supplies tended not to be as widely distributed and redundant as they used to be.

Rapp reached down and flipped the cable off the battery, plunging the cavern into darkness.

Shouts became audible almost immediately, but sounded more annoyed than alarmed. Rapp could tell that the voices belonged to two male Arabic speakers, but picking out exactly what they were saying was difficult with the echo. Basically a little name-calling and arguing about whose turn it was to fix the problem. When all your light came from a single improvised source, occasional outages were inevitable.

One of the men appeared a few seconds later, swinging a flashlight in his right hand but never lifting it high enough to give detail to his face. It didn't matter. From his youthful gait and posture, it was clear that it wasn't Halabi. Just one of his stooges.

Rapp aimed around the corner and gently squeezed the trigger. The sound profile of the crossbow and the projectile's impact were both outstanding. Unfortunately, the accuracy at this range was less so. The man was still standing, seemingly perplexed by the fletching protruding beneath his left clavicle.

Rapp let go of his weapon and sprinted forward, getting one arm around the Arab's neck and clamping a hand over his mouth and nose. The man fought as he was dragged back around the corner, but the sound of their struggle was attenuated by soft ground. Finally, Rapp dropped and wrapped his legs around him to limit his movement. There wasn't enough leverage to choke him out, but the hand over his face was doing a pretty good job of suffocating him. The process took longer than he would have liked and he was gouged a few times by the protruding bolt, but the Arab finally lost consciousness. A knife to the base of his skull finished the job.

Rapp slid from beneath the body and was recocking the crossbow when another shout echoed through the cavern.

"Farid! What are you doing, idiot? Turn the lights back on!"

Rapp yelled back that he couldn't get them working, counting on the acoustics to make it difficult to distinguish one Arabic-speaking male from another. He loaded a bolt into his weapon and ran to the battery, putting the flashlight facedown in the dirt before crouching. The illumination was low enough that anyone approaching wouldn't be able to see much more than a vague human outline.

A stream of half-baked electrical advice preceded the sound of footsteps and then another young man appeared. He didn't seem at all concerned, once again proving the grand truth of all things human: people saw what they wanted and expected to see.

Rapp let the terrorist get to within fifteen feet before snatching up the crossbow. This time he compensated by aiming low and left, managing to put the projectile center of mass. No follow-up was necessary. The man fell forward, landing face-first in the dirt.

Certain that he wasn't getting up again, Rapp reconnected the battery. He was likely going to need the light. Things had gone well so far but, in his experience, good luck never came in threes.

Support for that hypothesis emerged when a man who was apparently distrustful of the sound of falling sand bags sprinted around the corner. Rapp's .22 was in an awkward position to draw, so instead he grabbed one of the bolts quivered on the crossbow.

The terrorist had been a little too enthusiastic in his approach and his momentum bounced him off one of the cave's walls. Rapp took advantage of his compromised balance and lunged, driving the bladed head into his throat.

Not pretty, but effective enough to drop the man. As he fell, though, a small pipe sprouting wires rolled from his hand.

Not again.

Rapp used his boot to kick the IED beneath the man's body and then ran in the opposite direction, making it about twenty feet before diving into a shallow dip in the ground. The explosion sent hot gravel washing over him and he heard a few disconcertingly loud cracks from above, but that was it. The rock held. He rolled onto his back, pulling his shirt over his mouth and nose to protect his lungs from the dust. The smart money would be to turn tail and call in a few bunker busters, but he couldn't bring himself to do it. If Halabi was there, Rapp was going to see him dead. Even if they entered the afterlife together with their hands around each other's throats.

The sound of automatic fire started up outside but Rapp ignored it, pulling the Volquartsen and using a penlight to continue deeper into the cavern. Coleman and his boys could handle themselves.

The cave system turned out to be relatively simple—a lot of branches, but almost all petered out after a few feet. The first chamber of any size contained a cot and some rudimentary medical equipment—an IV cart, monitors, and a garbage can half full of bloody bandages. All of it looked like it had been there for a while.

The second chamber appeared to have been set up for surgical procedures but wasn't much more advanced than something from

World War I. A gas cylinder that looked like it came from a welder, a tray with a few instruments strewn across it, and a makeshift operating table streaked with dried blood.

And that was the end of the line. The cave system dead-ended just beyond.

"Shit!" Rapp shouted, his voice reverberating down the corridor and bouncing back to him.

The son of a bitch had been there. They'd brought him to treat the injuries he'd sustained in Iraq and to give him time to heal. A month ago, Rapp might have been able to look into his eyes, put a pistol between them, and pull the trigger. But now he was long gone. Sayid Halabi had slipped through his fingers again.

CHAPTER 2

AL MUKALLA
YEMEN

SAYID Halabi carefully lowered himself into a chair facing a massive hole in the side of the building he was in. Shattered concrete and twisted rebar framed his view of the cityscape stretching into the darkness. A half-moon made it possible to make out the shapes of destroyed vehicles, collapsed homes, and scattered cinder blocks. No light beyond that provided by God burned anywhere in sight. Power had once again been lost and the city's half a million residents were reluctant to light fires or use battery power out of fear that they could be targeted by the Saudis.

It hadn't always been so. In 2015, al Qaeda had taken advantage of the devastation brought by Saudi Arabia's air war in Yemen and mounted an attack on Al Mukalla. Government forces had barely even gone through the motions of fighting back. After a few brief skirmishes they'd run, abandoning not only a terrified populace but the modern weapons of war—battle tanks, American-made Humvees, and heavy artillery.

After that stunning victory, a glorious glimpse of what was possible had ensued. Strict Islamic law was imposed as al Qaeda took over the governance of the city. Roads were repaired, public order was restored, hospitals were built. Sin and destruction were replaced by order and service to God.

A year later, Emirati-backed soldiers had driven al Qaeda out, returning the city to the dysfunctional and corrupt Yemeni government. Since then, nothing had been done to rebuild, and the Saudis' indiscriminant bombing continued, slowly strangling hope. Hunger, disease, and violence were all that people had left.

A lone car appeared to the east, weaving slowly through the debris with headlights extinguished. Halabi followed it with his gaze for a time, wondering idly where the driver had managed to find fuel and listening for approaching Saudi jets. None materialized, though, and the car eventually faded from view.

The ISIS leader was finally forced to stand, the pain in his back making it impossible to remain in the chair any longer. Three cracked vertebrae were the least visible of his injuries, but by far the most excruciating. Mitch Rapp's attack on him in Iraq had taken its toll. Beyond the damage to his back, Halabi no longer had full use of his right leg and, in fact, had barely avoided its amputation. His left eye had been damaged beyond repair and was now covered with a leather patch. The shattered fingers on his left hand had been straightened and set, but lacked sensation.

He'd spent months hidden underground, submitting to primitive medical procedures, surviving various infections and extended internal bleeding. All the while wondering if the Americans knew he'd survived. If, at any moment, Rapp would once again appear.

After a time those fears had faded and he began to heal both physically and psychologically. Once he was able, he'd devoted himself to prayer and study. He'd spent endless hours watching newsfeeds from throughout the world, reading history and politics, and studying military strategy. During that time, he came to understand why God had allowed his most devoted servant to be attacked in such a way. Halabi had let his life become consumed with the battle. He'd pursued the fleeting pleasure of inflicting damage instead of dedicating himself to the far more arduous and unsatisfying task of securing a final victory.

Footsteps became audible behind him and he turned to watch his most loyal disciple approach.

Muhammad Attia was an American by birth, the son of Algerian immigrants. He'd expended his youth working at his parents' general store in New York and seeking the approval and acceptance of the Westerners around him. After high school, he'd attended a year of community college before taking a job as a civilian Arabic translator for the U.S. Army.

As a Muslim American, he'd already experienced the treachery and moral bankruptcy of his parents' adopted country, but it wasn't until he'd arrived in Iraq that he came to understand the magnitude of it.

His recruitment by al Qaeda had occurred less than six months into his tour and he spent almost five years as an agent for the organization before being discovered. He'd proved too clever for the Americans, though, and had escaped into the desert before they could come for him.

"Can we change?" Halabi said as the younger man approached. "Are my followers capable?"

"Everything is possible with Allah's help."

"But it's far more difficult than I imagined to garner that help."

"No man can see into the mind of God. We can only seek to play our small role in His plan."

Halabi nodded. "Are we ready?"

"We are."

The stairs had been cleared of debris, but the ISIS leader still needed help getting down them. The darkness deepened as they descended into what was left of the building's basement. Halabi felt a moment of panic when the door closed behind them and the blackness recalled the agonizing hours he'd spent dragging himself from the cavern in Iraq.

This time, though, the darkness didn't last. The dim glow of computer monitors coming to life pushed back the emptiness and he found himself standing in front of a series of screens, each depicting a lone male face.

The difference between this ISIS leadership meeting and his last one couldn't have been more stark. The former Iraqi soldiers who had lined up on the ground in front of him and the traitorous Aali Nassar were all dead now. Taken from him by God not as a punishment but because they were useless. He understood that and so much more now.

With his newfound clarity, Halabi saw his past actions as almost comically misguided. He'd put his faith in men who had already been defeated by the Americans once. They'd had no new ideas. No new capabilities. No knowledge or insight that hadn't existed for decades. The most that they could hope to do was bring order and discipline to ISIS's next failure.

A red light flashed on a camera in front of him and the faces on-screen gained resolve. Despite the hardening of their expressions, though, it was clear that none were soldiers. Some were well-groomed and clean-shaven while others had thick beards and unkempt hair. The youngest was barely twenty and the oldest hadn't yet reached his fortieth year of life. Two—one a pale-complected Englishman—didn't even speak rudimentary Arabic.

That diversity went deeper than appearance, extending to their areas of expertise. Computer programming. Marketing. Finance. The sciences. Perhaps most important was a young documentary filmmaker who had spent the last year working for Al Jazeera. The only common thread was that all had been educated in the West. It was something he now required of his inner circle.

While a far cry from the brutal and fanatical forces Halabi had once commanded, these men had the potential to be much more dangerous.

"There was a time when I believed that the movement had lost its way," Halabi said in English, his heavily accented words being transmitted over a secure satellite link. "But now I understand that there was never a path to victory. Osama bin Laden expected his actions in New York to begin the collapse of a society already faltering under the weight of its own moral decay. But what was really accomplished? Punishing but ultimately indecisive wars in Afghanistan and Iraq. A handful of minor follow-up attacks that were lost in America's culture of violence and mass murder. Bin Laden spent his final years bleating like a sheep and waiting for the Americans to find him."

Halabi paused and examined the faces on the screens before him. While these men were indeed different from the ones he'd commanded before, the fire in their eyes burned just as intensely. The movement was everything to them. It gave them purpose. It gave them a target for their fury, hate, and frustration. And it gave them peace.

"Al Qaeda failed because their leadership grew old and forgot what motivates young men," Halabi said flatly.

Osama bin Laden had feared the rise in brutality throughout the region, seeing it as counterproductive to recruitment. Unfortunately, he hadn't lived to see the truth. To see the slickly produced videos of chaotic, merciless victories. To hear the pumping music that accompanied them and the computer-generated imagery that enhanced them. To see thousands of young men, motivated by this propaganda, flood into the Middle East. Ready to fight. Ready to die.

"And ISIS did no better," Halabi continued. "I and my predecessors became intoxicated by the vision of a new caliphate. The Middle East was fractured and the West was tired of fighting wars that couldn't be decisively won. We deluded ourselves into believing that we were ready to come out of the shadows and stand against the U.S. military."

He paused, considering how much he wanted to say. In the end, though, this was the age of information. Withholding it from his inner circle would lead only to another defeat.

"It was all a waste of time and martyrs. The moment for that kind of action had not yet arrived."

"Has it arrived now?" one of the men said, his youthful impatience audible even over the cheap computer speakers. "America is as weak as it has been in a hundred and fifty years. Its people are consumed with hatred for each other. They see themselves as having been cheated by the rest of the world. Stolen from. Taken advantage of. The twenty-four-hour news cycle continues to reinforce these attitudes, as do the Russians' Internet propaganda efforts. And the upcoming presidential election is amplifying those divisions to the point that the country is being torn apart."

"It's not enough," Halabi said. "The Americans are people of extremes, prone to fits of rage and self-destructiveness, but also in possession of an inner strength that no one in history has been able to overcome."

The faces on the screens looked vaguely stunned at what they saw as adulation for their enemy. It was one of many lessons Halabi had learned in his time confined to a hospital bed deep underground: not to let hatred blind one to the strengths and virtues of one's enemies.

"If no one has been able to overcome it," the British man said, "how can we?"

It was the question that Halabi had been asking for almost his entire life. The question that God had finally answered.

"We'll continue to distract them by fanning the flames of their fear and division," he said.

"And after that?" the man pressed.

"After that we'll strike at them in a way that no one in history has ever even conceived of."

CHAPTER 3

AL HUDAYDAH
YEMEN

THE port city still had more than two million residents, but at this point it was just because they didn't have anywhere else to go. Some buildings remained untouched, but others had taken hits from the Saudi air force and were now in various states of ruin. Almost nightly, bombing runs rewrote the map of Al Hudaydah, strewing tons of rubble across some streets while blasting others clean.

Rapp walked around a burned-out car and turned onto a pitted road that was a bit more populated. Knots of men had formed around wooden carts, buying and trading for whatever was available. Women, covered from head to toe in traditional dress, dotted the crowd, but only sparsely. They tended to be kept squirreled away in this part of the world, adding to the dysfunction.

One was walking toward Rapp, clinging to the arm of a male relative whose function would normally have been to watch over her. In this case, the roles had been reversed. He was carrying the AK-47 and ceremonial dagger that were obligatory fashion accessories in Yemen, but also suffering from one of the severe illnesses unleashed by the war. The woman was the only thing keeping him upright.

He stumbled and Rapp caught him, supporting his weight until he could get his feet under him again. When the woman mumbled her thanks, Rapp figured he'd take advantage of her gratitude. The map he'd been given by the CIA wasn't worth the paper it was printed on.

"Do you know where Café Pachachi is?"

Her eyes—the only part of her visible—widened and she took a hesitant step back.

It wasn't surprising. As ISIS lost territory, a lot of its unpaid and leaderless fighters were turning to extortion, drug trafficking, and sexual slavery to make a living. Rapp's physical appearance and Iraqi accent would likely mark him as one of those men.

"Café Pachachi?" he repeated.

She gave a jerky nod and a few brief instructions before skirting him and disappearing into the glare of the sun.

It took another thirty minutes, but he finally found it. The restaurant was housed in a mostly intact stone building with low plastic tables and chairs set up out front. A few makeshift awnings provided shade, and improvised barriers kept customers from falling into a bomb crater along the eastern edge.

Despite the war, business seemed good. The patio was filled with men leaning close to each other, speaking about politics, God, and death. Waiters hustled in and out of the open storefront, shuttling food and drinks, clearing dishes, and occasionally getting drawn into one of the passionate conversations going on around them.

It was hard to believe that this was pretty much the sum total of the CIA's presence in Yemen. It was one of the most lawless, terrorist-ridden countries in the world, and the United States had ceded its interests to the Saudis.

America's politicians were concerned with nothing but the perpetuation of their own power through the next election cycle. The sitting president was playing defense, trying not to do anything that could cause problems for his party in the upcoming presidential election. The primaries were in full swing, with the sleaziest, most destructive candidates on both sides in the lead. And the American people were laser-locked on all of it, goading the participants on like it was some kind of pro wrestling cage match.

With no one watching the store in Yemen, ISIS was starting to find its footing again—using the chaos as cover to regroup and evolve. It was a mistake the politicians couldn't seem to stop making. Or maybe it wasn't a mistake at all. Terrorism was great theater—full of sympathetic victims, courageous soldiers, and evil antagonists. It was the ultimate political prop. Perhaps America's elected officials weren't as anxious to give it up as their constituents thought. Solved problems didn't get out the vote.

"Allah has delivered you safely!" Shamir Karman exclaimed, weaving through the busy tables to embrace him. "Welcome, my friend!"

Rapp didn't immediately recognize the man. Karman always carried an extra twenty-five or so pounds in a gravity-defying ring around his waist. It was completely gone now and his bearded face looked drawn.

"It's good to see you again," Rapp said in the amiable tone expected by the diners around him.

"Come! There's no reason for us to stand among this riffraff. I keep the good food and coffee in the back."

Laughter rose up from his customers as he led Rapp into the dilapidated building. The human element had always been Karman's genius. The native Yemeni had been recruited by the CIA years ago, but it had been clear from the beginning that he'd never be a shooter. No, his weapon was that he was likable as hell. The kind of guy you told your deepest secrets to. That you wanted in your wedding party. That you invited to come stay indefinitely at your house. All within the first ten minutes of meeting him.

"There was another bombing last night," he said as they passed indoor tables that had been set aside for women to sit with their families.

"Did they get close?"

The Agency was working to keep the Saudis away from this neighborhood, but no one was anxious to tell them too much out of fear of a leak. It was the kind of tightrope walk that was Irene Kennedy's bread and butter, but there were no guarantees. One arrogant commander or confused pilot could turn Karman and his operation into a pillar of fire.

"No. The bastards were just dropping random bombs to hide their real target."

"Which was?"

"The sanitation facility we keep putting back together with spit and chewing gum. We're already dealing with one of the deadliest outbreaks of cholera in history, and they want to make it worse. If they can't bomb us into submission, they'll kill us with disease and hunger."

The anger in his voice wasn't just for the benefit of his cover. In truth, Karman's loyalties were a bit hard to pin down, but that's what made him so good at his job. He sincerely cared about his country, and anyone who met him could feel that sincerity.

"Did you come with family?" the Yemeni said.

It wasn't hard to figure out what he was asking. He was worried that Coleman and his men were in-country and would stand out like a sore thumb. Rapp shared that concern and had sent them to Riyadh. They were currently floating in the pool of a five-star resort at the American taxpayers' expense.

"No. I'm alone."

"You'll stay with me, of course. I can't offer you much luxury, but there's not a lot of that to be had in Yemen anymore."

"Thank you. You're very generous, my friend."

They entered the kitchen and instead of the pleasant odor of boiling saltah, Rapp was hit with the powerful stench of bleach.

"My success isn't just about my skills as a chef and my consistent supply of food," Karman said, reading his expression. "With the cholera outbreak, it's all about cleanliness. No one has ever gotten sick eating at my establishment." He increased the volume of his voice. "And no one ever will, right?"

The kitchen staff loudly assured him that was the case.

"Seriously," he said, pushing through a door at the back. "Don't put anything in your mouth that doesn't come from here or you'll find yourself shitting and vomiting your guts out. And you'll be doing it on your own. The hospital's been bombed three times and still has hundreds of new patients flooding in every day. The sick and dying are covering every centimeter of floor there and spilling out into the parking lot. I don't know why. There's no medicine. Hardly any staff. Nothing."

The room they found themselves in was about eight feet square, illuminated by a bare bulb hanging from the celling. There was a folding table that served as a desk and a single plastic chair raided from the restaurant. Walls were stacked with boxes labeled with the word "bleach" in Arabic. A few notebooks that looked like business ledgers and a tiny potted plant rounded out the inventory.

According to Rapp's briefing, there was also a hidden chamber with communications equipment and a few weapons, but it was best to use it sparingly. If anyone discovered its existence, Karman's body would be hanging from one of his restaurant's ceiling beams inside an hour.

"Better than bleach . . ." the Yemeni said, rummaging in a box behind him, "is alcohol."

He retrieved a half-full bottle of Jack Daniel's and poured careful measures into two coffee cups before handing one to Rapp.

"Did your work go well?" he asked, keeping the conversation vague and in Arabic. He was well-liked and trusted in the area, but it was still a war zone. People were always listening. Always suspicious.

"No. I wasn't able to connect with our friend."

Karman's face fell. "I'm sorry for that. I did the best I could to schedule it, but you know how unpredictable he can be."

Rapp nodded and took a sip of his drink.

"I've become nothing more than a tea room gossip," Karman said in a hushed tone. "Trying to live off the pittance the restaurant makes and arguing politics with whoever sits down at one of my tables."

The message was clear. He was calling for resources. Unfortunately, the dipshits in Washington weren't in the mood to provide them.

"Really? Business looks good to me."

"An illusion. Customers are dwindling and talk has turned wild. Spies. Intrigue. Conspiracies. I spend my days listening to this and searching the sky for the Saudi missile that will kill me. Or looking behind me for the man who will put a knife in my back for the money in my pocket."

"Former ISIS fighters?" Rapp said.

Karman nodded. "They're heavily armed and purposeless. Young men full of hate, violence, and lust. All believing that their every whim is a directive from God. If Sayid Halabi is alive I would have expected him to move them toward the lawless middle of the country. But he doesn't seem interested. The rumor is that he's forming a much smaller group of well-educated, well-trained followers."

Karman brought his mug to his lips and closed his eyes as he swished the whiskey around in his mouth before swallowing. "People speak of him as though he's a ghost. As if he'd died and returned. They believe that God spoke to him and gave him the secret to defeating the infidels."

"Do you believe that's true?"

"No. But I think Halabi does. And I think that he's even more brilliant than he is twisted. What I can tell you for certain is that ISIS is evolving. And if he's behind that, I guarantee you he's not doing it for his entertainment. He's working toward something. Something big."

Again, Karman was using the cover of idle gossip to make a point: that something needed to be done before Halabi could assert his dominance over a reinvigorated jihadist movement. Unfortunately, he was preaching to the choir. Rapp and Kennedy spent a hell of a lot of time and effort making that precise case to politicians who seemed less interested every day.

Karman reached for a pack of cigarettes and lit one before speaking again. "There's nothing more for us here, my friend. I can't distinguish one day from another anymore. I serve food. I clean. I listen to loose talk. And I wait for death."

CHAPTER 4

CENTRAL YEMEN

THE boy curled up on the dirty cot, covering his mouth and bracing himself for the coughing fit that was to come. Dr. Victoria Schaefer watched helplessly as he convulsed, the sound of his choking muffled by the hazmat suit she was wearing. When it was over, he reached out a hand spattered with blood from his lungs.

She took it, squeezing gently through rubber gloves and fighting back the urge to cry. With the headgear she was wearing, there was no way to wipe the tears away. It was a lesson she'd learned over and over again throughout the years.

"It's going to be all right," she lied through her faceplate.

The respiratory disease she'd stumbled upon in that remote Yemeni village killed more than a third of the people who displayed symptoms. Soon he'd be added to that statistic. And there was nothing she could do about it.

He managed to say something as he pointed to another of the cots lined up in the tiny stone building. She didn't understand the words—bringing her interpreter into this makeshift clinic would have been too dangerous—but she understood their meaning. The woman lying by the door was his mother. After days of struggling for every breath, she'd lost her fight two hours ago.

"She's just sleeping," Schaefer said in as soothing a tone as she could manage.

The boy was young enough to have eyes still full of trust and hope. In contrast, the adults in the village had started to lose faith in her. And why not? Even before her medical supplies had dwindled, she'd been largely powerless. Beyond keeping victims as comfortable as possible and treating their secondary infections with antibiotics, there was little choice but to just let the virus run its course.

The boy lost consciousness and Schaefer walked through the gloom to a stool in the corner. The windows had been sealed and the door was closed tight against a jamb enhanced with rubber stripping. Light was provided by a hole in the roof covered with a piece of white cloth that was the best filter they could come up with.

The other three living people in the building were in various stages of the illness. One—ironically a man who estimated himself to be in his late sixties—was on his way to recovery. What that recovery would look like, though, she wasn't sure. Yemeni acute respiratory syndrome, as they'd dubbed it, left about thirty percent of its survivors permanently disabled. It was almost certain that he would never be able to work again. The question was whether he would even be able to care for himself without assistance.

The ultimate fate of the other two victims was unknown. They were in the early stages and it was still too soon to tell. Both were strong and in their twenties, but that didn't seem to make any difference to YARS. It was an equal opportunity killer that took healthy adults at about the same rate it did children and the elderly.

The boy started to cough again, but this time she didn't go to him, instead staring down at his blood on her gloves. She'd leave his mother where he could see her and take comfort from her presence. The heat in the building was suffocating, but it didn't matter. He wouldn't last long enough for her to start to decompose.

"Vick—"

The satellite phone cut out and Schaefer shook it violently. Not the most high-tech solution, but it seemed to work. She was able to make out the last few words of her boss's sentence, but ignored them. Ken Dinh was the president of Doctors Without Borders, a good man and a personal friend. But he was sitting behind a desk in Toronto and she was on the ground in the middle-of-nowhere Yemen.

"Are you listening to what I'm saying, Vicky?"

No one was watching, so she allowed herself a guilty frown. At forty-two, she'd already been through a number of husbands, all of whom had roughly the same complaints. The top of the list was that she was obsessed with her job. Second was that she was—to use her last husband's words—always camped out in some war-torn, disease-ridden, third-world hellhole. The last one was something about never listening and instead just waiting to talk. She wasn't sure, though, because she hadn't really been listening.

"I heard you but I don't know what you want me to say. No worries? Hey, maybe it's not as bad as it looks? And what do you want me to tell the people in this village? Take two aspirin and call me in the morning?"

"This sarcasm isn't like you, Vicky."

"Seriously?"

"No. Obviously that was a joke."

"So now we're going to sit around telling jokes?"

Even from half a world away she could hear his deep sigh. "But it's *isolated*, right? You haven't seen or heard anything that points to an outbreak outside that village."

She'd walked about a third of a mile to make the call, stopping partway up a slope containing boulders big enough to provide shade. It was the place she came when she needed to be alone. When she needed to find a little perspective in a world that didn't offer much anymore.

The village below wasn't much to look at, a few buildings constructed of the same reddish stone and dirt that extended to the horizon in every direction. She surveyed it for a few moments instead of answering. Dinh was technically right. The disease she'd discovered appeared to be isolated to this forgotten place and its forty-three remaining inhabitants.

And because of that, no one cared. It had no strategic relevance to the Houthi rebels or government forces fighting for control of the country. The ISIS and al Qaeda forces operating in the area didn't consider it a sufficient prize to send the two or three armed men necessary to take it. And the Saudis had no reason to waste fuel and ordnance blowing it up.

The disease devastating the village had probably come from one of the bat populations living in caves set into the slope she was now calling from. But the specialists she'd consulted assured her that their range was nowhere near sufficient to make it to the closest population center—a similarly tiny village over forty hard miles to the east.

"It's isolated," she admitted finally. "But I don't know for how much longer. I'm containing it by giving these people food and health care so none of them have any reason to leave. And I'm counting on the fact that no one from outside has any reason to come. Is that what you want to hang your hat on?"

"You also told me that you thought the whole thing was a fluke, right? The war cut off the village's food supply and they started eating bats for the first time?"

"That's just a guess," she responded through clenched teeth. "We can't get anyone with the right expertise to come here to do the testing. Look, Ken, I'm here with one nurse and a microbiologist who's only interested in getting his name in the science journals.

Twenty-five people in this village are dead. That's a third of the population."

"But you've stopped the spread, right? You've got it under control."

"We've got the last few identified victims quarantined and for now we've convinced the villagers to steer clear of the local bat population," she admitted. "But it's incredibly contagious, Ken. Not like anything I've seen in my lifetime. Even casual contact with someone who's sick comes with over a fifty percent infection rate. But the worst thing is how long the virus seems to be able to survive on surfaces. We have credible evidence of people getting sick after touching things handled by a victim seventy-two hours before. What if someone infected with this went through an airport? They could push a button on an elevator or touch the check-in counter and have people carry it all over the world. How could we stop it?"

"We stopped it last time," he said in an obvious reference to the SARS outbreak in the early 2000s.

"It's not the same thing and you know it! SARS is an order of magnitude less contagious and it broke out in Asia. We had time to mount a worldwide response in countries with modern medical systems. This is Yemen. They don't have the resources to do anything but stand back and pray. We could be talking about a pandemic that could kill a hundred million people. Are you a doctor or a politician, Ken? We—"

"Shut up, Vicky! Just shut your mouth for one minute if that's possible."

She fell silent at the man's uncharacteristic outburst.

"Do you have any idea what's happening in the rest of Yemen? Outside your little world? We're dealing with a cholera outbreak that's now officially the worst in modern history. NGOs are backing out because of the bombing and growing violence. Local medical personnel are either sick themselves or haven't been paid in months and are moving on to figure out how to feed themselves."

"Ken—"

"I'm not done! About a third of the country is slowly starving. We're seeing infections that none of our antibiotics work on. And there are rumors that there's going to be a major attack on Al Hudaydah. If that port closes, most of the imports into the country are going to dry up. No more humanitarian aid. No more food or medicine. No more fuel. On top of everything else, the country's going to slip into famine."

"But—" she tried to interject.

"Shut it!" he said and then continued. "All this and I can barely get governments or private donors to take my calls. Why? Because no one gives a crap about Yemen. They can't find it on a map and they're bone tired of pouring money into Middle East projects that get blown up before they're even finished. And that's leaving aside the U.S. presidential election that's already consuming every media outlet in the world. If an alien spaceship landed in Yemen tomorrow, it'd be lucky to make page nine in the *Times*."

"Ken—"

"Shut up, shut up, *shut up*!" he said. "Now, where was I? Oh, yeah. So, after all that's said, you want me to divert my almost nonexistent resources from the thousands of people dying in the cities to a little village of fifty people surrounded by an impassable sea of desert?"

"Screw you, Ken."

When he spoke again, his voice had softened. "Look. I really do understand what you're saying to me. Remember that before I sat down behind this desk I spent years doing exactly what you're doing. I want to help you. What you're dealing with terrifies me—"

"But you're going to do nothing."

"Oh, ye of little faith."

She perked up. "What does that mean?"

"I wish I could take credit for this, but in truth I had nothing to do with it. A couple weeks ago, a Saudi businessman I've never heard of contacted me. He said he'd seen something about you in a university newspaper and wanted to help. It kind of took me by surprise, so I just threw a number out there."

"What number?"

"Two hundred and fifty grand."

"And?"

"Long story, but he said yes."

"What?" Victoria stammered, unable to process what she was hearing after months of fighting for castoffs and pocket change. "I . . . I don't even understand what that means."

"It means that I've got a team putting together a drop for you. Equipment, food, medicine. I might even have someone from the University of Wyoming who's willing to look at your bats. We'll lower the supplies down to you from a cargo chopper so we don't have to get anywhere near your patients. I'm working on permission from the Saudis now."

"Why didn't you tell me this when we started talking?"

"Because I wanted you to make an ass out of yourself. Now, listen to me. This isn't a bottomless well. I don't even know how to get in touch with this donor. He wanted to be anonymous and he's doing a good job of it. Get that village healthy and figure out a way to keep them that way."

"Ken. I'm sorry about—"

The line went dead and she dropped the phone, leaning against the rock behind her.

It was hard to remember everything that had happened to get her to that particular place at that particular time. Her childhood outside of Seattle had been unremarkable. She'd never traveled much and she'd stayed in Washington through her early career as a physician. It wasn't until she was in her early thirties that she'd felt the pull of the outside world and the billions of desperate people who inhabited it.

Schaefer scooted away from the approaching rays of sun and

focused on the village below. The door to their improvised clinic opened and a man in protective clothing appeared, shading his faceplate-covered eyes as he emerged. Otto Vogel was her no-nonsense German pillar of steel. They'd met in Ghana seven years ago and had been working together ever since. Not only was he the best nurse she'd ever met, but he was perhaps the most reliable person on the planet. There was no situation that he couldn't deal with, no disaster that could ruffle him, no objective danger that could scare him. They'd been through Haiti, Nigeria, and Laos together, to name only a few. And now here they were in Yemen. The world's forgotten humanitarian disaster.

He scanned the terrain, finally finding her hidden among the rocks. She'd told him that she was calling Ken Dinh and it wouldn't be hard for him to guess that she'd do it from the shade of her favorite boulder.

Vogel made an exaggerated motion toward his wrist. He wasn't actually wearing a watch, but she understood that it was a reference to the tardiness of their third musketeer. A man who was less a pillar of steel and more a pile of shit softened by the heat.

When Vogel disappeared around the corner to begin removing his contaminated clothing, she stood and reluctantly started toward a building at the opposite edge of the village.

When she finally pushed through the door of the stone structure she found a lone man scribbling in a notebook. He was only partially visible behind the battered lab equipment she'd borrowed from fleeing NGOs. Usually while wearing a black turtleneck and driving a van with the headlights turned off.

"You were supposed to relieve Otto more than a half an hour ago," she said.

The initial reaction was an irritated frown—intimidating to the grad students who hung on his every word, but not as weighty in Yemen.

"I'm in the middle of something," he said. His English was

grammatically perfect, but he took pride in maintaining a thick French accent. "I need to work through it while my mind is fresh."

Gabriel Bertrand was a world-class prick but unquestionably a brilliant one. He'd started his career as a physician, but after discovering that he didn't like being around sick people, he'd moved into research and teaching.

"I appreciate that," she said, her good mood managing to hold. "But we've got people dying in that building. Otto and I can't handle—"

"Then let me help them, Victoria! You know perfectly well that we don't know how to save those people. What I'm doing here could prevent future victims. It could—"

"Get you a big prize and invitations to all the right Paris cocktail parties?"

That condescending frown again. This time aimed over his reading glasses. "If this disease ever defeats our containment measures, it's going to be *my* work that's important. Not what's being done in your little infirmary."

"Tell that to the people in the little infirmary."

"There's a bigger picture here. In fact, I'm guessing that a few minutes ago, you were trying to impress that very fact on Ken Dinh."

He stood from behind his improvised desk and moved a little too close, rubbing a hand over her bare shoulder. She was quite a bit older than the coeds he normally hit on, but she was still trim, with long blond hair and the tan that she'd always aspired to while growing up in the Pacific Northwest. More important, she was the only game in town.

"Your narrative can be featured prominently in my work. It would come off as very heroic. That wouldn't be bad for your career."

In her youth, she'd have probably gone for him. The brilliant, distinguished ones had always gotten to her. But not anymore. She'd seen way too much.

"Ten minutes, Bert," she said using the shortened version of his name that he despised. "After that, I'm going to have Otto drag you out of here."

CHAPTER 5

AL HUDAYDAH
YEMEN

"TWO orders of saltah," Shamir Karman shouted through the open door of the restaurant. "And do we still have any bottled cola?"

Rapp was sitting alone at one of the tables outside, drinking coffee and working through the pack of cigarettes he always traveled with in this part of the world. It was still early and the sun was at a steep enough angle to shade the improvised terrace. Around him, about a quarter of the tables were occupied by men sipping from steaming cups, gossiping, and shooting occasional jealous glances at Rapp's smokes.

If he ignored the bomb crater behind him and the collapsed buildings in front, it all seemed pretty normal. Not much different than a thousand other cafes Rapp had eaten in over the last twenty years of his life. According to Karman, though, the illusion of business as usual would disappear sometime around lunch.

Apparently, his restaurant—along with all the other struggling businesses in the area—was being shaken down by an organized crime outfit made up of former ISIS fighters. The gang had their hands in just about every dirty enterprise going on in Al Hudaydah, but that wasn't what had attracted Rapp's attention. No, his interest was in the whispers that they were still connected to Sayid Halabi.

The question was whether those rumors were true or just marketing. Staying in the glow of the ISIS leader's legend would be good for the images of men who were now nothing more than unusually sadistic criminals. Anything they could do to amplify the fear of the desperate people they preyed upon worked in their favor.

If it was true that Halabi was trying to build a smarter, more agile organization, it was possible that he'd completely severed his ties with the morons terrorizing Al Hudaydah. On the other hand, men willing to martyr themselves could be extremely powerful weapons. Maybe too powerful for Halabi to give up.

After four more hours, all the tables were full and the conversations had turned into an indecipherable roar. Waiters weaved skillfully through the customers, serving coffee, tea, and dishes prepared by Karman's harried kitchen staff. Tattered umbrellas had gone up and people huddled beneath them, trying to escape the increasingly powerful sun.

Rapp was almost through his bowl of marak temani when the buzz of conversation began to falter. He glanced behind him and quickly picked out the cause of the interruption: two hard-looking young men approaching. They were armed with AKs like just about every other Yemeni male, but these weren't fashion accessories. They were slung at the ready across their torsos with fingers on the trigger guards. That, combined with their sweeping eyes and cruel expressions, suggested they weren't there for the food.

Rapp waited for them to enter the restaurant before following. The sparsely populated interior had gone dead silent except for Karman, who was standing in the kitchen door inviting the men inside.

Again, Rapp followed, slipping into the hectic kitchen in time to see his old friend lead one of the men to his office. The other stood near the open door, chewing khat and scanning for threats.

Not ready to be identified as yet, Rapp angled toward an employee bathroom at the far end of the kitchen. After pretending to test the door and find it locked, he pressed his back against the wall and lit another cigarette.

It was hard to see into the office but there was just enough light for Rapp to make out Karman opening a small lockbox. The Yemeni started calmly counting bills onto the table as the other man speculated loudly about the success of the restaurant and whether he was being paid fairly. In the end, the calculations proved too taxing and he just snatched a little extra from the box before scooping up the stack Karman had dealt out. A hard shove sent the CIA informant stumbling backward into his chair with enough force that it almost flipped.

The kitchen staff bowed their heads as the two men left, careful to not make eye contact. Rapp didn't follow suit, instead staring intently at them. Neither noticed. They were too busy arguing about how they were going to split the unexpected bonus cash.

After they disappeared back out into the dining room, Rapp tossed his half-smoked cigarette on the floor and started after them. By the time he stepped into the blinding sun, the men had a twenty-yard lead. He let that extend a bit as he swung by his table and slammed back the rest of what might have been the best cup of coffee he'd ever had.

They led him through the sparsely populated maze of streets, finally arriving at a bustling market. The stench of sweat and raw sewage filled Rapp's nostrils as he watched the men work their way through the stands, extorting money from each of their cowering proprietors.

The sun was sinking low on the horizon by the time the men finished their rounds through the business district and started toward a more desperate area of town. Rapp was getting hungry and thirsty, but the occasional corpse of a cholera victim awaiting removal kept him from doing anything about it.

The dust caked in his throat and the empty stomach just added to the anger that had been building in him all day. Watching these men steal from people who had virtually nothing was something he'd seen before, but it never got any more pleasant. Rapp had dedicated his life to eradicating this kind of scum from the earth, but there seemed to be an endless supply.

They finally stopped at a house that had been repaired with tarps and other scrounged materials. Rapp assumed they were done for the day and had led him to their base of operations, but he turned out to be wrong.

A halfhearted kick from one of the men knocked in what was left of a wooden door and they disappeared inside. Weak shouts and the screams of children flowed through the empty window frames as Rapp moved into a shadowed position that still gave him a solid line of sight.

The ISIS men reappeared a few minutes later with a girl of about fourteen in tow. She was struggling and screaming, trying futilely to break free and retreat back into the house. A moment later a man Rapp assumed was her father came after her, grabbing one of the men, but then collapsing to the ground. The remaining glow from the sun glistened off his sweat-soaked skin, highlighting its pallor and dark, sunken eyes. Another victim of Al Hudaydah's nonfunctional sanitation system and lack of medicine. The ISIS men just laughed and continued dragging his daughter up the street.

What followed was easily predicted: the journey to a somewhat more affluent part of town. The dull stares of the people along the route, their lives too close to the edge to interfere. The delivery to a man who paid in cash. Her screams penetrating the walls of the house and echoing up the street.

Rapp followed the men, trying to block out the girl's cries for help. He'd been in a similar situation in Iraq and it was one of the few episodes in his life that wouldn't leave him alone. His stride faltered and he considered going back, but knew that it was impossible. She was one of thousands. The mission wasn't one girl. It couldn't be.

The night was starting to get cold when the two men led him to a block of commercial buildings that had been spared from bombing. They disappeared into a small warehouse and Rapp came to a stop, staring blankly at the stone structure. What he wanted to do was walk in there and execute every son of a bitch inside.

It would be so easy. Men like that had no real skill or training and they became accustomed to everyone being too afraid or weak to move against them. While they expected to die one day in a battle or a drone strike, the idea of one man acting against them was unfathomable. If Rapp's experience was any indicator, they'd just sit there like a bunch of idiots while he emptied his Glock into their skulls.

A beautiful fantasy, but like the empty heroism of saving the girl, an impossible one. This was the real world—a dirty, violent place, where wins came at a high price. Even capturing and interrogating them would be of limited value. Far more useful would be figuring out how many men were in there, getting photos that the CIA might be able to connect with names, and compromising their communications.

Halabi was out there and he was going to hunt that bastard down and stick a knife in his eye socket—even if it meant he had to do the thing he hated most in life.

Wait.

CHAPTER 6

CENTRAL YEMEN

THE late afternoon sun cast virtually no shadows because there was little to create them. The terrain here consisted of nothing but blunt ridges, rocky desert soil, and a single, poorly defined road disappearing over the slope ahead. Mullah Sayid Halabi didn't see any of it, though. Instead, he focused on the sky. The Americans were up there. As were the Saudis. Watching. Analyzing. Waiting for an opportunity to strike.

Normally he didn't emerge during the day. His life was lived almost entirely underground now, an existence of darkness broken by dim, artificial light, and the occasional transfer beneath the stars. The risk he was running now was unacceptably high and taken for what seemed to be the most absurd reason imaginable. One of his young disciples had said that this was the time of day that the light was most attractive.

It was indeed a new era.

He was positioned in the center of a small convoy consisting of vehicles taken from the few charitable organizations still working in the country. A bulky SUV led the way and a supply truck trailed them at a distance of twenty meters, struggling with the rutted track.

The Toyota Land Cruiser he was in was the most comfortable of the three, with luxurious leather seats, air-conditioning, and the blood of its former driver painted across the dashboard.

The men crammed into the vehicles represented a significant percentage of the forces under his direct command. It was another disorienting change. He'd once led armies that had rolled across the Middle East in the modern instruments of war. His fanatical warriors had taken control of huge swaths of land, sending thousands of Western trained forces fleeing in terror. He had built the foundation of a new caliphate that had the potential to spread throughout the region.

And then he had lost it.

That defeat and his months convalescing from Mitch Rapp's attack had left him with a great deal of time to think. About his victories. His defeats. His weaknesses as a leader and failings as a disciple of the one true God. Ironically, the words that had been the seed of his new strategy were said to have come from an agnostic Jew.

The definition of insanity is doing the same thing over and over and expecting a different result.

While his current forces were limited in number, they were substantially different than those that came before. All would give their lives for him and the cause, of course. But the region was full of such fighters. What set the men with him apart was their level of education and training. All could read, write, and speak at least functional English. All were former soldiers trained by the Americans or other Westerners. And all had long, distinguished combat records.

His problems had come to parallel the ones that plagued the American military and intelligence community: finding good men and managing them effectively. The well-disciplined soldiers with him today were relatively easy to deal with—all were accustomed to the rigid command structure he'd created. The technical people spread across the globe, though, posed a different challenge. They were temperamental, fearful, and unpredictable. Unfortunately, they were also the most critical part in the machine he was building.

The lead vehicle came to a stop and Halabi rolled down his window, leaning out to read a large sign propped in a pile of rocks. It carried the Doctors Without Borders logo as well as a skull and crossbones and biohazard symbol. In the center was text in various languages explaining the existence of a severe disease in the village ahead and warning off anyone approaching. Punctuating those words was a line of large rocks blocking the road.

Muhammad Attia, his second in command, leapt from the lead vehicle and directed the removal of the improvised barrier.

It was a strangely disturbing scene. They worked with a precision that could only be described as Western. The economy of their movements, combined with their camouflage uniforms, helmets, and goggles, made them indistinguishable from the American soldiers that Halabi despised. The benefits of adopting the methods of his enemy, though, were undeniable. In less than three minutes they were moving again.

The village revealed itself fifteen minutes later, looking exactly as expected from the reconnaissance photos his team had gathered. A few people were visible moving through the spaces between stone buildings, but he was much more interested in the ones running up the road toward him. The blond woman was waving her arms in warning while the local man behind her struggled to keep up.

She stopped directly in front of their motorcade, shouting and motioning them back. When the lead car stopped, she jogged to its open side window. Halabi was surprised by the intensity of his anticipation as he watched her speak with the driver through her translator.

Of course, Halabi knew everything about her. He'd had a devoted follower call Doctors Without Borders and, in return for a sizable donation to her project, the organization's director had been willing to answer any question he was asked. In addition, Halabi's computer experts had gained access to her social media and email accounts, as well as a disused blog she'd once maintained.

Victoria Schaefer had spent years with the NGO, largely partnered with a German nurse named Otto Vogel. Though she was a whore who had been through multiple husbands, there was no evidence of a relationship between her and the German that went beyond friendship and mutual respect. She was ostensibly in charge of the management of the operation there, but it was the as-yet-unseen Frenchman who was the driving force behind the research being done.

Her relationship with Dr. Gabriel Bertrand was somewhat more complex. Based on intercepted messages sent to family members, she despised the man but acknowledged his genius and indispensability. Bertrand's own Internet accounts were even more illuminating, portraying an obsessive, arrogant, and selfish man dedicated largely to the pursuit of his own ambition. He had no family he remained in regular contact with and was blandly noncommittal in his responses to correspondence sent by the various women he had relationships with in Europe.

Schaefer began stalking toward Halabi's vehicle with her translator in tow, apparently unsatisfied by the response she was getting from the lead car.

"We speak English," Halabi said, noting the frustration in her expression as she came alongside.

"Then what in God's name are you doing here? Didn't you see the sign? Why did you move the rocks we put up?"

Halabi gave a short nod and his driver fired a silenced pistol through the window. The round passed by the woman and struck her translator in the chest. He fell to the ground and she staggered back, stunned. A moment later, her instincts as a physician took over and she dropped to her knees, tearing his shirt open. When she saw the irreparable hole over his heart, she turned back toward them. Surprisingly, there was no fear in her eyes. Just hate.

Only when Halabi's driver threw his door open did she run. Chasing her down was a trivial matter, and she was bound with the same efficiency that had been deployed to clear the rock barrier. Once she was safely in the SUV's backseat, Halabi's men spread out, mounting a well-ordered assault on their target.

The handful of villagers outside realized what was happening and began to run just as the woman had. All were taken out in the same way as the translator—with a single suppressed round. It was an admittedly impressive display. The last victim, a child of around ten, was dead before the first victim had hit the ground. It was unlikely that America's SEALs or Britain's SAS could have acted more quickly or silently.

His driver stopped fifty meters from the first building and Halabi watched the operation through the dusty windshield.

Two men went directly for the building that their spotter confirmed was currently occupied by both Gabriel Bertrand and Otto Vogel. The other men penetrated the tiny village to carry out a plan developed by Muhammad Attia.

Each carried a battery-powered nail gun and they moved quickly through the tightly packed stone dwellings, firing nails through the wood doors and frames, sealing the people in their homes. As anticipated, the entire operation took less than four minutes. The muffled shouts of confused inhabitants started as they tried futilely to open their doors. One woman opened shutters that had been closed against the heat and was hit in the forehead by another perfectly aimed bullet. The round wasn't audible from Halabi's position, but the shouts of her husband and shrieks of her children penetrated the vehicle easily.

As the Frenchman and German were dragged from the lab, Halabi's men began prying open shutters and throwing purpose-built incendiary devices into the homes and other buildings, carefully avoiding the structure that had been repurposed as a hospital. The screams of the inhabitants became deafening as they began to burn.

Halabi finally stepped from the vehicle, walking toward the village as a man followed along, filming with an elaborate high-definition camera. He focused on Halabi's face for a moment, drawing in on the patch covering his useless left eye—a battle scar all the more dramatic for having been inflicted by the infamous Mitch Rapp. Halabi's awkward use of a cane to help him walk, on the other hand, would be artistically obscured. While that too was a result of Rapp's attack, it made him appear old and physically weak—things that were unacceptable in this part of the world.

Smoke billowed dramatically over him as he gazed into the flames. A woman managed to shove a crying child through a window but he was shot before he could even get to his feet. The Frenchman was blubbering similarly, lying on the ground in front of his still-intact lab while the woman and the German were pushed down next to him.

Halabi took a position next to them and his videographer crouched to frame the bound Westerners with the mullah towering over them. Halabi looked down at the helpless people at his feet and then back at the camera.

"Now I have your biological weapons experts," he said in practiced English. "Now I have the power to use your weapons against you."

The man with the camera seemed a bit dazed by the brutal reality of the operation, but gave a weak thumbs-up. In postproduction he would add music, terrifying stock images, and whatever else was necessary to turn the footage into a propaganda tool far more potent than any IED or suicide bomber.

A few moments later, Muhammad Attia took Halabi by the arm and helped him back to the vehicle. His driver already had the door open, but Halabi resisted being assisted inside.

"The smoke could attract the attention of the Saudis," Attia warned. "We need to be far from this place before that happens."

Halabi nodded as the medical people were dragged to another of the vehicles.

"Be that as it may, your men will stay."

"Stay? Why? I don't understand."

"Because he's coming, Muhammad."

"Who?"

"Rapp."

One of his men had survived the recent assault on the cave where Halabi had recovered from his injuries. The description of the attackers could be no one but Rapp and the former American soldiers he worked with.

"He missed you in the cave," Attia protested. "Why would he still be in Yemen?"

"Because he doesn't give up, Muhammad. He's still here. I can feel him. And when he finds out I was in this village, he'll come."

"Even if that's true, we can't spare—"

"Tell your men not to kill him," Halabi interjected. "I want him captured."

"Captured? Why?"

Halabi didn't answer, instead lowering himself into the Land Cruiser.

Why? It was simple. He wanted to break Rapp. Over months. Perhaps even years. He'd make the CIA man beg. Crawl. Turn him into a pet, naked and helpless in his cage, looking with fear and longing into the eyes of his master.

CHAPTER 7

THE CAPITOL COMPLEX
WASHINGTON, D.C.

SENATOR Christine Barnett continued to hold the phone to her ear but had stopped listening more than a minute ago. Instead she leaned back in her chair and gazed disinterestedly around her office. The heavy, polished wood. The photos of her with powerful people throughout the world. The awards and recognition she'd received over a lifetime of successes.

There was a pause in the dialogue, and she voiced a few practiced platitudes that set the man to talking again. He was an important donor who expected this kind of personal access, but also one of the most tedious pricks alive. He'd grown up in the shadow of World War II and was still a true believer—in America, in God, in objective truth. A doddering old fool trapped in a web of things that no longer mattered.

There was a no-nonsense knock on her door and a moment later someone more interesting entered.

Kevin Gray wore the slightly disheveled suit and overly imaginative tie that everyone in Washington had come to associate with him. He was only in his mid-thirties but still had managed to rack up a series of successes that nearly rivaled her own. A Harvard master's degree, a brief career with a top marketing firm, and finally a splashy entry into the world of politics.

He struggled sometimes to focus, but was unquestionably a creative genius—a man who could communicate with equal facility to all demographic groups and who always seemed to know what was coming next. Every new platform, every new style of messaging, and every cultural shift seemed to settle into his mind six months before anyone else even had an inkling. That, combined with his ability to act decisively on those abstractions, had made it possible for him to get a number of ostensibly unelectable people comfortable seats in Congress.

Her campaign was completely different, of course. The comfortable seat she was looking for was in the Oval Office and, with the exception of being a woman, she was eminently electable. A number of people in her party thought she'd been insane to hire Gray—dismissing him as a bottom feeder who relied on tricks and barely ethical tactics to salvage failed campaigns.

As usual, they'd been wrong and she'd been right. With a strong candidate to work with, the Gray magic became even more powerful. She was now thirty points ahead in the primary race and had become her party's de facto candidate for the election that was already consuming the nation.

A few of her primary opponents were staying in the race, but more to position themselves for a place in her administration than any hope they could overtake her in the polls. She would be the nominee. And based on the weakness of her likely opponent in the general election, she would become the first female president of the United States.

At least that was the opinion of the idiot pollsters and television pundits. But if she'd learned anything as a woman in the most cutthroat business in the world, it was to not take anything for granted.

Gray sat in front of her desk and crossed his legs, bouncing his loafer-clad foot in a way that she'd come to recognize as a sign of impatience. The call was winding down, but she asked an open-ended question to the man on the other end of the line to prolong it. This was her office and her campaign. Gray needed to remember that.

After another five minutes, she felt like she'd made her point and wrapped up the call. "I understand —exactly what you're talking about, Henry. It's why I'm running for president. And it's why I'm going to win."

Gray held up a thumb drive before she could even get the handset back in its cradle.

"Have you seen it?"

She had no idea what he was talking about but whatever *it* was must have been important. Normally the first words out of Gray's mouth when she hung up with a donor were "How much?"

"I haven't seen anything other than the inside of this office. And I haven't talked about anything but taxes, guns, and environmental regulations. What is it?"

"Mullah Sayid Halabi."

"What do I care about a dead terrorist?"

A smile spread slowly across his face. "You care that he's not actually dead."

"What are you talking about?"

He slipped the drive into his tablet and transmitted its contents to a television hanging on the wall.

Barnett watched in stunned silence as a slickly produced propaganda piece played out on the screen. Dramatic historical images of Halabi and ISIS victories accompanied by a voice-over diatribe about America and the West. In accented English and with a background of modern Arab music, he called on Muslim people throughout the world to unite against the infidels.

Just after that plea, the video stabilized, depicting him standing in front of a primitive village that was being consumed by fire. He appeared and disappeared in the smoke like a ghost, accusing the villagers of helping the Americans develop biological weapons to be used against the Muslim people.

Quick image cuts to bacteria squirming under magnification, overflowing hospitals, and diseased human flesh followed before returning to Halabi. Heavy-handed, but unquestionably effective.

The camera angle widened to encompass three people bound at the ISIS leader's feet.

"Now I have your biological weapons experts," he said, staring directly into the lens. "Now I have the power to use your weapons against you."

The screen faded to black and Christine Barnett just stared at it, her mind bogging down on the almost infinite political possibilities Halabi's survival provided.

"That video hit the Internet a few hours ago in Arabic and English," Gray said. "And it's expanding into other languages every few minutes."

"Are we sure that the footage of Halabi isn't old? From before Mitch Rapp supposedly killed him?"

"One hundred percent. According to the CIA, that video from that burning village was taken three days ago in Yemen."

Barnett felt her mouth start to go dry. "Who are the people tied up?"

"Doctors Without Borders. They were there treating the villagers for some respiratory infection."

"Do any of them really know anything about bioweapons?"

"One of them is a microbiologist from the Sorbonne in France. Obviously, his field isn't bioweapons, but he certainly has that kind of expertise. The woman is an American doctor and the other man is a nurse."

Barnett stood and began pacing around the spacious office. At this point the kidnapped doctors were a secondary consideration.

Window dressing for the real issue at hand. Mitch Rapp and Irene Kennedy had screwed up. Badly.

"So Halabi isn't dead like the Agency told us."

"Actually, they said that Rapp threw a grenade at him but they couldn't confirm the kill because of the collapse of the cave system."

"The American people don't do nuance and they have the attention span of a goldfish. What they're going to remember is President Alexander telling them that we hit him with a bomb and that we haven't heard from him since. Now we find out he's been around all along. Hiding. Planning. And now capturing a Frenchman capable of building a bioweapon. All right under the noses of Irene Kennedy and Mitch Rapp." She spun toward Gray. "I assume the video's starting to get traction in the media?"

"It started on the jihadist sites and now it's all over Al Jazeera. The U.S. stations are just starting to pick it up. Of course the Internet is way ahead of all of them. It's lighting up with hysterical predictions and partisan finger pointing. Half the trolls are saying we brought this on ourselves and the other half are proposing war with every country in the Middle East."

She started pacing again, turning what she'd been told over in her head. Alexander had been in power for almost eight years, with only one moderately successful attack on the United States and a number thwarted—largely by some combination of Rapp and Kennedy. The economy was solid with a deficit that was starting to decline. And the president was a generally well-liked former University of Alabama quarterback. It didn't leave much room to generate the kind of fear, rage, and sense of victimization that was necessary to win an election. Up to now, she'd been forced to focus on humanity's natural tendency toward tribalism to fuel her campaign. And while it had been effective thus far, it was really just smoke that could dissipate at the slightest breeze.

"Could this be it, Kevin? Could this be our issue?"

"It's not an attack, Senator. It's just a video. A good one for sure, but—"

"The danger exists now, though. It's not theoretical. It's right there. On TV. This administration failed to kill Halabi and now he has bioweapon technology. Maybe the only reason there hasn't been a successful attack on U.S. soil is because ISIS was concentrating on the Middle East. But now they're focused on us and the CIA has no idea what to do about it."

Gray folded his arms across his chest and stared out the window for a few seconds before speaking. "The American people like their safety. It's an issue that cuts across partisan lines and resonates with the undecideds. And it's something real to go after Alexander on. This happened on his watch."

She nodded. Alexander's vice president was likely going to be the nominee and he wasn't much of a threat in and of himself—a seventy-two-year-old blue-blood with an increasing tendency to babble about the past. It was Alexander's support for him that made the man dangerous. Halabi's survival, though, could take the president's legs out from under him. If he could be forced to focus on his own political survival and legacy, there wouldn't be much capital left for him to expend supporting his party's candidate.

"Can we use this to bring down Alexander? Maybe even make him a liability?"

"I'm not sure," Gray hedged. "There hasn't—"

"Bullshit, you're not sure. With the right message, repeated enough times on enough media outlets, you could turn the American people against Jesus Christ himself."

He frowned. "You shouldn't blaspheme."

"When did you turn into a Boy Scout?"

"One of these days you're going to slip and say something like that on a hot mike."

"Don't try to change the subject. How hard can this be? Halabi's churning out propaganda videos left and right. The media's going to eat it up and the Internet is going to turn it toxic. All we have to do is make sure it hits our target."

His enthusiasm for her idea seemed unusually muted. The man loved manipulating people. The strange truth was that he didn't care about the trappings of power, just the exercise of it. He wanted to bend people to his will. To force them to turn away from reality and replace it with his carefully crafted speeches, tweets, and ads. Instead of the calculating excitement she'd expected, though, he looked worried.

"What?" she said.

"Do you think Halabi could actually succeed in an attack?"

She didn't answer, instead walking to the window and pretending to look out. In truth, she was focused on her own reflection, searching her carefully curated appearance for anything that didn't seem presidential. At fifty-two, she was still an extremely attractive woman—a product of good genetics, a rigid workout schedule, and a few discreet cosmetic procedures. The blue suit was conservative in style but fit her curves in a way that treaded the line between sex and power. Her still largely unlined face was framed by dark hair that could be used as a surprisingly versatile prop depending on her audience.

As always, everything was perfect. Despite that, it was still almost impossible to believe that she was about to become the most powerful person in the world. She had been neither born to power nor groomed for it. Her entry into politics had been largely at the whim of her tech billionaire husband. It was he who had suggested that she leave her law practice and run for an open seat in the Senate.

His company had been under heavy scrutiny by the Securities and Exchange Commission and other regulatory agencies for improprieties that had the potential to cause both of them serious problems. He'd backed her candidacy with virtually unlimited funds, and when she'd won, she'd used her new political clout to make their problems go away.

But it hadn't ended there. Her gift for politics had been immediately obvious, and over the course of fifteen short years she'd risen to become the chair of the Senate Intelligence Committee. Now she was poised to take the Oval Office.

Her husband, on the other hand, had been relegated to an increasingly secondary role. While still successful as a venture capitalist, he now lived a relatively anonymous life in Chicago, where her two children were in college. They saw each other often enough to keep the press happy, but otherwise their family functioned more as a business than anything else. Her husband continued to provide her campaign heavy financial support in return for the quiet privileges she could provide and her daughters toed the line to keep their trust funds flowing.

"Your silence is worrying me," Gray said finally.

She turned back toward him. "Could Halabi succeed in an attack? I have no idea. Can I assume we're demanding a briefing?"

"I have multiple calls into the White House. They said they're working on it and they'll get back to us."

She returned to the window, this time gazing past her reflection and into the American capital. In reality, a limited biological attack would be an ideal scenario for her. There was no way Alexander and his party could ride something like that out this close to the election. It would be a deathblow.

"We're going to have to deal with the fact that you've always been strongly opposed to our involvement in the Middle East in general and Yemen in particular," Gray continued.

"Because I was told that Halabi was dead. That ISIS was defeated."

He looked skeptical. "You staked out that position before ISIS even existed and I don't remember Irene Kennedy ever saying that ISIS was defeated or confirming that Halabi had been killed."

She took a seat behind her desk again. "The American people don't give a crap about political positions and they care even less about the truth. What they want is fireworks. They want a show and we've just been handed the script. While the other side talks about health care and the economy, we'll be talking about Islamic terrorists unleashing a plague that could wipe our country out. About watching your children die while Irene Kennedy covers her ass and Mitch Rapp chases his tail. This is a gift, Kevin. Use it."

CHAPTER 8

**AL HUDAYDAH
YEMEN**

"BUT it's your last one," the man said, staring longingly at the slightly bent cigarette Rapp was offering him.

Over the last five days, Rapp had graduated from sitting alone near the edge of the terrace to being crowded around a long table near its center. In that time, he'd gone through more than thirty cups of tea, twenty cups of coffee, every food product Yemen had to offer, and way too many cigarettes. It was a good way to blend in and make friends, but at this rate cancer was going to kill him before ISIS did.

"You'd be doing me a favor, Jihan. My youngest wife has been begging me to quit."

"This new generation," the man responded with a disapproving shake of his head. "They think they can live forever."

There was a murmur of general agreement from the men around them.

"Tell me. How old is she?"

"Sixteen," Rapp responded.

After another few seconds of thought, Jihan accepted the cigarette. "Then I'll smoke it. You need your strength."

The table burst into laughter and Rapp joined in, crumpling the empty pack and tossing it on the ground as the conversation resumed. The men wandered through the topics of the day—the Saudi bombings of the night before. The Iranians' backing of the rebels. The continued spread of disease and famine. And, finally, America's role in it all. Rapp tuned it all out, watching the discarded cigarette pack blow around on sun-heated cobbles.

The Agency had implemented round-the-clock overhead surveillance on the building full of former ISIS soldiers that Rapp had found. And the NSA had cracked all their communications with the exception of a couple of burner phones they couldn't get a bead on. Unfortunately, all that had been accomplished was to confirm his first impression. Those men were nothing more than a bunch of violent dipshits whom Halabi would have no use for other than maybe to stop bullets.

Rapp let himself be drawn back into the conversation, but it was a waste of time. There was no solid intel to be gained from restaurant gossip—particularly in a country where no one drank alcohol. Either the politicians needed to let the Agency commit resources to this part of the world or they needed to get out. Half measures against a man like Sayid Halabi were pointless. He was all-in, and anyone going up against him had better be the same.

The conversation had just turned to Syria when the voices around Rapp began to falter. He followed the gazes of the men around him to an old CRT television set up in the shade. The endless stream of Arab music videos had been interrupted by something that seemed almost like a twisted homage to them. Images of young people dancing and singing were replaced by ones of violence and death, with a sound track voiced over by none other than Sayid Halabi.

Rapp had seen the prior version of the video, but not this update. The backing music was more somber and the footage of the assault on the village more extensive. Halabi droned on about Muslim unity and combining forces against the West, but Rapp focused on the footage of the ISIS team tearing through the village. The men couldn't have been more different than the ones he was keeping tabs on in Al Hudaydah. They moved more like SEALs than the undisciplined psychos he'd come to expect from ISIS. More evidence of Halabi's efforts to turn his organization into a tighter, more modern force.

The video ended and was replaced by a CNN interview with Christine Barnett. The men around him began an animated discussion of Halabi's role in the region but Rapp remained focused on the television. The flow of the interview was pretty much what he would have predicted, with the head of the Senate Intelligence Committee insisting that she'd been assured that Halabi had been taken out.

So after managing to flail her way to a massive lead in the polls, Barnett had finally found her message: that the current administration had lied about Halabi's death for political gain while leaving the American people completely unprotected from the threat ISIS posed.

It was a demonstrable lie, but she'd probably get away with it. Sure, there was endless footage of Irene Kennedy saying that Halabi's body had never been found, but why would the press want to dredge that up? They knew a ratings grabber when they saw one.

Barnett went on to blame the very security agencies she'd been hamstringing for failing to utterly eradicate terrorism from the face of the earth. And, of course, she rounded out the interview the way all politicians did—by implying that she, and only she, had the answer. All the American people had to do was elect her president and they'd be guaranteed safety, wealth, a hot spouse, and six-pack abs.

The scene cut again, this time to a couple of know-nothing pundits speculating about the type of attack that the kidnapped medical team could conjure up. The debate had devolved into nonsensical shouting about Ebola and plague when Shamir Karman came up behind Rapp and whispered in his ear.

"A call for you just came in. Use the phone in the office."

Rapp took a seat behind Karman's desk and made sure the door had swung all the way shut before he picked up the handset.

"Go ahead," he said in Arabic.

His greeting was met with silence on the other end and he suspected he knew why. Since taking over logistics for Scott Coleman's company, Claudia Gould had been diligently trying to learn Arabic. Unfortunately, she was still in the "See Dick run" stage. Partially it was his fault. She was also the woman he lived with, but he always found a reason not to get involved in her language education. Patience wasn't his strong suit.

"Hello," he said, simplifying his Arabic. There was no way he could use the English or French she was fluent in. One overheard word and he might as well tattoo *CIA* to his forehead.

"It's good to hear your voice, Mitch."

He hated to admit it, but it was good to hear hers, too. The soft lilt was a reminder that, for one of the few times in his life, he had something to go home to.

"First," she continued. "Are you okay?"

"Yes," he said, keeping his responses basic.

"Don't worry. I didn't call just to ask that question."

"Then why?"

"I assume you've been watching the news and you're aware of Halabi's videos?"

He grunted an affirmation.

"The Saudis have located the village he burned. It's in central Yemen about five hundred kilometers east of you."

"And the people?"

"The ones he kidnapped? The reporting has been pretty accurate about them. What *hasn't* hit the networks is that they were there caring for the victims of a respiratory disease similar to SARS. Based on the Agency's analysis of Halabi's videos, he must have known about it. He went in when none of the medical personnel were in the infirmary they'd set up and his people burned everything without coming in contact with the villagers."

"And?"

"The Saudis want to incinerate the village from the air as an additional safety measure. It appears that they're already making plans but they're not sharing the details with the Agency. I don't think there's any point to you going there. It seems high risk, low return."

While her assessment was hard to argue with, *high risk, low return* was a front-runner for the engraving on his tombstone. Currently in third place behind *Do you think they'll be able to stitch that up?* and *Does anyone else hear ticking?*

It was a thin lead but it was better than sitting around Al Hudaydah giving himself emphysema. There was always a chance that Halabi or one of his men had left something useful behind.

"Can I assume you disagree with my analysis and insist on going?" Claudia said, filling the silence between them.

"Yes."

"I thought you'd say that, so I sent the village's coordinates to Scott in Riyadh. They know a Saudi chopper pilot who's willing to pick you up and take you to the village."

"Where and when?"

"Before I tell you that, you have to listen me. I know you always want to charge in, but are you sure it's worth it to spend a couple of hours looking around a burned village? Al Qaeda and ISIS control that area. We have no eyes there and no idea of their strength or distribution."

"Understood," he said, swallowing his natural urge to just bark orders. It was the main drawback to having the woman he was sleeping with handling his logistics. The upside was that she was one of the best in the business.

"I'm not finished."

His jaw clenched, but he managed to get *go ahead* out in a relatively even tone.

"The Saudi pilot isn't one of ours. He has a solid reputation, but he's not Fred and he's not loyal to us."

"He'll be fine."

There was a brief pause as she translated his words in her head.

"One last thing. Doctors Without Borders gave us information about the virus that the medical team was dealing with and it sounds terrifying. Without going into detail—"

"This is your definition of not going into detail?"

She had no idea what he'd said but chose to ignore it based on his tone. "It's incredibly dangerous, Mitch. And more important, it can survive on surfaces for days. Don't take the idea that the fire killed it for granted. You need to use the biohazard protocols you've been trained in. I'm serious. If there's even a vague possibility that you or one of Scott's men has been exposed to this, you'll have to be quarantined and you'll probably die."

He was starting to think that she was enjoying his inability to give anything more than one-word answers. "Understood."

"So, you promise to be careful and not touch anything?"

"Yes."

"Okay then. The chopper will pick you up outside of town at exactly 2 a.m. I'll send the coordinates to your phone."

CHAPTER 9

WESTERN YEMEN

SAYID Halabi stood on the ancient minaret looking out over the landscape hundreds of meters below. The village's tightly packed stone buildings dominated the top of the peak, offering 360-degree views of mountains dotted with cloud shadows. Steep slopes had been terraced for agriculture over the centuries, and some were still green with the coffee plants that Yemen had once been so famous for.

Up until about a year ago, this place had been home to a community of farmers who had contracted with an American company to produce and export coffee beans. The hope had been that the industry would regain its economic foothold and stabilize the region.

The foreign businessmen had quickly recognized the realities of trying to carve a secular commercial paradise from this war-torn country and given up on the enterprise. Most of the farmers and other workers had moved on shortly thereafter, leaving a core group of thirty villagers who were either too rooted to this place to abandon it or had nowhere else to go.

Their bodies were now piled in a low building to the southeast. Halabi couldn't see it from his vantage point, but knew from reports that the work bricking up the windows and doors was nearly complete. By the end of the day, the godless collaborators would be sealed in the tomb where they would stay for all eternity. Forgotten by their families, by history, and by Allah.

He limped to the other side of the minaret and looked into the narrow street below. Two of his men were visible, one dressed in traditional Yemeni garb and the other in a chador. It was a bit of an indignity for the battle-hardened soldier, but an unavoidable one. The Saudis and Americans were always watching from above and they couldn't be permitted to see anything but the normal rhythms of rural Yemeni life.

The wind began to gust and he closed his eyes, feeling the presence of God on the cool, dry air. The path to victory became clearer every day as Allah blessed him with an increasingly detailed understanding of His plan. The objective, so indistinct before, now seemed as well defined as the landscape around him.

Halabi finally turned and began descending the spiral steps that provided access to the minaret. His injuries forced him to use the stone walls to steady himself, but he was grateful for the struggle. Every stabbing pain, unbalanced step, and constricted breath reminded him of his arrogance and God's punishment for it.

As expected, Muhammad Attia was waiting patiently for him on the mosque's main floor.

"What of Mitch Rapp?" Halabi asked as Attia fell in alongside him.

"There's still no sign of him, and our sources say that the Saudis are planning to bomb the area out of concern over the biothreat. I've been forced to move our men into the hills immediately surrounding the village."

"Do I detect disapproval in your voice, Muhammad?"

"Disapproval? No. But concern. Our resources are limited and risking the few reliable men we have in hopes that Rapp will appear in an empty, burned-out village . . ."

"He'll come," Halabi assured him.

"Even if he does, how much are we willing to risk over one man?"

Halabi didn't answer, instead exiting the mosque and winding through the narrow cobbled paths between buildings. Near the center of the village, they entered a tall, slender structure with rows of arched windows and a ground floor lined with diesel generators. After descending another set of stone steps, they crossed into a room that had been built inside a natural cavern.

Despite the fact that he'd been personally involved in its design, the environment inside the room was disorientingly foreign. It was a long, rectangular space, with smooth white walls and rows of overhead LEDs that glinted dully off stainless steel biotech equipment arranged beneath.

The machinery had been extremely difficult to acquire and transport but the effect was exactly as he'd envisioned. The impression was of a medical research lab that would look at home in London, Berlin, or New York. Videos made in this room would be disseminated online, fanning the West's fear into full-fledged panic and intensifying the chaos already present in America's political system.

He turned his attention to the only thing in the room that wasn't modern and polished—a sheep's diseased carcass lying on a cart near the center of the room. As promised, the matted hair and dried blood around its nose and mouth contrasted terrifyingly with the sterile environment.

Halabi's cane thudded dully as he walked the length of the room, finally finding the three Westerners near the back. They were huddled together on the floor beneath the watchful eye of an armed guard. None made a move to stand as he approached, instead staring up at him with expressions that were easily read. The German's face reflected calm resignation. Bertrand's, in contrast, projected desperation and terror. Finally, the American woman was consumed with hate.

It was exactly the reaction he'd expected. While social media was one of the most powerful weapons ever devised by man, it wasn't that platform's ability to disseminate false information that was useful to him at the moment. It was other people's willingness to use it to strip themselves of their secrets. The intimate knowledge he had of these three infidels would have been impossible only a few years ago. Organizations like the FBI, Stasi, and KGB had spent billions on wiretaps, physical surveillance, and informants to learn less than he could with a few keystrokes.

Halabi understood their hopes and motivations. Their strengths and weaknesses. Their allegiances and the subtle dynamics within those allegiances. Enough to assign each of them a very specific role in the drama that was unfolding.

"Who are you? Why are you keeping us here?"

As expected, Victoria Schaefer was the first to speak. And while he had a strong distaste for dealing with women, there was no alternative in this case.

"I am Sayid Halabi."

The recognition was immediate. Some of the defiance drained from the woman's eyes, and the Frenchman appeared to be on the verge of fainting. The German, as was his nature, seemed unaffected.

Halabi swept a hand around the room. "All this is for you. So that you can build a biological weapon."

"A biological weapon?" Schaefer said after a brief silence. "I'm a doctor. Otto's a nurse. And Gabriel's a scientist who researches how to *stop* diseases. Not how to cause them."

"The skills are the same," Halabi said, and then pointed at the dead sheep. "It was taken from a flock infected with anthrax. The bacteria are simple to incubate and weaponize. It's my understanding that a second-year biology student could do it."

She stared at him for a few seconds and then began slowly shaking her head. "No way in hell."

There was a time when he would have immediately turned to violence in order to coerce them. Now, though, he understood that this tendency was just another facet of his arrogance. Less an opportunity to carry out God's plans than to vent his own hate. And while the time for savagery would undoubtedly come, it hadn't yet arrived. Manipulation was the secret to victory in the modern world. Not force.

He turned his attention to Gabriel Bertrand, the weakest and most knowledgeable of the three. "I assume you're aware that while anthrax is a simple weapon to create, it's not particularly effective. In order to contract a deadly form of it, you'd have to inhale the spores and then not seek the widely available antibiotics capable of curing it. I'm a terrorist, yes? Isn't that how your government and media portrays me? If this is true, then it's my goal to spread terror, not death. I'll use you and this equipment to create propaganda videos—"

"Like the one you made in the village," the woman said, cutting him off. "You sealed innocent women and children in their homes and burned them alive. And now you want us to believe that all you want to do is a little marketing?"

"What you believe isn't important to me. Only what you do."

After a life dedicated to battle, the scene playing out in front of Halabi seemed laughably banal. The Crimean documentary filmmaker whose artistry had thus far exceeded all expectations was now entirely in his element. He had the three Westerners dressed up in elaborate hazmat suits and was orchestrating their every movement as they dissected the sheep. Lighting was constantly adjusted, camera angles were tested, close-ups were taken and retaken. He'd even experimented with some rudimentary dialogue, though it was unclear whether he thought it would be dramatic enough to make the final cut.

For their part, the three Westerners seemed content to play along. And why not? In their minds, nothing they were doing was real. Much of the equipment, while impressive looking, wasn't fully assembled or even relevant to the task of producing anthrax. The elaborate computer terminal they were pretending to consult wasn't plugged in. For now, they would be allowed to believe that they were nothing more than actors trading performances for survival.

The truth, though, was so much grander.

With biology, God had created a class of weapon infinitely more powerful than anything ever devised by man. Halabi now understood that pathogens and the skillful manipulation of information were the only weapons that mattered in the modern era. While the Western powers spent trillions maintaining massive armies and involving them in meaningless skirmishes, he had assembled the tools necessary to set fire to the earth.

CHAPTER 10

CENTRAL YEMEN

CONDITIONS were solid, with a half-moon, a sky full of stars, and light winds. Rapp's Saudi pilot was keeping the chopper high, making it unlikely that they'd be noticed by the scattered al Qaeda and ISIS forces that controlled the area.

Rapp scanned the dark terrain through the open door but couldn't pick up so much as a cooking fire. Maybe they'd get lucky and this operation would go quickly and smoothly. The best intel they had suggested that the village they were on their way to was completely devoid of human activity. Sayid Halabi's men had been admittedly efficient at turning it into a tomb, leaving nothing but the charred bodies of its inhabitants sealed in their burned homes.

The main dangers they expected to face were a few potential booby traps and the germs that Claudia was so afraid of. Time on the ground would have to be limited, so if they were going to come up with any clues as to where Halabi had taken the medical team, they'd have to do it fast. The Saudis were definitely committed to wiping what was left of this village off the face of the planet, but were being cagey as to exactly when. Better not to be standing in the middle of it when the bombers showed up.

The wind gusting through the door intensified and he pulled back, turning his attention to the dim cabin and the men sharing it with him. Scott Coleman, Joe Maslick, Charlie Wicker, and Bruno McGraw were all sitting calmly, lost in their own thoughts or lightly dozing. They'd been with him almost since the beginning. Long enough to accumulate a few too many years and a few too many injuries. It didn't matter, though. The kind of trust they'd developed over that time couldn't be replaced by one of the standout SEALs or Delta kids that Coleman occasionally got wind of.

This team had always been there for him and not a single one of them was replaceable as far as Rapp was concerned. He knew what they would do before they did it. He knew that every one of them was one hundred percent loyal to him and to each other. And he knew that not one of them would stop until five minutes after they were dead.

"Everyone's clear on the drill," Rapp said over the microphone hanging in front of his face. "We're looking for anything that could even have a chance of being useful—equipment left behind, shell casings, tire tracks. The guys in Langley said they'd take gum wrappers if that's all we can find. Get pictures of everything, and you're authorized to use flash. We don't have any choice, and I don't think anyone in that village is going to mind. The far building to the west is what they were using as a hospital. Don't get any closer than thirty feet. Hazmat protocols are in effect for the entire op, and anything we collect goes in the bags."

"What if we find a survivor?"

"Keep a twenty-foot interval and get 'em on the ground. We'll question them like that and call in an army medical team to make sure they're not sick."

"And if they don't follow directions?" Coleman asked.

"If they get inside that twenty-foot perimeter, give them one warning shot, and if they still don't get the message, put 'em down. Then we burn the body."

The shadowed faces around him seemed slightly more nervous than normal. Stand-up fights were one thing but bacteria and viruses were another. They'd all been there. Smoldering with fever in some godforsaken jungle. Trying to be quiet while puking your guts out behind enemy lines. Dengue. Malaria. Dysentery. Infected wounds oozing pus. Everyone's least favorite part of the job.

The nose of the aircraft dipped and the pilot announced that they were on their final approach. The plan was to never let the runners touch the ground. As soon as they were out, the chopper would climb to a safe height and wait for them to call it back in. There was no reason for ISIS or al Qaeda to be hanging around here, but it didn't make sense to take chances.

Rapp grabbed the edge of the door and hung partway out the side as they descended. The darkness was too deep to discern the charring on the walls of the stone buildings. The collapsed roofs and the inky graves beyond, though, were easy enough to pick out in the moonlight.

The Saudi did a respectable job of the drop-off and Rapp slipped the face mask off the top of his head and over his face. Coleman's men spread out, looking a little less smooth than normal in the chem suits designed to protect them from biological threats. Rapp positioned himself at the right flank of the formation, searching the darkness for human shapes as the chopper started to climb.

The beat of rotors began to fade like they had in so many ops in the past, but then were drowned out by the deafening crash of an explosion. He instinctively threw himself to the ground and trained his M4 carbine on the source of the sound. The sky to the northeast was lit up, and he watched through his face mask as the helicopter broke apart and flaming chunks of it started to rain down on the desert.

Predictably, the shooting started a few seconds later.

A disciplined burst from a tango to the south landed a few feet to Rapp's right and he rolled in the opposite direction, getting to his feet and sprinting toward the village, finally penetrating into the narrow streets as rounds pounded a stone wall to the east.

"Give me a sit rep!" he said over his throat mike.

Everyone sounded off as uninjured, reporting opposition east, north, and south. Rapp dropped behind a rock wall but it turned out to be a bad position when what seemed like a .50-caliber round pulverized a stone two feet from him. He flipped over the wall, sweat already starting to soak him in the poorly ventilated hazmat suit.

"Mitch!"

It took Rapp a moment to realize the shout hadn't come over his earpiece and he followed it through an empty doorway to his right. Coleman was inside with his back to the wall next to a window opening, occasionally peeking over the blackened sill to make sure no one was moving in on them.

Rapp took a similar position next to the door, peering out as he called for an update from Coleman's men.

"We're just inside the southwest edge of the village and we're in a position to cover each other," Maslick said over the radio. "No one's hit yet but we're taking heavy fire from the south and we're seeing sniper activity to the north. The low ground to the west looks clear. Can you reach us? We can cover you and then get out down the slope on our side."

"Rocket!" Coleman shouted.

They both threw themselves to the ground, anticipating an impact on the heavy stone walls of the building. The projectile went wide, though, and instead exploded in a narrow street just to the east. Flame billowed through the windows and door but didn't reach either one of them. The smoke was another story. Suddenly Rapp was thankful for the fogged face mask.

"If these assholes could shoot straight, this would kind of suck," Coleman said, moving back to his position next to the window.

The former SEAL's muffled words were intended as a joke, but it was a pretty good description of their situation. The problem was that from what Rapp had seen, their attackers *could* shoot. They'd hit the chopper. Fire discipline was good—with controlled bursts only when a viable target presented itself. And while they continued to miss, they seemed to always go just a little wide to the east.

They weren't going for kills, he suddenly realized. They were driving his team west, trying to draw them into the low ground. And it was working. He already had three men on that side of the village, and both he and Coleman were in a position where the smoke and fire were encouraging them to re-form with them.

"Why didn't they take the chopper out while we were on it?" Rapp shouted over the sound of gunfire starting to pound the walls around the window Coleman was beneath.

"Maybe we caught them by surprise."

"You mean the force dug in around a burned-out village in the middle of nowhere?"

Coleman looked back at him through his face mask as chunks of shattered wood and rock rained down on him. "It does seem a little far-fetched."

"But they forgot to put men to the west."

"You're thinking ambush? That they're driving us there? Why? If they want us dead, why not just surround us and do it?"

The answer was pretty clear: Sayid Halabi. The son of a bitch was holding a grudge. He didn't want to kill Rapp, he wanted to capture him. He wanted to throw him in a hole and spend the next five years working him over with a set of pliers and a blowtorch.

And if that was true, it was their ticket out of there.

"We're going east," Rapp said into his throat mike.

Not surprisingly, Joe Maslick's voice came on the comm a moment later. "Did you mean west, Mitch? The heaviest fire is coming from the east and it'd leave us climbing toward shooters controlling the high ground."

"You heard me. East. Come right up the middle of the main

street on Scott's orders. Leave your hazmat suits and face masks on. I repeat, biohazard protocols are still in effect. Understood?"

The response sounded hesitant but there was no question that Maslick, Wicker, and McGraw would follow his orders to the letter.

"What are you thinking?" Coleman said as Rapp slipped up next to him and took a quick look outside. The flames had managed to find fuel and the smoke was combining with the condensation on his face mask to make it hard to see.

"Halabi figured I'd come and he left men with orders to capture me. But they don't know which one of us I am because of the suits."

"So we're going to charge a bunch of guys dug in above us because you think he ordered them not to kill you?"

"You got it."

Coleman looked up at the missing roof and the flames starting to lap over it. "That's a lot to hang on a hunch."

Rapp nodded and moved to the door. "I'm going. If I'm still alive in fifty yards, follow me."

Before Coleman could answer, Rapp slipped out and started sprinting along the edge of the street. Incoming fire was intermittent and, as he'd hoped, always led him by a few yards, trying to drive him back. Another rocket was fired and he was forced to drop, but it struck a building well ahead. Halabi's men were playing it safe. None of them wanted to go back and give their dear leader a bucket containing what was left of the prize he so desperately wanted.

Rapp leapt back to his feet, charging through the scattered flames left by the RPG and starting up the slope on the east side of the village. He could make out five separate guns all sparking in the darkness ahead of him. Despite that, he fought his natural instinct to zigzag and vary his pace. Unpredictability was a good strategy when faced with an enemy that wanted to kill you, but counterproductive when facing an enemy dedicated to near misses.

He heard gunfire erupt from behind him and looked back to see four figures in hazmat suits falling in with him. The guns in front went dark, as did the sniper going for long shots from the south. Halabi's men had finally figured out what was happening and were having to recalibrate.

Rapp put the shooters to the north and south out of his mind for the time being. He could see lights coming on in his peripheral vision and assumed they were headlamps being used by the men as they ran to reinforce their comrades to the east. They were hundreds of yards away, though, crossing moderately difficult terrain. It was unlikely that they would figure in the fight over the short term.

Human figures rose up from the earth about fifty yards ahead, their outlines just visible in the moonlight as they began to charge. Based on the way they were holding their rifles, it appeared that they were planning to use them as clubs.

Completely insane, but pretty much what Rapp was counting on. While these men were a serious step up from the average terrorist psychopath, they were still ISIS. And that meant they'd follow the man they believed to be God's representative on earth right off a cliff. In fact, they'd be happy to do it. More virgins for them.

The men coming in from the sides started shooting again, but were still making sure not to hit anything. Coleman's team engaged them while Rapp focused on the men coming at him. Individual rounds from his M4 dropped the first two and left two remaining. They were running crouched now, zigzagging to reduce their chance of being hit. Rapp, still on a collision course with them, fired on the run at the man to the right. It took nearly his full magazine, but he finally spun him around with an impact to the right side of his chest.

Less than a second later, he collided with the last man. They went down locked together, starting to roll back down the slope. Some of the rocks beneath them were sharp and while the chances that Rapp had any deadly germs stuck to his chem suit were low, he wasn't anxious to puncture it.

He managed to arrest their momentum but ended up with Halabi's man on top. Predictably, he went straight for Rapp's mask so he could get a look at who he was fighting and thus determine the rules of engagement. While Halabi's orders would have been to keep Rapp alive, he doubted Coleman and his men would receive the same courtesy.

Rapp grabbed the man's finger just before it went under his faceplate, wrenching it hard enough to feel it snap. When he jerked back in pain, Rapp scissored a leg up and used it to slam his opponent to the ground. After a brief struggle, the CIA man managed to get hold of one of the rocks he'd been worried about a few seconds before and slam it into the man's forehead.

He was just getting back to his feet when a man went streaking by—undoubtedly Wick, a fast and light sniper who would be anxious to set up in the high ground before the men approaching from the north and south could close in.

Rapp let Coleman and the rest of his men pass by before he started up, protecting their flank. A few quick bursts in the direction of the headlamps emptied what was left of his mag. There wasn't much chance of hitting anything, but he might be able to persuade them to slow down.

By the time Rapp made it to the top of the slope, Wick already had his McMillan TAC-338 rifle set up on a bipod and was sighting through the thermal scope. He pulled the trigger and a single round exited the barrel.

"Hit."

A second shot followed three seconds later.

"Hit. They're taking cover."

Rapp lay down among Coleman and his men, glancing behind him and seeing a barely perceptible band of light on the horizon.

Rapp wiped the dust from his faceplate and watched the jet's angle of descent steepen. Contrails appeared, followed by a massive wall of fire rising from the earth. Another jet dropped a similar payload, spreading the firestorm.

Unfortunately, the air support had nothing to do with him. The Saudis had finally gotten around to incinerating the village, which was about four miles back now. The sun was still low on the horizon, but the heat was already starting to climb. In another hour, running in the chem suits they were still wearing would no longer be doable.

Rapp picked up a set of binoculars and scanned across the six ISIS operatives pursuing them, finally settling on a man using his hand to shade a similar set of lenses against the sun. They were persistent and well organized, but seemed content to prosecute their chase from just out of rifle range.

His earpiece buzzed and he picked up the satellite call. "Go ahead."

"Do you see the Saudi jets?" Claudia said.

"They're hard to miss."

"According to the pilots, you've got two groups coming in on you. One from the northeast and the other from the southeast. As many as twenty vehicles in total. Another seven vehicles are coming in from the west to reinforce the men chasing you."

That explained why their pursuers were keeping their distance. Halabi had called in the locals still loyal to him. Probably nowhere near the quality of the men they'd been dealing with so far, but it didn't matter. The terrorist leader's plan to capture him didn't really demand crack troops. Just a lot of warm bodies willing to turn cold in an effort to overwhelm them.

"ETAs?"

"Call it twenty-five minutes for the forces approaching from the east. A little longer for the western reinforcement because now they're going to have to go around the fire."

"Can the Saudis take them out?" Rapp asked.

"Irene's working on it and she's gotten the president involved. He's tried to contact the king directly, but he's sick and not taking calls. I don't think they're going to help us, Mitch. The people Irene has reached out to are angry that the Agency's operating in the area without notifying them and they're throwing up a bunch of red tape."

The fact that the two jets had turned back toward Saudi Arabia suggested that she was right. Yet another pain-in-the-ass development in what was turning out to be a serious pain-in-the-ass day.

"Mitch? Are you still there?"

"I'm here."

"What can I do to help?"

"You tell me."

When she spoke again she sounded like she was on the verge of breaking into tears. "I . . . I don't know."

"No problem. Can you do me a favor?"

"Of course. What?"

"Make us a reservation at that new Japanese place in Manassas for Saturday. I've had sushi stuck in my mind all day."

She actually managed a choking laugh. "You're getting better at this relationship stuff. I appreciate the effort."

"It's going to be fine," he said and then cut off the call.

When he walked back to Coleman and his men, he found them all crammed into a sliver of shade provided by a boulder.

Bruno McGraw was the first to speak. "What's the plan, boss?"

"We take off the monkey suits."

That order was met with more enthusiasm than probably any he'd given in his career. The strict protocols necessary for the safe removal of the suits felt painfully slow, but after ten precious minutes, they were down to their custom desert camo. Despite the fact that temperatures were already hovering around ninety, Rapp felt like he'd just plunged himself into a frozen lake.

He squinted into the sun and pointed at two dust plumes now visible to the east. "Twenty vehicles total with an unknown number of men. ETA to us is about fifteen. Seven more vehicles coming in from the west to reinforce the men chasing us. ETA's probably around twenty-five minutes."

"What about the Saudis?" Coleman asked.

"Forget them. We're on our own."

The mood that had been elevated a moment before by the removal of the chem suits started to slide again.

"We're limited on ammo and water," Rapp said. "And there's nowhere around here to get more."

"The nearest village is a long way away," Maslick pointed out. "And there ain't much in it."

"We could reverse course and charge the guys coming up behind us," Wick suggested. "If they still don't want to shoot us, it'll be easy to whack them and take their gear."

Rapp shook his head. "If they're smart—and I think there's a good chance they are—they'll just run and lead us straight into the reinforcements coming in behind them. If you figure five men per vehicle, we could be facing a force of over forty men. They'll blitz us and absorb whatever casualties they have to."

"And even if we kill them all," Coleman said, "by the time we do, we could have as many as another hundred men on top of us from the east."

"Well, we can't wander around on foot in the flats," Wick said. "They might just be a bunch of pricks in pickups but that's still cavalry as far as I'm concerned. And who's to say those are the only people coming to the party? There could be another fifty vehicles gassing up somewhere."

Rapp nodded. They were trapped on a narrow plain with a steep rocky slope rising about five hundred yards to the north and an equally steep and rocky one descending the same distance to the south.

"Seems like an easy decision," Coleman said. "We climb. We'll be way faster than the guys on foot, it'll give us the high ground, and it'll neutralize the advantage of the trucks."

"What then, though?" Rapp asked. "You saw the map. That slope tops out into a mesa that's about a quarter mile square."

"Chopper extraction?"

"Based on what I'm hearing, I don't think we can count on it."

The group fell silent as Rapp walked back to a vantage point that allowed him to see the men digging in to the west. He scanned with his binoculars again, and again found a man scanning back. Rapp lowered his lenses and let him get a good long look at his face.

"You all are going up the ridge to the north."

"What do you mean 'you all'?" Coleman replied. "What are you doing?"

"I'll head down the slope to the south. They don't care about you. Their orders are to capture me or die trying."

"Screw that," Coleman said, and his men mumbled their agreement with the sentiment. "We're not leaving you to roll down a canyon with a hundred guys coming in on you."

"You have your orders."

"Kiss my ass, Mitch. You don't give orders anymore. The Agency pays me and you don't even work there. As far as I can tell, you're just an unemployed tourist."

"Then let me put it this way," Rapp said, starting to gather his gear. "I'm going south and I'm shooting anyone I see behind me. If it's one of you guys, I probably won't go for center of mass. But I'm gonna make it hurt."

CHAPTER 11

WESTERN YEMEN

VICTORIA Schaefer leaned out the window and once again squinted into the sunlight. Nothing had changed. It probably hadn't for hundreds of years. Three- and four-story buildings rose across from her, separated by narrow dirt and cobble paths. Beyond, she could see the land drop off steeply and the terraced mountains beyond. The splashes of vibrant green created a stark—and strangely beautiful—contrast with the reddish brown that had made up her universe since arriving in Yemen.

For what must have been the thousandth time, she studied the sheer drop from the tower they were locked in and for the thousandth time calculated it at just over fifty feet. The nearest building was only about ten feet away, but instead of the empty arched window frames that dominated the village's architecture, it presented a blank wall. Signs of humanity were fleeting, and over the past few days she'd become convinced that all were men loyal to Sayid Halabi. What had happened to the original inhabitants, she could only imagine.

Schaefer turned and focused her attention on the room that they were imprisoned in. The entire space was no more than fifteen feet square, with rock walls and two heavy wooden doors. One led to the stairway they'd been brought up and the other was a mystery. The ceiling was supported by beams that had been darkened by what she suspected was centuries of cooking fires. Good for hanging yourself from if it became necessary. And it appeared that it might.

Since their star turn in Halabi's video three days ago, they'd had no contact with anyone. A water jug, now almost empty, had been provided but no food. The bucket they used for a toilet was in the far corner and was in danger of overflowing. She wanted to dump it on an unsuspecting scumbag who wandered beneath their window, but Otto kept stopping her. Always the voice of reason.

The worst, though, were the nights. The cold wind flowed freely through the windows, and the uninsulated stone turned the room into a meat locker. They slept—probably only a few minutes a night—huddled together in a corner. Gabriel Bertrand had finally gotten his chance to grind up against her but didn't seem to be enjoying it as much as he'd expected.

She turned her attention to the Frenchman, who was sitting with his back against a wall and knees pulled to his chest. She'd been doing her best to ignore him, and he took her flicker of interest as an invitation to speak.

"They're going to just leave us here to starve."

He was already cracking. Hunger, lack of sleep, and uncertainty were potent weapons against anyone. But they were particularly potent against a man who had led a charmed life since the day he was born. The only son of a wealthy Parisian family, he'd been gifted with an exceptional mind and spent his entire adult life coddled by top universities. His research in Yemen had been the hardest thing he'd ever done, and he wouldn't have lasted an hour if he hadn't been certain it was his path to blazing academic glory.

Otto Vogel, on the other hand, was an almost perfect counterpoint to the French scientist. He was sprawled on the floor, deftly spinning a twig on the tip of his index finger. As always, his armor seemed impenetrable.

"Anthrax isn't that dangerous," Bertrand continued as she turned back to the window. "And they filmed us. Why? So they can put the videos out on the Internet to scare people. But that will backfire, yes? People will be frightened, but they'll also be wary. If they have symptoms, if they come into contact with some unknown substance, they'll go to the doctor and get antibiotics. And the governments of the world can't allow the manufacture of weaponized anthrax. They have to come. They have to rescue us."

The suggestion that they should build a bioweapon to bring about their rescue prompted Victoria to look at him over her shoulder. He averted his eyes.

"I didn't mean it like that."

Vogel stopped spinning the piece of wood, a rare glimmer of anger crossing his face. He'd had enough of the Frenchman within an hour of their first meeting and now he was reaching his limit.

"The Americans were motivated to find Osama bin Laden, too. How long did that take? And even if they are able find us, what is it you think they're going to do? Send soldiers to assault this mountain in order to save us? Risk their men's lives and maybe give Halabi a chance to escape to save three people?"

"What are you saying?"

"I'm saying that they'll blow the entire top of this mountain off. You'll hear a slight whistle and then you'll explode into—"

"Otto!" Schaefer interjected. "You're not helping."

He frowned and went back to spinning his stick.

"They aren't going to be satisfied with making movies and they're not going to give us a choice," Bertrand said. "How long can we hold out? They'll starve us. Freeze us. Torture us. And finally, they'll kill us."

In truth, none of that would be necessary, Schaefer knew. It wouldn't take much more than a mild rash to get Bertrand pumping out every dangerous pathogen he knew how to create. Trying to get him to grow a backbone was a waste of time. As she saw it, there were two paths ahead of them. The first was to throw the man out the window and let his incredible knowledge of microbiology die with him. Undoubtedly, Otto would enthusiastically sign on to that strategy, but to her it was just an abstraction. She'd never knowingly harmed anyone in her life.

That left only one option: convincing him to focus that magnificent brain on something other than the hopelessness of their situation.

She sat next to the Frenchman and motioned Vogel over.

"Listen," she said, speaking quietly in case there were listening devices. "We're scientists, right? There's a lot of equipment in that room, and we can probably ask for more if we play our cards right. All we need to do is figure out how we can use it to get ourselves out of here."

"Agreed," the German whispered.

"Agreed?" Bertrand said, the volume of his voice high enough that Victoria clamped a hand over his mouth.

"Don't talk, Gabriel. Think. Gas? Poison? Explosives? You keep telling everyone you're a genius. Prove it."

Sayid Halabi climbed the stairs with Muhammad Attia hovering directly behind. The voices of his prisoners had dipped to below what his microphones could pick up, suggesting that it was time to pay them a visit.

Undoubtedly, they'd begun plotting. They would pretend to cooperate and use the equipment he gave them to create some kind of weapon. Perhaps a disease that they inoculated themselves against. Perhaps a poison. Perhaps even a way to contact the outside world. It was to be expected.

He pulled back the bolt and opened the door, watching the three Westerners leap to their feet as he entered.

"How long will it take to make weaponized anthrax in a quantity sufficient for multiple large-scale attacks?" he said.

They looked at each for a moment before the woman answered. "None of us have ever made anthrax. We have nothing to do with bioweapons research. Do you have an Internet connection? You can look it up and see that I'm telling the truth."

The Frenchman kept glancing over at her, drawing strength from his unwillingness to look weaker than a woman.

"Dr. Bertrand?" Halabi prompted.

He drew back at the sound of his name. "It's . . . It's not as easy as you think. That's why no one uses those kinds of weapons. It's not just that you could infect your own troops, it's that nature tends to take its own path. It's impossible to control and impossible to predict. And anthrax has its own unique problems that make it hard to weaponize. It—"

"I can assure you that I'm not stupid," Halabi said, cutting the man off. "We know that anthrax can be weaponized because it's been done before. By the Russians on a large scale and in 2001 by an American scientist with a background similar to yours. Now tell me how long and what additional equipment you will need."

None answered.

"Muhammad . . ." Halabi said.

Attia pulled a pistol from the holster on his hip and fired a single round into the German nurse's chest.

Victoria Schaefer managed to catch him before he hit the floor and Halabi watched a scene play out that was identical to the one with her translator. She tore open Vogel's shirt, looked at the wound over his heart, and realized that she was powerless.

This time, instead of running, she lunged with surprising force and speed. It wasn't enough, though. Attia caught her and dragged her toward the door at the back of the room. She screamed obscenities and fought violently enough that Attia was struggling to keep hold of her as he slid an ancient key into the lock. She actually managed to inflict a superficial wound on his neck before they disappeared across the threshold.

Her shouts and the sound of her beating futilely against Attia continued and Halabi examined Bertrand's reaction. The Frenchman's eyes flicked back and forth from the body on the floor to the open door the woman had been forced through. He was a surprisingly simple and transparent man. He showed no more empathy for his comrades than he had for patients. Instead, he seemed entirely focused on calculating how this affected his own situation.

The sounds of struggling faded and finally went silent. The woman, just out of sight in the room, would now be secured to the table at its edge. She managed to shout a few more epithets, but then her words became screams. Within a minute, there seemed to be nothing but her terror, pain, and hopelessness bouncing off the stone walls.

"How can you stand there and do nothing to stop this?" Halabi asked Bertrand. "What was it you said earlier? Anthrax isn't even dangerous. And, as you suspected, I've released videos with my plans. The Americans will know what's coming and be vigilant."

Bertrand didn't respond. He seemed to be slipping into shock as the screams of the woman echoed around them.

"I need to generate fear, Doctor. That's all. My goal is to convince the Americans that there's a price to be paid for continuing to create instability and suffering in the Middle East. We don't want to be murdered for our oil. We don't want our democratically elected governments to be overthrown and violent dictators to be inserted. In short, we don't want to live like you and we don't want to be your slaves. We just want to be left alone to find our own path."

It was a sentiment that he would undoubtedly be sympathetic to, because it had largely been gleaned from his own naïve political posts on Facebook. Still, he didn't answer immediately, holding out until the woman's screams took on a gurgling quality.

"I'll do it."

Halabi nodded and shouted to Attia in Arabic. "Finish her!"

A gunshot sounded and Halabi put a comforting hand on Bertrand's shoulder. "I'm sure she appreciated your mercy."

CHAPTER 12

AL HUDAYDAH
YEMEN

"THESE images are *garbage*, Irene!"

Scott Coleman had recon photos that covered a radius of twenty miles around the place where he'd split from Rapp, but they looked like they'd been taken through the bottom of a dirty Coke bottle.

"The wind's kicking up and the satellite can't penetrate the dust," Kennedy explained.

He ran a hand over the hazy eight-by-tens arranged on Shamir Karman's desk, leaving a streak of blood across them. The bandage on his forearm was so tight he could barely feel his fingers, but the wound just wouldn't stop seeping. It was hard to complain, though. He was lucky his arm was still attached. The fight to get back to Al Hudaydah had been nastier than he'd counted on.

Rapp had been right about most of the ISIS forces focusing on him, but that still left three vehicles full of terrorist pricks to come after Coleman's team. The climbing had been steeper and looser than it looked and they'd gotten pinned down in a cliff band about thirty yards up the slope.

With the crack troops concentrating on Rapp, the less disciplined fighters had unleashed as much ammo as they could in his team's general direction, underestimating how good their cover was. After ten minutes of setup, his guys had started to return fire—single rounds aimed at carefully selected targets. About half the ISIS force went down in the first two minutes, but then the rest got wise. After that, the skirmish had turned into a stalemate that wasn't broken until well after sunset. The injury to his arm, a set of bruised ribs, and a self-sutured gash over his kneecap were souvenirs of the two hours he'd spent silently climbing back down the dark slope.

The remaining ISIS forces had assumed Coleman would go up and try to escape over the top, leaving them completely unprepared when the four Americans walked into their camp with silenced pistols. Things had gotten a little hairy when the inexperienced force panicked and started shooting wildly in every direction, but eventually they all ended up dead.

By then, though, it was too late to do anything for Rapp. More ISIS troops had joined the hunt and there were headlights spread out in a search pattern that was probably five miles wide. Worse was the fact that a few of them noticed the shooting behind and reversed course to provide support for their comrades.

Piling into the ISIS pickups and turning tail was one of the hardest decisions Coleman had ever made. But with that many enemy fighters and no idea where Rapp was, there had been no other option.

"Screw the photos," Coleman said, sweeping them off the desk. "They're not going to tell us anything we don't already know. Mitch is out there and there's only so far he could have gotten in the last . . ." He paused and looked at his watch, cursing silently. ". . . forty-three hours. All we need is air support from the Saudis and to bring in—"

"It's not going to happen, Scott."

"What do you mean it's not going to happen?"

"America's role in the Middle East in general—and Yemen in particular—has come under a lot of scrutiny since the presidential primaries started. Christine Barnett is on the attack and everyone else is in defense mode. Getting anyone to authorize an operation in Yemen and trying to get any meaningful cooperation from the Saudis at this point is . . ." Her voice faded but the message was clear.

"So after everything Mitch has done for the president, America—and even Saudi Arabia—this is how they repay him? By abandoning him in the middle of the Yemeni desert? Because the optics might not be great inside the Beltway?"

"I'm afraid optics are all that's left inside the Beltway," Kennedy said. "But I'm not completely powerless. Not yet. I have a chopper pilot on his way to you and I'll find a way to borrow an aircraft. I've also contacted a number of private contractors who have worked with either you or Mitch in the past. We're bringing them in—"

"When?" Coleman said, cutting her off for perhaps the first time in his life.

"You should have one chopper and as many as ten men within thirty-six hours."

He did the math in his head. "By then he'll have been out there for more than three days with nothing but a half-full CamelBak, an M4, and a couple of spare mags."

"Christine Barnett has everyone on—"

"I don't give a shit about that crazy bitch!" he shouted but then lowered his voice after realizing he'd just yelled at the director of the CIA. "I'm sorry, Irene."

"I'm as frustrated and angry as you are, Scott. And I'm doing everything I can."

"I know. Keep me posted," he said and then disconnected the call.

He lowered himself into the chair behind him and looked down at the useless photos scattered across the floor. That was it.

Mitch Rapp had been abandoned. And not just by the American and Saudi politicians. By him. He should have told Rapp to shove his orders up his ass. He should be out there fighting with him. And if necessary dying with him. One last charge into a barrage of ISIS bullets would be a hundred times better than sitting in this room doing nothing.

His sat phone rang and he declined the call when he saw that it was Claudia. What could he tell her? That Mitch was somewhere in the desert with every ISIS fighter in Yemen either searching for him or on their way to search for him? That instead of helping, his team was sitting around with their thumbs up their asses?

"You should talk to her."

Joe Maslick was sitting on a stool in the corner of the tiny room, feeling as helpless as he was. The others were checking their weapons or catching some shut-eye on the building's bombed-out second floor, waiting for word that they were going back into action.

Coleman nodded and was about to reach for the sat phone when the door leading to the office started to swing inward. Instead of the phone he grabbed the SIG P226 next to it, while Maslick retrieved a similar weapon from his holster.

The man standing in the threshold had a bearded face almost completely obscured by the scarf wound around his head. Only two bloodshot eyes and the sun-damaged skin around them were visible. He was dressed in traditional Yemeni garb but it was so caked with dirt that it was impossible to even guess at the original color of the cloth.

He ignored the two men aiming guns at him, fixating on the bottle of water on the desk. Coleman watched as he pushed the scarf away from his mouth and drained the bottle in one long pull.

It took the former SEAL a few seconds to conjure the expected nonchalance. "What took you so long?"

Rapp tossed the empty container on the floor and used the

back of his hand to wipe the mud from his lips. "Stopped for lunch. Can I assume we're blown here?"

"Yeah. Four Americans in camo showing up at the restaurant hasn't been great for Karman's cover."

He nodded. "Tell him to gather up his people and get us some vehicles. We'll wait until dark and then make a run for the Saudi border."

CHAPTER 13

WESTERN YEMEN

SAYID Halabi began to stand, but the pain in his damaged spine prompted him to abandon the idea. Instead he settled back behind the desk that dominated the room. A Panasonic Toughbook computer sitting in front of him was connected to a series of satellite dishes that beamed signals horizontally for kilometers before finally pointing skyward. Maps of the Middle East, Europe, and America hung on the walls, allowing him to visualize how the world would be affected by his plans.

Thousands of miles to the west, Irene Kennedy was sitting at a similar desk, with a similar computer, considering similar maps. All more grand and sophisticated, of course. But fundamentally the same. If he was going to defeat America, he would have to learn to think like the woman charged with protecting it. Strategize like her. Use the high-tech tools at her disposal with equal dexterity.

During his time convalescing from the injuries Mitch Rapp had inflicted on him, he had come to accept that ISIS would never be a military force to rival the West. With that acceptance, though, had come the realization that it wasn't necessary. The era of traditional armies was over and had been for decades. For all its size and sophistication, even the American military was capable of little more than a lengthy string of elaborate failures.

The world was now defined by a complex web of interrelated cold wars. External battles between the Europeans, Americans, Russians, and Chinese raged just beneath the surface. But even more important were the internal battles—between the individual countries that made up the EU, between political parties, between races and economic classes.

The United States was as weak as it had been in human memory. Its people were unconcerned with anything but their own selfish needs and had turned their political system into just another source of cheap entertainment. Its defenses were still built around standing armies that had become little more than a way for the military-industrial complex to enrich itself. America's ability to adapt and reinvent itself had been stripped away by politicians who had trained their constituents to view change with fear and anger.

God had provided him with the right weapon at the right moment in history. Now his primary mission was to use America's internal tumult to keep Irene Kennedy and Mitch Rapp blinded, and to ensure that when the moment came, America would be too fractured to react. The world would be left rudderless.

So far, it had been child's play. Christine Barnett had latched on to the anthrax videos immediately, using them to attack her political opponents and the CIA instead of concerning herself with defending her country. Even more interesting was her willingness to go beyond accusations of incompetence and to insinuate that the Alexander administration's activities in the Middle East had brought about this attack.

Halabi had thought Barnett was going too far and might suffer backlash, but he'd been proven wrong. In an America trained to react only to partisanship, her message was finding an audience. It was human nature to hate the traitor more intensely than the enemy, and in America the two parties were increasingly using the language of treason when referring to each other. It had gone so far that an enterprising businessman was printing T-shirts that read "I'd Rather Be ISIS Than . . ." and then finished half with "Republican" and half with "Democrat." To Halabi's great amusement, he was having a hard time keeping them in stock.

He reached out and retrieved a worn notebook from his desk, flipping absently through it for a few moments. Gabriel Bertrand's elegant scrawl was all in French but it would have been equally incomprehensible in English or even Arabic. The complex analysis of the Yemeni respiratory disease contained in the text was currently being translated and put into layman's terms by a young Egyptian doctor.

The man's report would be delivered later that week, but Halabi didn't need it to know that the book contained the blueprint for overthrowing the world order that had persisted for centuries. That Gabriel Bertrand had unknowingly revealed the secret to inflicting suffering and death on a scale unimaginable in the modern era.

Muhammad Attia appeared in the doorway and Halabi returned the book to his desk. "What of Mitch Rapp, Muhammad?"

The man's brow furrowed, but he didn't speak.

The reaction was no surprise. Attia had always opposed his master's focus on the CIA man but hesitated to give voice to that opposition. Finally, he spoke.

"Our last confirmed contact with him was almost twenty hours ago."

Halabi leaned forward in his chair. "Does that mean you believe him to be dead?"

"No."

"Then I don't understand. He's one man alone in difficult, unfamiliar terrain. On the other hand, your highly trained men have now been joined by what? Two hundred additional fighters and more than thirty vehicles?"

Attia nodded.

"Your silence isn't an answer, Muhammad."

Finally, a hint of resolve became visible in his disciple's expression. "No one has even seen him since he descended into the canyon. Or, better said, no one who's survived. Twelve of our men are dead, including three of mine. He seems to be targeting our crack troops and leaving the others alone to the degree possible. He kills them, strips them of their food, water, and weapons, and then fades back into the desert."

"He'll become exhausted," Halabi said, the volume of his voice slowly rising. "He'll get sick or injured. He can't last out there forever. Bring in more local men loyal to us. Overwhelm him. Trap him like the animal he is."

"Trap him?" Attia said, the frustration audible in his voice. "We can't even *find* him. All we can do is make guesses based on the pattern of bodies he leaves behind. It's likely that he buries himself during the day to sleep and moves only at night. And he has an endless supply of food, water, and ammunition because it's being provided by his victims."

"The desert will—"

"The desert will do nothing!" Attia said, daring to interrupt him. "This isn't a hardship for him. It's his home. He's spent his entire adult life fighting in places just like this one. He could live out there for weeks. Perhaps months. Killing our people when they present an opportunity or when he needs supplies. But he won't have to, because his comrades won't leave him out there forever. They'll find men loyal to him and they'll find aircraft. When that day comes, our men will die without ever having laid eyes on Mitch Rapp. What is it you tell me every day? That with a thousand good men, you could bring America to its knees overnight? But you can't find a thousand good men. And now you're going to leave the few you *have* managed to find to be picked off one by one by a man who America's next president will likely put in prison."

Halabi felt the familiar hate well up inside him but then it faded into an unfamiliar sense of confusion and uncertainty. Had he fallen into the same trap that had snared him so many times before? Rapp's life had been his for the taking in that village. But instead of ordering the helicopter destroyed on its way in, he'd insisted on Rapp's capture. Why? Did it further the pursuit of Allah's will?

No.

He had failed to kill God's greatest enemy on earth because of his own desperate need to take revenge. To see the CIA man broken and groveling not at God's feet, but at his own.

Halabi understood now that Rapp wouldn't be caught in that desert, that God had put him beyond the reach of his men as a punishment. Once again, he could feel God's eyes on him. This time, though, they radiated something very different from the love and approval that he had become accustomed to.

"Pull our men out, Muhammad."

"All of them? There's no reason not to leave the local—"

"All of them. It's no use."

Attia gave a short, relieved nod before speaking again. "I assume you agree that we have to move out of Yemen immediately? It's unlikely that Rapp could have interrogated one of my men before killing him, but it's possible that he's learned about this place. Can I begin preparations to move our operations to our secondary site in Somalia?"

Halabi nodded and the man turned, disappearing through the door.

More retribution from God. They would trade a mountaintop fortress surrounded by people sympathetic to his goals for a maze of caverns surrounded by men whose allegiances changed like the direction of the wind.

Halabi closed his eyes and once again envisioned the dangerous path to victory. The greatest obstacle ahead wasn't the U.S. military or Irene Kennedy or even Mitch Rapp. It was his own arrogance.

Finally the ISIS leader pushed himself to his feet and limped to the far wall. There he retrieved a whip consisting of various chains attached to a worn wooden handle. He swung it behind him, feeling the metal bite into his flesh. The blood began to flow and the pain flared, but God remained agonizingly silent.

CHAPTER 14

WEST OF MANASSAS
VIRGINIA
USA

RAPP accelerated out of the trees and onto a flat summit bisected by a newly paved road. Below he could see the widely spaced dots of porch lights and, in the distance, the glow of Manassas reflecting off low clouds.

Their escape from Yemen had been surprisingly uneventful other than the number of people involved. Predictably, Shamir Karman had become emotionally attached to a number of his employees and had refused to leave them behind. It had taken a little creativity, but they'd managed to cram everyone into a five-vehicle motorcade and avoid getting strafed by the Saudi air force. By now Karman would be installed in a New York condo and the others would be getting fast-tracked through immigration.

Coleman and his men were at Walter Reed getting their wounds checked for the various antibiotic-resistant infections making their way around Yemen. And, of course, grumbling about the fact that Rapp's two days fighting his way through the desert had left him with nothing more than a moderate sunburn.

Empty lots started to appear on either side of the road, all owned by people loyal to Rapp. Near the center of the private subdivision, he passed a couple of completed foundations and a house surrounded by a yard strewn with toys and sports equipment. With all those kids, Mike Nash's place was always either descending into anarchy or recovering from it.

Creating a neighborhood full of shooters had been his brother's idea and, as usual, it had been a solid one. While the fortress of a house Rapp had built was capable of repelling pretty much any attack that didn't involve artillery, the fact that any fight would be immediately joined by a bunch of former SEALs, Delta, CIA, and FBI added to the deterrent.

And so he finally had a place he could let his guard slip a little bit. Maybe relax and have a couple of beers in a chair that wasn't backed up to a wall.

Or not.

Sayid Halabi was alive, pissed, and had apparently been doing some deep thinking. His propaganda videos were beautifully produced and perfectly targeted. His men were well trained and well disciplined. His use of technology was cutting-edge.

He seemed to have lost interest in futile attempts to take and hold territory in favor of embracing the concept of modern asymmetrical warfare. He'd identified the internal divisions tearing America apart and was using fear—amplified by Christine Barnett—to widen them.

It was hard not to give the terrorist piece of shit credit. The rage gripping Barnett's constituency seemed to become more powerful and more deranged every day. Her followers didn't seem to think Sayid Halabi carried any of the responsibility at all for the bioweapon he was cooking up. They were far more interested in blaming America's foreign policy for provoking jihad, the president's party for not anticipating the threat, and the CIA for not making it magically disappear. Trying to find a news program that even touched on the subject of stopping ISIS was an exercise in futility.

All they were talking about was how Halabi's videos were affecting the presidential primaries and how an attack might reshape the general election.

He used the controls on the steering wheel to turn up the stereo, filling the interior of the Dodge Charger with Bruce Springsteen's "The River." Not the most uplifting song, but it took him back to a simpler time. A time when America's enemies were external and could be eradicated with a gun.

A traditional red barn appeared on his left and shortly thereafter the white stucco wall surrounding his house began to emerge. Dim spotlights illuminated the copper gate, but also something else. A lone figure sitting on the ground next to it.

Claudia.

She didn't seem inclined to get up as he approached, so he stopped and stepped out of the vehicle. Despite the cloud cover, it was a beautiful night. There was a light breeze from the north and temperatures were hovering in the mid-seventies. Even so, she had her arms wrapped around her knees, pulling her thighs to her chest as though she was freezing. His headlights combined with the spots, reflecting off tears running down her cheeks.

He wasn't sure what to say. She'd been in this business a long time and knew the realities of his world. The likelihood of him living long enough to buy a set of golf clubs and retire to Florida was fairly low.

"You did everything you could," he said, finally.

"Which was nothing. No one returned our calls, Mitch. And the few who did gave nothing but excuses."

He pressed his back against the wall and slid down next to her. "At the end of the day, I'm at the sharp end of these operations. And I'm comfortable with that."

"Comfortable being abandoned by the country you spent your life fighting for?"

He considered her question for almost a minute before speaking again. "It's nice out there at night. You wouldn't believe the stars. And the quiet."

She just stared straight ahead, unable to meet his eye.

"In a way, I like it," he continued. "Being alone is simple. I like the freedom of knowing that I don't have anyone to rely on and no one's relying on me. There's a clarity to it that you can't get anywhere else."

She laughed and wiped at her tears. "You should never tell a psychiatrist that. They'll lock you up."

"Probably," he said. They sat in silence for a few minutes before she spoke again.

"It was a trap, Mitch. Halabi went after you specifically."

"Seems like."

"What terrifies me is that he didn't want to kill you. That he was willing to lose good men to capture you. I try not to, but I can't stop thinking about what would have happened if he'd succeeded. What he would have done to you."

Rapp shrugged. "There's no point in dwelling on things that could have happened. You take what lessons you can from them and you move on."

"And what did you learn out there, Mitch?"

He looked over at her. "I feel like we're beating around the bush here. If you have something to say, say it."

"Okay, I will. It's getting bad here, Mitch. America's changing. I think maybe you don't see it, because it's your country. But I do."

"It's just politics," Rapp said dismissively. "I've been dealing with this crap my entire career."

"No. It's more than that. You weren't here to see the brick wall Irene and I hit trying to get help for you. Most people believe that Christine Barnett will be America's next president and they're focused entirely on dealing with that fact. A lot of good people are getting out and a lot of bad ones are moving up. People are paralyzed. They don't know who they should ally themselves with. What positions they should take. No one can figure out exactly what she wants."

"Power," he said, standing and holding a hand out to her. "That's all any of them want."

CHAPTER 15

THE WHITE HOUSE
WASHINGTON, D.C.
USA

WHEN Irene Kennedy entered the Oval Office, the meeting's other attendees were just settling into the conversation area at its center. President Alexander was the first to notice her and he strode toward her with a hand outstretched.

"Irene. It's good to see you. As always."

His years in Washington had done nothing to diminish the southern gentleman in him, though they both knew he was lying. When they got together outside of their normal schedule, it meant something had gone wrong. A nuclear threat. A terrorist threat. A Russian leader gone mad. Or, in this case, a psychotic fundamentalist building a biological weapon.

"I think you know Senator Barnett?"

The handshake between the two women was coldly mechanical and accompanied by what must have been Barnett's thousandth attempt to stare her down. As chairman of the Senate Intelligence Committee, Kennedy was forced to interact with her much more than she would have liked. Barnett was a woman whose only true human emotion seemed to be ambition. She was interested solely in information that could advance her status, increase her personal wealth, or destroy the careers of her rivals. Everything else was just noise to her. And that laser focus had worked. It was almost certain that she would be the next leader of the free world.

"And I assume you've met Colonel Statham?" Alexander continued, picking up on the tension between the two women and trying to diffuse it.

"Of course," Kennedy said, turning with a genuine smile toward the army officer. Despite being a bit overweight and barely five foot four, he was in many ways the Mitch Rapp of deadly diseases. Statham had spent his career seeking out the most terrifying pathogens Mother Nature could dish out. Everything from Ebola to plague to rabies. He had endless stories about things like extracting a foot-long worm from his own leg, being swept over a waterfall while trying to reduce his runaway fever in an Asian river, and being chased through the bush by a hippopotamus. Not surprisingly, he was extremely popular at cocktail parties.

"Gary," she said as he took her hand warmly. "I thought you were in Africa."

His eyes lit up at the mention. "We're working on an Ebola vaccine. Just initial testing, but it's promising."

"Are we ready?" Alexander said, clearly feeling one of the microbiologist's infamous digressions coming on.

"Yes, sir," Statham said.

"Then you have the floor," he said, motioning for everyone to sit.

"I didn't bring the ISIS videos because I figure everyone's watched them too many times already. My team's gone over them with a fine-toothed comb and, combined with the Agency's analysis, I think we have a pretty good idea of what happened."

"And?" Christine Barnett said, already starting to sound impatient. Undoubtedly, she was looking for ammunition for another attack on the administration of the man sitting next to her.

Despite this, neither Alexander's expression nor his body language even hinted at his deep hatred for Barnett. He'd resigned himself to the fact that she would likely be his successor and he was committed to doing his best to make sure she was prepared for the job.

And while Kennedy admired his effort, she also understood that it was a waste of time. The presidency demanded less a specific skill set or background than it did a type of person. Unfortunately, Christine Barnett would never be that woman.

"Doctors Without Borders was working on an outbreak of a very dangerous SARS-like virus in the village," Statham continued, unflustered. "The three medical personnel that Halabi snatched had stopped the spread and had victims corralled in a building that they'd converted into a treatment facility. It's clear that ISIS knew about it and they sent extremely well-trained and well-prepared troops. Even our Delta guys were impressed by their plan and how it was carried out."

"What plan?" Barnett said.

"I was just getting to that. If you combine all the existing videos into one timeline, you can get a pretty good blow-by-blow. All of Halabi's men were wearing protective gear and they nailed all the doors in the village shut, starting with the treatment facility. They didn't touch anything and after the villagers were sealed up, they burned the buildings."

"Are we certain there were no survivors?" President Alexander asked.

"As certain as we can be," Kennedy responded. "As you know, Mitch took a team there and confirmed that the entire village was burned. Also, there's a significant amount of open desert around it, making it unlikely that a hypothetical survivor could have reached the next-closest population center. Having said that, we're monitoring all of them for unusual activity that could suggest the illness has spread."

"Is there any point to sending another team to have a more in-depth look?" Alexander asked.

She shook her head. "The Saudis obliterated that village five days ago."

"Nothing's certain in this business," Statham interjected. "But with the fire, the protocols used by ISIS, and the isolation, I think we probably dodged this bullet."

Barnett actually laughed at that. "So we don't have to worry about some village in the middle of nowhere with the flu. All we have to worry about is that ISIS now has a sophisticated bioweapons lab manned with Western experts. Is that how you define dodging a bullet? What were those people doing in a terrorist-controlled area of Yemen anyway?"

"Putting themselves in harm's way to help sick people and make sure a potentially catastrophic disease didn't spread," Statham said, no longer able to hide his irritation.

"It's a nice sentiment, but now look where we're at. If we hadn't allowed those—"

"They're from an NGO," Kennedy said, cutting her off before she could sidetrack the meeting. "Two of them aren't even American citizens. We weren't in a position to tell them where they can and can't help people."

"Well, maybe we should have been," Barnett shot back.

"Agreed. But your committee has been reluctant to support our operations in Yem—"

"I was told that Sayid Halabi was dead," she said, the volume of her voice rising. "If I'd known he was in Yemen looking to build a biological capability, I wouldn't have taken that position."

Kennedy wanted to remind her that the Agency had never confirmed Halabi's death and, even if it had, he was only one of a countless number of dangerous jihadists now taking cover in Yemen. But what was the point? This wasn't about truth. It wasn't about protecting America. It was about her installing herself in this office.

The uncomfortable silence that ensued was finally broken by Statham.

"Since you mentioned Halabi's biological weapons capability, let's talk about it for a second. The main purpose of those videos was to look scary. Basically, a lot of fancy stainless steel equipment and three people wandering around in biohazardy-looking clothes. But the truth is, most of that stuff has nothing to do with the production of bioweapons."

"What about the latest video?" Barnett said. "The one I just got a few hours ago? Halabi says he's got Gabriel Bertrand producing a half ton of anthrax."

"That video does suggest that he has the capacity to produce anthrax, but not in anywhere near those kinds of quantities. It's just propaganda."

"Whether it's a little anthrax or a lot doesn't matter," Barnett said. "People are terrified. And they should be. It's this government's duty to protect the country from these kinds of threats. And despite the billions we squander on homeland security, I have to spend my days sitting around watching a video of Sayid Halabi building bioweapons."

"How long before he has enough anthrax to attack us?" Alexander asked in an uncharacteristically subdued voice. He looked exhausted. Not only from his seven-plus years in office, but from the knowledge that everything said in this meeting would be used against him and his party in the evening news cycle.

"It depends on how much he plans on smuggling in," Statham said. "The amount necessary for a small-scale attack might already be available."

"Casualties?"

"Limited. Any biological weapon is serious and terrifying, but anthrax is hard to deploy. You have to get the granules small enough for inhalation and keep them from clumping. And then the victim actually has to breathe them in. It doesn't spread from human contact and it doesn't scale up well."

"The Russians did it," Barnett said.

"The *Soviets* did it," Statham corrected. "They bred a very deadly spore capable of being deployed as an aerosol. When it got through their lab's filtration system, it killed more than a hundred people. But we're talking about a massive effort by a major world power. This is different. Think about the Aum Shinrikyo cult in Japan. They put an enormous amount of money, expertise, and effort into trying to do the same thing and ended up abandoning the effort in favor of sarin."

"I keep being told not to worry about ISIS and I keep getting burned," Barnett said.

Kennedy frowned but, again, kept her mouth shut. The number of written warnings her office had provided about ISIS in Yemen would fill a good-size closet.

"The bottom line," Statham continued, "is that Halabi could kill a lot more people with a bomb or mass shooter. And it would be a hell of a lot less complicated."

"But not as terrifying," Kennedy said, turning her attention to Barnett and locking eyes with her. "The upcoming election's widening the already dangerous divisions in America. He understands that the fire's already raging and now he's passing out gas cans to anyone willing to use them."

As expected, Barnett glared back. What wasn't expected, though, was the nearly imperceptible smile.

"Irene," the president said, again trying to cut through the tension between the two women, "do we have any idea where Halabi and the French scientist are now?"

"That's why I was a little late arriving," Kennedy said. "We had a geological appraisal done on a cave wall visible in the last video. The general consensus is that it's consistent with what you'd find in Somalia. Unfortunately, a country where we have even fewer resources than in Yemen."

Again, Barnett laughed. "It's my understanding that we don't have *any* resources in Yemen. From what I've been told, Mitch

Rapp rolled into Al Hudaydah and started throwing his weight around, then flew into an ambush. We were forced to start mounting a rescue operation and in the process our operation's cover was blown."

It was a skillfully conceived piece of spin, typical of her and her office. Nothing she said was an outright lie, but it managed to tell a story that was more or less the opposite of the truth.

"The only lead we had was that village," Kennedy said calmly. "Mitch went in knowing full well that an ambush was possible. A chopper pilot was killed and Mitch spent two days fighting his way out of the desert. I wonder if you'd have done the same for your country, Senator?"

"I've devoted my entire life to public service," she shot back.

"And I'm sure we're all very grateful for the sacrifices you've made," Kennedy responded, but she was already starting to regret the exchange. All interactions with this woman were a bad combination of dangerous and a waste of time. Barnett placed everyone in two columns: useful to her and dangerous to her. Kennedy's designation had been determined long ago.

"And what exactly is Mitch Rapp's status with regard to the CIA?" Barnett asked.

Kennedy was surprised by the question. They were talking about a potential biological attack on the United States. What did Mitch's employment details matter? She glanced at the president but he seemed to be content to give Barnett some leash. Instead of intervening, he was scrutinizing the woman as though she were a toddler trying to learn a new skill.

"I'm not sure what you're asking, Senator."

"Does he work for you?"

"He no longer works directly for the government, if that's what you mean. He's a private contractor."

"Contractor," Barnett repeated. "Is that a way of saying that what little oversight we once had over him is gone?"

An expression of resigned disappointment appeared on Alexander's face and he finally stepped in. "I think we're getting a little off topic here, Gary. As much as I hate to even contemplate this attack happening, what if it does? What are we doing to get ready for it?"

"The most important thing we can do is get the facts out there and keep the hysteria down. Though that's easier said than done with everything getting stirred up by the media and the—" He managed to catch himself before saying *politicians*. "Uh, the medical community is prepared and looking for potential infections. If anything, we're going to end up with an overreaction. People thinking they have anthrax when they don't. But that's not a serious problem."

"Irene?" the president said.

"We're marshaling what resources we can in Somalia but, as I said, they're limited. And obviously we're coordinating with other areas of Homeland Security to do what we can to keep any biological agent from ever making it into the United States."

Joshua Alexander nodded. There wasn't much more he could do. He was at the end of his last term in office and it was likely that this disaster would land in his successor's lap. On one hand, he was incredibly thankful for that. Eight years in this job was enough for anyone and too much for most people. On the other hand, the idea of Christine Barnett taking the reins was terrifying.

"I want daily progress reports from both of you. And if anything significant changes, contact me immediately."

Kennedy and Statham—two of the most competent and reliable people he'd ever worked with—nodded and stood. After a few strained pleasantries, his three guests began filing out. Before Barnett could fully turn toward the door, though, Alexander put a hand on her shoulder.

"Could you hang back for a minute, Christine?"

When they were alone, Alexander indicated toward the sofa

Barnett had been sitting on. The senator looked a bit suspicious, but she sat and watched him take the chair opposite.

"I don't agree with the way you're running your campaign, but I'm a big boy and I understand that what you're doing is effective." He pointed to the Resolute Desk. "And that pretty soon that'll probably be yours."

Barnett tried to keep her expression neutral, but she was clearly pleased to hear that assessment from the leader of the opposing party.

"It's important to understand," Alexander said, speaking deliberately, "that the job of *being* president has very little to do with the job of *running* for president. When you sit down in that chair, you've won. There's nowhere else to go. You'll be there for a few years and then you'll retire and end up a few pages in a history book. While you're in this office, though, it can't just be about politics. You have the lives of three hundred and twenty-five million people in your hands."

Barnett nodded, considering his words for a few seconds before standing. "You rule your way, Mr. President. And I'll rule mine."

CHAPTER 16

WEST OF MANASSAS
VIRGINIA
USA

"I CALL her Betty, Mitch. Doesn't she seem like a Betty?"

Anna ran one of her tiny hands along the sheep's woolly back. It nuzzled her briefly and then went back to whatever it was that it found so fascinating in the dirt.

The sun was directly overhead and the humidity kept pushing higher, creating a haze on the mountains around them. The barn they were standing next to was designed to be shared by the homeowners in the subdivision and had been set up with stalls for horses.

Rapp's plan had been to rip them out in favor of a gym and shooting range. Unfortunately, Scott Coleman and his wily seven-year-old co-conspirator had commandeered the space while Rapp was in Iraq. He'd left for Baghdad with visions of a thirty-foot climbing wall and returned to a petting zoo.

"That animal's not a pet, Anna. Wouldn't a better name be something like Shank? Or maybe Stew?"

She spun, pressing her back against the sheep and spreading her arms protectively. "Betty's not dinner! And neither is Jo-Jo or Merinda!"

"He's just being a grouch," Claudia said. "Look how fluffy they are. Maybe we could shear them and make him a nice sweater instead."

Anna's eyes narrowed suspiciously and she pointed to another knot of animals near the south fence line. "The goats aren't fluffy."

"But they eat grass," her mother assured her. "We won't need to mow anymore."

Rapp frowned. Was he really destined to live in a subdivision with thirty people and two hundred ungulates?

"Scott told me people have ostriches."

And a flock of eight-foot-tall flightless birds.

"They make really big eggs," Anna said, picking up on his reaction. "You can have them for breakfast. Mom could make like a gallon of that eggs benny dick sauce."

"Benedict," her mother corrected.

Rapp's phone rang and he glanced down at the screen. "I've got to take this. Why don't you go see how Cutlet's doing?"

"Her name's not Cutlet!"

"Vindaloo?"

Anna wagged a finger at him in a gesture she'd picked up from her mother and then ran off to join her new friends.

"Hello, Irene," Rapp said, fighting off a vague sense of disorientation. Having one foot in two completely different worlds took some getting used to. But learning to switch immediately between them was even harder. "How'd the meeting go?"

"Not as well as I'd hoped."

He watched Claudia follow her daughter across the grass. She looked like a French fashion magazine's idea of a cowgirl. Spotless jeans and work shirt, straw hat, and a pair of boots that suggested ostriches weren't just good for eggs.

"What'd Gary say?"

"The anthrax threat is real. Halabi just needs a way to smuggle it in."

"Take your choice," Rapp said.

"We're ramping up border security on every point of entry in the country, but it's not an easy thing to intercept. We're not talking about a large package or a package with contents that would look particularly remarkable."

"I assume we still don't know anything about Halabi or the lab's location?"

"Probably Somalia. That's it."

"I killed a bunch of his people and he's going to have to replace them. Maybe we could get to him that way. I can go back and—"

"No, you can't."

"What?"

"Christine Barnett's blaming you for failing to kill Halabi in Iraq and then blowing the cover of our operation in Yemen."

"She was *opposed* to that operation in Yemen. And she made us starve it to the point that it was useless."

"I'm pretty sure that's not how she's going to portray the situation."

The malleability of truth was another disorienting thing that had crept into his world. There were hours of video and thousands of pages of documents demonstrating Barnett's history of opposing U.S. operations in the Middle East. But it didn't matter. All she had to do was get on TV and deny it. For her supporters, history would be erased.

"Barnett sees the intelligence agencies as a check on her power," Kennedy said. "And she's going to do everything she can to either weaken us or turn us into part of her political apparatus."

"What about Alexander?"

"He's reconciled himself to her being president and doesn't want to make any more waves than he has to. This election is tearing the country apart as it is."

"Rolling over for her isn't going to pull the country together."

"To be completely honest, I also think he's concerned about

becoming a target once he's out of power. At this point, I think he'd be happy to just ride off into the sunset, never to be seen again."

"So he's going to leave us hanging just like any other politician."

"Yes. The only difference is that he'll regret it."

"Doesn't mean much when you're swinging from a rope."

"Maybe not. But I'm more sympathetic to his position than you are. He's a fundamentally decent man in an impossible job."

Rapp moved into the shade of the barn. "I don't work for the Agency anymore. Seems to me that there's no law against a private citizen and a few of his friends going on vacation in Yemen or Somalia. And if in the course of that vacation Sayid Halabi were to get shot in the face or beaten to death with a hockey stick, no harm done, right? Better to stop the anthrax there than to hang your hopes on some TSA guy stumbling on it in a piece of luggage."

"That's the real reason I called, Mitch. President Alexander knew you'd say something like that and wants to impress on you that it's a nonstarter. He and his party are in defense mode right now and he doesn't want any explosions that Barnett could use to strengthen her position."

"You've got to be kidding me."

"I'm not. Do you see them yet?"

"See what?"

"Wait for it. They should be almost there."

Rapp looked around him and finally spotted what she was talking about. Two black SUVs with heavily tinted glass rolling up the street. They approached close enough to get a good view of his house and then parked by the still-unfinished sidewalk.

"They're FBI," Kennedy explained. "Alexander ordered round-the-clock surveillance on you to make sure you don't cause him any trouble."

He stared at the vehicles for a few seconds before responding. "So after more than twenty years that's how it is."

"I'm sorry, Mitch. And even though I know you won't believe it, so is the president."

He stepped out of the shade of the barn and started toward Claudia and Anna without bothering to look back.

"Good-bye, Irene."

CHAPTER 17

NORTH OF HARGEISA
SOMALIA

THE sandy earth allowed Sayid Halabi to move silently, even with the knurled walking stick that he now relied on. The cave's ceiling was low enough to brush the top of his head, a sandstone slab decorated with crude drawings that had been forgotten for thousands of years.

It was a less comfortable and versatile location than the one he'd been forced to abandon in Yemen, but in many ways far more secure. The area was remote enough to avoid prying eyes, but not so remote that the movements of his men would seem unusual. The cavern itself was in a strong defensive position with deep chambers and multiple widely spaced exits. Most important, though, Somalia's unfamiliar operating environment would degrade Mitch Rapp's effectiveness.

A glow ahead began to overpower the dim LEDs spread out on the ground, and Halabi increased his pace slightly. When he reached the end of the corridor, he stopped and silently scanned the semicircular chamber beyond. The nonessential scientific equipment had served its propaganda purpose and had been abandoned in Yemen. The lab was now less impressive to look at, but also far more functional—a space designed for nothing but the production of anthrax.

Photos of it had already been disseminated on the Internet, transforming the general threat to a specific one. Western experts had immediately identified the facility's purpose and capabilities, providing ammunition to the politicians and media companies. The airwaves were now filled with the most sensational and lurid depictions of a large-scale anthrax attack. Partisan disputes continued to grow in intensity, with Christine Barnett spinning the threat into a purely political issue.

America was nearing complete paralysis. Politicians were focused entirely on the battle for the White House. Homeland Security executives were scrambling to position themselves to survive the change in administration. And the American people were turning increasingly inward, focusing on imaginary internal enemies while largely ignoring the external forces bent on their destruction.

Halabi watched silently as Dr. Gabriel Bertrand moved from a stainless steel incubator to the table next to it. If it hadn't been for the stone walls, he could have been at home in France. The cool, dry environment inside the cave left his clean-shaven face without a hint of perspiration. Carefully combed hair hung just above the collar of a spotless lab coat and crisply creased slacks covered what was visible of his legs.

All very much intentional. The Frenchman had been provided a place to wash, living quarters far more luxurious than even Halabi's own, and a beautiful young Yemeni girl who had been instructed to attend to his every need. The more he had, the more he had to lose.

From Halabi's perspective, it was an unfamiliar and rather intolerable situation but one without a viable alternative. The physical coercion he would have normally used would be counterproductive in this case. While the anthrax was a simple matter,

Bertrand's role going forward was to become increasingly critical and complex. He needed to be healthy and clearheaded to complete the tasks ahead of him.

"I understand you've made a great deal of progress," Halabi said, moving out of the shadows.

Startled, Bertrand spun, pressing his back against the table and staring silently as Halabi approached.

"Am I correct that your first batch of anthrax will be ready for deployment later this week?"

The Frenchman nodded numbly.

"And you're aware that the effectiveness of our attack has bearing on your situation here? That I expect a number of Americans to be infected?"

"I can't guarantee that," he blurted. "I don't know how you're going to deliver it and to whom. And if people know they're infected they can get antibiotics to cure—"

"I'm not concerned about whether people are cured. Only that they contract the disease. I'm interested in causing panic, not in a specific death toll."

He didn't respond and Halabi smiled. What wouldn't this man do to protect his own life and comfort? Perhaps it was time to find out.

"Come with me, Doctor."

"Where?"

Halabi ignored the question and started back down the narrow corridor. Only a few seconds passed before the Frenchman's footsteps fell in behind. The circuitous route finally took them out into the starlight and they used it to cross to another cave entrance two hundred meters to the north. Halabi motioned the Frenchman inside and they began to descend.

"Where are you taking me?" he asked again, the numbness in his voice now replaced by fear.

This time Halabi answered. "To see if you can help me with a problem that's arisen."

They'd barely penetrated twenty meters when they came upon a computer monitor resting on a boulder. It was connected wirelessly to a camera set up in the depths of the cavern. Halabi pointed to the monitor and Bertrand's eyes widened as he looked at the two women depicted on it. One was lying motionless on a cot, so still that it was unclear if she was alive. The other was convulsing with a coughing fit violent enough that it caused her to vomit.

"One of my men was infected with the virus you were studying. Before he died, he infected his family. These are the two that are left."

It was a lie, of course. One of the infected villagers had been secretly taken from the makeshift infirmary before it was burned. She had died more than a week ago, but not before Halabi had used her to infect the martyrs on the computer screen.

"What about your other men? Or people you came across during the journey here?" Bertrand said, his fear turning to something verging on panic.

"We had no contact with locals on our way here and none of my other men are showing symptoms."

That was in fact true. They had been extraordinarily cautious transporting the infected villager there. Only one of his men—wearing the appropriate protective clothing—had come into contact with her, and she had traveled in a sealed van along roads far from population centers. The vehicle had subsequently been incinerated and the man who had handled her was quarantined in a separate cave system. Without symptoms thus far, thank Allah, but he would stay there another two weeks in an abundance of caution.

"It is impossible to overstate how dangerous this virus is," Bertrand said. "Are you certain none of your other people are showing signs of infection? And do you have a record of who your man and his family came into contact with after exposure? Have any of them left the area? Can you get in touch with them?"

The Frenchman continued to talk, but Halabi ignored his

words in favor of his tone. It was impossible not to savor the horror and desperation in it. Impossible not to revel in the fact that soon the entire world would share that horror and desperation.

"What can you do to help them," Halabi said, silencing the man's babbling.

"Help them? What do you mean?"

"It's a simple question, Doctor."

"Nothing. There's no cure or way to attenuate the effects of the virus. The only thing you can do is try to keep the victims breathing and hydrated, and possibly use antibiotics to ward off secondary infections. Then you wait and see if they survive long enough for their immune system to react."

"We have ventilators and IVs, as well as basic protective clothing. What we don't have are people with medical training." Halabi paused for a moment. "Other than you."

He examined the French scientist as he stared at the screen. What would the man do? Would he put himself at risk to help these people? Two apparently innocent women?

The answer came a few seconds later when Bertrand began slowly shaking his head. "Basic protective clothing isn't enough. You'd need state-of-the-art equipment and to follow very precise procedures. Otherwise there's a chance that we could lose containment."

"So we should let them die?" Halabi prompted. "Alone and suffering?"

"If this got out, there'd be no way to stop it. We could be talking about millions—maybe *hundreds* of millions dead. And why? Because one of the gloves you gave me had a hole in it. Or one of the shoe covers I wore wasn't properly disposed of."

"We're completely isolated in a sparsely populated region of Somalia," Halabi pressed, now just goading the scientist. "My men would gladly die for me and I'm willing to order them to seal us in these caves should the illness spread. Not only would it die here with us, but it would likely be centuries before our bodies were even found."

Bertrand's only response was to turn away from the monitor and stare off into the darkness of the cavern.

Halabi had wanted to get a measure of the man and that's exactly what he'd accomplished. The people depicted on that computer screen were nothing to him. Two poor, uneducated peasants who lived and would die like so many others before them. Anonymous and irrelevant.

Of course, Bertrand would care more about the outside world. But how much? What would he sacrifice to save millions of strangers and the morally bankrupt societies that they comprised? Discomfort? Perhaps. Pain? Doubtful. Death? Almost certainly not.

When Halabi finally led the Frenchman out of the cavern, he looked utterly broken. Any illusions he might have had about himself had been stripped away and now lay dying with the people in that chamber.

CHAPTER 18

**SAN YSIDRO
CALIFORNIA
USA**

IT was still impossible to believe this was really happening.

Holden Flores was crammed into the trunk of a mid-1970s Cadillac—the only vehicle the Drug Enforcement Administration could find with enough space for his six-foot frame, body armor, and weapon. Air was provided by a few holes drilled in what turned out to be less than optimal places. The only comfortable position he'd managed to work out covered about half of them, leaving him with a choice between agonizing leg cramps and suffocation. So far he wasn't sure which one was worse. More experimentation would be necessary.

Not that he had any real right to complain. He was only a few years out of college and everyone knew shit rolled downhill. Besides, a car trunk wasn't the craziest place a DEA agent had ever hidden. Not even close. That honor would probably go to a porcelain clown statue outside of Albuquerque back in the 1990s. What made Flores's situation unique was less the Caddy itself than where it was parked. Not in a remote desert clearing near the border. Not in some dilapidated neighborhood full of meth labs and gangbangers.

No, he was in the bottom level of a parking garage serving San Ysidro's newest boutique mall. Above him was a tastefully laid-out selection of fair trade coffee, locally made jewelry, sustainable clothing, and all manner of gluten-free, vegan, organic snacks. Normally, not his thing but after four hours in a trunk, a soy hot dog with some ethically produced sauerkraut was sounding pretty good.

Flores started getting lightheaded and he slid his ass off the ventilation holes, feeling a trickle of cool air as he glanced down at his phone. The screen was linked to cameras hidden throughout the space and he scrolled through the feeds. Tesla? Check. Another Tesla? Check. Spotless minivan with a sticker suggesting it had been converted to run on recycled cooking oil? Check. Young, affluent couple pushing a baby jogger toward the elevator? Check and check.

What wasn't visible was the improbably long tunnel leading from this garage to a far less impressive building on the other side of the Mexican border. In fact, it was so well hidden that no one in Homeland Security's entire network had ever found even the slightest trace of it. The tip had come from NASA, of all places. They'd been testing a new geological survey satellite when they'd stumbled upon an underground anomaly that traced a perfectly straight line from San Ysidro to Tijuana.

At first they'd thought it was a glitch in their equipment. Once that was ruled out, they started searching for evidence of a disused sewer line or power conduit. When that turned out to be a dead end, a tech in Houston had made a joke about it being a drug tunnel. Apparently, someone there had taken the idea seriously enough to send a few screen shots to her cousin at DEA.

And now there he was, sweating his ass off with a spare tire wedged against his spine. Probably because of some forgotten mine or collapsed well that would have been easy to check out with a little cooperation from the Mexican authorities.

Unfortunately, the chances of that happening were right around zero. Relations with America's southern neighbor were at an all-time low. The constant background noise about immigration, trade, and drugs had been bad enough, but with the upcoming election, it was all blowing up. Everything was about blame and politics. Us versus them.

Even the solid Mexican law enforcement guys were now either sitting on their hands or, worse, actively undermining DEA and ICE operations. They figured why should they die in gangland executions because the Americans like to get high, eat tacos, and have their lawns mowed on the cheap.

Flores watched the screen of his phone as a maintenance guy appeared on the north camera. It would have been nice if he'd been one of theirs, but they'd run into a suspiciously solid wall on that front. Normally, those kinds of jobs were abundant in this area and the DEA sent various applicants with nicely fabricated résumés. Not so much as a call back.

That had left them with a pretty complicated surveillance environment, but they'd finally figured out the narco trafficker's system. How were they getting in and out of the tunnel with enough product to make this enterprise worthwhile?

A fucking car elevator.

The very thought of it made Flores a little queasy. Not the elevator specifically, but everything around it. This mall had been built by an American-Mexican consortium. The city had provided incentives and tax credits. When it opened, the mayor and Arnold Schwarzenegger had cut the ribbon. That's right, Kindergarten Cop himself had shown up to open a drug trafficking front partially paid for by the state of California.

The maintenance man paused, glancing around in a way that was suspicious enough to get Flores's attention. This section of the garage was as far as you could get from the elevator leading up to the mall. Lighting was worse than in other areas and there was a slight choke point that formed a bit of a psychological barrier for all but the most intrepid parkers, mostly those who wanted space to let their overpriced rides breathe and to reduce the possibility of a door ding.

After confirming he was alone, the man slipped into a spotless Ford Escape and pulled it out of a space along the wall. Flores felt a burst of adrenaline and disbelief when the floor behind it dropped six inches and slid back. A moment later, a van rose from the ground so fast that it was almost thrown in the air when the platform reached ground level. But only almost. Clearly the weight and speed had been calculated to make sure it just bounced silently on well-oiled shocks.

And all this had happened with the Ford situated in a way that would completely block the view of anyone approaching. Fortunately, the DEA had managed to mount a camera on an overhead pipe, allowing everyone to watch this magnificent operation in full HD.

The van began pulling smoothly off the platform and the elevator immediately dropped again, allowing the asphalt cover to begin sliding back into place.

That, however, was exactly what this operation was designed to prevent. There was no practical way to get into that tunnel from the U.S. side once the cover was closed. It would take serious construction equipment and approvals that wouldn't go unnoticed by the drug lords. At best, everyone would be long gone before the DEA could get access. At worst, they'd blow it up and cave in half the town.

Everything had to go right and, for once, it did.

The Tesla directly across from the elevator was on remote and its DEA controller floored the accelerator. It collided with the van, forcing it back until its rear end dropped into the gap in front of the closing cover. At the same time, Flores leapt from the trunk, listening to the crunch of metal as the cover slammed into the rear doors of the van.

He sprinted to a predetermined position behind a pillar as the two men in the van struggled to open doors that had been jammed by the flex of the overloaded vehicle as it had dropped over the edge. The sound of distant screeching tires could be heard from above, suggesting his backup was on the way. Power should have already been cut to the passenger elevator leading to the garage and the lane down to this level would now be blocked by a Special Response Team.

"DEA! Put your hands where I can see them!" Flores shouted, aiming his weapon around the pillar.

There had been no way to put more men than him on this level. There were only so many 1970s Caddies you could pack into mall parking without someone taking notice. And while he agreed with that assessment, it didn't do anything to make him feel less alone. Particularly when the men, instead of following his orders, hunched forward and reached for the floorboards.

Flores held his fire. Maybe they were just scared and dazed from the impact of the Tesla. They could be cartel enforcers, but they might also just be twenty-dollar-an-hour drivers. No need to have soldiers pilot your transport vehicles. In fact, it would be worse, right? They'd look suspicious.

Unfortunately, his theory fell apart when the men's hands reappeared holding MP5s.

The weapon in Flores's hand wasn't what he would have liked. Something terrifying like the DEA's Rock River LAR-15. Or maybe a Daniel Defense DDM4 with a sweet integrated suppressor and an oversize mag. Nothing shouts *down on your knees* like thirty rounds of .300 Blackout ready to rock.

Instead, he had a punk-ass grenade launcher filled with tear gas rounds. The first two shots went in quick succession, and he pulled down the full face mask he had riding on top of his head. The gas was made even more effective by the confined, poorly ventilated space. Within a few seconds it was already getting hard to see.

That didn't bother the men in the van, though. They just started shooting on full auto through windows they'd unwisely rolled down. The haze around him lit up with the barrel flashes and Flores dropped to his stomach, covering his ears. Those assholes' eyes and noses would feel like they were on fire by now and it would be getting hard for them to breathe. At this point, they wouldn't be able to pick out targets smaller than a battleship if they were standing on a mountaintop on a clear day. He just needed to avoid getting tagged by a ricochet.

The guns went silent and he could hear shouting in Spanish as the men hunted blindly for fresh magazines.

Flores's position on the concrete was right where he wanted to be but he couldn't stay. His backup was going to come around that corner in a few seconds and by then the assholes in the van might have reloaded. If they weren't deaf from the shooting they'd done already, they could aim by sound at the approaching car. Not high percentage, but that didn't mean they wouldn't get lucky.

Flores toggled his throat mike. "I'm going for the van. Don't shoot me."

He pulled his sidearm and ran through the gas mostly by memory. It took less than five seconds to make it to the van's open window but he was having a hard time picking out what was going on inside. The click of a magazine being driven home made it fairly obvious and he slammed the butt of his pistol into the side of the driver's head. He slumped unconscious onto the steering wheel and Flores aimed his pistol at the man struggling to get the passenger door open.

"Hands up, dickhead!"

The man froze, trying to decide what to do. There weren't many options. He was out of ammo, blind, and his breathing was coming in choking gasps.

Flores's backup came around the corner and skidded to a stop.

Doors were thrown open and shouts drowned out the quiet hiss of one of the canisters still spewing hesitant streams of gas.

Confronted with all that, the man in the passenger seat finally raised his hands.

Flores kept his weapon trained on the drug runner's head as his team started moving cautiously toward the vehicle.

Holy shit. I'm a total badass.

CHAPTER 19

LOS ANGELES
CALIFORNIA
USA

RAPP'S limousine eased beneath the hotel portico behind a lemon yellow Lamborghini and an SUV adorned with an improbable amount of chrome. He watched a woman struggle from the low-slung sports car with the help of the doorman and then teeter toward the entrance tugging at a miniskirt that seemed to be half-missing.

"I'll get out here," he said, reaching for the handle.

"It'll just be another moment," his driver responded. "I can get you under cover and to the doors."

He appreciated the man's professionalism, but it was eighty-three degrees beneath a clear dark sky and the doors he was talking about were less than twenty yards away.

"I think I can make it."

Rapp stepped out under the watchful eye of a group of young people standing at the edge of the parking lot. He was wearing the new suit he'd found hanging in his closet and a clip-on tie that was signed on the back by some Italian guy. His hair was tied back and his beard trimmed, but that still left enough of his features obscured that they initially thought he might be a celebrity trying to fly under the radar.

By the time he made it to the sidewalk they seemed to have concluded that he was nobody and were turning their attention to an approaching Ferrari. Rapp entered the lobby and found a similarly well-groomed Scott Coleman motioning him toward a private elevator near the back.

"Thanks for bailing me out at the last minute, Mitch. The job offer in Iraq came out of nowhere. It's going to be really good for the company's profile but I need to be there personally and we're stretched a little thin."

Everything he was saying was complete bullshit, Rapp knew. This was almost certainly part of a plot by Claudia to convince him of the benefits of the private sector and to get his mind off the Agency, anthrax, and Sayid Halabi.

His initial reaction wasn't just to say no, but to say *hell* no. Then he'd remembered that those words had never come out of Coleman's mouth in their entire relationship. Even when the job description ended with "and then we'll probably all die," the former SEAL charged in without question. How could Rapp do any less?

"Why don't I just go with you to Iraq," Rapp suggested. "Mas or Bruno can handle this."

Coleman smiled as he used a key to access the elevator. "I can't put you on a protection detail, Mitch. My client would end up getting killed by someone trying to get to *you*."

"Uh huh," Rapp said, following his friend into the elevator and resigning himself to the fact that there was no escape.

"Trust me, you don't want to go to Iraq. I guarantee you this is going to be the best job you've ever had. KatyDid bought up the entire top floor and they've locked themselves in the presidential suite."

"A venereal disease bought up a hotel floor?"

"That's chlamydia. Katydids are grassh—" He fell silent before finishing his sentence. "For God's sake, Mitch. It's what the press call Didier Martin and Katy Foster."

"Who?"

Coleman looked at him sideways as they began to rise. "Martin is pretty much the biggest singer in the world. He's been a household name since he was, what? Fourteen? His girlfriend Katy is an actress and model. Probably the most popular person on social media for two years running. I mean, I know you spend a lot of time in caves, man. But come on."

"What's this to me?"

"That's the best part. All you have to do is sit in a comfortable chair outside their door. They never leave the room. Basically, they eat, screw, get high, and watch TV. Almost always in that order. Two days from now, he's doing a concert and once he leaves the hotel, the venue's security takes over. And for this—wait for it—I'm jacking him for fifty grand a day."

"Visitors?"

"Not unless Martin calls you and tells you they're coming. Oh, and don't go inside unless he specifically tells you to. And if he does, don't talk to either one of them unless they ask you a question. Also, it's better if you don't look at them directly."

"Seriously?"

"Doesn't matter," Coleman said as the elevator opened and they stepped out. "He's not going to call, and the only time you're going to lay eyes on them is when you turn them over to stadium security. No one's going to try to kill them. No one's going to shoot at you. Just sit in the comfy chair, play Angry Birds on your phone, and collect twenty grand a day."

"I thought you said you were charging him fifty."

"I gotta cover my overhead," Coleman said and pointed to a chair set up next to a set of opulent double doors. Rapp lowered himself into it.

"What do you think?"

"It actually is pretty comfortable."

"Here's the key to the elevator and a key to the room that you won't need. Enjoy and don't forget to remind Claudia to water my plants. I'll see you when I get back in a couple weeks."

"So that's the chef's salad to start, the filet with french fries instead of baked potato, and a Coke." The room service guy lifted a silver cover off the plate and snapped out a napkin before dropping it in Rapp's lap.

"Did you forget the cheesecake?"

"Of course not. It's on the lower shelf. Best in the city. Did you want this on Mr. Coleman's account or on the room?"

"Definitely the room," Rapp said, reaching for his silverware.

"Anything else I can do?"

"Put a thirty percent tip on there for yourself."

"Thank you very much, sir."

Rapp expected him to disappear down the hallway like Coleman had a few hours ago, but instead he just stood there.

"Problem?"

"What are they like?"

Rapp shrugged and cut into the steak.

"Didier's music makes my ears bleed, but Katy . . ." His voice faded for a moment. "That woman is *smoking* hot. Wouldn't it be nice to be in there with her instead of out here?"

Rapp shoved the bite of steak into his mouth and grunted noncommittally. In truth, he had no idea what either one of them looked like. Though it probably wouldn't be a bad idea to check Google since he was supposed to be protecting them.

The man stared at the doors longingly for another couple of seconds and then started back for the elevator.

Rapp watched him go and then returned his attention to his filet. It was good, but not good enough to distract him from the fact that his life suddenly felt foreign to him. Normally, he savored boredom. It generally went hand in hand with his time between operations, and it gave him a chance to sleep, heal, and plan the next mission. This was different. He wasn't tired, he didn't have any injuries, and there *was* no next mission.

A stream of screamed curse words managed to filter through the door, breaking the hours of silence. He ignored them, taking a thoughtful sip of his Coke.

The fight against Islamic terrorists had been, in many ways, easy. The enemy was a bunch of religious fanatics perpetrating unprovoked attacks on civilians with no real purpose other than to create suffering. There were white hats and there were black hats. And while the tunnel was long, it was also straight. When you killed all the people in the black hats, the job was done.

The muffled crash of shattering glass became audible as he popped another piece of steak in his mouth.

Now the operating environment was changing. More and more, threats seemed to come from within. He'd been dealing with corrupt politicians his entire life, but there had always been the cover of a few good ones. Now they were running for the exits. In a few months, Christine Barnett could be the president of the United States. Kennedy would be out, as would pretty much every other person he respected in Washington.

What then? Comfortable chairs in hotel hallways?

The crash that came next was a hell of a lot louder—like a piece of furniture being thrown through a plate glass window. Had to be something else, though. Architects had gotten wise to celebrities throwing things through penthouse windows and had made them shatterproof.

Rapp leaned back in his chair, chewing thoughtfully.

Where did he fit into a world where the definition of "enemy" was becoming a constantly shifting matter of perspective? Where people were judged by their words and not their actions? Maybe nowhere. Maybe it was time to hand things over to the younger generation.

The next time the woman screamed, it wasn't to swear. Her voice was filled with fear and pain, and was partially drowned out by an enraged male voice making incoherent accusations. Rapp frowned as he sliced off another piece of steak. It was a perfect example of everything he'd been thinking about. He was happy to risk his ass saving people from ISIS or the Russians or al Qaeda. But when had he signed on to stop people from inflicting wounds on themselves?

Finally, the sobbing started. Terrified and barely audible through the door, it sounded so pathetic, Rapp figured it'd calm things down. Instead, it had the opposite effect.

Listening to that asshole tear around the room made Rapp think about other people he'd tried to protect over the years. And about how many were dead now. The innocent women and children guilty of nothing but being born in the wrong part of the world. The men who just wanted to make a life for themselves and their families but who found themselves conscripted into terrorist groups. The soldiers who did everything they could with the shit sandwich they'd been handed.

And now here he was sitting in some swanky hotel listening to two pampered screwups try to kill each other. They might as well have been spitting on those people's graves.

When something hit the door hard enough to knock off part of the molding, Rapp finally stood. His preference would have been to let them finish each other off, but one of them ending up dead wasn't going to reflect particularly well on Coleman's organization. He owed the man too much to let his company's name get splashed across every newspaper in the world.

Rapp tapped his key card against the lock and pushed reluctantly through the door. The scene inside was pretty much what he'd expected. Martin was in the middle of the room in his boxer shorts, high as a kite and slurring some nonsense that Rapp didn't bother to listen to. His pale skin was covered in tattoos and a baseball hat turned sideways completed the impression of a suburban kid playing gangster.

At his feet was a skinny young girl wearing nothing but panties and a cut-off T-shirt. She was beautiful in that over-the-top reality star kind of way, but the blood flowing from her nose and the heavily dilated pupils didn't enhance the package. When her gaze shifted to Rapp, Martin spun.

"What the fuck are you doing in here?" he screamed.

"I keep asking myself that."

Rapp was surprised when the little prick grabbed a lamp and rushed him. He deflected the lamp with one hand and rammed the other into his stomach, leaving the singer spewing his dinner all over the marble floor.

Then it was the girl's turn. She leapt to her feet with energy Rapp would have bet she didn't have and mounted a similar charge. This time he just stepped aside. Her momentum took her right past him but then she hit the vomit. Her feet went out from under her and she landed hard, cracking the back of her head on the tile.

Rapp looked down at them for a few seconds and then went back out into the hallway, closing the door behind him. He sat and pulled the cheesecake from the lower shelf of the cart before digging his phone from his pocket. Coleman picked up on the first ring.

"What? Why are you calling me?"

"There's been a problem," Rapp said through a mouthful of dessert.

"You didn't kill them. Please tell me you didn't kill them."

"No, I didn't fucking kill them." He paused to swallow. "But you might want to call an ambulance."

CHAPTER 20

NORTH OF HARGEISA
SOMALIA

WHILE his objective was still within sight, the vantage point from which Sayid Halabi was viewing it had changed significantly. The Western-style office he'd constructed in Yemen had been left far behind. He was now sitting on a broken stool behind a desk constructed of scavenged plywood. Lighting was minimal—an exposed bulb dangling from a spike driven into the rock overhead. It provided barely enough illumination to see a map of North America similarly anchored to the cave's wall. The few creature comforts they'd managed to bring into Somalia had been given to the Frenchman to keep him motivated.

In many ways, Halabi welcomed the change. The laptop on his improvised desk remained turned off. His worldly belongings were contained in a modest wooden crate in the corner. A prayer rug, faded and worn, was neatly rolled at his feet. The austerity made him feel closer to God, though he recognized that the sensation was a false one. In order to succeed in a world ruled by the enemies of Islam, he would have to return to the sophisticated tools they so deftly wielded. But for now, he'd allow himself to revel in the stillness.

He pushed himself to his feet and limped over to the map. It was difficult to make out detail in the dim light so he leaned in close, examining the line depicting the border between the United States and Mexico.

America's refusal to deal with its addiction to narcotics and cheap labor was yet another gift from God. Instead of creating a coherent framework to provide those products and services, the very country that demanded them insisted that they be illegal. Predictably, the result was a spectacularly profitable black market that had generated a smuggling infrastructure unparalleled in human history.

Halabi had recently partnered with a Mexican drug cartel that was desperate for a reliable Middle Eastern heroin supplier. It was a business he knew well, having used the trade to destroy the lives of millions of Westerners while using the profits to wage war on their countries.

In their first, tentative transaction, a small package that supposedly contained heroin had been hidden in a shipment of Mexican cocaine four days ago. The stated goal was a proof of concept—to ensure that Esparza's cartel could circumvent border security and deliver the package as promised to one of Halabi's representatives in California.

The weaponized anthrax that the package actually contained would then be deployed where it would have the biggest impact: politicians who backed Middle East intervention, business and tech leaders, the celebrities who were worshipped as though they were gods. And, of course, Mitch Rapp.

Delivery vectors would be far more sophisticated than the anonymous delivery of suspicious white powder that the Americans had experienced before and were expecting again. Careful profiles had been made of desirable targets, with ones that were difficult to access being ruled out. In truth, though, he'd been forced to discard surprisingly few. Politicians and captains of industry tended to be creatures of habit, and with America's low unemployment, getting ISIS operatives into kitchens, behind service counters, and even in the business of repairing sensitive HVAC systems was laughably simple.

More complicated, but in the end perhaps more fruitful, were the celebrities. Physical access to them, their food, and their homes tended to be more difficult. In the end, though, the answer had been obvious: identify the ones who were drug users and infiltrate their supply chain.

If all went well with the anthrax delivery, shipments of actual Afghan heroin would ensue, cementing his relationship with the Esparza cartel and providing a reliable means of getting whatever and whomever he wanted across the U.S. border.

Halabi stepped back from the map, continuing to contemplate the blurry image and wondering idly where the anthrax was now. An empty Mexican desert? Hidden in an innocuous vehicle waiting to cross a U.S. checkpoint? Already in California and on its way to his representative there?

How long until he saw the fruits of his labor? Reports of famous and powerful Americans being rushed to hospitals. Images of men in hazmat suits searching opulent mansions, glass office towers, and cordoned sections of the Capitol Building. Distant shots of elaborate funerals and furtive video of intensive care units.

Of course, Christine Barnett would not be targeted. She was too useful. He relished the thought of her using the attacks to further undermine the intelligence agencies that were her country's only hope. She would turn the American people against them, replacing their leadership with people whose only qualification was loyalty to her. Soon the organizations that had been America's first line of defense would exist only to protect and augment her power.

Muhammad Attia appeared at the cavern's entrance and pointed to the computer on Halabi's desk. "You have a call from Mexico. It's urgent."

The ISIS leader nodded and Attia disappeared again.

Even deep in the Somali cave system, it was impossible not to turn his gaze upward when he turned on the device. The assurances he'd been given by his communications experts were of little value. No one could fully grasp the evolving technology of the Americans. It was a never-ending arms race—terrorist groups discovered how to hide their networks and the Americans learned how to find them.

Unfortunately, the only way to know for certain where that arms race stood was to test it. To flip a fateful switch and wonder if somewhere overhead a warning light had begun to flash in one of America's drone fleet.

Halabi returned to the stool, reminding himself that his future was in God's hands. Only Allah had the power to decide whether he lived or died. Whether he would usher in a new age or disappear in a cloud of fire and dust.

He entered his password and waited for the secure call to connect. When it finally did, the accented voice of Carlos Esparza filled the confined space.

"Have you been following the news?"

"Of course."

The delay created by the signal bouncing all around the world was infuriating, but unavoidable.

"Did you see the DEA grandstanding about their big bust in San Ysidro?"

"The shopping mall," Halabi said. He'd made note of the story in passing but was more focused on the presidential election and the coverage of the anthrax threat. "Why should this be of interest to me?"

"Because your product was in that shipment."

Halabi felt the breath catch in his chest.

"Hey. You there?" Esparza prompted. "This connection isn't worth shit."

"You told me you had the most sophisticated smuggling network in existence. That the Americans—"

The Mexican talked over him, causing their voices to garble for a moment. ". . . kidding me? We had a German-engineered tunnel running to a mall with a fucking Whole Foods. Do you have any idea how hard it is to get those holier-than-thou vegan pricks to open a store in your property?"

"The engineering of your tunnel and your tenants aren't my concern," Halabi said, beginning to sweat despite the cool temperatures. "The fact that you lost my product is."

"Cost of doing business."

The ISIS leader opened his mouth to speak but then caught himself. Esparza believed that the package he'd been given was nothing but a trivial amount of heroin. A display of concern and irritation would be expected. But outright anger might be met with suspicion.

The scientific equipment necessary to make another batch of anthrax was there with them in Somalia. In the end, though, the anthrax was little more than a distraction designed to keep Irene Kennedy blinded and the American people at each other's throats. It was the fatal blow that mattered.

"I have people that you've assured me you can get across the border," Halabi said finally. "They're not as easily transported as a small package of heroin and they're not as expendable."

"Stop breaking my balls," Esparza responded. "Have you not been paying attention? It took *NASA* for those assholes to find my operation. Fucking NASA. Your people will be fine. In fact, it's getting easier to smuggle people every day. That nut bar putting out those anthrax videos has border security pulling resources from human trafficking and focusing on intercepting product."

"And if I send you another package? Can I expect you to lose it again because of this increased focus?"

"Remember what I said about those assholes needing NASA

to do their job for them? That intercept was a fluke. I've got a thousand ways across the border, and I hired a kid from MIT to tell me if we've got any more orbiting telescopes getting into our business. Send me another package and I guarantee it'll get through."

"What will happen to the heroin?"

"What heroin?"

"*My package that was confiscated*," Halabi said, trying to control the frustration in his voice.

"Who gives a shit? I told you already. These kinds of losses are just the cost of doing business. Once we get this partnership up and running, your problem won't be interceptions, it'll be what to do with all the money you're making."

"You didn't answer my question."

"You want an answer? Fine. Nothing's going to happen to it. Those DEA pricks will take some pictures of themselves with it to try to convince people they're actually earning their paychecks and then they'll put it in an incinerator and it'll all just go up in smoke."

CHAPTER 21

THE WHITE HOUSE
WASHINGTON, D.C.
USA

IRENE Kennedy had been directed to a conference room instead of the Oval Office, where she usually met the president. She'd been told nothing of the meeting's agenda, nor why it was urgent enough to force her to cancel a long-planned meeting with the director of the Mossad. Unusual enough to take note of, but hardly unprecedented. The president of the United States could call meetings however and whenever he wanted.

When she entered, she saw Christine Barnett sitting near the back of the long table that dominated the room. She didn't rise, instead glaring at Kennedy and giving her an almost imperceptible nod. In contrast, the other man in the room strode over to take her hand. Robert Woodman had been the director of the DEA for just over two years but Kennedy didn't know him particularly well. He was something of an enigma in Washington—a former lawyer who had known the president since college but who had few other contacts inside the Beltway. His leadership at the DEA had been competent, but cautious. Her gut feeling was that he was a smart, patriotic man who just didn't have much passion for his organization's mission.

"It's good to see you, Bob," Kennedy said, still in the dark as to the purpose of the meeting. Of course, she'd been briefed on the well-publicized bust in San Ysidro, but that was very much outside of her sphere of influence. When the army's diminutive bioweapons expert entered, though, her heart sank.

Gary Statham's face held none of the warmth or inquisitiveness that it normally did. He remained silent as he shook hands with Kennedy and Woodman. A moment later, he was seated at the table, staring down at it as though it held some secret.

When the president entered, Kennedy chose a seat as far from Christine Barnett as possible. Not only because of her personal distaste for the woman, but in hopes that some physical distance would keep the senator focused on the subject at hand and not her hatred of the CIA.

"I'm sure all of you are aware of the recent drug bust at that mall in California?" the president said.

"It'd be hard to miss," Barnett said, responding to what was obviously a rhetorical question. "What's next? Are we going to find levitating subterranean trains? The fact that our borders—"

"I'm sure we're all looking forward to you solving America's drug problem," Alexander said, cutting her off. "Robert? Could you bring us up to speed?"

Woodman nodded. "The truck that came through that tunnel was carrying roughly four hundred kilos of cocaine in two hundred separate packages. As a matter of procedure, we select a random sampling of them to test for purity, contamination, and to get an idea of where it came from. When our analysts opened the bags, it was clear that one of them didn't contain cocaine or any other narcotic. In light of everything that's been going on, we closed it back up and called Gary's people."

The president turned his attention to the army colonel, who immediately picked up the narrative.

"It contained anthrax," he said simply.

"How much damage could it have done?" the president asked.

"That depends on how it was deployed. To be clear, there's no way to make this some kind of weapon of mass destruction. It can't, for instance, be put in a crop duster and flown over New York. And with all the publicity, I imagine anyone opening an envelope full of suspicious powder would get in touch with the authorities pretty quickly. Having said that, Gabriel Bertrand knows what he's doing. This is finely ground, weapons-grade stuff. Obviously it could be put in food or drinks, but a much worse scenario would be if someone who knew what they were doing got it into a building's ventilation system. You wouldn't know it until people started coming down with symptoms and then it would be too late for many of them."

"How many casualties are we talking about with the quantity that was found?"

"The nature of this pathogen is that most of it is going to be wasted. Absolute worst case, you could have seen as many as a couple of hundred people infected, with casualty rates probably around fifty percent."

"Are we just going to assume that package is all that's out there?" Barnett interjected. "The fact that the DEA tripped over this one doesn't mean there aren't a hundred more that made it through." She pointed to a vent near the ceiling. "It could be coming through there right now."

"I don't think so," Statham responded. "Based on the equipment we've seen in the ISIS videos, this is about all the product they could have produced in the time they've had."

"What if they have equipment that wasn't in the videos?"

"Unlikely," Kennedy said. "Halabi is going for maximum emotional impact. He knows that the strength of anthrax as a weapon isn't its ability to generate a high body count. It's its ability to generate fear. Showing off his biological weapons capability is in many ways more important than the attack itself."

Barnett laughed. "That's what I'm supposed to tell my constituents?"

"Senator," the president cautioned, but Barnett ignored him.

"Are we at least assuming that Halabi's making another batch? And that we can't count on NASA to find it for us again?"

"I am," Statham admitted.

"Then what are we doing about it?" the president said. "Irene?"

"Since he can't go for big numbers, I think we can count on Halabi focusing on high-value targets. Politicians and business leaders concentrated in technology and defense. Maybe even celebrities. Among other things, we've already spoken with potential targets about securing the ventilation systems in their buildings. We've also tried to get our political leadership to randomize their habits, particularly where they eat and shop. We'll go back and impress on them again the importance—"

"So are we going public with this?" Barnett interrupted.

"I'd strongly recommend against it," Robert Woodman replied. "Based on what our informants are saying, the talk south of the border is about the loss of the mall, not the coke. That's about what we'd expect with a twelve-million-dollar bust like this. The lack of concern about the contents of that truck suggests that either the traffickers aren't aware that the anthrax was in their shipment or they assume we won't find it."

"You're trying to tell me that the drug traffickers don't know what they're transporting?" Barnett said incredulously.

"It actually makes perfect sense," Kennedy responded. "There's no profit in terrorism, and they run the risk of bringing an enormous amount of heat down on themselves. A likely scenario is that one of Halabi's Middle Eastern drug operations has partnered with a Mexican cartel and he slipped the anthrax into that shipment."

Woodman nodded in agreement. "We're trying to trace back the owners of that mall but, as you can imagine, it's a web of shell corporations and foreign partnerships. Based on the ambition of it all, we believe that it was a joint project between a number of different trafficking organizations. We've seen them spread their risk like that before on big projects. Also, we have the two men who were driving the van in custody. We're interrogating them and hoping to figure out which cartel they're working for. Bottom line is that if we go public with the anthrax, everyone in the supply chain is going to scatter. Our chances of tracing this package back to its source will go to zero before the first news show even finishes its report."

"Is your interrogation getting results?" Barnett said.

"Not yet. These are hard men, Senator. And the consequences of them talking to authorities is high. But we're continuing to work on them."

"I feel safer already," Barnett said sarcastically.

"If you have any thoughts on a course of action, Christine, I'd love to hear them," Alexander said.

Typically those kinds of questions had the power to shut her up for a while. Barnett was a prodigy at tearing down the efforts of others, but her policy proposals tended to be smoke and mirrors—designed more to pump up her base than to actually solve the complex problems facing America. This time, though, she wasn't so easily silenced.

"Get the hell out of the Middle East. That's my thought. We're spending the better part of a trillion dollars a year on a military that can't win wars against insurgencies and won't fight nuclear-armed countries—basically everyone we'd ever want to fight. The record's clear. Vietnam. Iraq. Afghanistan. We're not gaining anything. We're just whacking away at a hornet nest and then acting surprised when we get stung."

"I think that's a naïve view," Kennedy responded.

The senator's eyes narrowed at the insult but Kennedy couldn't bring herself to care. In the very likely event that Barnett became president, her first order of business would be to put someone loyal to her in as head of the CIA. And more than that, she'd almost certainly try to make an example of Kennedy by tying her up in years of bogus Senate investigations. There was little Kennedy could do or say at this point that would make her future any darker.

"Sayid Halabi's endgame isn't to use anthrax to kill a few hundred—or even a few thousand—Americans," Kennedy continued. "And while I agree that he wants us out of the Middle East, it's not so he can create a peaceful Islamic paradise there. No, he needs a refuge to build his capability to make war on the West. We learned this lesson in Syria, where we left a vacuum that ISIS exploited, and we've just learned it again in Yemen. Don't be fooled, Senator. Halabi will offer easy, seductive solutions and short-term political wins. But he won't stop until he's destroyed or we are. And in a world of runaway technology and political division, it might be us."

CHAPTER 22

WEST OF MANASSAS
VIRGINIA
USA

ONE last shove and the massive filter finally snapped into place. Rapp stepped back, wiping the sweat from his forehead and examining his handiwork. According to Gary Statham, the upgrade would filter most biological agents, complementing the existing system designed to combat gas attacks. The drawback—and there always seemed to be one—was that the motors in his ventilation system would no longer be powerful enough. Based on the manufacturer specs, they'd burn out after less than forty-eight hours under the additional load. So they'd have to be replaced, too.

Rapp tossed his screwdriver on a greasy rag and took a seat on an ammo box. The safe room hidden in his basement was about the size of a single garage bay. Constructed entirely of reinforced concrete and steel, it included two huge batteries for storing energy from the rooftop solar panels, filtered water drawn from a well beneath the building, bunk beds, and a full bathroom. The cheerful yellow on the walls was a gift from the interior designer he'd hired to deal with the details of the house. She'd said something to the effect of "if the wolves are at the gate, a little hygge will go a long way." What that meant, he had no idea.

Based on the theory "two is one and one is none," he'd had the space ridiculously overbuilt. At the time he'd figured the most dangerous thing he'd have to face was a coordinated attack by a well-trained, well-armed terrorist cell. In that scenario, all he really needed was solid blast resistance, a few weapons, and breathable air. The food, bathrooms, and well water were complete overkill in a neighborhood where a bunch of Arabs shooting rockets would be dealt with pretty quickly.

Now, though, it all seemed ridiculously inadequate. At this point his best-case scenario was that Sayid Halabi had weaponized anthrax and that Rapp was number one on his hit list. Worst-case was . . . What? Sayid Halabi was a terrorist piece of shit, but it would be a mistake to deny that he was a brilliant and ambitious one.

So now Rapp had biofilters in place and the already confined space had been turned claustrophobic by boxes of provisions stacked to the ceiling. Still, he only had enough to keep the three of them fed for five months and his goal was six. So much for the shower. And he might have to give up the minigun. It wasn't the most mobile or practical weapon in his arsenal and took up a lot of space. Having said that, there were some problems that could only be solved by six thousand rounds per minute.

He heard footsteps above and reached for a beer while Claudia came down the ladder.

"You here to help?"

"I don't think I'm qualified," she said. "But I know a very good psychiatrist who is."

"Funny."

"Every reasonable report I've seen says that the anthrax isn't a large-scale threat, Mitch. I agree that he'll try to target you if he can, but it looks like you're preparing for the apocalypse down here."

Rapp took a pull on his beer. "I don't trust him. Anthrax is easy to produce. He could have hired a third-year biology student to make it.

But he didn't. He took Gabriel Bertrand. My gut says there's more to this than the anthrax."

"What?"

"I don't know. But what I do know is that the U.S. isn't ready. If Halabi's figured out a way to hit us with something big—something biological—what's our reaction going to be? The politicians will run for the hills and point fingers at each other. And the American people . . ." His voice faded for a moment. "They faint if someone uses insensitive language in their presence and half of them couldn't run up a set of stairs if you put a gun to their heads. What'll happen if the real shit hits the fan? What are they going to do if they're faced with something that can't be fixed by a Facebook petition?"

"Then what are we doing here, Mitch? I have a house in South Africa that no one knows about. Let's go there. Make a life for ourselves and never come back."

"What are you talking about?"

There was a glint of sympathy in her eyes that bordered on pity. Like she was talking to a child who'd lost his favorite toy.

"The country you love is gone, Mitch. Christine Barnett is going to be the next president and she hates the CIA. She hates *you*."

He opened his mouth to respond, but she kept talking. "Look at yourself. You're not twenty-five anymore. You've been stabbed, shot, blown up. And nobody cares. Everything you've done, everything Irene's done. Barnett sees your success and the loyalty people have to you as a threat. She'll drag you in front of congressional hearings and twist your words and actions. Politicians who've never sacrificed anything for America will question your patriotism. Their followers will post lies about you on the Internet and the Russians will amplify them. Then the media will smell ratings and join in. They'll call you and Irene traitors and cowards and demand that you be prosecuted." She waved a hand around the room. "How is your fancy bunker going to protect you from that? Halabi doesn't need to kill you or anyone else. He just needs to keep fanning the flames that have taken hold here. Then you'll destroy yourselves."

"That was quite a speech," Rapp said when she finally fell silent. "Been practicing long?"

She ignored his jibe and dropped onto a box of dried pinto beans. "This is a battle you don't know how to win, Mitch. For the first time in your life, it's time to retreat. Let's go so far away that you'll be forgotten. You've earned that."

"Listen to what you're asking, Claudia. You want me to let myself be run out of my own country by a politician and a terrorist."

"It's over!" she said, the volume of her voice rising in the tiny space. "Not only have you been told to back off, there are guards parked in our neighborhood enforcing it! And Irene's next. After her, it'll be everyone else. Everyone who won't bow down and kiss Christine Barnett's ring."

"What do you want me to say, Claudia? That you hitched your wagon to the wrong man? I've been telling you that from day one."

"Don't you dare try to take the easy way out of this conversation."

"Then what? You tell me what you want to hear."

"I want to hear about our future, Mitch. I want to hear about the path forward that you see but I'm blind to. Where will we be in a year's time? Here? Barricaded in this room? Sitting with Irene in a Senate hearing? Meeting with the team of lawyers trying to keep you out of jail?"

His phone rang and he glanced over at it. The number was immediately recognizable but not one he would have expected to see. President Alexander's encrypted line.

"Don't even *think* of picking that up while we're fighting."

She would have been surprised to know that it never crossed his mind. While Claudia could be a monumental pain in the ass, she was one of the few people in the world who actually gave a shit about him. She wasn't there to bask in his notoriety or for protection or to use him as a weapon. She was just . . . there.

"We could have a life, Mitch. If you get bored, you can do some jobs with Scott. You could finally get your knee worked on. Heal. Maybe do a triathlon again." She leaned forward and gazed intently at him. "I admire everything you've done. You're the best at what you do. Maybe the best who ever lived. But there has to be an end to it one day. And that day seems to have come."

A ringtone sounded, but this time it wasn't his cell. He glanced at a bank of security monitors and saw one of the FBI agents charged with surveilling him. He was standing at the front gate, repeatedly pressing the call button. After thirty seconds or so, it became clear that he wasn't going to give up.

Rapp stood and opened the intercom. "*What?*"

The man's expression turned a bit sheepish. "The president requests that you take his call, sir."

Then he got in his SUV and drove off. But not back to his normal post at the edge of the road. Instead, he and his colleagues disappeared down the hill.

Rapp's cell started ringing again and this time he picked up. Claudia normally left the room when Irene or the president called, but this time she stayed put.

"Yeah."

Normally, his greeting would be one more respectful of the office, but on that particular day he couldn't conjure it.

"Has Irene briefed you on the latest developments?" Alexander asked.

"Why would she? I'm out and you posted guards to make sure I stay that way."

Alexander ignored the comment. "The DEA found a shipment of anthrax mixed in with the drugs they confiscated at that mall in San Ysidro."

"Nice work. Give Bob Woodman my compliments," Rapp said, hovering his thumb over the disconnect button.

"It's just blind luck that we intercepted it," Alexander rushed to say. "NASA stumbled on it. And it's even luckier that one of the random samples they took was from the package containing anthrax."

He could feel Claudia's eyes drilling into him. "That's very interesting, sir, but with all due respect, what's it to me?"

"We're not going public," the president said, clearly committed to dragging this out for some reason. "The hope is that we can trace the drugs back to the traffickers Halabi's using."

"Good luck," Rapp said, but again Alexander spoke before he could disconnect the call.

"You understand my position, don't you, Mitch? A few days ago, Halabi's anthrax was nothing but a bunch of propaganda videos on the Internet. On the other hand, I see Christine Barnett as a clear and present danger to the country. Now the situation's changed. We've been attacked with a biological weapon and it's not going to be the last. All other considerations—including doing something that could inadvertently help Barnett get into the White House—are secondary. And that's the kind of playing field you work best on."

"Is it? Next year you'll be playing golf and signing a multi-million-dollar book deal. Irene and I will be running from five different Senate investigations."

"Maybe. But you're not going to turn your back on your country. And neither am I."

Before he could answer, Claudia did it for him. Her shrill scream nearly shattered his eardrums in the tiny bunker.

"He doesn't want your fucking job!"

Both he and the president fell into stunned silence as she climbed the ladder and disappeared through the hatch.

Alexander was the first to speak. "Is that true?"

Rapp sat back down. In many ways everything Claudia had said to him that day was right. America was tearing itself apart with hate and rage that had no basis in reality. Christine Barnett would be the next president of the United States and come out gunning for Rapp, Kennedy, and anyone else she couldn't control. What Claudia couldn't see, though, was that America's core was unchanged. The United States was a country of extremes. It had moods. Phases. Eras. But in the end, it always eventually got its shit together and remembered what it was.

"Mitch? Are you still there?"

"Yeah, I'm here. But I've got a question."

"Ask it."

"How much is it worth to you?"

"What do you mean?"

"We had a conversation just like this one a while back. You made it clear that it was my neck on the chopping block, not yours. I'm not in the mood to play that game again."

"I assume you have demands?"

"You assume right. I want a pardon."

"You haven't done anything yet."

"Then just start it with 'I pardon Mitch Rapp' and end it with your signature. The middle can be blank. And you should probably leave a fair amount of space."

When Alexander spoke again, his voice had turned a bit cold. "Anything else?"

"A letter saying that you were kept fully informed of my actions and approved of all of them."

"Are you actually going to?"

"What?"

"Keep me informed."

"No."

"Then how can I sign documents like that?"

"That, sir, is not my problem."

CHAPTER 23

SOUTHERN CALIFORNIA
USA

THE road's dirt surface was rutted to the point that Rapp could barely get the SUV to forty miles per hour. In the east, the rising sun was illuminating the mountains and creating a blinding glare on his windshield. The desert in this part of California didn't look much different than Yemen beyond the addition of a few scattered cactus and Joshua trees.

After another ten minutes and two dry river crossings, a building started to separate itself from the heat shimmer to the north. No photos had been available, but it was pretty much as Claudia described—a dilapidated wood and stone structure that had served various purposes over its sixty-year history: storage facility for the forest service, barracks for construction crews, and a temporary holding facility for captured illegal immigrants. Now some of the windows were missing glass, part of the roof was bowing, and the chain-link fence surrounding it was streaked with rust.

The two Mexican traffickers caught at the San Ysidro mall were being held there, but they couldn't be kept incommunicado for much longer. The cartels had eyes and ears everywhere and this would already register as unusual to them. A few more days would blow past unusual and move into the territory of suspicious.

There was a partially collapsed wall about twenty yards from the fence and he pulled into the shade it offered. Claudia hadn't called yet, so he grabbed a greasy paper bag from the passenger seat and got out, jumping up onto the vehicle's hood and lying back against the windshield.

The Coke he extracted from the bag was a little warm, but the burrito wasn't bad. He watched the sun climb into a cloudless sky as he chewed, finally turning his attention to the building when a man in his early thirties appeared and approached the fence. They looked at each other for a moment and then Rapp went back to his breakfast.

According to the intel he'd been provided, the man's name was Holden Flores. He was a relatively new recruit to the DEA, well liked and in possession of a spotless record. It had been he who'd captured the two men being held in that building and for his first time at bat, it had been a solid performance.

A tiny dot became visible in the sky to the south and Rapp shaded his eyes to watch it approach. The radio-controlled plane set a course straight for him, finally circling at an altitude low enough to show off its six-foot wingspan, cerulean paint scheme, and video equipment. Apparently the cartels had started using these things to keep their eye on American law enforcement.

By the time he finished his burrito, another man had appeared at the fence. Thomas Braman was in charge of this operation and his reputation was more mixed than that of the young man he was now barking at. Not completely useless, but one of those arrogant government assholes who reveled in throwing around whatever scrap of weight they had. This was just the kind of situation that would drive a man like Braman crazy. He hadn't been told about the anthrax, he had no idea why he'd just spent the better part of a week living in an abandoned maintenance building, and he was completely in the dark as to the identity of the man lying on the SUV outside his gate.

Apparently he'd already called headquarters demanding information nine times and was currently dialing for an even ten. Rapp watched him jab Flores in the chest while he waited for the line to connect. A moment later he was pacing across the dusty enclosure, pointing in Rapp's direction as he spoke urgently into the phone.

Rapp went back to watching the drone, following it lazily for a couple of minutes before his own phone rang. The number that came up was a string of zeros ending in the number four, indicating an encrypted call from Claudia.

"Yeah."

"I have them."

"And?"

"One blank pardon and one letter saying that the president is aware of and has approved all of your actions. Both with original signatures."

"Any loopholes?"

"They were too complicated for my English but Scott read them . . ." She paused a moment to recall his exact words. "He said you could 'drive-by a bunch of nuns and walk.' I'm not sure what that means exactly, but I gather it's what you wanted."

Rapp nodded. "And he's got them now?"

"Yes."

Coleman was going to put Rapp's presidential get-out-of-jail-free cards in an airtight lockbox that would then be buried somewhere along the remote trail system they ran on. Alexander was a decent enough man for a politician, but it didn't stretch the imagination to think he might get cold feet and want those documents back.

"And you're set on your end?" Rapp said.

"Yes," she said reluctantly.

"Then let's do it."

He hung up and slid off the hood, striding toward the gate. Flores just watched and Braman disconnected his call, moving to within a couple of feet of the chain link.

"What's your name?"

"Mitch."

"You got ID?"

"No."

This was just a bullshit dance and everyone knew it. Braman had been told someone of Rapp's description was coming and that once he arrived, it was his operation. But the DEA man wasn't going to cede authority without at least a show of defiance.

Rapp pointed to the chain around the gate and Flores unlocked it, letting him through.

"Anything I should know?" Rapp said as he walked toward the building with Braman hurrying to catch up.

"They're typical cartel soldiers. We're in the process of interrogating them, but they're not talking. They know their rights. And they know that if we keep them here much longer without charging them, their lawyers are going to eat us for lunch."

They entered the building and Rapp looked around the room he found himself in. Debris had been pushed to one side and the floor had been swept to the degree possible. To the right was a smaller room stacked with rusted tools and, incongruously, millions of dollars' worth of cocaine.

"Are they down there?" Rapp said, pointing to a narrow hallway.

"Yeah. But I don't know what you're going to do with that information. I told you, we've been interrogating them nonstop since we got here, and tomorrow we have orders to get them and their product into the system. I don't know where the hell you came from, and frankly I don't care. But I guarantee you've never dealt with psychos like these. They're the kind of people who throw bags of human heads into nightclubs. And they know exactly what's going to happen to them if they say one word to us. So you're wasting your time. And worse, you're wasting mine."

Rapp nodded and started down the hallway, pushing through a metal door at the back. The room on the other side was probably twenty feet square, furnished with a single chair and illuminated by sun filtering through holes in the roof.

The two men handcuffed to an overhead pipe were pretty much what he'd expected. Muscular, late twenties or early thirties, with tattoos visible through sweat-soaked shirts. Their shoes were missing and they had a few minor scrapes, probably from their capture and not their interrogation.

The younger of the two had hard eyes, but the older one had crazy eyes. He lunged pointlessly in Rapp's direction, before being stopped by his handcuffs. The motion was violent enough to open a cut on his right wrist and the blood began sliding down his wet forearm.

"Fresh meat!" he shouted in heavily accented English. "Another DEA pussy? You got a woman at home? Would she like a real man? How about a daughter? You know I like them young. I show them a real good time before I slit their throats. We know who you are, little boy. We're watching. We're always watching."

"Shut the fuck up!" Braman shouted, trying to take control of the situation.

"Your family's first," the man said, fixing on him. "You think we don't know where they live?"

The DEA man couldn't hide that he was a little unnerved by the man's words. And, in truth, he had every right to be. The cartel's use of drones, hackers, and highly paid informants made it pretty credible that they really did know where his family lived. To date they hadn't acted much on that kind of information on the U.S. side of the border, but it was just a matter of time.

As the drug trafficker's diatribe slipped into unintelligible Spanish, Rapp turned toward his compatriot. The younger man's resigned expression suggested that he figured his future was pretty well laid out: Keep his mouth shut. Go to jail for a few years under the protection of cartel-sponsored gangs. Lie around, lift some weights, eat three squares a day, and finally get out and go back to work.

When he eventually got around to meeting Rapp's eye, though, he seemed to recognize that his situation had changed. He wasn't sure how yet, but he looked worried. Maybe this wouldn't be as long a day as Rapp had expected.

"Let me go," the crazy one said, switching back to English and refocusing on Rapp. "You could both just say I escaped. Then my friends won't have to visit your families."

Rapp thought about the offer for a moment and then retreated back through the door. Flores jumped to his feet when he entered the outer room, but Rapp went straight for the storage area. He had to climb over the coke and a few shovels, but he managed to retrieve a large bolt cutter that he'd noticed earlier.

When he returned to the interrogation room, Braman looked at him like he was nuts. "What kind of idiots is Washington sending me? If you're too scared of this guy to be here, then go back home to the suburbs."

The cartel man's face broke into a smug smile when Rapp lifted the bolt cutters toward his handcuffs.

"Stop!" Braman said, reaching for his sidearm.

Rapp opened the cutters, but at the last second diverted them to the man's wrist. They were likely too old and dull to cut through the steel of the cuffs, but they didn't have any trouble taking off a hand.

The man screamed and dropped to his knees as Braman drew his pistol. The problem was that the DEA man wasn't sure whom to point it at, and his hesitation gave Rapp time to swing the bloody bolt cutters into the weapon. It flew across the room as Rapp slammed his foot into Braman's chest, sending him toppling back through the door.

The DEA man just lay there on the floor, staring wide-eyed while Rapp slammed the door shut. As anticipated, there was no way to lock it from the inside, so he slid a rubber doorstop from his pocket and shoved it under the gap in the bottom.

When Rapp finally turned back around, the small room looked like a slaughterhouse. Blood had spattered the walls and was pooling beneath the man staring at his severed hand.

Then he was in motion. Rapp dodged right when he lunged, letting him pass by and collide with one of the room's concrete walls. The second attack came almost immediately and was accompanied by a moaning scream that didn't sound entirely human. This time Rapp went left with roughly the same result.

Someone started banging on the steel door from the outside but the specially designed doorstop didn't budge. The cartel man's attacks continued for another minute or so, becoming slower and clumsier as the blood loss took its toll.

Finally, he couldn't rise. He tried to crawl in Rapp's direction but only made it a few feet before collapsing facedown on the floor. The pounding on the door stopped around the same time, undoubtedly because Braman was on the phone, desperately trying to connect with the DEA director's office.

The sudden silence was surprisingly pleasant, and Rapp wiped some of the blood off the only chair in the room before sitting.

The surviving cartel man looked a little shell-shocked.

"How's your English?" Rapp said.

The man's eyes locked on his colleague and the blood flowing from the stump where his hand had been a few minutes before. "It's good."

"All right then. Let's talk about how the rest of the afternoon's going to go. You're going to die. There's nothing that's going to change that. If you tell me everything I want to know, it'll be quick. If you don't, I'm going to use those bolt cutters to remove your balls.

And if you don't tell me after that, things are going to get serious. Do you understand?"

"Don't tell him anything!" the man on the floor gurgled.

Rapp retrieved his Glock from a holster hidden beneath his shirt and shot him in the temple.

"Do you understand?" he repeated, laying the weapon in his lap.

The man managed to nod.

"Good. What's your name?"

"Miguel Arenas."

"There was a specific package in that shipment of coke, Miguel. It was different than the others. What do you know about it?"

When Arenas responded, his voice sounded a bit distant. Exactly what Rapp had been going for. People facing certain death tended not to concern themselves with their professional obligations or the problems of their multimillionaire employers.

"There was one packet with markings that could be seen with black light. We were told to separate it out and deliver it to a different contact."

"Who?"

"I don't know."

It was undoubtedly true. Cartels ran a lot like the CIA—need to know was one of their main mantras.

"You have a description though, right? You had to be able to identify him to meet him."

"Six feet. Dark hair and skin. Beard. He doesn't speak Spanish." The man nodded toward his dead friend. "That's why Paco and I were chosen for this job. We speak good English."

"Where?"

"In the desert. The coordinates are on our phones."

The NSA had the phones, but hadn't been able to crack them yet.

"What's the password on your phone?"

"Calvillo386. All capital letters."

"When are you supposed to meet?"

"Four days ago."

Rapp swore under his breath. Not that he was surprised, but he'd been hoping to get lucky. The goal had been to deliver a package of harmless simulated anthrax to the contact and then follow him as he distributed it to his network. And if it hadn't been for all the grab-ass going on in Washington, he might have had time to pull it off. Now, though, he was screwed.

"What cartel do you work for?"

"Lacandon."

"Any other orders?"

"No. Just make the delivery and cross back into Mexico."

Rapp picked up his pistol. "Then I only have one more question. Head or chest?"

The man sagged against the handcuffs securing him to the pipe. "Head."

Rapp aimed and squeezed off a single round. Predictably, someone started pounding on the door again, but it lasted only a few seconds.

He leaned back in the chair, contemplating the two dead men. As usual, options were pretty much nonexistent. He was either going all in on this thing or he was getting on a plane to South Africa with Claudia and letting the world go to shit without him.

Maybe she was right. Maybe it was inevitable. He and people like him had managed to hold back the tide for this long, but the modern world was generating too many threats coming from too many different directions. Eventually he or someone else was going to miss. Did it really matter if it was now or a year from now? Maybe it was time to hit the reset button on the world. Make people see that there were consequences to their actions. Make them remember what they had and value it enough to protect it.

Who was he kidding?

He dialed Claudia and, not surprisingly, she picked up on the first ring.

"Are you all right?" she asked in a tone that was impossible to read. The hat she was wearing now was that of Scott Coleman's logistics director, and it meant her personal feelings for Rapp had to be temporarily put aside. At least that was the theory.

"Yeah."

"How did it go?"

"We're shit out of luck on the meet. It's come and gone."

"You weren't able to get anything on the contact?"

"He didn't know anything. The password on one of the phones is Calvillo386 in all caps. It has the coordinates of the meeting place. Worth checking out, but I'm guessing you'll just find a piece of empty desert."

"What about the cartel they work for?"

"Lacandon. Do you know anything about it?"

"Of course."

It was to be expected. She'd made extensive contacts in the underworld during her time working with her husband in the private contracting business.

"Don't keep me in suspense."

"It's operated by Carlos Esparza."

"Never heard of him."

"Years ago when he was still an up-and-coming trafficker, one of his competitors tried to hire my husband to deal with him."

"He didn't take the job?"

"No. Even by cartel standards Esparza is extremely violent and volatile. He's also smart and obsessed with security. I was struggling to even locate him, let alone get enough information to plan a successful hit."

"So you decided the risk and amount of work weren't worth the reward?"

"We probably would have come to that conclusion. But about

a month into our initial legwork, Esparza caught up with our client."

"And?"

"Our best information was that he tortured him and his family for months and then ground them up and fed them to his men."

"Outstanding."

"He's our nightmare scenario, Mitch. Some cartel leaders get where they are because they're careful and methodical. He's the opposite. His success is based on the fact that he's unpredictable and brutal. The smaller operations are afraid of him and the larger ones don't think it's worth going to war with him. And he's greedy to the point of self-destructiveness. He wants to run the biggest cartel in the world. Be the richest and most powerful man in the world. Based on my research into him, nothing will ever be enough."

"Okay. Get me whatever updated information on him you can."

"Mitch . . . This isn't going to work. The plan you've come up with isn't a plan. It's—"

"If you have any better ideas, I'm listening."

"You know my answer to that."

"I'm not walking away, Claudia. But you're free to. Anytime you want."

"You say that so often, sometimes I wonder if it's what you want," she said coldly.

He considered his next words more carefully than he would have thought given his current situation. "It's not what I want. But I understand what I'm dragging you into here. You like to control things, and this isn't that kind of an operation. If it goes to shit, I don't want it to blow back on you and I don't want to leave you thinking it was something you did or didn't do."

She was silent for long enough that he started to wonder if they'd been disconnected. Finally, she responded.

"I don't want to be involved. I admit that. But I'm not going to trust your life to someone else. There's no room for error here, Mitch. Nothing can go wrong. Not one thing."

And yet something always did.

"Where do you stand on your end?" he said, changing the subject.

"I spoke with your brother. He said he can bankrupt you and involve you in as many illegal financial schemes as you like."

"Will it look real?"

"He says yes, but he asked me to tell you that you're an idiot, suicidal, and that whatever you think you owe to America, you've already paid back a hundred times over."

"But he'll do it?"

"He said he'd handle all the arrangements personally."

Rapp nodded. Steven was a financial genius who hadn't made a mathematical error since he was seven years old. And as an added bonus, he liked his big brother and would be disappointed to see him made into hamburger patties.

"Mitch, I still think we should bring Irene in on this. With her power and experience we could be much more thorough."

"No. She'd shut us down the minute she heard the plan. And even if she didn't, she'd be obligated to tell the president. With everything that's going on in Washington, I don't trust him. We'll hold her in reserve. Nothing we do is going to fool her. She'll know what's going on and she'll be there for us if we need her."

"What about Scott and his men? We need them to get talk going in the spec ops rumor mill."

"No problem. Tell them whatever you need to."

Coleman and his boys were one hundred percent loyal and none of them gave a flying fuck about what was going on in Washington. They'd gun down everyone in Congress before they left him hanging.

"Even if everything goes right, Mitch . . ." Her voice faltered.

"It'll be fine. All I have to do is be convincing."

When she came back on she spoke so softly he could barely make out her words. "Not too convincing, though, right, Mitch? Not too convincing."

CHAPTER 24

THE CAPITOL COMPLEX
WASHINGTON, D.C.
USA

"IF I didn't know better, I'd think there was a god," Senator Christine Barnett said.

Her campaign manager looked up at her with a deep frown.

"What?" she said.

"I've warned you about this before, Senator. . . . If you ever slip and someone records you—"

"It wouldn't matter."

"You're not bulletproof."

"Pull your head out of your ass, Kevin. I hired you for your cynicism and now you're finding Jesus on me?"

"I'm not finding Jesus. But there are people out there who have. And you need their votes."

She smirked and started pacing around her office again. "You're thirty-five years old and already living in the past. The American people don't give a shit about God. They don't care about the environment or the deficit or health care. And they couldn't find Iraq or Yemen on a map."

"What do they care about?" Gray said coldly.

"Should it worry me that I'm having to tell you?"

"Anytime you think you can find someone better, I'll be happy to step down."

Barnett was always on the lookout, but the truth was that there wasn't anyone even close. She wasn't sure if that spoke to Gray's brilliance or the fact that everyone else out there was a drooling idiot, but at this point it didn't matter.

"What they want—what they thirst for—is to hurt the people they hate. They don't want a politician droning on about unemployment. They want a general. They want to blindly follow someone who can provide them an enemy and lead them to victory against that enemy. Someone who can give their lives purpose." She leaned back against her desk and glared down at him. "If you spend your time and my money finding ways to help people, we're going to lose this election. But if you can find me ways to inflict damage, we're going to run away with it."

"And you think making anthrax your signature issue is the right weapon?"

"I'm not sure yet. It has potential, but like all good weapons it's dangerous if you don't use it right." She smiled, recalling yesterday's meeting. "You should have seen Irene Kennedy. She was sweating bullets. And Alexander just looked lost. He's done and just wants to avoid any fireworks on the way out. The DEA head, though . . ."

"Woodman?" Gray said.

She nodded. "He doesn't seem stupid. We should be reaching out to him and letting him know there's a place for him in my administration if he plays ball."

"Agreed. I'll take care of it."

"The question is whether we leak the fact that the anthrax made it across the border. Then we'd have a clear message: Sayid Halabi isn't bluffing and we can't keep counting on blind luck and NASA. Next time this administration lets someone stroll over the border with a bioweapon, people are going to die."

"I'd advise caution, Senator. If that leak were ever traced back to you—"

"Then we'd have to make sure that doesn't happen. It's not the first time we've leaked something and it's never been tracked back to us before."

"What about the fact that we'd be jeopardizing an ongoing terrorism investigation? ISIS will pull back if they know we're onto them. Halabi will disappear and they'll switch to another smuggling route. Our chance of stopping them will be even worse."

"That's the story Alexander and that bitch Kennedy will tell, but no one's going to listen. After the fact, it'll just sound like an excuse. What the American people would take away is that the White House and CIA were keeping a serious threat secret so they wouldn't look bad during the election season."

"What if this goes beyond politics, Senator? What if our actions actually *do* help the terrorists?"

She shrugged. "How would that hurt me?"

"I don't understand."

"You read the briefing. It's anthrax. It can't be used as a weapon of mass destruction. We're talking about a few high-profile targets. Hysteria grows and Alexander's administration gets the blame."

"People will die."

"According to Gary Statham, fewer than a hundred. What would be much worse for us is if Alexander's people actually succeed. What I don't need to see on television is a bunch of spec ops guys busting up terrorist cells. Or even worse, one of them putting a bullet in Sayid Halabi. That could give Alexander's party a bump at the worst possible moment."

"And what do you think the chance of that is?"

"Of them pulling off something big? Low. And even lower now. My understanding is that Mitch Rapp is out. Alexander's afraid of letting him off the leash during the election cycle."

Gray didn't look as happy about that as he should have.

"Relax, Kevin. I've got Secret Service and thirty private contractors working my security."

"Yeah, *your* security. But nobody's looking for suspicious white powder in my mailbox."

She waved a hand dismissively. "ISIS isn't going to bother with you."

"You have no idea what ISIS is going to bother with."

"Fine," she said. "Figure out what security you're comfortable with and set it up. Happy now?"

Based on his expression, happy was an overstatement. But he gave a short nod. "So what do you want to do, Senator?"

She fell silent for almost a minute as she considered the question. "Right now? Nothing. But we need to be ready. Start looking into how we can leak with zero chance of it being tracked back to us. If I decide to move on this, I want to be able to move fast."

"Fine," Gray started. "But laying the groundwork is very different than acting on it. We've got a lead in the primary that's looking unassailable and your numbers against your likely opponents in the general are just about as good."

"Don't start resting on your laurels, Kevin. We need to stay on the offensive."

"Are you sure? Risk and return, Senator. What we don't need right now is an unforced error."

"Hell yes, I'm sure!" she said, the volume of her voice rising. "Those poll numbers aren't worth the paper they're printed on. People will say they'll vote for a woman, but when they actually get in the booth, will they? Or will I go into the general with a twenty-point lead and come out giving a concession speech? When Election Day comes, Alexander, his party, and whatever idiot they run against me have to have been destroyed. Do you understand me? When we're done with them, their own mothers are going to question voting for them. And if you're willing to do what it takes to get me there, then you've got a very bright future ahead of you. If you're not, then not only will I replace you, but I'll make sure you never work in politics again. Am I being clear?"

"Senator, we—"

"Am I being clear?"

Gray stared back at her for a couple of seconds, but finally diverted his gaze and stood. "Crystal."

CHAPTER 25

SOUTHERN CALIFORNIA
USA

A FEW hard kicks got the sticky rubber doorstop free and Rapp pulled the door open. Thomas Braman and Holden Flores spun toward him, along with another man who hadn't been in evidence when Rapp arrived. All had donned bulletproof vests and the new man was holding a Remington 870 shotgun. Flores immediately put his hand on his sidearm but didn't draw it, instead leaning left to get a look at the blood-splattered room and the two corpses. For a second it looked like he might throw up.

Braman's eyes remained locked on Rapp, but most of his attention seemed to be focused on the phone plastered to his ear. It wasn't hard to guess what was happening on the other end: absolutely nothing. His bosses in Washington would be hiding in their offices while their assistants provided excuses and transferred him to another unavailable executive.

And Braman, while a pain in the ass, wasn't an idiot. He knew that the music was winding down and that he was going to be the only one left without a chair. If he stopped Rapp and that created a backlash from the White House, he'd be crucified for not following orders to hand over authority. On the other hand, if he let Rapp walk, he could be charged as an accessory to the murder of two Mexican nationals.

Welcome to the current state of American politics, Rapp thought. Everyone who didn't have a place at the very top of the political food chain was expendable. No loyalty. No gratitude. No courage. Braman was an arrogant prick looking to move up in the world, but there was nothing in his record that suggested he'd ever screwed his men in pursuit of that goal. He probably figured he'd been an honorable soldier in the war on drugs and didn't deserve to be hung out to dry for something that wasn't his fault.

And he was right.

Rapp passed silently by them, leaving bloody footprints on the concrete floor. He pushed through the door and felt the morning heat hit him. The sky was devoid of clouds and bleached yellow by the dust and the sun. Despite the situation, he had a sudden craving for an icy beer. Something to help him contemplate a future that was now so dark he couldn't even penetrate its edges.

The DEA men spread out behind him, and for the better part of a minute he stood there listening to Thomas Braman desperately try to get someone to take his call. The man's voice rose to a shout, dominating the small enclosure as Rapp watched the cartel's surveillance drone circle overhead. Whoever was operating that plane had already been taking particular interest in this situation and now he had a blood-splattered man staring up at his cameras.

"Don't even think about transferring me again," Braman said. "If he's in a meeting, get him out!"

This wasn't how this was supposed to go down. He'd figured on waiting until they were on the dirt road leading out. There was a dry wash that he'd identified as being a perfect spot for what had to be done. He'd purposely bog the truck down, and then when the DEA men were gathered in a tight group looking at the buried tires, he'd make his move. It would be about as controllable a scenario as he could create.

Now, though, he had the drone overhead and the three DEA men standing right behind him. Braman, the most experienced, had a phone instead of a gun in his hand. A glance back confirmed that Holden Flores had his hands at his sides instead of on his weapon. The other DEA man still had the shotgun but was holding it across his chest aimed at the sky.

Bird in the hand.

"Don't hang—!" Braman fell silent for a moment. "Shit!"

Rapp waited until the man was consumed with redialing before he turned, walked a few steps, and slammed a fist into Flores's jaw. The kid crumpled, but before he even hit the ground, Rapp had drawn his Glock and pumped a round into the sternum of the man holding the shotgun. He jerked back and fell, his weapon bouncing from his hands and spinning through the dirt.

Braman dropped his phone and went for his pistol, but then went down when he took a bullet to the chest.

Rapp kicked the weapons away from the men and surveyed their condition. Flores was out like a light, so Rapp started with the first man he'd shot, rolling him on his stomach and using the flex cuffs hanging from his bulletproof vest to bind his wrists behind him.

Out of the corner of his eye, he saw Braman starting to reach for his weapon.

"Don't do it, asshole . . ."

When he didn't listen, Rapp shot him in the ribs. That seemed to put an end to his plans.

The drone swooped in even closer when Rapp started dragging the men inside the building. Flores didn't regain consciousness, but the other two moaned and swore under their breath at the pain of being moved. The ballistic vests had saved their lives, but between them they had more than a few broken ribs and probably one cracked sternum.

Braman was last, and by the time Rapp dropped him into a

puddle of blood in the interrogation room, he'd gotten enough wind back to make some fairly graphic accusations regarding Rapp's mother. He fell silent when Rapp hovered the barrel of his Glock an inch from his forehead.

"I don't need your commentary, Braman—I just need the drugs. I'm having a few financial problems and this is going to take care of them."

"Screw you!"

Rapp had to admit that this guy was starting to grow on him. Despite that, he slammed the butt of his Glock into Braman's nose and walked out, bolting the steel door behind him.

Rapp straightened, stretching his back and looking around him at the cluttered storage room. Fortunately, it had a set of rolling doors that the DEA had put back in working condition. He'd been able to back his SUV up to them and load about five hundred pounds of coke, which was now covered by a dirty tarp weighted down with a couple of shovels. In the unlikely event he got pulled over, he'd just look like he was on his way back from Home Depot.

He finished changing into clean clothing while the dull ring of metal started on the other end of the building. Apparently, at least one of the three DEA men had recovered enough to free himself and go to work on the door imprisoning them.

Rapp slipped into the vehicle and pulled out, accelerating to a speed that allowed him to crash through the chain link gate. Not surprisingly, Carlos Esparza's surveillance drone wasn't far behind.

CHAPTER 26

NORTH OF HARGEISA
SOMALIA

SAYID Halabi shut down the computer on his improvised desk, watching the cave descend into gloom as the screen went black. He had scoured every report about the drug operation at the San Ysidro mall and found nothing even hinting that something unusual had been found among the confiscated drugs. Now most of the stories were about the sophistication of the tunnel structure and the profitability of the narcotics trade.

It was exactly what Carlos Esparza had told him to expect. A few of the individual packages would be randomly selected for testing and then the entire shipment would be destroyed. The chances of the brick containing anthrax being chosen were diminishingly small. But small was very different than nonexistent.

If the bioweapon *were* found, it was extremely unlikely that the discovery would be reported to the public. Kennedy would maneuver from the shadows, using the information she gleaned from the intercept to trace the bioweapon back to its source. And when she succeeded, she would send Rapp. It was how they operated. And it was how so many of his brothers had been martyred.

The Frenchman was completing another batch of anthrax, but

Halabi had begun to question whether it had ever been important. He'd told himself that it was a necessary distraction to keep Kennedy blind to his real goal.

But was it?

He wanted so desperately to outsmart Irene Kennedy. To outfight Mitch Rapp. To ensure that the American people knew, as they slowly suffocated, how easy it had been to defeat them. He wanted Kennedy and Rapp to understand that he had been pulling their strings the entire time. That they had been the defenders of the walls when they had finally fallen.

Ironically, the semidarkness allowed him to see with unprecedented clarity. In Yemen, he'd already made the mistake of not striking when the moment was at hand. Allowing Rapp to escape had been an inexcusable tactical error, and he wouldn't compound it by underestimating the threat the man posed. Halabi knew that every moment he hesitated was a moment the CIA man could use to destroy him.

The cave that housed the weapon that would annihilate the West was within the reach of America's specialized weaponry. A single bombing run could incinerate the deadly virus incubating in his people's bodies. And he would likely die with them, arriving at the feet of God having failed once again.

There was no choice but to accelerate his timetable forward. Rapp was coming. He could feel it. Speed was the critical component now. Not complexity.

Halabi reached for the notebook at the edge of his desk, opening it and running his fingers across Gabriel Bertrand's elegant script. He had read the annotated Arabic translation that had been prepared for him, but there was something about seeing the original that created a compelling sense of history. Would this book one day be enshrined in a holy site commemorating the fall of the West?

Bertrand called the disease he'd discovered Yemeni acute respiratory syndrome, a laughably innocuous name for something that was about to reshape the world. Symptoms typical of a mild flu tended to appear within two days of exposure. Onset was fairly slow, with the illness generally not turning severe for another five days. For those who reached that point, around seventy percent would be dead within a week, a mortality rate thirteen times higher even than that of the Spanish flu, which decimated the world population in the early twentieth century.

Even more unusual was how easily it spread. Under normal conditions, the pathogen could survive on surfaces for as much as seventy-two hours. And, according to Bertrand's extensive calculations, even relatively trivial contact with the virus produced an infection rate of over fifty percent.

It was incredible how clumsy and ineffective the armies of the West now seemed. In comparison to the weapons created by God, they were nothing. Even the nuclear arsenals that so terrified the world were pitiful by comparison. Used against a major population center, they could achieve little more than a sudden blast, a few hundred thousand casualties, and a lingering radiation zone that could be easily contained or avoided.

The careful and purposeful release of YARS would spread through the highly mobile and densely populated West like a wildfire. Casualties would be tens—perhaps hundreds—of millions. The highly integrated and interdependent modern world would collapse as the specialized people who kept it running fell ill.

The medical system would be the first to be overwhelmed as workers abandoned it out of fear of being infected. Then law enforcement, who were critical to holding back the violence and avarice simmering just beneath the veneer of Western civilization.

Power grids would falter, as would the elaborate transportation systems that brought food and other critical products. Militaries would be called back from their imperialist missions in the Middle East and Asia to try to control the upheaval, but their close living conditions and contact with the public would make them even more susceptible than the general population.

Even after the contagion had run its course, the long-term effects would be immeasurable. The West's entire economic system, based on the slow growth of populations, would collapse. Homes, businesses, and entire cities would be abandoned. Open democracies, utterly incapable of returning their countries to order, would be replaced by insular dictatorships.

Of course, the death toll in the Middle East would be significant as well, but the effects would be less far-reaching. Larger cities like Cairo and Riyadh would be wiped out, but they had become godless cesspools and deserved their fate. Disconnected rural areas would take fewer casualties and were far less reliant on the complex web of technologies that kept the modern world functioning. Once free of the oppressors and colonists, the Muslim people would unite in the service of Allah. They would wage jihad on a mortally wounded West and extend the new caliphate across the globe.

The law of God, and not that of man, would once again reign supreme.

CHAPTER 27

SOUTHERN CALIFORNIA
USA

THE GPS on Rapp's phone called out the next turn and he veered left onto a dirt track that wound through Joshua trees and flowering ocotillo. There was still about an hour of sunlight, which would be just about what he needed.

It was a little more than a mile to a stucco building whose ochre color and organic shape allowed it to blend into the desert landscape. Probably a little bigger than he needed and in terrain that was a little more open than he would have liked, but beggars couldn't be choosers.

He stepped out of the SUV and glanced at the sky, struck by the irony that it was his turn to worry about overhead drones. Nothing. The cartel's model plane had followed him from the DEA outpost to the pavement but had been behind when he'd accelerated to highway speeds.

Rapp retrieved a remote from a lockbox near the front door and used it to access the garage. Mixed in among the beach chairs, mountain bikes, and coolers were a number of brand-new shovels and picks, as well as a locker filled with enough military-grade weaponry to take over a small African nation.

He pulled the SUV in and entered the house to see if Claudia's thoroughness extended to the fridge. As expected, it did. One of the benefits of having a French logistics coordinator was that you always got the good stuff. High-end cheese, homemade pasta sauces, fresh bread . . .

And alcohol-free beer.

He swore under his breath and explored the house while dialing his phone.

"Are you there?" Claudia said, by way of greeting.

"Yeah."

"What do you think?"

"Could be worse. The walls are thick and the windows are either glass block or barred. Power's off-grid and batteries are topped off. Kind of a complicated interior layout, which would work for me if I was planning on staying inside, but I'm not. It'd be too easy to get trapped in here and a few Molotov cocktails would be enough to set the place on fire."

"It was the best I could do at the last minute. You said you wanted remote and it doesn't get much more remote than that."

"Since I can't stay in here, where do I go?"

"Scott's men have you set up on the perimeter. There are diagrams on the tablet on the counter. The usual password."

"What about the DEA guys?"

"I called in an anonymous tip to the police. They're on-site now and have called ambulances for three injured men. So at least we know they're all alive."

He'd been careful with the placement of his shots and had chosen frangible ammunition that would hit like a ton of bricks but not penetrate their vests. Of course, the science of shooting people in the torso and not killing them was a fairly inexact one. In fact, he might have just invented it.

Rapp grabbed one of the nonalcoholic beers and sat down at the kitchen table. "Any luck setting up a drug deal?"

"No bites yet, but I set a good price and the word's getting around. I wouldn't be surprised if we have at least one offer by tomorrow morning."

He nodded and took a pull on the watery beer substitute. Claudia was using her old contacts to let people know that a couple hundred kilos of high-quality coke had just come on the market. The fact that the seller was an unknown necessitated a discount deep enough to get fringe players involved. The sale, though, wasn't the point. The goal was to get enough chatter going that Carlos Esparza found out that his stolen product was on the auction block.

While it was true that government confiscation was just another cost of doing business, the theft and attempted resale of his property was an entirely different animal. When a government agent turned criminal, the rules changed. The kid gloves came off and Rapp would now be treated just like anyone else who had stolen from the cartels.

"Do they know where I am? I lost the drone when I got on the highway."

"I imagine they have a pretty good idea. They have people all up and down these roads that they could have called on. And I wouldn't be surprised if they're doing something similar to what I just did—looking online for properties that were recently rented for the short term. I'm still gathering intel on Esparza's cartel, but it seems to be much larger and more sophisticated than when Louis and I dealt with them. About half their business is in marijuana trafficking, though, and they're getting hurt badly by legalization."

"So a perfect candidate for a business partnership with Middle Eastern heroin traffickers."

"Very much so. The cartels see this as their primary avenue for growth. As the U.S. cracks down on oxycodone, those addicts are looking for a replacement. Esparza's cartel is targeting the middle-class suburban market—painkiller addicts who have no contact with the underworld or drug dealers. He seems to be trying to create a reliable product that looks and works very much like pharmaceutical-grade oxycodone. But for his plan to work, he needs a reliable supply of high-quality opiate."

"That actually sounds like a pretty solid business plan. You should turn Steven on to it. He'll probably want to buy stock."

"Like I said, Mitch, Esparza's a psychotic. Not an idiot."

"And how's *my* life going?" he said, changing the subject.

"Poorly. Your brother's put you at the center of a massive web of illegal and collapsing investment schemes. You've got inexplicable inflows and outflows of tens of millions of dollars, a huge mortgage on your house, and involvement in a Russian real estate scam that implicates you in the death of Tarben Chkalov. Many of these things are actually real and currently under investigation by the authorities in various countries. What Steven's managed to accomplish in such a short time is incredible. He's a true genius. Did you know he can multiply four-digit numbers in his head?"

"Yeah. He's always been able to do that. Who knows about this?"

"I've anonymously sent files to the FBI, CIA, SEC, IRS, and a few congresspeople, including Christine Barnett."

"So, in a nutshell, I'm broke and under investigation for a bunch of illegal activities that I'm not smart enough to understand."

"Yes. But that's not all."

"No?"

"No. When I found out what you've been up to, I drained what few bank accounts you had left and ran. I'm now hiding out in southern Texas, fearful of your reprisal."

"That *is* pretty bad," he said, feeling more ambivalent than he should have about Claudia and Steven's thoroughness. His survival unquestionably depended on the convincing destruction of his life, but hearing it laid out in black and white was pretty sobering.

"There's more."

"More?" he said, feigning enthusiasm. "Really?"

"I'm not alone here in Texas. I left you for another man. In fact you know him. Scott Coleman. After working so closely together, a relationship evolved between us. He's here now ready to protect me should you ever find us. In fact, he and Anna are out back grilling dinner. Would you like to talk to him?"

"No." Rapp looked around the empty kitchen, trying not to think about her and Coleman flipping steaks while he waited for either the FBI or a cartel hit squad to show up on his doorstep.

"Mitch? Are you still there?"

"Yeah."

"You asked me to do this to you."

"I know."

"And the moment you shot those DEA agents, you passed the point of no return. There can't be any holes in your cover or questions about your motivations."

"It had to be done," he reassured her.

"No, it didn't," she said, some of her carefully constructed calm starting to crack. "We could have—"

"Claudia . . . Not now, okay? I don't have much light left and I have a lot of work to do. For all I know, Esparza has fifty men sitting at the end of my driveway waiting for sunset."

"I'm sorry, Mitch. I shouldn't have said anything. I was being selfish."

"Don't worry about it. We'll talk later."

He disconnected the call, wondering if what he'd just said was true. If they would ever talk again.

Rapp tossed the bottle into the sink, hearing it shatter against the porcelain. He'd made his decision and there was no changing it now. Time to focus.

CHAPTER 28

THE CAPITOL COMPLEX
WASHINGTON, D.C.
USA

IRENE Kennedy felt her pace slow as she approached Senator Barnett's office. The emergency meeting was originally scheduled to take place in the White House but when rumors about Mitch Rapp had begun circulating, the location had abruptly changed. And when those rumors had turned toxic, the president suddenly discovered a conflict that wouldn't allow him to attend. Not surprising, but disappointing. And a bit foreboding.

She passed through Barnett's outer office and was motioned to an open door at the back. Inside she found Barnett standing in the middle of the imposing space, speaking quietly with the head of the DEA.

Her handshake with Woodman was tense and perfunctory, but Barnett dispensed with the pleasantry entirely, instead walking to a small conference table. Kennedy was surprised, having assumed that the politician would take a position of authority behind her desk. The purpose of the move became clear when Woodman took a seat to the right of her. The only remaining chair was a rather austere wooden one directly across from them.

The battle lines had been drawn.

"When was the last time you spoke to Mitch Rapp?" Barnett asked.

"I'm not sure exactly. A few weeks? Around the time the president asked him to stand down."

Barnett made a show of writing her response down. "You're certain?"

"If you need a precise date and time, I can check my phone records and provide you with one."

She didn't seem that interested. "Are you aware that Mr. Rapp was sent to interrogate the two men who smuggled the anthrax across the U.S. border?"

"Sent? By whom?"

"I assume by you."

"I can assure you that isn't the case, Senator."

"So you're saying you had no involvement in those orders?"

"I think we've already established that."

Clearly Barnett was less interested in what was happening with the DEA and ISIS than she was with understanding who could be blamed and how it could help her quest for the presidency.

"Are you aware of what happened during Rapp's questioning of the two suspects?"

"I'm not."

It was actually true. There was a significant amount of loose talk swirling around the Beltway, but it would have been unnecessarily dangerous for her to look into it. For the first time in her career, ignorance seemed to be the best course.

"The police received an anonymous tip about gunshots at the facility where the men were being held. When they arrived, they found the suspects dead and three DEA agents gravely wounded."

Barnett leaned back in her chair, a satisfied smile exposing overwhitened teeth. She motioned to Woodman, who finally got an opportunity to talk. He didn't seem happy about it, though.

"Rapp tortured at least one of the suspects and murdered both. Then he attacked my men and stole a significant portion of the narcotics being held on-site."

Kennedy paused to consider what she had just heard. Conclusions weren't hard to come to. Rapp had wanted answers from those drug traffickers that the DEA weren't able to get. A murkier question, though, was on whose authority? Was he working under political cover that she wasn't aware of? The president had gone directly to him before. Was this another case of that?

"Are your people going to be all right?" Kennedy asked finally.

"They sustained substantial injuries, but I'm told they'll recover."

"Thanks to their body armor and training," Barnett cut in. "Otherwise they'd be in the morgue with those two suspects."

Woodman's face was expressionless. He knew full well that if Rapp had wanted those men dead, they would be.

"Please continue, Bob."

His expression suggested continued reluctance. What was causing that reluctance, though, was difficult to say. Even if Kennedy had known the man well, it was hard to predict how someone would react to a situation like this. He was smart enough to know that something didn't smell quite right. But he was also smart enough to know that Barnett was likely to be his boss in a few months.

"Rapp also said something."

"Yes?" Kennedy prompted.

"That he had financial problems and needed the drugs to settle his accounts."

"Are you aware of Mr. Rapp's financial situation?" Barnett interjected.

Kennedy folded her hands in front of her on the table. "Yesterday, my office received a file that seems to detail a number of financial improprieties on Mitch's part. It's my understanding that the FBI and IRS received similar files. Of course, we're looking into the allegations, but they're complicated and far-reaching, so I don't have anything to report yet."

"Financial improprieties," Barnett repeated incredulously. "My people's initial review of that file suggests something more like an organized crime syndicate that would put Al Capone to shame."

It was an exaggeration, but not an outrageous one. The maze of hidden accounts, foreign partnerships, and shell corporations had almost certainly been created by Rapp's brother Steven. And if that was the case, it would take years—perhaps decades—to get to the bottom of it. His gift for complex financial transactions rivaled his older brother's abilities with a gun.

The question was why? Rapp had very little interest in money and was already worth millions—as was Claudia Gould. Why had he created a phony financial crisis and then purposely told the DEA that he was stealing the drugs to deal with that crisis? The answer was as obvious as it was dangerous. He was trying to make contact with the cartel that had smuggled the anthrax and infiltrate them.

"As I said, Senator, we're looking into the allegations. But I'd urge caution. That file gives every impression of having been compiled by a hostile foreign government."

Of course, that was completely nonsense. The faint whiffs of Russia and Iran were much more likely Claudia's doing. She was an extremely clever woman.

"An ad hominem attack, Dr. Kennedy? I would have thought that was beneath you. It doesn't matter *where* the information came from, only whether or not it's true. And even if it isn't, Mitch

Rapp murdered two drug trafficking suspects in cold blood as well as—"

"They weren't drug trafficking suspects, Senator. They were transporting a bioweapon across the U.S. border. The rules of engagement are different for men like that."

Barnett laughed. "Ah, yes. That's the comic book, isn't it? Mitch Rapp, the great patriot, desperately interrogating two hardened terrorists in order to save us all. Don't insult my intelligence, Doctor. The questions Rapp was asking those men had nothing to do with America. More likely he wanted to know how to get top dollar for the coke he stole and how to stay ahead of the cartel he stole it from. And now while you sit there trying to spin the situation, he's using the skills you taught him to disappear."

She didn't respond, prompting Woodman to speak up.

"We have two separate informants saying that an unknown party has put word out on the street that he's got a couple hundred kilos of quality product and he's looking to unload it fast. There's no question in my mind that this is your man, Irene. There's a possibility that we can track—"

Barnett put a hand on his arm, silencing him. Clearly, she believed that any information Kennedy gained in this meeting would be passed on to Rapp. The human species' ability to believe whatever it wanted was truly incredible. Barnett would overlook everything Rapp had done for America and believe any attack on him—no matter how far-fetched—without question.

"I think we've said enough on that subject, Bob."

And then something completely unexpected happened. Woodman glanced at Barnett and moved his hand to scratch his left temple. When he was sure the senator wasn't looking, he raised his middle finger.

Kennedy barely managed to suppress her smile. The DEA chief

would be fully aware of what went into creating an undercover legend sufficient to get close to a major cartel. At a minimum, he would keep his mouth shut. With a little luck, he could be counted on for some minor assistance if it could be kept under the table. Kennedy gave him a nearly imperceptible nod as Barnett started into one of her infamously indignant speeches.

"It's hard for even me to believe that this is happening, Dr. Kennedy. The two men that Mitch Rapp murdered were our only lead in finding Sayid Halabi and intercepting the next package of anthrax that's probably already on its way. This is your fault and the fault of your agency. The fact that for twenty years you haven't noticed that you have a psychotic working for you is hard to believe. That you didn't notice the multimillion-dollar house of cards he'd built, though, frankly suggests more than incompetence."

And there it was. Barnett was going to play this as complicity. She was going to drag Kennedy in front of an endless string of congressional hearings in an effort to find something that could be used to prosecute her criminally. And to send a message to anyone else who might be feeling defiant.

Barnett let the accusation hang in the air, hoping to coerce Kennedy into responding to it. Instead the CIA director reached for her briefcase and stood.

"If there's nothing more, I obviously have a lot of work to do."

She turned and went for the door, barely getting her hand around the knob before Barnett spoke again.

"Have you heard about Rapp's partner Claudia? Apparently she left him for Scott Coleman and they're now in hiding because they're afraid that he'll kill them."

The malignant glee in Barnett's voice was clearly audible and Kennedy took comfort in it. The senator wasn't as calculating as she was given credit for. At her core, she was at the mercy of her infinite greed for power.

This was going to get ugly and no one was going to escape without getting bloody. But, as Stan Hurley had been fond of saying, it's not how you play the game, it's whether or not your opponent ends up dismembered in the woods.

CHAPTER 29

SOUTHERN CALIFORNIA
USA

WHERE *were these assholes?*

It was Rapp's second night sleeping in a foxhole stacked with five hundred pounds of coke. And while the drugs themselves were surprisingly comfortable, the impermeable tape wrapped around them left him wallowing in a shallow pond of sweat.

Even worse was the tree above him. Coleman had undoubtedly chosen that location for the additional cover the foliage provided, but hadn't considered the sizable spines that constantly dropped from it. So while he was all but invisible and had a good line of sight to the house, his back and ass were covered with tiny, infuriatingly itchy wounds.

How hard could it be for Esparza to find him? Maybe Claudia had overestimated the capabilities of his outfit. At this point, she'd dropped enough hints to lead a nine-year-old to his door.

Rapp looked past the offending tree at the stars and then glanced over at the vague outline of the house. It contained a comfortable bed, a well-stocked fridge, and satellite TV. Just twenty-five yards of dead-flat terrain away.

When he was in similar holes in the Middle East, he never thought about creature comforts. He was almost always in the middle of nowhere, often surrounded by people who had never even seen a microwave or automatic coffeemaker. But lying there within earshot of the air-conditioning unit somehow made every cactus spine, scorpion, and tarantula that much more irritating.

Not that there was anything he could do about it. Esparza's men were coming and there was no way to be certain from what direction or in what kind of numbers. The design of the house made it more of a trap than a viable defensive position, and if the team the cartel sent was smart enough to surround it, he'd have a hell of a time fighting his way out. Particularly if they brought anything heavier than the expected handguns and assault rifles.

He moved the M4 carbine to one side and tried to find a slightly more comfortable position. Six more hours to dawn. With a little luck, he could get some sleep.

The quiet crunch of tires or approaching footfalls that Rapp expected didn't materialize. Instead, two massive SUVs roared up the road and skidded to a dramatic stop in front of the house before firing up their light bars. He pushed himself to his elbows, peering over the top of the hole as an improbable number of men poured from the vehicles. Despite all the weapons and the glare of the lights, it had kind of a clown car quality to it.

They started firing at the house on full automatic as one of the vehicles' powerful sound systems started blasting something that to Rapp's ear sounded a little like polka music. He reached for his rifle and slid into a position that allowed him to keep an eye on his six, concerned that the fireworks at the house had been designed to cover the approach of foot soldiers from behind.

He decided he might be overestimating the enemy when one of them abandoned his position behind the SUVs and sprinted toward the front door. His comrades didn't have time to divert their fire and the man was cut down before he could even make it to the porch. His body skidded to a stop by the porch steps as the others focused their fire on the windows.

In a somewhat better-organized move, two men pulled a tactical battering ram from the back of one of the vehicles and managed to lug it onto the porch without getting shot. They struggled to coordinate their efforts, but on the second swing the door flew open. When they disappeared inside, their comrades reluctantly stopped shooting.

Everything went silent, but it lasted only about five seconds. A muffled explosion flashed in the empty window frames and Rapp figured it was from the grenade he'd wired across the hallway. Though it could also have been the mine he'd put under the carpet behind the sofa. It was pretty obvious in good light, but with all the dust and half the bulbs shot out, you never knew. These assholes didn't seem to be the sharpest knives in the drawer.

That assessment was confirmed when the men reacted to the explosion by running to the windows and door in order to randomly spray the interior. The fact that one or both of their men might have survived the blast didn't seem to concern them.

Some were running out of ammo and struggling to get new mags in weapons that they clearly weren't familiar with. Rapp considered picking off a few with his silenced Glock, but it seemed unnecessary at this point. Better to just settle in and watch the show.

Two more men ran inside, but the ones shooting through the windows didn't seem aware of it. Rapp assumed they'd get gunned down in a few seconds but he was proven wrong. The garage door suddenly billowed outward, sending a cloud of dust drifting lazily through the spotlights. One of them had gotten far enough to find the charge he'd hidden beneath the owner's stash of lawn furniture.

Rapp took the foil off a home-baked cookie and shoved it in

his mouth as a man with an impressive collection of tattoos finally managed to get everyone to stop shooting. A moment later, all that could be heard was the polka music and the dull hum of a model plane circling above.

The tattooed man started shouting at someone standing near one of the windows and pointing at the doorway. Rapp didn't speak Spanish, but it wasn't hard to figure out what was being said. Tattooed Guy wanted Guy By The Window to go inside. And Guy By The Window, not being quite as stupid or high as some of his companions, wanted to stay where he was.

The conversation ended abruptly when Tattooed Guy shot the man in the chest. That lit a fire under the others, and a few moments later, three men were crossing the threshold. Their cautious movements suggested that the group's initial enthusiasm was fading.

Rapp finished his cookie and reached for a box of Pop-Tarts. Popcorn probably would have been more appropriate, but how could Claudia have known?

Four relatively uneventful minutes passed before an explosion blew off part of the back of the house. He'd gotten pretty artistic with that charge. It had been hidden in an AC vent with the tripwire woven through the top of a shower curtain.

It took another three minutes or so before the surviving two men reappeared in the doorway and began giving their report. Again, Spanish fluency wasn't necessary to understand what they were saying. They'd found neither the man nor the coke they'd come for.

There were five men left outside and their discussion quickly went from heated to a full-blown shoving match. For a moment, Rapp thought they were going to start shooting at each other, but he didn't get that lucky. Tattooed Guy managed to get control and dialed a phone while the others huddled in tight around him. They looked like they were working out the next play in MS-13's annual football scrimmage. Did these people receive no training at all?

Rapp picked up the suppressed M4 and fired at the tightly grouped men on full automatic. Not surprisingly, they were all down before half his magazine was expended.

He stepped out of the hole, ducking under various low-hanging tree branches as he approached the men on the ground. All were dead or headed in that direction so he glanced up at the circling drone and raised one of his hands, palm up. The sentiment would be clear in any language.

Is that all you've got?

One of the men on the bottom of the pile started moving and Rapp shot him in the side of the head. He wasn't going to get anywhere with these soldiers. That had already been proved during his interrogation of the men the DEA had picked up. He needed to talk to the man in charge.

Rapp walked over to the nearest SUV and turned off the music. At this point, there wasn't much he could do other than load the product and drive off in one of Esparza's pimped-out vehicles. If that didn't piss the man off enough to reach out, nothing would.

He was about to climb in when the ring of a cell phone became audible. Rapp had to search through the pile of men, but finally found the phone in Tattooed Guy's lifeless hand. The blood on the screen confused its touch sensitivity but Rapp finally managed to pick up.

"What?"

The screaming on the other end started with what he assumed was a stream of Spanish epithets.

"Speak English, dipshit."

"I'm going to carve you up and feed you to my dogs, you . . ."

The sentence devolved into Spanish again.

"Who is this?" Rapp said, crafting his tone to sound vaguely irritated. "Lorenzo Varela? Why don't you shut the fuck up and let the big boys work."

The name belonged to the leader of an upstart cartel run by a college-educated kid from Mexico City. Just the kind of guy someone like Carlos Esparza would despise.

"Varela? You stupid piece of shit! This is Carlos Esparza!"

Rapp didn't respond immediately, instead glancing nervously up at the drone. "Bullshit."

"You want me to prove it? How about I send a hundred men with pliers and blowtorches up to you? I'm going to—"

And more with the Spanish.

Rapp waited for the cartel boss to run out of oxygen before he spoke again. "Look, man. The DEA said this was Varela's shipment. They didn't say anything about you."

More Spanish. Rapp was starting to regret not paying more attention in high school.

"I don't want a war with you, Carlos. I just needed some money to disappear with. Your product's in a hole to the northeast of the house. Why don't you send some guys over to get it."

"And are you still going to be there when they show up, *pendejo*?"

"I could be, but I don't think you can afford to lose any more men."

"Fuck you!"

Rapp didn't respond immediately, making a point to look thoughtfully up at the drone he hoped Esparza was watching from in real time.

"Maybe we can make this work for both of us," he said finally.

"What?"

"I need money and to get as far from U.S. law enforcement as I can. And you clearly need men who can tell one end of a gun from the other."

Esparza laughed hard enough that Rapp thought he might

choke. "You just stole my drugs and killed eighteen of my men. Now you're asking me for a job?"

"Why not? I said I'd give the coke back." He thumbed at the bodies behind. "And you're suddenly light on personnel."

"Then why don't you get on a plane to Mexico and we can have a talk face-to-face."

"Okay."

Esparza started laughing again, this time sounding less enraged and more incredulous.

"What's so funny?"

"You're either crazy or you've got balls too big to fit on a plane."

"Probably a little bit of both," Rapp said honestly.

CHAPTER 30

ABOVE CENTRAL MEXICO

NORMALLY Rapp slept like a baby on planes. Today, though, he was in an economy class seat wedged between a woman who weighed north of three hundred pounds and a man who let out brief, choking snores every twenty seconds or so. If he'd been on a C-130 over Afghanistan, he'd be spread out on a pile of cargo netting, dead to the world.

It wasn't just the seat, though. That imaginary C-130 would land in a country where he'd spent much of his adult life. In the Middle East, he knew the players, had access to highly trained backup, and spoke the language. He understood the culture and had a deep understanding of his enemy's capabilities and motivations.

When he touched down this time, he'd have none of those advantages. His Spanish was barely good enough to order a Coke. And worse, this wasn't one of the simple search-and-destroy missions he'd become so good at over the years. Killing Carlos Esparza wasn't the objective. In fact, the opposite was true. He needed to ingratiate himself with the man. To use him to learn about the ISIS network and follow it back to Sayid Halabi.

Unfortunately, endearing himself to people had never been Rapp's forte. Kind of the opposite, actually.

Not that any of this was likely to matter. Esparza was probably just flying Rapp to Mexico so he could put a bullet in his head personally. The timing was kind of a shame. He finally had the blank presidential pardon he'd always dreamed of, and instead of taking it out for a spin, he was going to end up buried in the jungle.

And while that was all bad, it wasn't enough to keep him awake on a plane. No, that went deeper, to a question that was easy to ask but hard to answer.

What the hell was he doing there?

He'd given Claudia's diatribe more thought than she'd probably give him credit for and come to the conclusion that she was largely right. Christine Barnett was going to be the next president of the United States and she'd use that position to destroy him and anyone else who refused to kneel.

Best-case scenario, Rapp would survive this mission and be forced out of government service by her. Much more likely, though, was that Barnett would dedicate a significant amount of government resources to seeing him and Kennedy enjoying adjoining cells in a maximum security prison.

And it wouldn't exactly be hard. Rapp had just killed—technically murdered—two drug smugglers, and forced his brother to create a web of illegal transactions that spanned the globe. Even if Steven sat down in front of a Senate panel and demonstrated that it was all smoke and mirrors, it wouldn't be enough. Rapp would end up being used as a weapon in Christine Barnett's war against the intelligence and law enforcement communities that she saw as a check on her power.

The plane finally touched down, and Rapp remained in his seat while the rest of the passengers rummaged around in the overhead bins. He'd leave the plane without the carry-on he'd brought. It was just a prop to make him look less suspicious to the people at the airline desk. At this point, his only meaningful possessions in the world were a fake passport, a GPS watch, a phone, and a wallet containing five hundred U.S. dollars and a couple of high-limit credit cards.

When Rapp stepped into the terminal of Angel Albino Corzo International Airport, he immediately noticed the man flicking his gaze nervously from his phone to the crowd. He likely had nothing but a hazy drone photo to work with, so Rapp decided to help him out. He adjusted his trajectory toward the casually dressed Mexican and pointed to the exit.

"That's me. Let's go."

The man led Rapp out of the building and they crossed to the parking area under clear skies and temperatures in the mid-nineties. Rapp's thin linen shirt was already starting to soak through by the time they reached a large black SUV parked at the far end of the lot.

Tinted windows made it impossible to see inside, but when Rapp climbed in the back, he found pretty much what he'd anticipated. Two men who looked like former Mexican soldiers frisked him and shoved him to the floor, pulling a cloth bag over his head and closing a set of handcuffs around his wrists. He resisted his natural urge to snap their necks. Driving around in an SUV full of corpses asking random people if they knew where Carlos Esparza lived wasn't going to get him very far.

It was impossible to measure the passing time, partially because his watch was secured behind him and partially because the warmth and vibration of the vehicle's floorboard finally put him to sleep. For some reason, lying there with two cartel killers' feet on his back was a lot more relaxing than the time he'd spent getting sucked into his own mind on the flight. There were no longer options to consider. No secondary concerns. No political agendas. His only job now was to survive long enough to find Sayid Halabi and kill him.

The trip started out on smooth pavement, eventually degenerating into rough asphalt and then a dirt track that jerked him fully awake. In the last half hour or so, they crossed two streams deep enough for water to seep under the door and a few ruts that seemed even deeper.

After what Rapp guessed was somewhere between three and four hours, they finally came to a stop. He was immediately dragged from the vehicle and shoved to his knees on the damp ground. Voices speaking Spanish swirled around him for a few minutes before the bag was pulled off.

He squinted into the filtered sunlight and counted eight guards within his field of view. All were wearing camo, all were armed with AKs, and all had the look of former Mexican cops or army. Nothing special, but head and shoulders above the men he'd killed in California.

Much more interesting was the house intermittently hidden by the jungle in front of him. From the exterior, it had the look of a primitive village, with clapboard sides, scavenged materials, and a roof of corrugated tin and palm fronds. From the air, it would be completely indistinguishable from the other tiny villages in the area, but from where Rapp was kneeling, it was quite the architectural marvel. Massive windows revealed a luxurious modern interior of marble and glass. A swimming pool was hidden under a roof held up by pillars designed to look like trees. Behind and to the north, some kind of crop—food, not drugs—had been planted in a way that suggested subsistence farming.

A man in slacks and an open-collared shirt appeared from the house and approached to within ten feet of Rapp. He was probably in his early thirties, with vaguely stylish glasses and an expensive haircut. Certainly not Esparza. More likely some kind of business advisor. Rapp ignored him, craning his neck to get a better feel for his operating environment. It wasn't too complicated. Jungle. Men with guns. Big house.

Another five minutes or so passed in silence before a second man appeared. He was probably in his mid-forties, with medium-length hair that was a little wild, a gold and diamond watch that looked like it weighed as much as a brick, and clothes that seemed to have been chosen based on the number of digits on the price tag. It was one of the strange things about these cartel bosses. They spent half their time obsessing over accumulating obscene amounts of money and the other half trying to figure out what to do with it.

"We had a bet whether you'd come," Esparza said in solid English. According to Claudia he'd spent a fair amount of his youth in Arizona.

"Who won?"

The man just smiled and pulled a gold .44 Magnum Desert Eagle from his waistband. He aimed it at Rapp, who began instinctively running through the sequence of moves necessary to survive: Drop the cuffs that he'd picked in the first few minutes of the drive there. Roll forward, letting the round go harmlessly over his head. Get hold of the man, disarm him, pull him in close enough that no one would dare take a shot . . .

That was a good way to kill Esparza and escape into the jungle, but Rapp had to remind himself again that that wasn't why he was here. He was here to make friends and figure out how to get close to Sayid Halabi.

"Seems like we've both gone through a lot of trouble for you to just shoot me," Rapp said.

"Oh, I'm not going to shoot you. I'm going to torture you. For months. Until there isn't anything left of you that can even feel pain. Until you don't even know you're *human* anymore. Then I'm going to feed you to my dogs."

"I feel like that would be a mistake," Rapp said, slipping the cuffs off and getting to his feet.

The familiar sound of weapons being slammed to shoulders momentarily drowned out the hum of jungle insects. Esparza thrust his weapon out in front of him but wouldn't allow himself to take a step back in front of the men. His assistant, who was apparently less concerned with machismo, retreated a few feet.

"You're pulling in what?" Rapp said, dusting off his pants. "Seventy-five million a year on a gross of a hundred and ten?"

Claudia had given him the number, and based on Esparza's expression she'd gotten pretty close. "You're heavily extended in pot, but legalization in the U.S. and Canada is starting to bite. So, you're looking to replace that business with Middle Eastern heroin. You want to take advantage of the crackdown on oxycodone and replace the pharmaceutical industry as the supplier of choice. The bottom line is that you want to move up and you figure this is the play that can get you there."

Rapp fell silent and was surprised when the next man to speak wasn't Esparza but the preppy sidekick. His accent was more highbrow.

"And what do you think of that plan?"

"I think you've got a good shot," Rapp responded. "But it's going to be complicated. Not only because the DEA knows the cartels are going to take this opening, but because working with the Arabs can be . . ." His voice faded for a moment. "Let's say challenging."

"I have hundreds of people on my payroll," Esparza said. "Police, intelligence operatives, judges, military officers. And I have enforcers. You're not the only man in this business who's good with a gun."

Rapp looked around him at Esparza's guards. "Are you sure? From where I'm standing, your talent pool looks a little shallow."

Esparza aimed directly between Rapp's eyes, but again his assistant cut in.

"I assume you think you have something to offer us?"

"I can provide extensive knowledge of the operations of the U.S. government. CIA, NSA, FBI, and DEA. You name it. Even the White House."

"I have contacts in these places, too," Esparza said, not wanting to be upstaged.

"I also have a lifetime of experience dealing with the Middle East and speak native-level Arabic and fluent Dari. Those are pretty dangerous waters, and I know how to navigate them. You're not just having to get around the Agency and the U.S. military. They're the least of your problems. You've got a hundred different terrorist groups, tribes, and other factions—all of whom are involved in pissing contests that go back a thousand years. And if you manage to cut through all that, then it's going to be time to deal with the Pakistanis and the Russians."

"And you expect me to believe that a crooked cop can, as you say, navigate those waters?"

"Better than anyone on the planet."

"Better than anyone on the planet?" Esparza mocked. "You're confident for a dead man."

"What's your name?" the assistant asked.

"Mitch Rapp."

It clearly didn't mean anything to the man, but Esparza's face went blank for a moment before he burst out laughing.

"This is your story," he barely managed to choke out. "That *Mitch Rapp* stole drugs from DEA and then came here to ask me for a job? For a moment, I thought you had balls. But now I see that you're just crazy."

He summoned one of his guards, but then held out a hand when Rapp spoke again. Apparently he was finding the whole thing pretty entertaining.

"You say you have highly placed contacts. Use them. My story isn't going to be hard to confirm. Unless I miss my guess, this is blowing up all over the Beltway right now. And if you find out I'm lying, it's just as easy to start cutting me up tomorrow as it is today."

CHAPTER 31

SOUTHERN MEXICO

AFTER almost two days, Rapp had his accommodations feeling pretty homey. The rusty steel cage itself measured about six feet long by three feet wide, by four feet high. It was located back far enough into the jungle that he could see the dim glow of Esparza's complex in the evening but nothing more than foliage during the day.

He'd managed to pull up the tall grass that grew around the cage and use it to create a fairly comfortable surface to stretch out on. A stick secured to one of the bars above him created a convenient stream of drinking water when it rained, which seemed to be about two hours every night. Bugs were plentiful, but a little too juicy and a touch bitter. Better than the lizard he'd caught last night, though. That thing had been dead hard to choke down. The bottom line was that the Lacandon jungle didn't seem to have anything with the pleasant texture and slight nuttiness of an Iraqi scorpion.

He'd been stripped of everything he'd brought with him and was now wearing a bright orange jumpsuit reminiscent of the ones ISIS passed out to their beheading victims. It was soaked through to the skin and covered with mud, but the material was still capable of keeping him comfortable through the relatively warm nights.

So he wasn't going to starve or freeze. The question was no longer whether he could survive out there; it was how long he was going to have to do it. So far, no one had come to visit and while the cage's lock was old and unsophisticated, it was solid. In the end, it might be boredom that got him.

Based on the temperature and the sound of the jungle, it was probably an hour from dawn when he heard soggy footsteps coming in his direction. Someone to let him out, hose him off, and give him a job? Someone to put a bullet in his skull? In the end, there wasn't much he could do about it either way. He had to fight his instincts and remain passive. He was there to win a popularity contest, not perform a bunch of executions.

The man who appeared wasn't Esparza, which was probably a good sign. If it was going to be the bullet in the head or the blowtorch, the cartel leader would want to do it personally.

He stopped in front of the cage, backlit by the light bleeding from the compound. A little shorter than Rapp, with a scraggly beard and a gut straining against grimy fatigues. Weaponry consisted of an AK slung over his shoulder and a Bowie knife sheathed on his right hip.

"What?" Rapp said.

The gun came off the man's shoulder and he leaned it against a tree before using the knife to hack off a thick branch. When he returned, he came a little closer, but stayed out of reach.

"California," he managed to get out through a barely comprehensible accent. "My cousin."

The fact that he then shoved the branch through the widely spaced bars and into Rapp's ribs suggested that one of the corpses currently ruining Claudia's Airbnb rating had been a relation. Rapp feigned pain, covering his side and cramming himself into the back of the cage.

As anticipated, the display of weakness encouraged the man. He rammed the branch in over and over as Rapp slapped ineffectually at it. The fact that this asshole hadn't been smart enough to trim the leaves was making it impossible for him to build enough momentum to do any real damage. He seemed to realize this and instead of stepping back to fashion a more effective weapon, he decided to go for a gravity assist.

He took a step forward and went in from the top, jabbing Rapp in the chest. The force increased a bit, but was still nowhere near what would be necessary to cause injury. Having said that, the guy seemed to just be warming up, and lying in the mud getting poked with a stick was already getting old.

He was now only about a foot or so out of reach. The opportunity was there, but Rapp couldn't decide if it made sense to take it. Esparza's assistant was probably still checking out his story and getting too aggressive might be a mistake. On the other hand, letting himself get trapped in a cage for days on end might suggest that he wasn't worth hiring.

Rapp suspected he was just talking himself into it, but he quickly decided that killing this piece of shit was definitely the right course of action. He waited for the stick to come down again and instead of slapping it away, he grabbed it and pulled. The already off-balance man pitched forward, struggling to keep his footing in the slick mud.

His right leg came into range and Rapp yanked it through a gap between the bars. The cartel enforcer made the mistake of bending at the waist to try to free himself and Rapp got hold of his beard, using it to slam his face into the top of the cage.

Unfortunately, there wasn't enough leverage available to do any real damage. A thumb in the eye socket was an option, but sound was the main problem at this point. Rapp managed to use his beard and hair to spin him around and clamp a hand over his mouth. At that point, it was just a matter of getting hold of the knife.

Ten more seconds and it was over. Rapp kept the back of the man's head pinned securely against the bars as blood cascaded from the gash in his neck. When he finally went still, Rapp let the body slide into the mud and turned his attention to the lock. The mechanism wasn't particularly sophisticated, but the overall build quality was depressingly solid. Prying it open with the knife wasn't going to happen and a search of the dead man turned up no keys. Just a half a pack of cigarettes and a lighter.

Rapp needed something stiff enough to work the lock mechanism but soft enough that he could fashion it with the knife. Materials at hand were limited. Rocks were hard, but not easily carved into a pick. The jungle foliage was easy to carve, but too flexible to move the heavy tumblers.

He pulled off one of the man's boots and pried apart the sole, hoping to find some kind of plastic stiffener, but it was just rubber and leather.

Why did everything have to go the hard way?

He pulled the man's leg inside the cage and yanked back on it, using one of the bars as a fulcrum. The quiet snap of bone sounded immediately, but he kept pulling until the jagged fracture popped through the skin.

Surprisingly, the knife was razor sharp, and it took only about fifteen minutes to fashion part of the man's fibula into the appropriate tools. Once the lock had dropped off, Rapp swapped clothes with the corpse and shoved it in the cage. It wouldn't fool anyone who was really interested, but it'd be enough for someone casually glancing through the trees as they passed.

A quick recon of the compound confirmed his first impression—minimal physical or electronic security, but a lot of armed guards. None looked particularly attentive, but their sheer number made getting by them unlikely even in the remaining darkness. Quietly killing a couple more was definitely doable, but how high a body count could you run up in a popularity contest? It wasn't really his area of expertise, but he guessed that anything over zero was a move in the wrong direction. So he waited.

Dawn brought what he was looking for: a fairly sloppy changing of the guard. Taking advantage of a temporary gap along the northeast corner of the compound, Rapp slipped out of the jungle and through a door partially hidden by foliage.

It opened to a storage room and probably provided access for deliveries. Past the well-stocked shelves was another door that led to a spacious industrial kitchen. There were a couple of pots steaming on the stove but no sign of the cook, so he crossed the tile floor into an airy dining room.

Human activity continued to be nonexistent as he crossed a surprisingly tasteful living room and entered a hallway at the back. Most of the doors were open and led to stylish bedroom suites that looked like they'd never been used.

He slipped into one of them and locked the door. A quick search turned up a closet full of designer clothes, some of which still had the tags hanging from them. As luck would have it, he and Esparza were around the same size. The loafers looked a little small but would undoubtedly be more comfortable than the guard's damp, torn-up boots.

The bathroom was behind a massive stone barrier that doubled as the headboard of the bed. The back wall was constructed entirely of glass and looked out into dense, flowering jungle. Rapp spotted a switch set apart from the ones for the lights and flipped it. The glass turned opaque.

This was more like it.

CHAPTER 32

RAPP pushed his hair from his face and examined himself in the still steamy bathroom mirror. With a belt, Esparza's designer slacks stayed up and the fact that he wore his shirts loose allowed them to accommodate Rapp's broad shoulders. The loafers were definitely on the tight side but that was probably a good thing—they'd stay on if he had to run. But that wasn't the goal. If there was any running happening today, his mission had failed.

Satisfied that he was appropriately groomed for a job interview, Rapp strode back out into the hallway. It was still empty and he headed unchallenged toward the large, palm-frond-covered terrace he'd noticed when he arrived.

On his way across the living room, a plump woman in her fifties appeared from a door to the right. She stopped short, giving him a quizzical look as she wiped her hands on an apron that appeared to have seen some serious action. Just the person he was looking for.

"Breakfast?"

Her eyes narrowed as she tried to decipher what he'd said.

"Comida?" he managed to dredge from his memory.

That got a nod.

"Cómo se llama?"

"María, señor."

"María. Café?"

That got another nod, but he wasn't through his Spanish repertoire yet.

"Huevos rancheros?"

"Sí, señor."

"Perfecto. Y orange juice." He pantomimed holding a glass. "Uh, naranja. Sí? Muy grande. Mucho hielo."

"Entiendo. Tortillas de harina o maíz?"

He had no idea what she'd just said, but on the subject of food his instinct was to just agree with whatever this woman recommended. "Sí."

She didn't seem to fully understand his response, but he wasn't worried. "Dónde está Señor Esparza?"

She pointed. "En la terraza."

Esparza was right where María said he would be, sitting at a table with a plate of fruit and a newspaper in front of him. The entire terrace—including the fountain and massive fireplace—was shaded and protected from overhead surveillance by foliage. The bugs were a little thick, but at least they weren't for breakfast anymore.

The cartel leader didn't look up until Rapp sat down across from him. His confused expression only lasted a split second before recognition set in. He looked like he was about to shout for help from the surrounding guards, but Rapp spoke first.

"I figured you'd probably heard something back from your contacts by now."

There was a place setting in front of him, so Rapp shook out the cloth napkin and set it on his lap.

Esparza was frozen, eyes flicking to the knife near Rapp's right hand. His body language suggested he was going to throw himself backward and call in a little machine gun fire, but then María appeared with a cup of coffee and a pitcher of icy, fresh-squeezed orange juice.

"Gracias," Rapp said, accepting it with a disarming smile. Esparza's desperation to escape seemed to wane as Rapp poured himself a glass of juice and downed it in a few gulps.

"I see you're making yourself at home," he said, examining the clothes Rapp was wearing.

"I figured you wouldn't mind," Rapp responded, testing the coffee. Not surprisingly, it was top-notch. "What have you been able to figure out?"

Esparza remained silent for a few seconds before finally speaking. "That it's possible you're who you say you are. There's a surprising amount of information available on the recent activities of Mitch Rapp but getting confirmation is difficult. My assistant is supposed to have a more thorough report for me this morning."

María returned with the huevos rancheros and Rapp dug in as the cartel leader looked on.

"It appears that you stole a fair amount of money over your career."

"Stole, my ass."

"So you deny the accusations your government is making?"

"I took money from terrorists and the people who funded them. I've been hanging it out there for America for twenty fucking years and my annual salary wouldn't cover the clothes I found in your guest bedroom. And what if one of my enemies came after me and I had to run? You think the politicians would help me out? I sure as hell wouldn't bet my life on it. So, sure. I had a few rainy day funds."

"Invested stupidly, apparently."

"I got some bad advice. Not really my area of expertise."

"A man with friends like yours could make these kinds of problems go away with the snap of a finger."

Rapp shoveled another forkful of María's amazing eggs in his mouth and shook his head. "*Could* is the operative word there, Carlos. Past tense. President Alexander isn't going to get anywhere near a scandal during this clusterfuck of an election. And Christine Barnett wants nothing more than to hang me up by my balls."

"An uncomfortable position."

"You think?" Rapp said, letting the volume of his voice rise. "I've been shot, stabbed, set on fire, and blown up. Twice. All in the defense of the Stars and Stripes. And all I asked in return was enough money to survive my retirement." He was almost shouting now, demonstrating the kind of passion that a man like Esparza would appreciate, but not so much that it would worry the guards. "But what am I looking at instead? A jail cell and a piece-of-shit president who's never lifted a finger for anyone but herself."

It was pretty much a retread of all the things Claudia had been telling him, but there was no reason it wouldn't work as well on Esparza as it had on him.

"And your woman? My people tell me she left you for a friend of yours."

"Her boss and my backup man Scott Coleman," Rapp spat out. "Who knows how long that's been going on? Turns out that when the money and power goes away, so do they."

"It seems you'd want to kill them," Esparza said, interested enough to keep probing, trying to find a crack in Rapp's story.

"I wouldn't mind. Believe me. But Scott's a dangerous son of a bitch and the Agency's going to be looking for me to make a move like that. For now, I'm just going to have to let it go. When all this dies down and I get my feet under me, though, you can bet your ass I'm going to be paying them a visit."

Esparza fell silent, watching the man in front of him. As insane as it seemed, all indications were that he really was Mitch Rapp. And that created both opportunities and dangers that he never thought he'd be contemplating. Over the years, he'd managed to put many important people on his payroll. But Mitch Rapp? None of his competitors—even those with revenues that would get them on a *Forbes* list—had anyone who could compare.

Vicente Rossi appeared, took a few steps across the terrace, and stopped dead. It was an understandable reaction, but one that Esparza couldn't be seen sharing. Instead, he cut a slice of the pineapple on his plate and casually waved his business advisor over.

"I don't think formal introductions have been made. This is Vicente."

Rapp nodded in the man's direction but otherwise didn't acknowledge him.

"What do you have for me?" Esparza said, taking a bite of fruit to cover his nervousness. He had killed countless men. Tortured them and their families. Built a cartel that commanded fear and respect that far outstripped the scope of its operation. He refused to allow his fear of this unarmed American to show.

Rossi, still standing, had no similar qualms. "Perhaps this is something that would be better done in private?"

Had he discovered something that would cause the CIA man to go for the knife still within his reach? Esparza met Rapp's dead gaze, refusing to turn away. "Now."

Rossi gave a reluctant nod. "I'm satisfied that this is indeed Mitch Rapp."

It wasn't a surprising conclusion at this point, but still the cartel leader felt a surge of adrenaline. "And the DEA men?"

"We were able to get people into the hospital where they're being treated. There's no question that they were shot, but because of their body armor, their injuries are relatively minor." He paused. "Unlike our men, who are dead."

Esparza leaned back in his chair, gazing up at the younger man. The reason the DEA men had survived was obvious. There would have been no reason for Rapp to antagonize the Americans any more than necessary. And the reason so many of his men were dead was equally obvious.

"Did my men talk?" Esparza asked.

Rapp shook his head. "That's why I didn't know the shipment was yours. My compliments on your management style. I took off one of their hands with a set of bolt cutters and they were still more afraid of you than they were of me."

Esparza smiled at that. In the end, he and Rapp were much alike. Two predators who got what they wanted. "Go on, Vicente."

"Mr. Rapp seems to have left his official capacity at the CIA some time ago to pursue what appears to be a vendetta in Saudi Arabia, though it's impossible to know how much Agency involvement there was. Irene Kennedy is quite clever at covering her tracks. He was recently in Yemen, most likely working as a private contractor in her employment."

"And now?" Esparza said.

Rossi seemed reluctant to continue but understood that he had no choice. "The allegations of long-term financial impropriety combined with the shooting of the DEA agents and the murder of two Mexican nationals has very much changed his status. Not surprisingly, everyone is backing away from him as quickly as they can."

"Including Kennedy?"

"Unclear. But her ability to support him at this point is nonexistent. People are abandoning her almost as quickly as they are Rapp. If Senator Barnett wins the presidency it's hard to see how she'll escape being indicted."

"So you can see my problem," Rapp interjected. "And why your organization is an interesting solution. Half those politicians would be dead if it weren't for me. But now they're turning on me without a second thought. You, on the other hand, have a reputation for loyalty and rewarding competence."

Esparza watched María approach and begin collecting their

empty plates. "I think you'd find working for drug traffickers much more predictable than working for politicians."

"I don't doubt it."

"Why don't you go with María. Since my men can't perform the simple task of keeping you in a cage, you might as well stay in the house."

Rapp stood and Esparza studied his confident gait as he retreated across the flagstone patio.

"Thoughts?" he said when the CIA man had disappeared through the glass doors.

"Kill him now."

The cartel leader laughed.

"I'm serious, Carlos. You can't trust this man."

"Didn't you just tell me that you confirmed his story?"

"He and Irene Kennedy have the capacity to create any illusion they want."

"But why? I think your lack of balls might be clouding your vision, Vicente. The CIA doesn't give a shit about drugs, other than maybe to sell them to finance their black ops. And I think it's unlikely that the rise of Christine Barnett is just a trick to allow Mitch Rapp to infiltrate a medium-sized Mexican drug operation. And then there's the matter of the DEA agents. Even with the vests, one could have easily been killed. The Americans don't take those kinds of risks. And they don't torture drug traffickers to death."

"But—"

"The timing of this couldn't be better for us, Vicente. We're in a dangerous position because of the loss of the San Ysidro mall, and there's no question that someone like Rapp could help with the Arabs. He speaks their language. He understands how they do business and what scares them. . . ."

"The timing of this couldn't be better for us," Rossi repeated. "You don't find this at all suspicious? That a man dedicated to fighting Middle Eastern terrorists arrived on our doorstep right after we sent through our first shipment of Middle Eastern heroin?"

Esparza frowned and took a sip of his coffee. "Heroin has been flooding out of the Middle East for years. Between that and Saudi oil, the Americans finance virtually every terrorist operation in the world. And even if they *did* care, why would they come after us? There are cartels with longer-standing relationships with the Arabs."

"What about our exposure to American retaliation?" Rossi countered. "Mitch Rapp probably has more ugly secrets in his head than anyone but Irene Kennedy herself. You say the CIA doesn't care about us and you may be right. But the day they find out we've taken on Mitch Rapp, we move directly into their crosshairs."

Esparza nodded thoughtfully. This was perhaps the most compelling argument for killing Rapp. The risks of having him there were incredibly high. Probably too high.

Rossi sensed that he'd gained an advantage in their discussion and decided to press. "I can figure out how to deal with heroin, Carlos. There are a lot of Arab immigrants in Mexico, some of whom are already involved in the drug trade. We can hire as many as we need."

Esparza tapped his index finger absently on the tabletop. Summarily executing Mitch Rapp seemed like an incredible waste. Both of talent and opportunity for sport.

Everyone he hired into a position of authority had to pass a test. Depending on the specific demands of the job, that test might relate to skill, toughness, loyalty, or intelligence. Some were relatively easy. María had been hired based on her ability to make food indistinguishable from Esparza's own mother's. For others, failure had meant death.

"We'll test him," Esparza said, finally.

"Carlos, I don't—"

"Relax, Vicente. We'll create a test that's impossible for him to survive. Do you have no curiosity at all? No interest in seeing Mitch Rapp in action? In seeing what he would do and how long he could last against impossible odds?"

"What if he beats those odds?"

Esparza considered the question for a moment. "Then we'd have to consider the possibility that the rewards of employing such a man might be worth the risks."

CHAPTER 33

RAPP followed two armed guards through the house in the direction of the front door. With the exception of his phone, all the possessions he'd arrived there with had been returned. The green cotton slacks and brown shirt supplied by Claudia had been cleaned and pressed but would still allow him to blend into the jungle if necessary. The gray trail-running shoes were less stylish, but sturdy, light, and possessed a tread designed for soft surfaces.

The barking of dogs became audible when they stepped into the humid morning, ahead and to the right but hidden in the foliage. They skirted the clearing that stretched along the front of the house, staying beneath the jungle canopy in an effort to foil possible overhead surveillance.

The scene they finally came upon was, unfortunately, about what Rapp had expected. Two dirt bikes and three 4x4s sprayed with matte camo paint—one with a mounted machine gun heavy enough to nearly bottom out the suspension. The sixth and last vehicle was a spotless Humvee painted British racing green. Like Rapp's clothes, designed to blend in anywhere.

Seventeen men were either in the vehicles or standing around them. All were wearing full camo and equipped with assault rifles, sidearms, and light packs with water bladders. The exception was

Esparza himself, who was wearing his typical five grand worth of designer linen. The only obvious change was that he'd traded his calfskin loafers for a sturdy pair of hiking boots.

Worse were the six dogs. In Rapp's estimation dogs were usually smarter than their human masters and always more motivated. The mix of breeds was designed more for intimidation than tracking but despite being heavy on the Rottweilers and pit bulls, the pack would still be effective. Particularly if they managed to catch what they were chasing. In this case, him.

"Everyone who works for me has to pass a test first," Esparza said, speaking in a voice loud enough to be heard over the frenzied dogs. "This will be yours."

"You're getting a little ahead of yourself, aren't you?" Rapp said. "We haven't talked money."

The man bristled, unaccustomed to being challenged. But none of his men seemed to speak English, so he was the only one who registered Rapp's attitude.

"How much do you think you're worth?"

"Two hundred and fifty grand seems about right."

The cartel leader laughed. "A quarter million a year? I don't even pay Vicente that much."

"A month, Carlos. Two fifty *a month*."

The cartel leader's bemused expression spoke volumes. He was going to agree. But probably not because he was willing to pay that amount. More likely, he'd created a test that he was certain Rapp wouldn't survive.

"Done," he said, pointing to a primitive road leading into the jungle. "All you have to do is make it to a small village twelve miles to the north. Actually, *village* might not be the right word. It's just three houses. But one of them has a covered porch and operates as an informal restaurant for the local farmers. Meet me there and you'll get your first month's payment."

Rapp was fairly sure he knew the place—a crossroads where the crappy dirt road met a slightly less crappy dirt road that ran from east to west. The bulky GPS watch on his wrist contained a color screen and was full of topographical maps that he'd downloaded during his layover in Mexico City. And while the tiny screen didn't have the resolution to depict buildings, the distance and direction was right, and businesses tended to set up at crossroads.

"What if I don't make it?" Rapp said.

"Then you'll be dead."

Rapp scanned the men around him again. Some were overweight, others looked like the run-of-the-mill psycho cartel enforcers, and a few looked like solid former Mexican soldiers. All the gear was well maintained and top-of-the-line. They had weapons, vehicles, dogs, and the home field advantage. In his column, the heat wasn't too bad this time of the morning and the sky suggested rain was coming. Likely a lot of it.

"Do I get a head start or does everyone just start shooting now?" Rapp asked.

"Ten minutes."

"That seems light."

"This isn't a negotiation," Esparza responded, retrieving an old-fashioned stopwatch from his pocket and making a show of clicking the button on top. "Your precious minutes are already running out."

Rapp toggled the timer on his own watch and started to run. The roadbed was soft and a little slick, limiting him to a seven-minute-mile pace. The goal was a stream just over a mile from there. Based on what he'd been able to make out on the topo, it was steep and narrow enough to neutralize even the dirt bikes, and the reliable water supply gave him a decent chance of running into a human settlement where he could scrounge supplies.

The critical component at this point was to stay ahead of his pursuers until the rains came and reduced the effectiveness of the dogs. Probably doable as long as the handlers kept hold of them. If they got close enough to release them, though, things were going to get exciting.

He notched his pace upward to the very edge of what the surface would safely allow. The idea that Esparza would live up to his word on the ten minutes seemed a little far-fetched.

After six minutes of running, he activated the screen on his watch to check his position with regard to the stream. In the end, it turned out to be unnecessary. The water from recent rains had swollen it to the point that it had washed out part of the road. Rapp slid down an embankment into the muddy creek, alternating between it and the banks, depending on which maximized his speed. After about a hundred yards he heard the distant whine of the dirt bikes starting up. The timer on his watch read eight minutes and four seconds. Frankly, a minute longer than Rapp had figured. Apparently, that was what passed for honor among thieves.

If they weren't complete morons, it would take only about three minutes before they found the place where he'd ducked into the jungle. At the pace he'd set, his footprints were clearly visible, though it would be impossible to determine whether he'd headed upstream or downstream. Best bet, the dirt bikers would radio it in and split up to chase. The dogs would be put in vehicles and driven to the place where Rapp had abandoned the road. So call it another five before he had an organized chase coming up behind him.

Not surprisingly, the microscopic topographical map hadn't provided a very accurate picture of the terrain. Instead of narrowing into a tiny scar cut through the jungle, the stream kept getting wider, deeper, and more powerful. Cascades that were half waterfall and half mudslide fed it from the canyon walls, making it increasingly hard for Rapp to keep his footing.

Overhead, the clouds were building, but at a pace that was slower than he'd hoped. The rain he was counting on to save his ass from the dogs seemed a long way off.

When the pack become audible again, they were going nuts.

The question now was, would their handlers try to keep them under control or would they let them run?

The answer came about a minute later when the sound of their barking suddenly diminished. They were no longer straining against their handlers. They were loose.

The jungle at the edges of the now thirty-foot-wide river was too dense for a human to move through, but the dogs would manage it pretty well. Rapp abandoned the shallow water on the right bank and went for the deeper center. He selected a thick, leafy tree from the floating debris and tangled himself it in. A branch behind his head kept his nose and mouth out of the water while the rest of him floated along beneath the surface.

Because he'd traveled mostly in the water, the dogs wouldn't have much to work with. They'd have to move along both banks, trying to pick up a scent. As long as the river kept moving and he stayed submerged, he'd probably be all right.

Probably.

After an hour of floating along at a less than thrilling three or four knots, the situation started to deteriorate. On the positive side, his femur wasn't yet a dog toy. On the negative side, it was potentially a few seconds from becoming one.

There were two pit bulls on the east bank, staying roughly even with him. They seemed to sense that their prey was close but hadn't yet focused on the tree he was hidden beneath. A Doberman was on the opposite bank, hanging a bit farther back with its handler alongside. Two soldiers were visible in the shallow water to the west, scanning the dense jungle around them with assault rifles gripped tight.

One got a call on his radio and he spoke into it for a few seconds. His words were unintelligible, but his tone and gestures weren't hard to decipher. They figured Rapp was in the river because the dogs couldn't pick up his scent, but they had no idea where. The response was also audible, a static-ridden jumble of anger and frustration from Carlos Esparza. He wouldn't be too worried yet, but he'd be looking up at the same darkening clouds as Rapp was.

When the clouds finally opened up, they did so with no warning at all. One minute Rapp was floating along with an overheated Rottweiler swimming about ten yards in front of him and the next he was fighting to breathe as water came at him from every direction.

The shouts of the soldiers were swallowed by the downpour, as were their outlines. Shots rang out but it was impossible to know if they thought they'd spotted a target or were just using the sound to locate each other. The Rottweiler, again proving its intelligence, made a beeline for the nearest land bank as the river began to swell.

Rapp stayed put, struggling against a current that kept pushing him under. He was finally forced to unhook his feet from the trunk and let them dangle in the deepening water. His head was still among the tree's leafy branches, but now high enough to get a few breaths between waves crashing over him.

From the impact of the stationary objects he was colliding with, he could tell that the speed of the water had picked up significantly. He held on, knowing that he was leaving his pursuers well behind. Soon, though, it became too dangerous. The water was filling with larger, more jagged debris, and the current was becoming impossible to fight. Ahead, the channel narrowed enough to give him a shot at reaching the east bank.

Despite his having a gift for swimming that had helped him win the Iron Man in his youth, the fifteen-foot trip turned out to be harder than it looked. He took a few good hits from deadfall, one particularly large tree sending him to the bottom and dragging him across the rocks for almost a minute.

When he finally came up, he found himself only a few yards from the edge of the jungle. A few hard strokes put him in range of a partially submerged tree and he managed to use it to pull himself to safety. After crawling onto the muddy bank, he lay there vomiting what felt like a tanker truck full of muddy water. Finally, he pulled himself beneath a bush, using the leaves to protect himself from the pounding rain while he got his breathing under control.

Images of carving Carlos Esparza's heart out with a dull stick flashed across his mind, but he reminded himself again that wasn't the mission. No, that'd be too easy.

Rapp had been out of the water for just over two hours when the dogs became audible again. Someone on Esparza's team was a pretty functional tracker and was using his canine teammates to maximum effect.

A temporary hole in the cloud cover had tipped the advantage back to the chasers, leaving Rapp with very little time. The handlers would soon get close enough to release the dogs again and then he'd have five hundred pounds of muscle, teeth, and claws bearing down on him like scent-seeking missiles.

He was currently lying in a large field of surprisingly healthy-looking coca plants. Typically, the Mexicans imported their coke from farther south, but Esparza seemed to be trying to integrate his supply chain. The plants were harder to spot from the air than marijuana, but it was doubtful that anyone was even trying. With the relationship between the United States and Mexico being what it was, the government would probably be happy to overlook this fledgling cash crop.

The compound in front of him contained four modest buildings—most notably a two-story structure that seemed to be the Mexican answer to a barn. It would have come off as a typical subsistence farm if it weren't for a few details to the contrary. The coca plants were a pretty clear tip-off, obviously. As were the well-camouflaged fifty-five-gallon drums that likely contained the chemicals necessary to refine Esparza's experimental crop. Most interesting to Rapp, though, were the two guards.

Both were armed with AKs, but older and more poorly maintained than the ones carried by the men pursuing him. Neither had sidearms, opting instead for knives sheathed on their hips. One was sitting on a log with his back to Rapp at a distance of about fifteen feet. The other was twenty feet farther, leaning against the barn and facing his companion. Every once in a while they spoke to each other, but neither seemed particularly interested in the conversation. Other than that, there was no sign of personnel or activity.

The sound of the dogs was getting closer. When they were released, it would be a matter of minutes before they were on top of him. And this time, he didn't have a whole lot to work with to escape them. While he'd made significant progress toward the village that was his objective, he was currently stuck in relatively flat terrain with no rivers nearby. The patch of blue sky above him was shrinking fast, though, suggesting the weather might be turning back in his favor.

No more time for fancy strategies or precision. It was time to pull out the hammer.

He dug the toes of his shoes into the soft earth, putting himself in a position similar to that of a sprinter in a starting block. He wanted to wait until the man against the barn wasn't looking in his direction, but the strained barking of the dogs suddenly became less frustrated. They'd been turned loose again.

He shot forward, snatching the knife from the first man's belt and dragging the blade across his throat. The guard near the barn grabbed his weapon and leapt to his feet just as Rapp threw the knife. While it was still in the air, the man caught his foot on something and pitched forward. It changed the range between them just enough that instead of penetrating his chest, the blade hit hilt-first.

Again, Rapp charged, but he was forced to drop and slide when the man got his finger on the trigger. A spray of rounds filled the air over his head as they collided. The guard's feet went out from under him and they wrestled for control of the weapon. Rapp had nearly gotten into a position to choke him out when he heard something burst from the coca plants behind him. He stopped fighting and let the guard roll on top of him just as the Doberman reached them. The man screamed when it clamped its jaws around his shoulder, and Rapp slid from beneath him as more crashes sounded.

The AK was out of reach and there wasn't time to go for it. Instead Rapp bolted for the barn with an unknown number of dogs chasing. He sprinted through the door, leapt over some rusting fifty-five-gallon drums, and landed three rungs up a ladder that led to a loft. There was no time to climb, so he just jumped, using his momentum and arm strength to flip himself onto the rickety platform.

At least one dog slammed into the base of the ladder, and Rapp heard the claws of others as they tried desperately to reach him. Rapp immediately got into a position that would allow him to kick any that made it to the top, but, as impressive as they were at moving through the jungle, climbers they were not. Every few seconds, a paw or snout would appear, but then it would disappear again as the dog lost purchase and fell back into the crazed pack.

Once he was reasonably satisfied that none were going to get lucky, Rapp looked around him. No weapons or even respectably sharp farm implements were in evidence. Instead, the space was neatly stacked with duct-tape-wrapped bricks. He ripped one open and tried a small sample of the cocaine he found inside. Apparently Esparza's botany experiment was succeeding. It was seriously good shit.

Rapp moved back to the edge of the loft and the sight of him got one of the pit bulls excited enough to make the top rung. Rapp kicked it in the side of the head, sending it cartwheeling back into the pack completely unfazed.

He ripped open the kilo brick in his hand and then did the same to a few others. While he was working, two more dogs took a shot at climbing the ladder. Their muzzles, necks, and chests were covered in the blood of the guard they had just torn apart.

All six were now present—enough that they could functionally climb on top of each other to try to get at him. It was an unexpectedly effective strategy and their barking turned deafening as Rapp kicked at them.

There was a brief lull as a falling Rottweiler knocked them back and Rapp took advantage of it to chuck the open kilo bags on top of them. They were momentarily enveloped in an impressive cloud that, when it dissipated, left them all a ghostly white. Predictably, their barking and attempts to get to him increased in intensity. He started to regret the light running shoes he'd chosen as he kicked at them, trying to protect his ankles from fangs coated in foaming saliva.

As the coke went to work on them, though, they lost their focus. Some started fighting. Others just ran around in circles or attacked the walls. One bolted out into the rain that had started up again.

While they were distracted, Rapp went to a window on the eastern edge of the loft. He stood to the side of it, gently pushing the wood shutter open and taking a look outside. The downpour had reduced visibility to less than twenty feet.

He climbed down the front of the building with the water pounding on him from above. About halfway to the ground, the force of it became too much for the slick handholds he was improvising and he lost his grip. Fortunately, the landing was soft—about three-quarters mud and one-quarter what was left of the guard the dogs had taken out. Rapp scrambled for the AK and, when he found it, ran for the cover of the coca plants.

CHAPTER 34

NORTH OF HARGEISA
SOMALIA

"I . . . I couldn't make as much. You didn't give me time."

Sayid Halabi looked over his laptop at Gabriel Bertrand standing in the rock archway. The package in the Frenchman's hands seemed to glow in the dull light. Vacuum packed and covered in duct tape, it was indeed smaller than last time. The anthrax it contained could be augmented with other materials to mimic the kilo packages expected by the Mexican smugglers. And, with luck, it would be deployed in America to some minor effect. But the handful of victims it would produce no longer mattered.

Halabi continued to silently watch the scientist as he shifted his weight uncomfortably from one foot to the other. The goal had been to keep him ignorant of the reality and scope of the upcoming attack, using him only to fill in critical pieces of information not available elsewhere. But this was now impossible. The complexity of accelerating the timetable on a biological attack of this scale made continued efforts at subtle manipulation impractical. Halabi would get only one chance. If he failed and was discovered, the entire world would line up against him. Militaries and intelligence agencies that had spent decades battling each other would join forces, coordinating their massive resources with the goal of exterminating both him and the organization he led. The next week would decide whether ISIS reshaped the planet or disappeared from its surface.

"It will be enough," Halabi said finally.

The Frenchman approached cautiously, leaving the anthrax on the plywood desk. He was a comically weak man. Ruled by cowardice and arrogance. Devoid of a belief in anything greater than himself. But unquestionably in possession of a magnificent mind.

Bertrand had written extensively on the history of contagions spanning from early Egypt to the outbreak of SARS in the modern era. He'd studied the spread of pathogens, examining how they initially took hold, modeling their paths, and scrutinizing their aftermath. Even more interesting, he'd done a great deal of work detailing how epidemics of the past had been made worse and how those mistakes had the potential to be repeated on a much grander scale in the future.

Halabi rotated his laptop so the man could see the screen. "Do you know what this is?"

Bertrand squinted at it for a moment and then shook his head.

"It's a population map of the United States, with transportation infrastructure overlaid—airports, bus and train routes, major highways . . ."

Not surprisingly, the man didn't understand. And there was no delicate way to remedy his ignorance.

"I intend to infect five of my men with the virus you discovered in Yemen and transport them across the U.S. border," Halabi said bluntly. "From there, they'll spread the disease throughout the country and the industrialized world."

Bertrand's expression went blank. "I . . . I don't understand. What are you saying?"

"I don't know how I can be more clear."

He stood frozen for a time before taking a few stumbling steps back. "You . . ." he stammered. "It's . . . It's not possible."

"It's not only possible, it's quite simple. YARS is extraordinarily contagious, so infecting my people will be a trivial matter. And I have a group of smugglers in Mexico willing to transport them across the border."

"You can't do that."

"I assure you that I can, Doctor. In fact it's already in motion. I just need you to help me with a few final details."

Bertrand squinted through the semidarkness as though he were looking at a child unable to grasp a simple concept. "This isn't anthrax. It's a highly contagious, extremely deadly disease with no effective medical treatment. Even Spanish flu . . ." His voice faded for a moment. "In 1918 and 1919 it killed more than thirty million people worldwide."

"I'm aware of the history of the Spanish flu," Halabi said calmly.

"All evidence suggests that this disease is even more contagious and has a significantly higher mortality rate. Add to that the rise in long-distance travel and the increase in the world population, and you could be talking about casualties in the hundreds of millions."

"That's my estimate as well."

Still, Bertrand's' expression suggested that he believed he wasn't being clear. "This can't be controlled. It won't just kill people you think are your enemies. It won't be just Americans. Or Christians. It'll come here. It'll spread across the Middle East. It'll kill your men, members of your family. Maybe even you."

"If that's God's will."

"Are you out of your mind?" the Frenchman said, finally starting to grasp what they were talking about. "If it was God's will, he'd do it himself. This isn't a bullet or nerve gas or even a nuclear bomb. You can't target an opposing army or country. You can't predict what it will do. And you can't stop it once it's started. It's impossible to win because winning doesn't exist."

"You're wrong, Doctor. With its complexity, interconnectedness, and reliance on technology, the industrialized world will completely collapse. It won't just be disease that kills them. It will be starvation. Cold. Darkness and chaos." He waved a hand around him. "Certainly, millions will die in this part of the world, but that isn't enough to destroy us. It's the way we've lived for millennia."

Bertrand took another step back. "You think . . . You think you can level the playing field?"

Halabi smiled. "I'd forgotten that idiom. Thank you. It encompasses my goals perfectly. The West's financial, human, and military resources will simply cease to exist. As will their desire and ability to interfere in the affairs of others."

The Frenchman had finally retreated far enough that his back hit the cave's stone wall. He seemed to be trying to speak but found himself unable to do so. Halabi filled the silence.

"As I said, infecting my men and getting them into America is relatively simple. As is selecting the cities they'll be sent to. Based on population density, location, and airport activity, the obvious choices are Chicago, Houston, Los Angeles, New York, Seattle, and Atlanta. My men will have no problem finding menial work—cleaning, food service, and the like. The details, though, are somewhat more difficult. How would this best be done? Transportation hubs seem obvious. But what about theaters where people are in very close contact and the virus wouldn't be subject to direct sunlight? What about cashiers who handle money for hundreds of customers a day? And what about when my people begin displaying symptoms? Perhaps nightclubs where the disorienting environment would make those symptoms less noticeable to the people around them?"

"Are you . . . Are you asking me to help you?"

Halabi ignored the question. "Another issue is how to protect my American disciples who will be hosting these people. They're all anxious to be martyred, of course, but it seems that it would be most advantageous not to infect them until my other people are near death. That would create a second wave of infection before the CDC and other authorities fully grasp what's happening."

"I made the anthrax," the Frenchman responded. "And that was probably a mistake. But if you think I'm going to help you do something like this, you're insane."

"Am I?"

"Yes," Bertrand responded. "Once this is put into motion, I'll no longer be of any use to you. You'll kill me. And even if you don't, there's a good chance the disease will."

The scientist fell silent and looked around him, peering into the shadows as though there was something meaningful hidden there. Halabi had seen it many times before. He was experiencing the confusion that all nonbelievers suffered when they realized their lives would soon end. The only thing ahead of him now was a dark, empty eternity.

"Come," Halabi said, standing and walking past Bertrand into the passageway. With no other option, the Frenchman followed. As they approached the end of the corridor, two men appeared and dragged him into a chamber to the left. A strangled scream rose up and then died in Bertrand's throat when he saw what was waiting for him.

Much of Victoria Schaefer's body was rotted away and what was left had been mummified by the dry conditions. Her face was mostly skeletonized, with missing cheeks exposing the roots of her teeth and empty eye sockets staring out through strips of leathery skin. In truth, it was only her clothing and long blond hair that identified her.

"No!" Bertrand finally got out.

Halabi's men forced him onto the table next to the corpse and secured him there with straps. His screams quickly turned to convulsing sobs and he began begging pathetically in French.

Halabi approached and leaned over him as one of his men ignited a blowtorch. Bertrand's face and the rotted one next to it turned bluish in the light of the flame.

"Now let's discuss the fine points of my plan."

CHAPTER 35

SOUTHERN MEXICO

CARLOS Esparza glanced back at the terrified family behind him and slapped a hand on the table. "Otra cerveza!"

They were huddled near the kerosene lamp throwing shadows across what passed for a kitchen. This was the building that was Mitch Rapp's goal, an improvised restaurant that was little more than a clapboard shithole with enough solar panels sufficient to keep a refrigerator running. Outside was a broad porch where local farmers gathered on weekends, but now the plastic furniture on it was in danger of being washed away by the pounding rain.

The husband retrieved a beer, but Esparza shook his head and pointed to the man's fifteen-year-old daughter. She took the bottle and approached hesitantly, holding it out in front of her.

She was a sexy little thing, with thick hair, coffee-colored skin, and a body that was still a bit awkward. He gave her a hard swat on the ass when she put the beer on the table and then watched her scurry off. Normally, he'd be laying plans to have her brought to his compound for a few interesting evenings, but tonight she was nothing more than an afterthought. Something to briefly distract him from the matter at hand.

They'd begun Rapp's test at 9 a.m. and it was now 3 a.m. the next day. One of the dogs had been recovered but the others were still on the loose, running off thousands of dollars' worth of his product. The heavy rains and loss of their tracking ability was allowing the CIA man to move through the darkness with impunity—an opportunity he was taking full advantage of.

At least seven of Esparza's men were dead. Some from bullets, others from knife wounds, and one who had been found with a tree branch wedged in his eye socket. So much equipment had been stripped from the bodies that it seemed certain Rapp was creating caches in the jungle. Preparing to survive and fight for as long as was necessary to reach his objective.

A burst of automatic fire erupted outside and Esparza swore loudly before edging toward the open doorway. He had four vehicles at the crossroad out front, two of which were idling with their headlights on. The rain had slowed and there was enough illumination to see the five men who had taken refuge behind them. All efforts to bring in further reinforcements had gotten bogged down in the mud miles from there.

The shooting stopped and, predictably, the shouting started. Fucking idiots. If they saw or heard something, it was a guarantee that Rapp wasn't there. Terrified for their own lives and enraged at the loss of their comrades, they'd begun shooting at ghosts and fighting among themselves. Exactly what the CIA man wanted.

Esparza stayed hidden behind the doorjamb as he scanned past the vehicles into the darkness. Was he kilometers away, planning his next move? Had he decided to run and take his chances as a fugitive? Or was he out there just beyond the circle of light?

The sound of a struggling vehicle became audible to the east and Esparza reluctantly crossed the wood deck, descending into the mud. Headlights began playing off the trees as his men dug in further. As though Rapp would just get in a car and drive up the road to them.

Idiots.

He took a position in the middle of the crossroad, shielding his eyes as the pickup drew near. One of his enforcers was driving and there were no passengers. At least no living ones. The vehicle stopped and Esparza looked at the man in the bed. He was stretched out in a bloody pool of rainwater, with his throat slashed from ear to ear.

"Find this motherfucker and bring me his head!" Esparza screamed as the rain gained force again. "Do you understand? Bring it to me now!"

No one moved. Finally, one man inched forward. "The dark and the rain are working against us, señor. Maybe we should try to get back to the compound. It's supposed to clear tomorrow and when the sun—"

Esparza pulled a pistol from the holster on his hip and shot the man in the chest. "Does anyone else have something to say?"

None seemed to, so he stalked back toward the building and the cold beer waiting for him there. How much was he paying to be surrounded by a bunch of weaklings? If this was the best they could do, he was a dead man. The other cartels would run over him like he wasn't there. Rapp was *one man*. One fucking man bumbling through jungle terrain he knew nothing about.

He stepped back onto the porch and went for the open doorway. Maybe he'd invite the girl to join him for a drink. His anger and nerves were building to the point that his head was starting to pound. It seemed almost certain that she could find some way to help him relax.

When he entered, Esparza saw a man in fatigues sitting at the table where he had left his beer. He was backlit by the kerosene lamp, but wore an immediately recognizable bandolier. Hand-tooled leather with a holster on one side and a similarly ornate scabbard for his silencer on the other. Pedro Morales had always seen himself in the romantic terms of a nineteenth-century Mexican bandit. But he'd served Esparza well. That is, until his naked body had been found in a ditch six hours ago.

"So if I remember right," Mitch Rapp said, "our agreement was for two hundred and fifty grand a month."

Esparza noticed that the holster was empty and Morales's nickel-plated Colt Government Model 1911 was lying on the table inches from his hand.

"That's your agreement with *me*," Esparza said, having a hard time thinking clearly under the American's stare. "But I'm not sure about my men. You've killed a lot of their friends."

Rapp remained motionless for a moment but then began screwing the matching silencer onto the pistol. He stood and Esparza silently cursed himself for his own stupidity.

Rapp walked past him and the cartel leader heard the sound of his footsteps on the wood porch. He didn't bother to turn, though. It was clear what was coming. His words had condemned what was left of his men to death. They'd see the camouflage-clad man coming from the restaurant and assume he was one of theirs.

Esparza could shout a warning of course. Or even pull out his own weapon and shoot. But then his role in this would fundamentally change. At that moment, he was the man with the job and money Rapp so desperately needed. All it would take was one sound, though. One wrong move. And then he would become just another of the CIA man's victims.

So he remained silent, imagining the scene playing out behind him. The silencer and the rain would keep his men from knowing what was happening until two of them were already dead. One more would die in the ensuing confusion. And the last would be shot in the back as he fled in panic.

Esparza's gaze moved again to the family huddled at the back of the building. They flinched noticeably at a brief burst of automatic gunfire outside. A lone shout rose above the rain and then everything went silent until the sound of footfalls on the porch became audible again.

"You're running out of guys, Carlos."

CHAPTER 36

THE CAPITOL COMPLEX
WASHINGTON, D.C.
USA

"To be clear, this isn't a formal hearing," Senator Christine Barnett said, doing a good job of sounding magnanimous. "We're here to talk without cameras and get an understanding of where we stand in this matter."

Despite her empty assurances, this felt very much like a formal hearing to Irene Kennedy. Barnett was in an elevated position flanked by congresspeople loyal to her. A number of aides were ensconced behind them and the gallery was scattered with people Kennedy assumed were political operatives.

"As you answer our questions, Dr. Kennedy, please keep in mind we're performing our own investigation into these matters."

The implication, of course, was that she'd lie. And that was exactly what she was there to do, but not for the reasons Barnett thought.

Kennedy leaned into the microphone on the table in front of her. "Thank you, Senator. I'll keep that in mind."

Kennedy's initial reaction had been to find a way to avoid this kangaroo court, but it had been impossible. Barnett's power was growing, and with it the upheaval inside the Beltway. Predicting people's shifting loyalties was becoming impossible as they positioned themselves for what was to come next.

"What was your involvement in sending Mitch Rapp to California to interrogate those drug traffickers?"

Word was that Barnett's inquiries into that subject had hit a dead end. The further she tracked the chain of command back, the murkier it got.

"As I've told you in the past, I had no involvement."

"If you're denying that it was you, then who was it?"

It was a question that literally might be the most dangerous in the world. According to Scott Coleman, the president of the United States had not only personally given the order, but had also signed papers giving Rapp carte blanche.

Again, Kennedy leaned into the microphone. "I don't know who authorized Mr. Rapp's involvement, though my people are continuing to look into the matter. Has your office's investigation been able to shed any light on the issue?"

"I'm asking the questions in this hearing!"

Kennedy poured herself a glass of water. The truth was that this meeting served no real purpose. It was a fishing expedition. Barnett was trying to find something explosive for the very public hearing she was undoubtedly planning. But she wasn't going to get it.

"Let me make another clarification, Senator. Mitch Rapp doesn't work for the Central Intelligence Agency and hasn't for some time. He functions as an independent contractor. The last contract the Agency had with him was in relation to tracking Sayid Halabi in Yemen."

"Is it possible that he acted alone?" another one of the senators offered.

The fury registered on Barnett's face before she could prevent it. She was there to gather ammunition against Kennedy and the intelligence community as a whole, not just one man.

"It's absolutely possible," Kennedy responded, deciding to take the gift. "Mr. Rapp is well known in the upper echelons of law enforcement and intelligence. He could have used his reputation and contacts to convince people that he was operating under the authority of the CIA when that in fact wasn't the case."

"In order to murder two drug traffickers, shoot three DEA agents, and steal millions of dollars' worth of narcotics," Barnett interjected.

"That appears to be correct, Senator."

It was an uncomfortable position for Kennedy. Any defense of Rapp could weaken the undercover legend he'd created and get him killed. She wasn't just there to stand by and let the Senate throw Mitch Rapp under the bus. No, she needed to be behind the wheel pushing the accelerator to the floor.

"And this all relates to his illegal financial dealings?" Barnett said, continuing to probe.

"Our investigation is in its initial stages, but that also appears to be correct. Mr. Rapp had a number of foreign accounts and investments of questionable legality. One of his main investments—a financial services company in Poland—collapsed and came under the scrutiny of EU officials. That created a cascade effect."

"Meaning the house of cards he'd built came tumbling down, prompting him to steal those drugs in order to put together enough money to run."

"That's a reasonable conclusion based on the facts that we have at this time, Senator."

"Where did he get all the money to invest, Dr. Kennedy? And how long have those investments existed? We all know what the man does for a living and we're now very aware that he doesn't have any qualms about shooting innocent people."

"If you're suggesting he was taking contract killing jobs on the side, Senator, I doubt that's the case. Much more likely, he simply siphoned funds from the terrorist organizations he broke up. They themselves have extremely complex financial structures and it wouldn't be hard to hide those kinds of transactions."

"But this house of cards he built," Barnett said, still trying to find her footing. "It was constructed while he was officially working for the CIA. Isn't that right? While he was under your supervision."

Kennedy took a sip of water and focused on staying in character. Avoiding personal responsibility and abandoning Mitch Rapp were two things antithetical to who she was. But, for now, there was no other way.

"Obviously, I'm the director of the CIA, so everything that happens there is within my purview. Having said that, the monitoring of our agents is largely the responsibility of an independent division within the Agency. They work under a very specific set of parameters, all of which were adhered to in this case. The problem seems to be that Mr. Rapp covered his tracks extremely well. His money was held in countries that we have a hard time seeing into, and his ownership interests in foreign businesses were hidden behind a maze of offshore shell corporations and partnerships."

"So, you're saying that, as the director of the CIA, you take no responsibility for any of this?"

"The Agency's oversight infrastructure works independently from the office of the director. That independence is critical to their success and credibility. In light of what's happened, though, I'd agree that the system needs to be reviewed."

Christine Barnett entered her office, nearly catching Kevin Gray's leg when she slammed the door.

"Backstabbing bitch!"

"Calm down, Senator. It may—"

"Calm down? What the hell are you talking about, Kevin? Everyone in town whispers about Irene Kennedy like she's Joan of Arc. We went in there counting on the fact that she'd fall on her sword for her lifelong friend, the great Mitch Rapp. And what do we find out? She's just another politician covering her ass."

"We've still got—"

"And then that dipshit Hansen hands her the keys to the handcuffs!" She imitated the man's buttery drawl. " 'Is it possible that he acted alone?' "

"Mitch Rapp was the CIA's top operative for years, Senator, and in that time he stole millions of dollars. The fact that he was technically a contractor when he murdered those two men—"

"Were you not listening, Kevin?"

"Of course I—"

"Rapp killed two *terrorism suspects*. And his money didn't come from stealing from the government, it came from stealing from extremists. Why would voters give a shit about that?"

"He didn't kill those men to stop a terrorist attack, Senator. Like you said in your last meeting with Kennedy, he probably did it to figure out how to get top dollar for the drugs he was going to steal. And he didn't take the money from those terrorist organizations to starve them of funds. He took it to line his own po—"

"Too complicated!" she shouted. "The average American is barely smart enough to tie his own shoes. Do you really expect them to follow complex motivations and offshore shell corporations? In order for them to know who to hate, we need to tell them in a way they can understand. A strong, simple narrative. One sentence. No words more than two syllables."

"We weren't going to get hold of the news cycle anytime soon anyway. This morning's school shooting is sucking all the air out of the room."

"How many kids?"

"It's bad. Twenty-one dead and another seven wounded."

"So we get backseated and the anthrax story—"

"—was already starting to fade," Gray said, finishing her

sentence. "The videos ISIS is putting out are just remixes of footage everyone's seen before."

"If we're going to keep people focused on this administration's inability to protect them, Halabi's going to need to get off his ass and do something more than make movies."

"I'm not sure we should be wishing that on ourselves, Senator."

She dropped into the chair behind her desk. "Don't turn into a Boy Scout on me again, Kevin."

"You're way out in the lead, Sen—"

"I don't want to be in the lead!" she shouted. "I want to win the election in such a landslide that everyone in Washington drops to their knees and kisses my ass. Do you understand?"

Judging by his expression, he didn't.

Kevin Gray was a hell of a political operative but, like everyone in his profession, he saw the winning of the presidency as an end, not a beginning. A seat in the Oval Office was a guarantee of pomp and circumstance, but not the guarantee of real power that most people suspected. As a woman, she'd have to fight for that. She'd have to tear it from the hands of the powerful men who had dominated the country since it was founded.

"The shooting of those DEA agents got some coverage," Gray said. "But because they survived and the identity of the shooter hasn't been released, not as much coverage as we hoped. We could leak that the perpetrator was a former CIA operative and that he also murdered two drug traffickers. Maybe hint that Kennedy could be involved. Everyone knows how close she and President Alexander are. It could get us—"

"Absolutely nothing," Barnett said, finishing his sentence. "In the current news cycle, that story wouldn't make an AM radio station in Bumfuck, Kansas."

"Then we wait," he said, not bothering to hide his frustration. "When things slow down, a story like that could get some traction. No question it'll get the attention of conspiracy theorists and

Russian Internet trolls. They're always looking to give the Agency a black eye."

"We're losing control of this thing, Kevin. We've got a story about incompetence and corruption in this administration that we can spin into full-on hysteria. We can't let it get hijacked by some basement dweller who walked into a school with a gun. We're going to end up spending the next month running in circles debating gun control."

"I don't know what you want me to do," Gray said. "I can only work with what I've got."

She remained silent for almost a minute, calculating the pros and cons of every possible action. Finally she spoke.

"For now we forget about trying to tie Rapp to Kennedy. Instead we leak that the DEA intercepted the anthrax. We show the American voter that this administration allowed ISIS to transport a biological weapon across the U.S. border and the only thing that saved us was dumb luck. We tell them that Halabi's making another batch and that the administration has been keeping it secret from the American people. That Alexander's preventing our citizens from taking steps to protect themselves because he doesn't want to look bad in the press."

"I strongly disagree with that course of action, Senator. Leaking a former CIA agent's involvement in what happened in California is one thing. But this is an ongoing terrorist investigation. That's why the administration is keeping it secret—they're trying to track the supply line back to Halabi. If he discovers that the authorities know about the anthrax he could—"

"He could what? Run? How does that hurt me? The last thing I need is Alexander standing on a podium saying that he tracked down Halabi and put a bullet in his eye."

"Senator, this is—"

"Shut up and do it, Kevin."

"It's going to take some time. We'll use the same procedures as before, but this leak is a whole other level. If it were ever traced back to us . . ." He fell silent, leaving the ramifications to her imagination.

CHAPTER 37

SOUTHERN MEXICO

"IT'S all opportunity now," Esparza said, swerving his custom Humvee around a rut in the dirt road. "Your politicians are just actors. They shout all day about drugs and illegal immigrants but they don't want to fix the problem. They just want to keep their voters angry while not pissing anyone off by taking away their coke or maid. All that shit you talk about us up north . . . separating children from their parents, the wall . . . it's a perfect storm. It puts our politicians in a position that they have to push back. And that doesn't just mean they look the other way. These days I've got more government assistance than I know what to do with. I mean, I pay. Don't get me wrong. And the last local government piece of shit who turned on me got to watch my guys gang-rape his daughter. But even if I didn't do any of that, a lot of our bureaucrats would screw the Americans for the hell of it."

Rapp focused on the edges of the jungle from the passenger seat. In all likelihood it didn't contain any imminent threats, but there was no way to know that for sure. He had no sense of his operating environment, no sense of Esparza's position in the current drug trafficking hierarchy, and no idea what was happening in America or the rest of the world.

"So you're looking to take the opportunity to expand," Rapp prompted. Esparza had been running his mouth nonstop for the entire drive, but so far hadn't said anything useful. Mostly bragging about his business genius and the meteoric growth of his operation.

"Hell yes, I'm going to take advantage. The Arab heroin is going to be big for us. The American government's doing its normal screwup job dealing with your oxycodone problems—half because your politicians are morons and half because they've got their heads completely up the pharmaceutical companies' asses." He paused for dramatic effect. "And you saw the coke plantation."

Rapp just nodded. He'd spent the better part of the week roaming around Esparza's compound, eating María's food, and drinking fresh-squeezed fruit juice. He had no access to phones, television, or computers. Discussions with Esparza tended to be centered on his excessively ambitious business plans and his passion for young girls. Unfortunately, the former subject tended to be overly vague and the latter overly detailed.

"That crop has been even more successful than we thought," Vicente Rossi said from the backseat. "It's obviously a long-term investment but within ten years we expect to have converted it into a significant profit center."

Again, Rapp didn't respond. The trail that led to Sayid Halabi was getting colder every day. He just didn't have the patience for this undercover shit.

"You didn't bring me out here to talk about profit centers," Rapp said finally. "Where are we going?"

Esparza glanced at his assistant in the rearview mirror. An out-of-character nervous tic.

"A meeting."

"Details, Carlos. Give me details."

The cartel leader's jaw tightened in anger, causing his response to sound a bit strangled. "We negotiated the terms of it more than a month ago, but since then things have gone to shit. The asshole we're going to see is named Damian Losa. He's an arrogant, aristocratic prick who's huge but flies way under the radar. He's doing probably a little over a billion U.S. dollars a year gross between blow, heroin, and weed. And that doesn't include his aboveboard businesses. He's got car dealerships in Iowa and factories in England. Son of a bitch gives money to museums and shit."

"What's he to me?" Rapp said.

When Esparza didn't answer, Rossi stepped in. "Losa was one of the main investors in that mall in San Ysidro. It's one of a number of projects financed and operated by a cooperative of cartels presided over by Mr. Losa. His idea was to reduce the fighting between individual organizations by creating joint enterprises. As you can imagine, he isn't happy about it being discovered."

"Didn't NASA find that tunnel?" Rapp said. "How can he blame you for that? Shit happens."

Again Esparza didn't respond, instead concentrating on avoiding the branches on either side of the dirt track.

"The construction of the San Ysidro mall was overseen by our organization," Rossi said.

"So? From everything I heard, you knocked it out of the park. The DEA was talking about that tunnel like it was the eighth wonder of the world."

"Yes," Rossi said, drawing out the word. "But the mall was meant to be a money-laundering operation."

Rapp considered that for a moment. "So you're telling me that the tunnel was something you added without telling Losa and the other cartels?"

"That's correct."

"So a megamillion-dollar money-laundering operation just went up in smoke, a number of American politicians have been exposed for taking cartel money, and a huge number of offshore corporations are now being investigated because you decided to add a smuggling operation on the down low."

"I think that's a fair summary," Rossi said in a tone that suggested he'd disapproved of their little improvisation. "We—"

"It was sitting there like a fat whore!" Esparza shouted suddenly. "If I don't take opportunities like that, someone else will. Where would that leave me?"

"Alive," Rapp said, turning his attention back to a jungle that was suddenly looking a lot more threatening than it had thirty seconds before. "Tell me about the meet."

"It's in a natural clearing in neutral territory. The land around it is mostly open and we've had drones flying overhead for two days now. No suspicious activity. Each of us can bring two men. It'll be fine. And this'll give you an opportunity to get a good look at Losa."

"Why?" Rapp asked, though he suspected he knew the answer.

"Because you're going to kill him. He's not going to let this go and I'm not going to wait for one of his people to slit my throat in my sleep. We need to move first."

"Are you saying you want to do this today? At the meeting?"

"No. The area's controlled by another cartel that's guaranteed our safety. If we move against him here, we might not make it home. Next month will be soon enough."

"Next month," Rapp repeated.

"Is that a problem? I hired a miracle worker, right? Isn't that what you told me? You didn't think I was paying you three million dollars a year to eat my food and work out in my gym. My *private* gym."

Rapp let out a long breath. This was bullshit. He was getting no closer to Halabi and now he was being driven into a possible ambush orchestrated by a man who sounded more like the CEO of General Motors than a drug lord. Time to end this.

He reached for the Glock 19 he'd been provided, keeping his movements slow and casual. He'd find a place for them to pull into the jungle, locate a quiet spot, and go to work on these two pricks. Rossi would crack at the first face slap and, for all his swagger, Esparza wouldn't last much longer. In an hour, Rapp would be using the late cartel leader's bejeweled sat phone to send Irene Kennedy everything the two men knew about ISIS.

"But first I need some help with the Arabs," Esparza said.

Rapp hesitated, finally withdrawing his hand from the weapon and returning it to the armrest.

"I'm listening."

"The first shipment from our Middle Eastern supplier got confiscated in the mall bust. It was actually part of the shipment you stole—a dry run to show them what our distribution system could do."

"And?"

"The towelheads have access to good product but they're complete assholes to deal with. They don't understand shit about the smuggling business and got all twisted up over us losing their package."

I'll bet they did, Rapp thought.

When Esparza spoke again, his voice had lost some of its bravado. "Look, this heroin angle could mean a lot of money for me, and with what happened in San Ysidro, it needs to work."

"Meaning?"

"Meaning, you understand them, right? You speak their language and everything."

"Yeah."

"Then you could explain that what happened is just part of doing business and that no one else could do any better. Make sure they're not trying to find another organization to partner with."

After a week of feeling Halabi slipping away, Rapp could suddenly picture his head in the sights of his Glock again. "Sure. I could fly over and tell them how things work in the real world. Maybe help coordinate their shipments."

"That won't be necessary," Rossi said, leaning up between the seats. "They're flying in a representative with another small shipment."

"Right. All you need to do is talk his gibberish, kiss Allah's ass, and whatever else it takes to get his confidence. This time the product will get through. I guarantee it."

Rapp nodded and further relaxed his gun hand. While it wasn't Sayid Halabi's home address and a spare cruise missile, it was enough to work with. Esparza and Rossi had just earned themselves a temporary reprieve.

Esparza pulled into a gap in the foliage that looked like it had been recently cut. Beyond there was a small clearing with three men visible in the shade of its northern edge.

"That's him," Esparza said, without looking. "In the middle."

Damian Losa looked to be in his mid-fifties, with a trim waist, nice but not over-the-top clothing, and immaculate gray hair. The men on either side of him were just muscle, but even at a distance it was clear they were high-class muscle. Probably Eastern European. Almost certainly former spec ops. Whether there were a hundred more like them in the trees was yet to be seen. Relying on Esparza's surveillance team wasn't all that comforting but there wasn't a choice at this point.

They got out of the vehicle and Esparza indicated for him and Rossi to hang back while he started for the center of the clearing. Losa began to do the same but then one of his men grabbed his arm. Rapp moved a hand closer to his weapon, but it seemed that all he wanted to do was whisper in his boss's ear. He gave a brief response before walking to meet Esparza.

The conversation seemed to go about the way Rapp had imagined. Esparza was animated, waving his hands around and speaking in a loud voice, while Losa nodded and answered too quietly to be heard at a distance.

More interesting was that one of Losa's guards had broken away from his companion and was edging around the clearing. Again, Rapp moved a hand toward his weapon, but then the man got close enough to make out his features.

"How've you been, Andraž?"

"Good, Mitch. Mr. Losa would like a word with you after he's finished."

"Why?"

He just shrugged and started back the way he'd come.

The discussion between the two cartel leaders went on for another fifteen minutes before Esparza spun and began stalking back in their direction. Losa, on the other hand, stayed put and turned his gaze toward Rapp.

Screw it. Why not?

He started forward and Esparza waved him off. "We're leaving."

Rapp ignored him and passed by without speaking. When he got close to Losa the man offered a hand and he took it.

"Andraž recognized you," he said in lightly accented English. "I heard about your problems in America but I'm surprised to see you here. Can I assume that the drugs you stole belonged to Carlos?"

"Yeah," Rapp said, glancing back to see Esparza glaring at him and questioning Rossi in a low voice.

"And what exactly is your interest in all this?"

"I don't understand the question."

"I think you do."

Clearly Losa wasn't buying the legend Rapp had created to explain his sudden entry into the narcotics business.

When he stayed silent on the subject, Losa just smiled. "Even if everything you've done recently is a smoke screen, I believe that

Christine Barnett's animosity toward you is real. You're going to have a hard time going back."

"Are you coming to a point?"

The man pulled out a business card and slipped it into Rapp's shirt pocket. "When you've killed Carlos—and I assume that will be in the next week or two—call me. I think you'd find working for my organization very rewarding."

Rapp nodded and turned, but then paused when Losa spoke again. "And if your friend Irene Kennedy finds herself needing to make a quick exit from the United States, my offer extends to her as well."

Rapp walked back to the Humvee thinking that maybe Coleman and Claudia were right. In the private sector all you had to do was stand around while people threw money at you.

"What the fuck was that all about?" Esparza said.

"He figures I'm going to kill you in the next couple of weeks and wants to give me a job after I do." Rapp slid into the passenger seat. "Now let's get the hell out of here before someone changes his mind and starts shooting."

CHAPTER 38

NORTH OF HARGEISA
SOMALIA

SAYID Halabi embraced the last person in line and stepped back as all six filed away. Allah had provided a rare overcast night, blinding any U.S. surveillance that might be overhead and extinguishing the stars. He was standing at the edge of the hazy ring of light created by a bonfire some fifty yards away. The light breeze swept the smoke toward him, bringing with it the sensation of warmth and scent of charred wood.

Near the fire a young girl lay on a cot, deathly still between violent coughing fits. From a safe distance, a man filmed the towering flames that framed her. He followed the embers swirling through the air for a moment and then focused on the six martyrs approaching the girl. Each wiped a hand across her face, smearing their fingers with saliva, blood, and phlegm, and then rubbing it into their eyes and noses.

When it was done, two of the men threw the cot and its dying occupant into the fire. Her screams filled the air for a moment before going silent forever.

Gabriel Bertrand looked on from beneath the tree he was chained to, watching in horror as the girl's body writhed and blackened. Finally, he turned toward the people stripping off their clothing and cleaning themselves with powerful disinfectants. Halabi didn't want them to leave a trail of disease that Western authorities could follow to him in Somalia. But more than that, he wanted the infection to appear in America as though it had come from nowhere. As though it was a punishment from God's own hand.

Tears reflected on the Frenchman's swollen cheeks and he began to sob. Whether he wept over his own fate or that of the world was impossible to know. Of course, he had broken easily. The removal of one of his fingernails had gained his cooperation and a few minor burns near his groin had ensured that it would be enthusiastic.

Halabi now had an optimized plan for spreading YARS throughout the West while sparing the Middle East to the degree possible. Individual targets had been identified, protocols had been refined, and timetables had been developed. Using software downloaded from the Internet, they had run a number of simulations based on different variables.

Even if nearly everything went wrong during deployment and the West's reaction was more robust than anticipated, the death toll would be no less than ten million, centered on major cities in America and Europe. If everything went to plan, though, the outcome would be very different. The disease would run out of control, creating a pandemic that would fundamentally change human existence for generations.

The computer application that they were relying on had originally been designed to research the spread of the Spanish flu. Comparing that disease with YARS was a fascinating exercise, as was comparing the world it devastated to the one that existed today.

The very name "Spanish flu" was just another lie foisted on the world by America. The truth was that the disease had first taken hold in Kansas City military outposts. It killed more U.S. troops during World War I than combat, spreading easily in the cramped conditions that prevailed on ships, battlegrounds, and bases.

The initial reaction of the medical community had been slowed by its focus on the war, but when the scope of the threat was recognized, the country had pulled together. Surgical masks were worn in public to slow the spread of the disease. Stores were prohibited from having sales to prevent the congregation of people in confined spaces. Some cities demanded that passengers' health be certified before they boarded trains.

There was no denying that the United States and its citizens had been strong in the early twentieth century—accustomed to death and hardship, led by competent politicians, and informed by an honest press.

So much had changed in the last century. The American people were now inexplicably suspicious of modern medicine and susceptible to nonsensical conspiracy theories. They were selfish and self-absorbed, willing to prioritize their own trivial desires over the lives of their countrymen. Their medical system, designed less to heal people than to generate profits, would quickly collapse as it was flooded by desperate patients and abandoned by personnel fearful of being infected.

And during all this, America's politicians and media would use the burgeoning epidemic to augment their own power and wealth. That is, until the magnitude of the crisis became clear. Then they would flee.

The sound of a truck engine pulled him from his contemplation and he turned. His people, disinfected and wearing clean clothing, climbed into the vehicle and set off into the darkness. Halabi bowed respectfully in their direction, acknowledging their sacrifice and the enormity of the journey ahead of them. After the long drive to Mogadishu, they would board a private jet that would take them to Mexico. From there they would be smuggled across the northern border.

And then everything would change.

As he stared into the darkness beyond the fire, he recalled the black-and-white images he'd seen of the Spanish flu epidemic. The most striking, as always, were those that contained children. Like the little ones of the Middle East, they stared out from the photograph with a mix of ignorance, hope, and misplaced trust in the adults around them.

On a blurred portrait taken in a hospital ward, someone had scrawled a nursery rhyme created by minds too young to understand the collapse of their world but desperate to somehow acknowledge it.

I had a little bird,
Its name was Enza.
I opened the window,
And in-flu-enza.

CHAPTER 39

SOUTHERN MEXICO

RAPP paused to check his reflection in the glass door before exiting onto the terrace.

The set of clippers provided by María only had one setting so his previously long hair was now a uniform three eighths of an inch. The beard was completely gone, leaving smooth, slightly pale skin in its wake. A pair of aviator sunglasses hid his eyes and the sun damage around them.

Combined with clothing loose enough to obscure his muscular physique, it was a pretty effective disguise. Esparza and his people had been warned not to use his name around the Arab who was about to arrive. There was a good chance Rapp had killed someone he knew at some point.

An SUV appeared to the west as Rapp came up behind Esparza and Rossi, who were already waiting. Their impeccable clothing and expectant expressions once again demonstrated the importance of this deal to them.

The vehicle pulled up and a man carrying a large courier bag immediately stepped out. Rapp remained outwardly serene but his heart rate notched higher.

He and Muhammad Attia had never been face-to-face but Rapp knew everything about him. His height and weight. His U.S. passport number. Even the name of his first girlfriend in high school. Attia's family had immigrated to America as refugees when he was still a toddler and done well for themselves, providing their son a life of middle-class security.

What had turned him against his adopted country was something that the Agency's psychologists speculated on endlessly. As far as Rapp was concerned, all that mattered was that he was a smart, fanatical son of a bitch who could blend effortlessly into American society. A man that Rapp had spent a lot of time trying to hunt down and kill.

Resisting the urge to jam a thumb into his eye socket, Rapp instead gave him a stilted greeted that would camouflage his real ability with the Arabic language. Westerners with native-level fluency were unusual enough that they tended to generate questions.

"I speak English," Attia replied.

Esparza smiled and offered his hand. "That's excellent. I'm Carlos. This is my assistant Vicente."

Attia shook hands a bit reluctantly, more interested in scanning his operating environment just as Rapp had been when he'd arrived.

Esparza pointed at Rapp. "Don't just stand there. Take his bag."

The cartel leader had been expecting all communication to have to be translated and was clearly enjoying being in a stronger position than expected. His curt order was intended as a reminder. *You work for me.*

Attia held the satchel out as Esparza put a friendly hand on his back. "Come. We have lunch prepared. I'm certain you're going to enjoy it." He glanced back at Rapp as they started toward a dining table decorated with fresh-cut flowers. "Take that to his room. And then you're dismissed."

Instead of going to Attia's room, Rapp ducked into his own and locked the door. A quick search of the courier bag turned up what he was looking for: a duct-taped package about the size of a building brick.

He laid it in the bottom of the bathtub before digging a box of scrounged supplies from beneath the vanity. The sunglasses, a pair of kitchen gloves, and a scarf tied over his nose and mouth was the best he was going to do for protection. Better than nothing, but he imagined that it would get a disgusted face palm from Gary Statham.

Using a pocketknife, he carefully peeled back the tape to expose a shrinkwrapped core. The color and consistency of its contents were exactly like the pictures he'd seen of the intercepted anthrax. Lady Luck was with him. Or not, depending on whether he started coughing up blood in the next few weeks.

He filled the bathtub and worked beneath the surface, slitting the plastic and emptying it into the water. When it looked pretty well cleaned out, he drained the tub and washed both it and the bag with a bottle of high-end tequila that was the most reliable disinfectant he'd been able to turn up. It took another ten minutes to mix a decent facsimile of the anthrax with stuff raided from the kitchen.

He was forced to replace the shrink-wrap cellophane from María's personal stash, but the original tape was salvageable with the help of a little superglue. It likely had hidden markings and their absence would be noticed by men down the supply chain.

Finally, Rapp patted the package with a bath towel and used a blow dryer to eradicate any remaining moisture. The finished product wasn't bad. Someone would have to be paying serious attention to attribute the damage to anything more than normal wear and tear.

He put it back in the bottom of the bag and then carefully replaced the clothes and other items in the order they'd been removed. Now all he needed to do was take it to Attia's room, trace him back to wherever he came from, find Halabi, kill him, and wipe out his operation. Preferably before Attia's contacts in the United States noticed they were trying to destroy the great Satan with a mixture of flour, cornstarch, and dried mustard.

What could possibly go wrong?

CHAPTER 40

CENTRAL IOWA
USA

"I WANT you all to look around," Christine Barnett said, gazing out over the crowd. "Let what you see really sink in."

As was their custom, they did as they were told. Almost two hundred people, mostly men wearing work clothes despite being unemployed, craned their necks to examine their surroundings.

The building was cavernous and filthy. Disused machines stood silent and rusted. Spotlights had been brought in and were focused on the stage, leaving her audience illuminated only by what sunlight could filter through broken windows.

America was booming economically. The stock market was rallying, unemployment was under four percent, and corporate profits were near record highs. But none of that mattered as long as there were a few crumbling factories and pockets of forgotten citizens like the ones before her. Their confused, angry faces made all those statistics meaningless. And more important, it made Joshua Alexander's affirmations of his administration's success look callous and out of touch.

When attention turned back to her, she leaned closer to the microphone. "We have the world's biggest economy. We have the most powerful military in history. We invented pretty much everything worth having. Cars. Electric light. Personal computers. Smartphones. The Internet. *We* push the world forward. *We* keep it safe. How did this happen? How did we *allow* this to happen?"

The inevitable applause started and she stepped back to gaze benevolently over the crowd. Of course, the answers to her question were well known. Mechanization had made many factory jobs obsolete. Others had inevitably—and, in truth, irretrievably—flowed overseas.

The world was changing at an ever-increasing rate and that was a trend that couldn't be stopped. These people were the ones who had been left behind. The ones who steadfastly refused to leave the dead cities they had been born in. The ones who saw themselves as America's backbone but who survived on government aid and disability checks. Drug addicts, drunks, and halfwits incapable of performing anything but the simplest of tasks.

Ironically, it was those self-destructive traits that made them so useful. Their inflated sense of worth and victimization was easy to manipulate. When asked what exactly it was they wanted, they either didn't know or weren't willing to make the sacrifices necessary to get it. What they did know—with burning certainty—was what they hated: the world that had stolen everything from them.

"You didn't lose your way of life," Barnett said. "It was *taken* from you. The incompetence and corruption in Washington has gotten so bad that an honest hardworking person can't succeed in this country. That's not the America I know. It's not the America we grew up in. The country I remember was one where being honest and hardworking *guaranteed* success. It guaranteed that you could provide for your families and that your children could expect to do even better."

She waited for another wave of applause to die down.

"Instead, we spend trillions sending our brave men and women to fight and die overseas. For what? To spread peace and democracy? The people in those countries don't *want* peace and democracy. And even if they did, why is this our job? Why aren't we using that money and our incredible military to fix the problems we have here? Why are we building bridges and power grids in Afghanistan while we watch ours fall apart? They told us these wars and all this nation building was going to keep us safe, but trillions of dollars later, it's done the opposite. Now we have a madman threatening us with a biological attack. And what's this administration's response? To keep doing the same things that haven't worked in the past."

She pulled the microphone off its stand and began pacing across the stage. "America's the strongest country in the history of the world. But even it can't take this kind of incompetence year after year. Nothing's unbreakable. So now it's up to us. This is a democracy. It's our responsibility to turn this around. To protect our country and change it back into one where good, hardworking people aren't taken advantage of. They're rewarded."

"You were on fire today," Kevin Gray said as Barnett slid into the back of the limo across from him. "Reactions look good."

"Are we going to get decent television coverage?"

"I'm pushing, but political speeches in Iowa aren't exactly ratings grabbers. One of the British royals just announced she's pregnant and President Alexander's out there stumping hard for your opponent. His rally in Texas was quite a bit more successful than we'd anticipated. After almost eight years, he can still pack 'em in."

"We've got to choke him off, Kevin. He's the past. We have to *own* the media on this. I don't want to see that man's face or hear his redneck drawl on any outlet in America."

"Alexander was the clear star of the show, Senator. But that's a good thing. You're not running against him. Col—" He caught himself before uttering the name of the man who was now almost certain to be her opponent in the general election. She'd forbidden the speaking of it out loud in her presence. "*Your opponent* looked like a sidekick."

"Where are we with the anthrax story?" she asked.

The glass separating them from the driver was soundproof, but Gray still leaned forward and lowered his voice. "Our contact in the press has the information. He's gone through it, and my understanding is that he's satisfied."

"So he's going to run with it."

Gray nodded, looking a little queasy. "In the next forty-eight hours, the equivalent of a nuclear bomb is going to go off in the press. Mexican cartels smuggling anthrax. NASA and dumb luck keeping it from hitting the street. A former CIA operative shooting DEA agents. It'll be splashed across virtually every news outlet in the world."

"And none of it can be traced to us."

"If anything, it's going to look like it came from somewhere inside the DEA."

"You're sure? That bitch Irene Kennedy has eyes and ears everywhere."

"She'd have to be psychic. I used a brand-new laptop running a secure, open-source operating system. Heavily encrypted email from anonymous account to anonymous account. And now the laptop's crushed and lying in a landfill."

Barnett nodded. In truth, the weak link was the reporter himself. Alexander and Kennedy would unquestionably accuse him of collapsing an ongoing terrorism investigation, but the clock was ticking. Even if they threw him in jail, he'd be watching the poll numbers and know that all he had to do was wait. In a few months Barnett would be president, Alexander would scramble for anonymity, and Kennedy would be on her way to prison.

Of course, it would have been neater to have the reporter killed after his story broke and to use his death to feed a conspiracy theory implicating the CIA. But that had the potential to light a fire that she didn't have the power to control.

At least not yet.

CHAPTER 41

SOUTHERN MEXICO

RAPP stepped out of the air-conditioning and into the late morning heat. The sun was in the process of clearing last night's rain from the jungle, creating a palpable cloud of humidity. Esparza and Vicente Rossi were on the terrace, sitting at a shaded table.

Security was unusually heavy, with no fewer than twenty camo-clad men in view. Many were new, raided from other cartel operations to replace the men Rapp had killed. He memorized their positions and weapons as he strode toward the table. There was an empty place setting for him, but instead of sitting at it Rapp took a position that would allow him to keep his back to the building. He wasn't normally invited to these meetings and that, combined with the heavy security, was putting him on guard.

"Not hungry?" Esparza said, shoveling some pineapple in his mouth.

Rapp just shook his head and continued to watch the guards through dark sunglasses. They didn't seem to be paying much attention to him and most didn't look smart enough for tricks. If he was the target, he'd be getting furtive glances and Esparza wouldn't be sitting so close.

"Things keep getting worse for your friend Irene Kennedy. Our informants say there are a lot of rumors floating around Washington that she knew about your financial dealings and might have been involved."

"She can handle it. In the end, Irene always comes out on top."

"The story about what you did to those DEA agents still hasn't broken. Maybe I should send CNN my drone footage. Throw a little gas on the fire."

Rapp just shrugged. "Why am I here? Problems with the Arabs?"

There was a flash of anger in Esparza's eyes. He was a man accustomed to deference, but he was also a man backed into a corner. A corner that he thought Rapp could get him out of.

"If you're worried about losing that package again," Rapp continued, "I could take it over the border myself. I'll guarantee its delivery."

He made certain to sound bored at the prospect of acting as a delivery boy, but beneath his vague frown, he felt very much the opposite. If he could make contact with even one of Halabi's men in the United States, Kennedy could put multiple surveillance teams on him. Combined with penetration into phone and Internet communication, they could have eyes on the entire network within a week.

"Fuck the Arabs," Esparza said. "I should lose their shit again on purpose. Teach those whiny little assholes that they can't start crying like women every time the cops get lucky."

"Why don't I have a conversation with the guy that came in yesterday? I could give him a lesson on the facts of life."

"He's gone," Rossi said, searching Rapp's face for a reaction to his statement. The former CIA man didn't give him anything, keeping his expression dialed to bored irritation while running through a string of screamed curses in his mind.

"Back to the Middle East?" he said, sliding an empty plate toward him and scooping some bacon onto it.

"We're not that lucky," Esparza replied. "Those assholes won't stop riding me about their lost product. They're bringing men into a private airstrip about an hour from here. That asshole went to pick them up. He wants us to smuggle them into the U.S. to keep an eye on my distribution network."

Esparza slammed his fork down on the tabletop as his voice became a shout. "Piece of shit! He's bringing in men to watch *my* operation? They don't know dick about what I deal with here. They just run around the desert picking poppies and fucking goats. I have to deal with border security, the cops, the FBI, the DEA, and those pricks at the IRS. And if that wasn't enough, now I've got NASA poking its nose into my operation. Fucking *NASA*! What do these assholes think they're going to do about that? Attack Cape Canaveral on camels?"

Esparza's face had turned bright red and the sweat was starting to run down his forehead when he finally fell silent. The question seemed rhetorical but his intense gaze suggested that an answer was required.

"I don't know," Rapp said honestly.

Halabi would have already had a network in place for the first shipment of anthrax. Why bring in more people now? It was a huge risk with no apparent payoff.

"That's it?" Esparza said. "*I don't know*? You told me you were the world's great expert on these people."

"I can't read their minds, Carlos. When he gets back, hand him over to me. I'll get you your answers."

Esparza contemplated Rapp's clean-shaven face for a moment

and then slid a manila envelope across the table. "We have bigger problems than a bunch of towelheads spying on my operation."

"What?" Rapp said, ignoring the envelope and instead stabbing a slice of pineapple with his fork.

"Damian Losa is trying to put the screws to me on this mall thing. He and my other partners already made enough off that deal to pay back their investment but now they want more."

Rapp opened the envelope and thumbed through its contents. Pictures of Losa, his houses, his security. Bios on his bodyguards, information on his family and the school his kids went to. Even a copy of the itemized bill for armoring his Range Rover.

"Not an easy job," Rapp said, speaking on automatic as his mind tried to make sense of Halabi's latest move. "Losa's got more security than the president."

"I'm paying you a lot of money and you don't do anything but eat my food and kill my men. Time to step up."

"You want it to look like an accident? Or would you ra—"

"I want a fucking *fireball*! I want people scraping him and his family off the sidewalk with a toothpick. I want to send the message that anyone who screws with me is a walking dead man."

"I don't do families."

"You work for me."

"It's unprofessional, Carlos. And I have a reputation to protect. If you want his wife and kids taken out, get one of your other people to do it. His oldest son's nine and his wife wears three-inch heels. You must have *someone* who can shoot straight enough to hit targets that slow."

Esparza opened his mouth to respond but Rapp cut him off. "I'll need a team. Two men should do it. I have people in mind."

"A team? That comes out of your pocket."

Rapp smiled and dabbed his mouth with his napkin. "Not how it works, Carlos. Expenses are yours."

"You're not the only killer in the world."

"Then bring in a second-stringer who'll work on the cheap. But if they screw up—if Damian Losa survives—he's going to come down on you like the wrath of God. You've got one chance at this and you can afford precisely a zero percent chance of failure. I—and only I—can provide that."

Esparza's temper flared again and again he managed to control it. The man was in an even tighter box than Rapp had imagined. Losa and the other cartels were breathing down his neck, his marijuana operation had hit serious headwinds, his cocaine cultivation initiative was years from providing any real benefit, and his foray into Middle Eastern heroin was bogging down. The cartel leader was stretched to the breaking point and he knew it.

Before anyone could speak again, the sound of a motor started to separate itself from the hum of the jungle. The guards all straightened and pulled their weapons off their shoulders.

Esparza walked to the edge of the terrace, watching a white panel van approach from the west. It went as far as it could on the worsening road, finally pulling beneath the trees at the edge of the compound. Attia jumped out of the driver's side and went to the back, opening a set of double doors to let the passengers out.

Rapp took a position next to Esparza and examined them as they began filing up the road. Six in all, no fighters. Two were probably in their mid-fifties, another in his late teens. There was even a woman—hunched as she covered her mouth and tried to suppress a cough. These weren't people trained to keep tabs on Esparza's operation. They had been chosen for their ability to blend in—to move through America unchallenged. But to what end? Suicide bombers? That seemed a little mundane after all the trouble Halabi had gone through to hype his biological attack.

"These are the people they sent to spy on your ops?" Rapp said, trying to prompt Esparza to break his silence. When it didn't work, he pressed a little harder.

"These aren't traffickers. Look at them. There's something going on here and we need to figure out what it is."

"I don't give a shit what they look like. I just want this deal done."

"I don't think—"

"I didn't ask you what you think!" he shouted. "They told us we're supposed to keep our distance and that's what we're going to do."

"What do you mean 'keep our distance'?"

"I don't know. Maybe they think we're going to corrupt them. Give them a drink and some pork or something. Either way, no one's supposed to get any closer than ten meters and they wanted them to be housed as far from the compound as possible. Fuck 'em. I just cleared out the main equipment shed. If they want to sleep on the ground in there, let 'em."

Just as he finished speaking, one of the older men started coughing. It wasn't the light hack the woman had displayed a few moments before, though. The convulsions doubled him over. Two men grabbed him by the arms and kept him moving forward as the pieces began clicking together in Rapp's mind.

Halabi's men hadn't killed all the people in that Yemeni village like their propaganda films depicted. They'd taken them and used them to keep the virus alive. And now this innocuous group of people would be smuggled across the border where they'd infiltrate airports and stadiums and restaurants—anywhere people gathered in large numbers.

He remembered the briefing he'd gotten on the YARS virus before he'd gone to that village. The warnings about touching even the charred remains of the buildings. The fear in the voice of the famously unflappable Gary Statham.

"Mitch . . ." Esparza said. "Mitch!"

Rapp finally tore his gaze from the place where the Arabs had disappeared into the jungle, fighting to keep his expression neutral. "What?"

"Forget these pricks. They're just noise. Losa's the only thing you need to worry about right now. Once he's gone, I'll be back in the driver's seat."

CHAPTER 42

A HAND gripped Carlos Esparza's shoulder and gave it a weak shake. He came out of his light sleep but didn't bother opening his eyes. He could neither feel the heat of the sun angling through the windows nor hear the sounds of the staff preparing for the new day. It was still the middle of the night.

"Go back to sleep or get out."

The girl was young, beautiful, and blessed with an unusual level of sexual enthusiasm. Other than that, though, she was a complete pain in the ass. Sleep was hard enough to come by these days without some seventeen-year-old whore jabbing at him.

It seemed that everything that could go wrong *had* gone wrong over the course of just a few months. On the positive side, though, problems that arose so quickly could recede at a similar pace. He'd get the Arabs and their product into the United States without incident this time and then the heroin profits would start flowing. Rapp would deal with Losa. And then he would deal with Rapp. It would be a shame, but unavoidable. When Christine Barnett became president of the United States, she would make Rapp public enemy number one. It would be too much heat for his organization to bear.

The question was whether to kill Rapp or make a deal with the U.S. government to turn him over. His impression of Barnett was that she was even more corrupt and power hungry than the Mexican politicians he dealt with on a day-to-day basis. And while the mundane bribes he was accustomed to paying out wouldn't interest her, Mitch Rapp in chains was another matter. Certainly there could be little harm in having the gratitude of the world's most powerful leader.

He let his head sink deeper into his pillow, putting the matter out of his mind and starting to drift again. One problem at a time.

The hand gripped him again, this time tighter. He was about to swat at the girl but then heard a harsh whisper.

"Carlos! Wake up!"

The sound of Vicente Rossi's voice jolted him awake. What was the man doing in his bedroom? Instinctively, he reached for the bedside lamp, but Rossi slapped his hand away.

The girl next to him rolled onto her back. "Carlos, are you—"

Rossi lurched forward and clamped a hand over her mouth. "Be silent, bitch! Stay still and don't speak! Do you understand?"

Esparza saw the vague outline of her head move up and down before his assistant pulled back.

"What the fuck are you doing in here?" he whispered, trying to get control of the situation while his heart pounded uncomfortably in his chest. "Is it Losa? Are we—"

"Shut up!" Rossi said, pulling a phone from his pocket. The screen lit up, bathing the gaunt face of his assistant in a dull blue light.

"What—"

"Read it," Rossi ordered.

Esparza looked at the phone, scanning a headline about the interception of anthrax on the U.S. border. "A news story? You woke me up for this? What the—"

"Don't talk. Read!"

Esparza took the phone and scanned through the story, his anger flaring when he reached the part stating that the intercept had been made at the San Ysidro mall.

"Those motherfuckers," he said under his breath.

The Arabs he was dealing with weren't heroin traffickers. They were terrorists trying to use his network to smuggle a bioweapon into the United States.

"Tell the guards to go to the shed and kill every one of—"

"Forget the Arabs!"

Esparza fell into confused silence.

"You trusted Mitch Rapp enough to hire him based on one thing and one thing only. You believe that a man like him doesn't care about drug trafficking." Rossi tapped the screen. "But he does care about this."

Mitch Rapp stood motionless and listened to the jungle around him. The hum of insects. The quiet rustling of leaves created by a breeze too light to feel. The rhythmic dripping of water.

The only practical way out of Esparza's house without being seen was through a narrow strip of bushes that extended all the way to the walls. Rapp had climbed out a window when two guards briefly abandoned their posts to share a cigarette. Slipping beneath the foliage, he'd spent the next hour and a half inching along the power conduit it hid. Finally, he'd made it to the jungle.

And that's where he was still, looking back at the dark compound. Esparza ran his security in two twelve-hour shifts, with all posts manned around the clock and three additional roaming guards at night. The problem was that none of those men were currently visible. All posts now appeared to be empty and everything was silent. On the surface, that lack of guards would seem to be a good thing. But it was unexpected. And he hated unexpected.

Coming up with a coherent strategy to handle this situation had turned out to be harder than he'd anticipated. His first plan had been to get to Rossi's phone, but it was an idea that didn't hold up under examination. Assuming he could get into Rossi's room undetected and assuming Rossi had a phone capable of connecting internationally without Esparza's authority, what then? Call Kennedy for the cavalry? Based on his last conversation with Esparza, she was fighting for her political life. And he wasn't in Iraq or Afghanistan. This was Mexico, a country that wouldn't take kindly to a bunch of U.S. troops rolling in unannounced.

Further, the threat he faced wasn't just a shed full of bioweapons; it was a shed full of bioweapons that could think and move on their own. If they made it out of here, the shit was going to hit the fan in a way that no one had seen for more than a century.

In light of all that, there was no point in trying to get fancy. Better to just shoot them all, close their bodies up in the shed, and set it on fire. Nice and neat on the bioweapon front but it did leave one small loose end.

Him.

He didn't need Gary Statham to tell him that if he went into that building and started splattering blood around, he had a high probability of being infected. So when this was over, he couldn't risk any human contact at all. No going back to the house. No fighting with guards. No getting to a phone. At best, his next two weeks would be spent living barricaded in a muddy cave in the mountains. At worst, his next two weeks would be spent dying barricaded in a muddy cave in the mountains.

Another careful scan of the compound didn't turn up any sign of the missing guards, so he started forward again. Staying silent in the dense foliage forced him to move at a crawl but he finally came alongside the shed housing the Arabs.

All the equipment and supplies the clapboard building had once contained were now piled haphazardly around it. Rapp dropped to his stomach and slithered across the damp earth, aiming for what appeared to be a small tractor stacked with rakes and shovels.

The tractor likely contained the gasoline he needed, but accessing it would be more than he wanted to deal with. Fortunately, just past a pile of rotting pallets, he found a much more convenient five-gallon gas can. A gentle nudge confirmed that it was almost full, prompting him to start screwing the suppressor to his Glock. Once secured, he weaved back through the equipment toward the front of the building.

The plan had been simple. Kick in the door. Shoot everyone inside using muzzle flashes for illumination. A little gasoline. A match. And then run for the hills.

Unfortunately, that plan broke down before he even made it to step one. When he arrived at the door, it was wide-open.

Rapp pulled his T-shirt over his nose and mouth before edging toward the threshold. He flicked a lighter, letting the brief spark illuminate the interior.

Empty.

The shooting started a moment later. He spun instinctively but then realized it wasn't coming from anywhere near him. Through the trees, he could see that the side of Esparza's home was lit up with the wavering light of automatic fire. And while it was impossible to determine how many guns, their location was easy to pinpoint. His bedroom.

Rapp retrieved the gas can, emptying its contents on the shed's exterior walls. When he reached the door again, he tossed the empty container inside and then circled again, this time with his lighter. By the time he was finished, the flames on the far side were already ten feet high.

The sound of gunfire at the house had stopped and the shouting had begun. He couldn't understand any of it, but the tone suggested that they'd finally realized they were shooting at an empty bed.

CHAPTER 43

"BACK up, idiots!"

As the tight group of guards lurched back into the hallway, Esparza made sure to stay slightly lower than the men surrounding him. The one exception was Vicente Rossi, who looked like he wanted to drop to his knees and crawl.

The morons he was currently using for cover had fired on an empty bed, most completely emptying their clips in one terrified burst. Now they were retreating down the hall toward an exit on the south side of the compound. Everyone remembered what Rapp had done to their comrades and the few who had been unwise enough to leave themselves without ammunition looked like they were ready to break ranks and run.

"Stay together!" Esparza shouted. "If we separate, he'll pick us off one by one."

It was a lie, of course. Mitch Rapp had no interest in the guards that Esparza was using as a human shield. In fact, it was possible that he wasn't interested in any of them. It was the Arabs he wanted. The fucking lying towelheads who had—

The deafening roar of automatic fire suddenly filled the hallway and Esparza stumbled as the men in front of him began to fall. A few tried to return fire, but their position crammed together in the corridor caused them to jostle each other to the point that accuracy was impossible. Esparza could see muzzle flashes around the far corner of the hallway, but most of the body and face of the shooter was obscured. The men behind Esparza began to flee and he followed, shouting at them to cover him from the rear, to no effect.

The two guards just in front of him went down and he felt a searing heat in his right ear as a bullet grazed him on the way to tearing through another of his men.

The shooter—almost certainly Rapp—turned his attention to the overhead lights and Esparza was showered with glass as the corridor turned to shadow. Next to him, Rossi tripped but managed to stay on his feet as the men in front disappeared around a corner.

Instead of following, Esparza ducked into an expansive, unused library. He began shoving the door closed, but was stopped when Rossi slammed into it from the other side. The younger man fought his way through the gap, gasping for air as Esparza slammed the bolt home. Outside, everything had gone silent. Only the stench of gunpowder remained.

"It's not going to stop him!" Rossi said, stumbling down a short set of stairs that allowed him to reach the far side of the room. The floor had been sunken almost two meters in order to create a dramatic sense of space beneath an open-beamed ceiling. Walls lined with unread books towered over the only furniture in the room—an ultramodern acrylic desk and leather chair. Rossi took cover behind the latter, his university-educated brain unable to comprehend that it would offer little protection.

Esparza was wearing nothing but a pair of sweatpants, loafers with no socks, and a shoulder holster containing his Desert Eagle. He pulled the weapon and aimed it at Rossi.

"What are you—"

Esparza fired a single round into the top of the chair, punching a hole in it and showering his assistant with vaporized leather.

"Go out there and talk to him, Vicente."

"No! He'll shoot me!"

"Why would he do that? He doesn't care about drugs, right? Just explain to him that we knew nothing about the anthrax. Find out what he wants."

"We just tried to kill him, Carlos. *You* just tried to kill him. He—"

Esparza fired another round into the chair, causing Rossi to dive to the floor. "Stop shooting!" he screeched.

"The next one's going in your face, you useless piece of shit! Now get out there!"

The younger man remained frozen for a moment but then seemed to process the fact that his boss wasn't bluffing. He moved reluctantly back up the stairs as Esparza watched over his sights.

"Mr. Rapp!" he shouted through the door. "It's Vicente. We just read the news about the anthrax. This is the first we heard of it. You must know that's true. Why would we get involved in an attack on America? All we want to do is provide a safe, high-quality product to people who want it. No different than your alcohol, tobacco, and pharmaceutical companies. We're in the business of making money. We talked about this. It's the only reason we're working with the Arabs."

"Open the fucking door," Esparza said, continuing to aim the pistol at Rossi. "Do it now."

The younger man complied, sliding back the bolt and letting the door drift back a few centimeters. When nothing happened, he pulled it fully open and took a hesitant step into the hallway.

"This is terrible for our business and we want to help you. We can—"

The sound of automatic fire erupted, drowning him out. Esparza jerked back with the pistol held out in front of him, but immediately recognized that Rapp wasn't responsible. If he'd wanted

Rossi dead, it would have been a single shot between the eyes. More likely a guard who had glimpsed the American when he broke cover to make contact.

Rossi threw himself toward the door but missed and slammed into the jamb instead. The collision caused him to lurch back into the middle of the hallway, where he was hit by at least two rounds. The force of them spun him around and he landed flat on his back, staring sightlessly at the ceiling.

Esparza sprinted to the door, slamming it shut and throwing the bolt again. It wouldn't hold for long if Rapp got to it, but with the guard covering the hallway it would be enough. He retreated down the steps and cut left, feeling for a hidden switch behind a bookcase. Once toggled, the entire shelf assembly swung away. The hidden passage was something he'd insisted on not because he thought he'd ever need it, but because he'd always wanted one. Now it was going to be the thing that saved his life.

Esparza turned sideways, slipping inside and pulling the shelf back into position. The sensation of claustrophobia quickly took hold as he inched through the dim light sandwiched between concrete walls. The architect had insisted on shrinking the size of the passageway to provide a more elegant shape to the library and Esparza silently cursed himself for agreeing.

The sharp corner near the middle almost stopped him. His stomach had expanded over the past few years but panic and a lubricating film of sweat got him through.

Then the lights went out.

Esparza froze, the blood pounding in his ears interfering with his ability to pick something out of the silence. But there was nothing. No gunshots. No shouts. Just the labored rhythm of his own breathing.

In the end, it wasn't his ears that discerned something, but his nose. Smoke. A burst of adrenaline surged through him and he felt his mouth go dry. Had Rapp set fire to the house to flush him out?

He started moving again, panic starting to take hold. Finally, he reached the end of the corridor and searched blindly for the latch. Where was the fire? Where was Rapp? Had he gained access to the library and found the passage? Was he moving silently down it at that very moment? Maybe only a few meters away?

The latch! Where was it?

On the other side of that wall was freedom, Esparza told himself. Rapp, for all his skill, was just one man and the compound was enormous. He couldn't kill what he couldn't find.

His fingers finally grazed a recessed metal handle and he twisted it. The muted click seemed dangerously loud as he twisted his body into a position that would allow him to push the panel open a few centimeters. He was rewarded with a rush of humid, smoky air and the flickering glow of flames. Rapp was a formidable killer, but he wasn't a magician. There would be no way for him to know the passage was there. No way for him to find the exit behind the cascade of vines camouflaging it.

The truth was that while the CIA man had been admittedly good in the jungle, he was out of his element. He didn't speak the language, he wasn't familiar with the territory, and he had no backup or communications. Esparza, on the other hand, suffered from none of these disadvantages. All he had to do was get to his vehicle. Once out of immediate danger, he could call in reinforcements. This time Rapp wouldn't be up against a handful of men. He'd be hunted by military, police, and even local farmers. There would be no escape for him.

The cartel leader inched along the wall with his Desert Eagle held out in front of him. When he came to the edge of the vines, he was finally able to pinpoint the source of the smoke. It wasn't the house that was on fire, it was the shed where the Arabs had been housed.

Esparza finally broke cover near the east side of the building, weaving through widely spaced trees toward a freestanding garage fifty meters away. When he reached the side door, he pressed his back against the wall next to it. His hand was shaking and slick with sweat, but he finally managed to turn the knob. The door swung open on well-oiled hinges and he slipped inside. The dim outline of his Humvee was only a few meters away.

It was heavily armored, with bullet-resistant glass, run-flat tires, and a supercharged engine. There were no weapons Rapp could get his hands on that would be capable of stopping it and no vehicles in the compound that could chase it down.

He crossed the concrete floor in a crouch, peering through the SUV's windows to ensure that Rapp wasn't waiting for him inside.

Empty.

The wave of elation felt similar to the one he'd experienced when he'd escaped the hidden passage. Maybe Rapp wasn't even hunting him. Or, better yet, maybe the traitorous piece of shit had been shot by one of the guards. Anything was possible.

Esparza climbed inside the vehicle, retrieving the key from a hidden compartment beneath the dashboard. The garage door was closed and it would take too much time to raise. While he was confident in the Humvee's armor, it made no sense to gamble his life on it. Better to just ram the door, spin the wheel, and present Rapp with nothing but a set of receding taillights. He twisted the key in the ignition and hovered his foot over the accelerator.

Nothing.

A second twist produced a similar result and he suddenly realized that the interior lights hadn't come on when he'd opened the door. He toggled the switch that controlled them to no avail.

His emotional state swung violently back to terror when he popped the hood and went around to look at the engine. The workings of car engines were a complete mystery to him, but the problem was still immediately evident. The battery was missing.

Esparza sank down behind the driver's-side tire, losing control of his breathing again. It was Rapp. The CIA man was toying with him, trying to make him panic. Trying to make him do something to reveal where he was in the sprawling compound.

Esparza left through the same door he'd entered, holding the gun shaking in his hands. He thought he saw movement in the wavering firelight but managed to keep from squeezing the trigger. Stealth was his only hope now. The slightest sound could lead to his death.

He crept into the jungle, moving through the wet leaves in search of the service vehicles parked seventy-five meters to the east. The darkness deepened and his eyes hunted for human shapes in the trees. Every few seconds he was forced to freeze when his mind tricked him: Rapp coming up from behind. Rapp in a tree waiting to drop. Rapp's mud-streaked hand snaking out from beneath a bush.

He made it to the access road and stayed near its edge, watching silently for movement. All but one of the vehicles—an open Jeep—was gone. Fucking cowards. The surviving guards had taken them and fled.

He remained perfectly still, scrutinizing the vehicle. Normally the keys were left in it, but were they there now? Rapp had no reason to have ever come back there. Would he even be aware that this vehicle storage area existed? No, Esparza tried to convince himself. The CIA man would focus on the compound and the more obvious escape routes.

He tried to stay put but with every passing second he became more impatient. The Jeep was right there. Only a few meters away. He'd drive it up the poorly maintained but passable dirt road that would eventually lead him to civilization. There he could gather his forces and plan his next move.

Finally, he jogged silently across the road and leapt into the lone vehicle. When he reached for the ignition, instead of finding the key he was hoping for, he felt something smooth and wet. Leaning forward, he was able to make out its vague outline. A severed hand still clinging to the key.

Esparza's ability to think abandoned him and he jumped from the Jeep, running up the road away from the compound. After less than twenty-five meters, a searing pain flared in his right leg and he collapsed in a shallow puddle. His mind was struggling to comprehend what had happened and he ran a hand down his leg, stopping at the shattered kneecap.

He screamed and tried to stand, but just went down in the puddle again. A moment later, something got hold of his ankle and began dragging him into the trees.

CHAPTER 44

NORTH OF HARGEISA
SOMALIA

"WE'RE safe."

The words coming over Sayid Halabi's headset were badly distorted but still intelligible. He let out a long, relieved breath, leaning back against the cavern wall and staring blankly into the semidarkness.

He had more than a hundred people throughout the world monitoring the news twenty-four hours a day. Thank Allah they'd discovered the mention of the anthrax interception within minutes of its first posting and he'd been able to get through to Muhammad Attia.

"Esparza's guards didn't try to stop you?"

"We were scheduled to leave around sunrise. The fact that we left early didn't seem to concern them."

"Where are you now?"

"We're in the van on the 307 west of Juncaná. Our GPS says we're approximately nine hours from the warehouse where we're to pick up the truck. What are your orders?"

The plan was for them to drive to Córdoba, where they'd transfer to a semitruck with a hidden compartment designed to smuggle them over the border. The question was how much had their situation changed? Was it necessary to radically alter his plans in light of this leak from the U.S. government? He could have Attia drop off individuals in various towns on the route north, but what would that accomplish? They didn't speak Spanish, they had no safe haven in or paperwork for Mexico, and they had only ten thousand dollars in cash among them. The disease would spread, but slowly and through a sparsely populated region thousands of kilometers from America's southern border. The world would recognize what was happening and would have time to stop it like they had SARS in Asia.

"What is the condition of your people?"

"Two are showing minor symptoms. One is fairly sick, but still able to function."

"Do you foresee a problem getting to the truck?"

"No. We have good roads and dry weather. Traffic is virtually nonexistent this time of the morning and we've seen no police. My only concern is that Esparza might have contacted his people. That his cartel might be working against us now."

Halabi stood and began limping back and forth through the small chamber. In fact, it was possible that Esparza still knew nothing about the anthrax report. And even if he did, why would he care enough to devote significant resources to finding Attia? Esparza's concern would be damage control—protecting himself not only from U.S. authorities who would label his cartel a terrorist organization, but from the Mexican government and other drug traffickers.

"What are your orders?"

Halabi didn't answer immediately, though his decision was made. In truth, it always had been. God had provided this crossroad in history—a span of a few short hours when a handful of people could dismantle everything the West had built over the last two thousand years.

The arrogance that had corrupted men's hearts would disappear. Once again, humanity would prostrate itself at the feet of God and beg for his mercy. Once again, they would understand that nothing they had done—nothing they had built—meant anything.

"We move forward as planned," Halabi said finally. "But be cautious."

"Understood."

Halabi disconnected the call and looked around him. They were already in the process of fleeing. While their communications were relatively secure, he couldn't risk trying to stay in contact with Attia from a fixed position. No communications were invulnerable, and there was no telling from day to day what new capabilities the Americans could bring to bear.

He walked to a plywood box on the floor and retrieved the pistol it contained. A Glock 19. The same model that Mitch Rapp used.

By the time he exited the chamber, the activity in the rest of the cave system had reached a fevered pitch. Evidence of their time there was being erased, equipment was being dismantled, and supplies were being transferred to trucks waiting outside. Once loaded, the vehicles would scatter, staying on the move for some time before crossing into Ethiopia. A storm system was forecasted, bringing periods of rain and critical cloud cover over the next three days. They would take advantage of it to foil Western surveillance before finally converging on a similar cave system to the west.

Halabi turned right when the corridor split, finally arriving at the chamber he sought.

Gabriel Bertrand looked very different than he had only a week before. The relatively opulent surroundings he'd been provided were gone now, replaced with . . . nothing. He was sitting in the dirt with one wrist handcuffed to a bolt driven into the stone. His body and hair were filthy, streaked with mud, blood, and what appeared to be his own excrement.

The man turned toward Halabi but his dull eyes didn't seem to understand what they were seeing.

"I thought you'd want to know before you die that the plan you devised is in motion." Halabi raised the Glock. "Nothing can stop it now."

CHAPTER 45

SOUTHERN MEXICO

"BUT you're all right?" Kennedy said, her tinny voice emanating from the satellite phone lying on the Humvee's fender.

"Yeah," Rapp said, opening a cabinet at the back of the garage and fishing the vehicle's battery from it. "For now."

"And you're sure that anthrax shipment's been neutralized?"

On the floor near the open bay door, Carlos Esparza craned his neck, trying desperately to see what was happening. He was bound with items Rapp had found in a drawer—hands with a length of framing wire and feet with a colorful bungee cord. The bleeding in his leg had been slowed with a greasy rag and roll of duct tape.

"Yeah, but it doesn't matter. That was never Halabi's play—it was a diversion."

"A diversion? From what?"

"He didn't kill all those sick villagers in Yemen. He took at least one of them and used him to infect his people with YARS. You've got six of them headed for the border with Muhammad Attia."

There was a brief pause over the line. When Kennedy came back on, she sounded uncharacteristically shaken.

"I'm showing a roughly thirty-hour drive time to get from your position to Texas. Do you know where they are now? What their plans are?"

"No," Rapp said, finishing reinstalling the battery. "But I'm about to find out."

Esparza tried to scoot away, making it only a few centimeters before Rapp crouched down and grabbed him by the hair.

"I don't know anything about anthrax or Yemen!" he said in a panicked shout. "You know this. I just wanted to partner with—" His words turned to shrieks when Rapp clamped a hand around his shattered knee.

"The only thing that comes out of your mouth from now on is answers to my questions. Is that clear?"

"Yes! Yes, it's clear. But I—"

Rapp gave the wound another squeeze and once again the garage echoed with the man's screams.

" 'Yes' was the only answer required."

Esparza clamped his lips together, muffling himself.

"The Arabs, Carlos. Where are they?"

He looked legitimately confused. "What . . . What do you mean?"

Rapp reached for the man's knee again and he tried to jerk away. "Stop! You killed them! You burned them."

"I burned an empty shed. They were already gone when I got there. And so is the van they came in."

"I . . . I don't know."

Rapp retrieved a set of vise-grips off the floor and closed the jaws around the middle joint of Esparza's right index finger. He nearly choked himself screaming as the bone was crushed flat.

"Wrong answer, Carlos."

The cartel leader's face turned pale and his eyes started to roll back in his head as he teetered at the edge of unconsciousness. He'd undoubtedly done similar things to countless men, women, and probably a few children over the years. But he wasn't doing so well being on the receiving end. Rapp walked out of the garage and found a flowerpot that was partially full of rainwater. Emptying it onto Esparza's head brought him back around.

"Do you expect me to believe that your guards just let them drive out of here without your approval?"

"Why wouldn't they?" Esparza said, his voice barely a whisper. "I gave them a safe point of entry to Mexico and the contact information for a few coyotes who could help them cross the border. They said they wanted to handle the arrangements themselves and why wouldn't I let them? I didn't want them here. There was no reason for me to take on the risk of smuggling Arabs over the border. And I didn't want them in the U.S. watching my operation."

"Names, Carlos. What coyotes did you put them in touch with?"

"I . . . I don't know for sure," he replied, having a hard time getting in enough breath to speak. "Vicente handled those kinds of details."

Rapp pulled out his gun and pressed it to the man's head. "Then I don't need you anymore."

"Wait!" he shouted. "I have names. I have all of them! I just can't tell you for sure which ones Vicente passed on. Please, Mitch. Please. Why would I lie? They used me. I want them dead as much as you."

Rapp holstered his weapon and went back to the Humvee to close the hood.

"Irene. What kind of help can you get me from the Mexican government?"

"I'm sorry, Mitch, but the answer is none. Even if our relationship with them was good at this point, the Mexican government is flooded with drug money. If we try to involve them, those coyotes are going to hear about it. And even if that wasn't the case, their local police don't have biohazard protocols in place. If they were to intercept Halabi's people, how many of their personnel would be exposed? Would we be able to stop them from putting Halabi's men in a crowded jail? What if they kill them in a public area and there's a significant amount of blood? What if they botch the operation and scatter them? The spread of the disease isn't stopped by borders. If this gets out it'll—"

"What about Gary Statham and his guys?" Rapp interjected.

"Are you suggesting we send a U.S. military force across the Mexican border?"

"From where I'm standing, it doesn't seem like a bad option."

"Even in the most cooperative political climate imaginable that would take weeks of negotiations. And that's not the environment we're working in. Mitch, it's a little after five in the morning here and the anthrax story is about to break hard. The White House is already all hands on deck trying to figure out how to mitigate the damage. In fact, I'm in a car on my way there now."

"Can I assume that Christine Barnett's people are going to be doing the opposite?"

"I think that's a safe assumption. When the morning news shows get into full swing, all hell is going to break loose inside the Beltway."

Rapp grabbed Esparza by the collar and dragged him toward the vehicle. The cartel leader started to cry out in pain, but Rapp clamped a hand over his mouth.

"What about Scott? Can you get him and his people over the border?"

"They're in Texas. Fully equipped and waiting for your orders."

"Brief them and tell them we're a go," he said, stuffing Esparza into the backseat. "And use whatever magic you've got left to get Gary's team in a position to move fast."

"I'll do what I can, Mitch."

He grabbed the phone off the Humvee's bumper and a roll of duct tape off the floor.

"I'm putting Esparza on."

Rapp leaned through the open rear door, pressing the phone to the cartel leader's ear and securing it there with a few winds of tape.

"There'll be a survey at the end of this call, Carlos. I suggest you make sure you have a very satisfied customer on the other end."

Esparza nodded weakly, looking increasingly dazed. Part of it was blood loss, but the other part was probably the shock from how fast his life had turned to shit. Only a few hours ago, he'd been lying on satin sheets with one of his underage whores, dreaming of the billions he was going to make in the heroin business. Now he was slowly bleeding out with a phone taped to his head.

"Mr. Esparza?" Rapp heard Kennedy say as he slammed the door and walked around to the driver's side. Her voice was firm, but soothing. Just the tone necessary to give the man the illusion of hope.

"I'm sure this has been a very difficult night for you, but I have some questions that need to be answered."

CHAPTER 46

ARLINGTON
VIRGINIA
USA

"THAT'S a lie!" Senator Christine Barnett shouted, wielding the television remote in her hand as though it were a weapon.

There was no doubt that she was right, Kevin Gray knew. The DEA man being interviewed could barely meet the interviewer's eye. But this was politics. Truth and lies were irrelevant. All that mattered was what people believed.

He had arrived at Barnett's house around 4:30 a.m., just as the Internet was starting to light up with rumors about an anthrax shipment being intercepted on the U.S. border. Now the sun was up and the newspaper article filled with the lurid details he'd leaked was in the wild. As expected, it had caught fire and was burning bright on virtually every news outlet worldwide. But like all infernos, it was proving impossible to control.

Joshua Alexander was once again demonstrating the political cunning that had made his meteoric rise to the presidency possible. He and Irene Kennedy weren't satisfied to absorb—or even deflect—the political blow. They were trying to turn it to their advantage.

"Can we see?" the reporter said over the television's speakers.

The DEA agent grimaced in pain as he lifted his shirt and showed the deep bruising on his chest.

"So that's where the bullet hit your vest?"

He nodded. "One round here and another in my back."

"And you were sure the vest would stop the round?"

"Yeah," he responded, lowering his shirt again. "Well, pretty sure anyway."

"That seems like an incredible risk to take."

An uncomfortable smile played at the edges of his mouth. "The cartels have millions of dollars to spend on technology and they spend a lot of it on surveillance. In this case, it was something we could use. It can take years to penetrate a trafficking organization with an undercover agent, but with the biothreat we didn't have years. We had to make sure another attack wasn't carried out and try to trace the supply chain back to ISIS. Like the old saying goes, desperate times call for desperate measures."

Based on the reporter's expression, she had lost all objectivity. "I never thought I'd be sitting across a kitchen table from a card-carrying hero. But here I am."

The DEA man shook his head. "The American people pay my salary. It's the job."

Barnett started jabbing in the air with the remote again. "Look at that son of a bitch! He's eating this up! He and his people just went from being the morons who let someone walk away with their coke to being America's darlings."

Gray felt like he was going to be sick. He didn't have any idea how to talk his boss down and, for one of the first times in his career, he had no idea what to do.

Barnett began compulsively changing channels, finding pretty much the same story on every one. While she was distracted, Gray pulled the phone from his pocket and pretended to check texts. In reality, he was turning on a recording app.

Barnett landed on a station with a former FBI executive speaking to a roundtable of pundits. Even more ominous was the tiny picture-in-picture at the bottom right corner of the screen. It depicted people shuffling into the White House Briefing Room.

". . . next time you complain about paying taxes or start talking about how the government can't get anything done, I want you to remember those guys getting shot for the benefit of a cartel surveillance drone."

"So you're saying that CIA operative's financial problems—his motivation for stealing those drugs—were fabricated," the man next to him said.

"Of course they were. The Agency would have used the IRS, SEC, and probably a number of foreign intelligence agencies to create an ironclad legend for his guy. They had to make it *absolutely* convincing that he'd resort to something like this. After that, I can only speculate. My best guess is that he used this to make contact with the cartel that transported the anthrax and made a case for them to hire him. It's really incredible. This is dangerous to the point of being insane. I mean, we're talking a ninety-nine percent chance the cartel just tortures him to death for stealing their product."

"Bullshit!" Barnett shouted. "That asshole isn't just coming up with all this on his own. He and Kennedy have been friends for years. She fed it to him and sent him out on a media tour."

"And where do you think this man is now?" one of the interviewers asked.

"Dead," the FBI man answered, genuine anger audible in his voice. "If he actually managed to succeed in getting inside that cartel operation, they would have executed him the second that story leaked."

"And our ability to track the terrorists and cartel operations died with him," the host said by way of a quick summary. "We're being told that the White House press conference is about to start."

The screen shifted to a view of the briefing room, and Gray watched Alexander's press secretary stride onto the podium.

"This is going to be short," he said and then began reading a prepared statement. "The events described in the *Post* this morning are largely accurate. We did intercept an anthrax shipment in San Ysidro and a CIA operative did assault three DEA volunteers in an attempt to infiltrate the cartel that had partnered with ISIS. What you don't know is that the operation was successful. Our man was able to access the top echelons of that cartel and was using those contacts to locate Sayid Halabi and the rest of the ISIS hierarchy. He was also able to thwart a second attempt to smuggle a quantity of anthrax across our border. However, as of this morning, we've lost contact with him and he's now presumed dead. Unfortunately, the information he was able to gather to date wasn't specific or conclusive. Having said that, our law enforcement agencies are doing what they can with it. Further, the FBI has picked up the reporter who wrote the article and are questioning him about his source. There's not much more to say at this point, other than to thank the men and women who have risked everything to keep this country safe. They won't be forgotten."

Hands in the audience immediately went up and he pointed to one of them.

"Do we know if we've intercepted all of the anthrax or if there could be additional attacks in process?"

"We're reasonably certain that the anthrax threat has been neutralized," Alexander's press secretary said. "But without a man inside, we can no longer monitor the situation on an ongoing basis."

He pointed again.

"Can you tell us more about the operations you're carrying out with regard to ISIS and the cartels?"

"No," he said and indicated another reporter.

"Was Christine Barnett aware of the existence of this undercover operative?"

Kevin Gray stared at the television screen and held his breath. The Alexander administration tended not to like to politicize these kinds of things. Would he stay that course?

"We had no choice but to brief the senator about the initial anthrax attack," he said, and Gray felt his heart sink.

Leave it there. Please, God, just leave it there.

"She was *not*, however, aware of the existence of our undercover agent. That information was shared on a need-to-know basis. For reasons that should now be obvious, we were concerned with leaks."

Gray squeezed his eyes shut and let out a long, shaking breath. There it was. The press secretary for the president of the United States had just implied that Barnett couldn't be trusted with sensitive information out of fear that she would leak it. And now that leak had happened.

He barely heard the rest of the news conference or Barnett's increasingly deranged ranting, only opening his eyes when the screen turned back to the roundtable of pundits.

"They didn't say their man was dead," the host said. "Only that they lost contact with him."

The former FBI man shook his head in disgust. "Losing contact with an undercover agent almost always means the same thing. Take it from me—because of this newspaper article, that magnificent bastard is lying in a ditch somewhere with his throat cut." He leaned forward, planting both elbows on the table. "I've been enforcing the laws of this country my entire life. But as far as I'm concerned, the law is too good for the person who leaked this. Their head should be put on a pike and marched through the streets."

Barnett threw the remote at the television, missing by a couple of feet and hitting the wall instead. The TV went silent and Gray focused on not throwing up. Finally, he managed to speak.

"That's my head he's talking about."

"Quit whining," Barnett snapped back. "That computer operating system is a hundred percent secure. God himself couldn't trace it. What we need to focus on now is damage control. Where do we stand?"

"Where do we stand?" he said, squinting in her direction. "We stand in the middle of a complete clusterfuck. We were going to walk away with the nomination and were way ahead in the general election polls. You could have coasted right into the Oval Office. But that wasn't good enough for you. How long is that reporter going to hold out before he gives up his source? This isn't a story about the Alexander administration covering up their incompetence anymore. He got an undercover agent killed and collapsed a bioterror investigation. He—*we*—could actually be responsible for the U.S. getting attacked."

Barnett stared at him, the fury disappearing from her face in favor of a dead expression that was somehow much worse. Gray wondered if, for the first time in their relationship, he was seeing the real woman behind the façade.

Of course, she was bat-shit insane. The truth was that they all were now. There had probably been a time when politicians achieved this level of success because of patriotism or a deep sense of responsibility to their countrymen. But now it was just about power. In fact, crazy seemed to have become a prerequisite. The American people demanded it.

He suddenly wanted to disappear. To storm out of the room, get on a plane, and get the hell out of the country. To go to work for some multinational corporation marketing soap. Or perfume. Or blood pressure pills. To leave this life behind forever.

But he was scared shitless. The woman staring lifelessly at him from across the room was smart, ruthless, and driven. Even with everything happening—even if he walked out the door—she would likely be the next president of the United States. And the first thing she'd do with the power of that office was destroy everyone who hadn't supported her. Anyone she perceived as a threat. Would he end up in jail? In Guantánamo Bay? Drugged and seat-belted into a car careening down the side of a cliff?

"Okay," he said, struggling to keep his voice even as he recited his mantra. "There are no disasters. Just opportunities we haven't found yet."

Barnett's expression reverted to the more familiar—and now oddly comforting—one of rage.

"Where do we stand?" Gray said, repeating his boss's question of a few moments ago. "If anyone asks—and they will—you deny you had anything to do with that leak and point out that there isn't even a shred of evidence to the contrary. And the fact remains that the first anthrax shipment *did* make it across the border and it was pure dumb luck that it was found. On the other hand, criticizing guys who let themselves get shot to protect the country isn't going to poll well with anyone." He fell silent, rubbing his temples and trying to think the situation through. It wasn't hard.

"We only have one option, Senator. We play it down as hard as we can and try to change the narrative. Like you've said before, the public has the attention span of a goldfish. And this doesn't really have anything to do with you. You kept the anthrax intercept secret from the public against your will at the order of the president and on the advice of Irene Kennedy. As long as no one ties the leak to you, this'll eventually blow over."

"Blow over?" Barnett said. "You think I'm just going to let this go? Slink away and let Irene Kennedy make a fool out of me?"

"Ma'am, Rapp's dead and—"

"He's not dead!" Barnett shouted. "That son of a bitch has more lives than an alley cat. He's alive and they're not telling us. That means he's out there, still working on this operation. Waiting."

"Waiting? Waiting for what?"

"For me to win the primary. Then, at just the right moment, he's going to reappear and save the day. Alexander and Kennedy will be heroes and I'll be standing there looking like a fool."

Gray just stared at her. How could he have not seen this before? The presidency wasn't an end for Barnett, it was a beginning. She wanted the power to close her fist around everything and everyone. She saw Kennedy and Rapp as beneath her—meaningless government workers who existed to do her bidding. Their defiance was stoking her hatred to the point that she was slipping into paranoia.

"Senator, the idea that Mitch Rapp is involving himself in some kind of complex political game is—"

"He sees me as a threat," Barnett said. "Just like Kennedy. They're going to use this to come after me. We have to find out what's happening in Mexico. We have to get ahead of it."

"We have no way of finding out what's happening," Gray said, becoming increasingly alarmed at Barnett's erratic demeanor. "No one's going to tell us anything, and if we try to twist arms at the intelligence agencies, it's going to go public and blow up in our faces."

"Not the *American* government," she said. "We can use our contacts in the Mexican government. They want us to get off their backs regarding immigrants and drugs, right? Well, as president, I can make that happen. And all I ask in return is a little cooperation and information."

"Now hold on, Senator. If Rapp's alive, it's possible that he's actually still on the trail of ISIS. We—"

"I'm not going to sit on my hands and see that son of a bitch shooting it out with terrorists on television!" she screamed.

Gray tried to stay calm, but he was starting to feel the honest-to-God beginnings of panic. This was the first time he'd ever seen Barnett under real stress. She'd lived a charmed life—an obscenely wealthy husband, children willing to toe her political line, and a career that went nowhere but up. What would happen when she got backed into a corner like all presidents did? What would happen if she was in charge when there was a real national crisis?

"We're in a hole, Senator. It's time to stop digging. This is about damage control now. You need to go out there and praise those DEA guys for their heroism. But then you remind voters that we can't count on NASA and government employees willing to get shot every time there's a threat to America. That this isn't a failure of the men and women in the trenches, it's a failure of leadership. Then we'll start talking about the economy. Or Russia. North Korea. Guns. It doesn't mat—"

"They're not going to allow it," she said, cutting him off. "This is going to be about a bunch of big strong men on the front lines while I'm back in my office hiding. The weak woman. I'm not going to let that happen, Kevin. We're going to get in front of this."

"That's crazy," he said, the words coming out of his mouth before he could stop them. "You can't control the Mexicans, Senator. They have no loyalty to you and no particular love for the U.S. right now. If you ask them to dig up information on Mitch Rapp, the first thing they're going to do is contact the cartels and—"

"Make it happen."

"Excuse me?"

"Call them, Kevin. Call the Mexicans. Find out what's going on. We can still head this off. If there really is something happening down there, we might be able to get the Mexican authorities to deal with it and keep Rapp and Kennedy from getting the win. If it works out, we might even be able to take some credit. Show the American people that I can stop threats *before* they make it to the United States."

Gray remained silent. He'd already allowed himself to be dragged into the leak that was turning into a disaster. He was already in deep and it was time to take his own advice and stop digging. The hole was starting to feel like a grave.

Gray picked up his coat and started for the door. "If you want to call the Mexicans, Senator, call them yourself."

CHAPTER 47

EL PASO
TEXAS
USA

SCOTT Coleman let the minivan drift forward, coming to a stop again behind the Prius he was trailing. Farther up in line, an SUV was passing through the border checkpoint and into Mexico.

He had the windows down and was enjoying cool temperatures that wouldn't last long after the sun rose in about an hour. The news station playing on the radio was focused on the only story that anyone cared about—the anthrax that had crossed the border and the anonymous CIA operative who had been tracking it. The anonymous CIA operative that he was now on his way to meet.

"Mas is through," Claudia said, staring down at her phone from the passenger seat. "Bruno's next. He's three cars from the checkpoint."

Coleman wasn't particularly worried about the team getting across. While it was true that they were lone, dangerous-looking men in pickups and SUVs, they were completely clean. Perfect IDs, backdated resort reservations, and nothing in their vehicles but suntan lotion and swim trunks.

His situation was somewhat different. On the positive side,

couples in late-model minivans tended not to raise a lot of red flags with border security. Less ideal, though, was the fact that they were carrying enough weapons to launch a pretty respectable coup attempt. Hidden beneath piles of luggage, for sure, but not enough to fool anyone who decided to do more than glance.

"Bruno's through," Claudia said, finally putting down her phone and looking up. "Mitch is on the road and he'll rendezvous with us at the airfield."

"Assuming we make it across the border," Coleman said.

"Are you worried?"

"Nah. God wouldn't let me get gunned down in an Izod shirt. He doesn't hate me that much."

Ahead, next to the open gates that led into Mexico, a green light kept flashing on and off. It was random and every once in a while it turned red, indicating that the car going through would be searched by customs. Normally the Agency would have rigged the game, but Kennedy was dead set against notifying the Mexican authorities. So they were just rolling the dice.

Claudia seemed to be feeling the pressure too, because she suddenly snapped a hand out and changed the radio station—as though listening to a news story about anthrax would give away their involvement with it. The green light flashed and the car two ahead rolled through. The Prius ahead of them was next, gliding through without incident. And then . . .

Green.

Coleman let out a quiet breath and pulled through, but they weren't out of the woods yet. There was a secondary military checkpoint ahead specifically set up to look for weapons being transported into the country. According to Claudia's smuggling contacts, they were typically interested in pickups and SUVs piloted by one or two men between the ages of twenty-five and forty. However, if they spotted someone driving a larger vehicle that looked a little too innocuous, they sometimes pulled that over, too.

It was those same smugglers who had recommended the setup they were using. Red minivan loaded with options. "Baby on Board" sticker, but no baby. White couple, not too young, not too old. The smuggling Goldilocks zone.

And they turned out to be right. The soldiers by the side of the road didn't even look up as they passed.

Claudia turned the radio back to an analysis of the presidential nominations through the lens of the anthrax leak. Christine Barnett was fighting like a junkyard dog, of course, but the fact that she'd been out of the loop was making her look weak. There was also a fair amount of speculation flying around that she might have had something to do with the leak, but no evidence. The spin machines on both sides were running full speed and it was getting harder and harder to tease truth from bullshit.

Coleman tuned out the voices as he accelerated up the road. It was just a distraction at this point. His role in all this was simple: shoot in the direction Mitch told him to.

Claudia's phone rang and she picked up, channeling it through the vehicle's sound system.

"I understand everyone's through," Irene Kennedy said over the speakers. Her voice was distorted by the encryption they were using, but still intelligible.

"Yeah, we're clear," Coleman said. "We'll make it to the airfield around eleven thirty tonight. Where do you stand?"

"Our worst-case scenario timing-wise is that the terrorists left Esparza's compound at one a.m. and are driving roughly thirty hours to the closest border checkpoint. If that's the case, they could be as far as Coatzacoalcos. Twenty-two hours from the border."

He consulted the GPS in his dash. "Then I'm starting to question our strategy, Irene. It looks like we're going to pass them on the road."

"We don't think so," Kennedy said calmly. "They appear to have contracted a smuggling organization and it's likely they're planning on changing vehicles. That's going to take time to deal with."

"Do we have a line on their coyotes yet?" Coleman asked.

"We're running down the names Carlos Esparza provided, but haven't come up with anything solid. We're also searching the roads in southern Mexico, but that's going to be low percentage. It's a lot of road and our satellite coverage is spotty."

"And if you do manage to find us a target?" Coleman said. "What are our marching orders?"

The fact that she didn't respond immediately worried him a bit.

"As of now, this is an unauthorized private operation on foreign soil. I've talked to the commander at Luke Air Force Base who's a personal friend of mine and he's agreed to put the appropriate aircraft on alert, but he isn't going to do anything more than that without a direct order from the president."

"Do you think you can get that?" Claudia asked.

"I'm meeting him in an hour, but a military incursion over the Mexican border involving a bombing run against a moving target is a big ask. The amount of ordnance necessary to ensure that the virus is completely eradicated is fairly shocking. I'm not hopeful."

"Great," Coleman said. "So you're saying we should just handle this on our own with a handful of people and a minivan with a few guns in it. And if we make the slightest mistake, no big deal. Only a few hundred million people will die."

"I'm doing everything I can, Scott. Alexander's a good man and he's been a good president. But politicians aren't built for these kinds of all-or-nothing decisions."

"What about going around him?"

This time the pause was long enough that Coleman thought they might have lost the satellite link. Finally she came back on.

"I had an informal conversation about that with a few highly placed people I won't name. What I can tell you is that no one has the stomach for what would essentially be a coup. In a way, it's comforting that our institutions are holding strong even in the face of something like this."

"It doesn't feel comforting from where I'm sitting, Irene."

"I know. And I'm sorry. Claudia? Are you there? How are you holding up?"

The question was understandable. While Claudia Gould was a logistics genius, she'd spent most of her career supporting her private contractor husband. Her definition of failure had involved things like missing the target, getting arrested, and not being paid. Now she was getting a crash course in the difference between that world and the one inhabited by Mitch Rapp.

Her eyes narrowed and the expression on her youthful face hardened. She had a daughter to protect and, at thirty-six, a life left to live.

"If you say we're the only people who can deal with this, then that's what we're going to do. Deal with it."

CHAPTER 48

OUTSIDE OF SAN LUIS POTOSÍ
MEXICO

RAPP stopped and examined the chain link gate illuminated in the Humvee's headlights. The sign on it was badly faded, but he could still make out the cheerful logo of a company that had once offered sightseeing flights over a nearby national park.

He dug a couple of antibiotic pills from his pocket and popped them in his mouth. A couple hours into his drive he'd spotted a pharmacy and made a quick stop. The man behind the counter had been oddly unfazed by Rapp's demand for an anthrax remedy, but in retrospect it wasn't so surprising. The American people were panicked over Halabi's threats and loved buying cheap pharmaceuticals in foreign countries. There was a good chance that he wasn't the first gringo to stop at that drugstore on his way home.

The bitter taste of the pills was strangely comforting. He had no idea if he'd inhaled any spores while emptying that bag into his bathtub, but chances were high. There was probably a reason the CDC didn't issue kitchen gloves and tourist bandannas as standard protective gear.

He spotted movement out of the corner of his eye and inched a hand closer to his Glock before registering the blond hair of Scott

Coleman. The gate opened and he pulled through, idling while the former SEAL relocked the barrier and slipped into the passenger seat.

"I haven't talked to Irene in more than two hours," Rapp said, accelerating. "Give me a sit rep."

"We got here about a half hour ago and I have a chopper inbound. The tarmac's in worse condition than we thought so we can't land planes. We should be able to get two private ones in the air from the local airport, though. Irene's scrambling basically everyone the Agency has in-country—including a few people who retired down here. Not the most organized or well-trained force we've ever worked with, but at least we have warm bodies."

"And your team?"

"I left them closer to the border to form a defensive line. If we get a target, they'll be in a position to intercept from the north. But so far we've got nada."

A dark, wooden crate of a building appeared in the headlights and Rapp pulled around behind it, parking next to a minivan with a "Baby on Board" decal. There was a generator humming outside and a couple of extension cords running through the wall.

"What about Esparza?" Coleman asked, glancing at the empty backseat before jumping out.

"He didn't make it."

Technically accurate, but not the entire story. In truth, the man had stopped bleeding and was doing pretty well by the time he'd finished his conversation with Kennedy. When Rapp reached pavement, though, he'd decided that driving around with a bound cartel leader in the backseat was all risk and no reward. He'd pulled off into the trees and left Esparza there with his head twisted backward. With a little luck, his bones were already being picked clean by scavengers.

Coleman just shrugged and went for the building's only door.

The interior was painted in the same colors as the logo on the gate, but much of it was peeling or stained from leaks in the roof. Two windows had been covered in a mix of plywood and canvas to keep light from bleeding through and a bathroom with a collapsed sink was visible in the corner. Other than that there wasn't much—not even a table. The operation was being run from the floor.

Claudia was at the far end of the building, staring at a map and talking excitedly into the phone. "Where? Yes, I understand. And how good is this information? Fine. Yes. Get back to me as soon as you can."

She hung up and spun, fixing her almond-shaped eyes on him. The relief was clear in them but she let it show for only a moment. "We may have a functional lead. One of the coyote organizations Esparza gave us runs their operation out of a warehouse in Córdoba, southeast of Mexico City. That warehouse burned down three hours ago."

"Kind of weird," Coleman said. "But why risk setting it on fire and attracting attention? Are we sure it's not just a coincidence?"

"It's not a coincidence," Rapp said, running a finger along a map hanging on the wall. "The one thing we have going for us is that Halabi fucking *despises* the United States. I know this asshole better than he knows himself. This isn't about God. It's about him. He doesn't want to infect a bunch of coyotes with YARS and have them running around Mexico randomly spreading it. He burned that warehouse for the same reason he told Esparza to keep his men at a distance. Because he wants this to come from America. He wants everyone to think Allah himself slapped down on us. That *we* brought this on the world. Not Mexico."

"If you're right, then things might be finally moving in our direction," Claudia said. "The coyotes that operated out of that warehouse were a boutique organization specializing in smuggling contraband in refrigerator trucks. Flawless paperwork and hidden compartments that are almost impossible to detect without cutting the trailer apart."

"They're moving slower than we thought," Rapp said, continuing to study the map. "I'm guessing they stuck to back roads on their way to Mexico City and then hit traffic. After that, they had to load their people and fill the trailer with frozen food. Claudia, if we figure they rolled out of there around the time it burned, where could they be now?"

"Likely somewhere just to the east of Mexico City."

Rapp used a pencil to create an arc centered on that area of the map. Then he traced multiple similar lines above at roughly fifty-mile intervals, labeling each with a time.

He pointed to the gap between lines marked 12 a.m. and 1 a.m. "The way I see it, we have a fully loaded refrigerator truck somewhere in this band. Claudia, tell the Agency to create a map that'll give us real-time animation of the sections of road we need to focus on."

"That shouldn't be a problem," she said.

"Scott—what about the people you told me we have in-country?"

"I'll get Bruno, Wick, and Mas moving south. Two prop planes can be in the air in forty minutes searching the roads in your target area. And we've got around another twenty people spread out across the roads from the U.S. to Guatemala. Like I said, no one special, but all perfectly capable of looking for a truck. We've also got clear skies and some satellite coverage. But someone's going to have to tell us how to differentiate a refrigerated truck from a regular one."

Rapp nodded. "Claudia. Have Irene pull together all her Spanish speakers. If we spot a truck that looks like a good candidate, we'll phone in a plate number and description. Then Irene's people can call the company that owns it, confirm it's theirs, get a final destination, and make sure it's where it's supposed to be. How much time do we have?"

"If you're right about where they are now, it'll take them at least ten hours to cross into the U.S."

Rapp finally turned away from the map. There weren't many things that could make the sweat running down his back turn cold, but this was it. They were trying to cover thousands of square miles in a country where they'd never operated with a team made up of people who had little or no operational experience. No military support. No support from local law enforcement. And a Mexican government that vacillated between useless and openly hostile.

"Should we be putting U.S. authorities on alert that they might have to close the border?" Coleman asked.

Rapp thought about it for a moment and then shook his head. "Once that word goes out, how long until the press gets hold of it? We've already had one leak and we know how Halabi reacted. If he gets spooked and turns those people loose in Mexico, we're screwed."

"What about additional inspections for refrigerator trucks?" Claudia suggested.

"Same problem," Rapp said. "There's no way ISIS doesn't have people watching the border crossings, and it's hard to imagine they'd miss our guys going over every refrigerated truck with a fine-toothed comb. Halabi desperately wants to believe this is working. All we have to do is not convince him otherwise."

"So let's say we get lucky and find that truck," Coleman said. "We've got RPGs, but that's going to make a mess. We'll have half-burned bodies and thawing frozen food all over the place. There'll be civilians, cops, maybe army. Can we control that?"

Rapp didn't answer. He'd had a number of strategy sessions with Kennedy on his drive, and neither one of them had come up with a workable plan to keep this in Mexico. It went against every instinct he had, but he'd finally had to resign himself to the fact that the border was just a meaningless line on a map. Attia and the six terrorists he was transporting weren't the enemy. It was the billions of germs they carried.

"No," Rapp said finally. "We can't control it. And that's why we're going to let them through."

"Repeat that?" Claudia said, obviously thinking her less than perfect English had failed her.

"Gary Statham's got a team standing by in New Mexico. We need that truck to roll across the border without any fireworks. He'll be waiting for it on the other side."

CHAPTER 49

WEST OF MONTEMORELOS
MEXICO

RAPP held the hand pump on top of a fifty-five-gallon fuel drum while Coleman worked it. Their pilot had the nozzle inserted in their rented chopper and was encouraging them with nonstop updates on their progress.

They'd set down on a remote dirt track fifteen minutes ago and, after a fair amount of searching, located the fuel cache left for them. The foliage was thicker and the terrain more undulating than Rapp had expected in this part of Mexico. Mountains were visible in the distance and they'd flown past cliffs that looked to be more than a thousand feet high. Population centers were pretty spread out and largely connected by two-lane rural highways. Road surfaces weren't bad, but inconsistent enough that the myriad transport trucks traveling over them were doing so at fairly conservative speeds.

The phone in his pocket started to vibrate, and he squinted at the screen through the midmorning sun.

"Go ahead," he said, picking up and leaving the former SEAL to complete the job.

"We've got a good candidate," Claudia said.

"Another one?"

They had nine cars on the road, looking for refrigerator trucks, supplemented by two private planes and the chopper they were currently refueling. At first he'd thought it wasn't enough, but now he was wondering if it was too many. Passing plate numbers and transportation company names to Agency analysts had turned out to be an inexact science. They'd already had three false alarms—one caused by some misfiled paperwork in Guadalajara, one by a simple transposition of a number, and one that probably was a smuggler, but not the one they were after.

"This is solid," she said. "We have circumstantial evidence that it originated in Córdoba around the same time that warehouse burned."

Rapp nodded. Soft, but at least it was something.

"Do we have anyone in contact with it?"

"One car ahead. He's stopped and will be in a position to get photos in about ten minutes."

"What about Scott's guys?"

"Bruno's about half an hour from the target. Mas and Wick are probably more like an hour and a half out."

"Understood."

"Gary Statham's waiting for your orders, and we have spec ops teams keeping a low profile at all the viable crossings. But this is starting to get tight, Mitch. Based on the maps we're using, Halabi's people could be within three hours of the nearest border. According to Irene, the president's starting to panic. He wants to close them."

Rapp looked out at the landscape surrounding him. The plan was still to let ISIS roll onto American soil unchallenged. Once they were on the U.S. side, a sniper would pump a single round into the driver and the army's biohazard team would basically put a plastic bag over the entire site. On a gut level, it was a terrifying scenario, but it got better the more he thought about it. A semi at a border crossing was easily controlled—one car in front and one in back were enough to completely immobilize it. The driver was easily taken out and his body would be contained inside the cab. The likelihood that the people in back would have the ability to escape the trailer on their own was pretty remote, but even if they did, they wouldn't make it two feet before they took a bullet to the chest.

"Tell her to hold him off. Right now we're in reasonably good shape. We might not know for sure where Halabi's people are but we're fairly certain they're contained and all together. If we lose that, we're screwed."

"I'll relay the message."

He heard a shout and saw Coleman waving him over. They were done refueling and the chopper's blades were already starting to rotate.

"Send me the coordinates of that truck. We'll be in the air inside of two minutes."

"Did you say Grupo Amistoso?" Rapp shouted into the microphone hanging in front of his mouth.

Coleman, who was sitting next to him in the back of the chopper, gave him the thumbs-up. Rapp focused a pair of binoculars on a distant semi, but the trailer didn't carry the logo they were looking for.

"That's not it, Fred," he said. "We're still too far south."

"Roger that," their pilot said.

Coleman nudged him and slid a portable computer onto his lap. Rapp clicked on the file Claudia had sent and was rewarded with a series of high-resolution images depicting a truck driving along a straight stretch of highway. He enlarged one and focused on the windshield. Whoever had taken the photo was smart enough to use a polarizing filter, giving detail to the inside of the cab.

Muhammad Attia.

The surge of adrenaline that he expected didn't materialize. The opposite, really. All he felt was a profound sense of relief.

"This is our guy."

Coleman pumped a fist in the air.

"Fred, get eyes on him, but stay way back. We don't want to get made. We need to find out where the closest exits off that road are and make sure they're covered. Pull the planes back and keep our guy on the ground with him. Scott, what's Bruno's ETA?"

"Call it five minutes. Mas and Wick are still about an hour out."

"Okay. We need to line up people and vehicles along every possible path so we can keep staggering them. We're just here to keep an eye on him and stay invisible. Make sure everyone's clear. No interference and nothing that could call attention to us."

"Roger that," Coleman said before isolating his radio to start coordinating their effort.

Rapp responded to Claudia's email and then used his binoculars to scan the road again. Traffic was light—probably an average of two hundred yards between cars. The terrain continued to be rolling, with distant mountains now starting to soften in a dusty haze.

Another minute went by before their pilot's voice came over Rapp's headphones. "That's gotta be him at eleven o'clock."

He banked the chopper east so that Rapp could get a better look. Blue cab towing a yellow trailer with GRUPO AMISTOSO stenciled on the side. Exactly like the pictures.

Attia was staying just below the speed limit, driving smoothly and trying to keep a decent interval between his truck and the other vehicles moving in his direction. The closest was behind, a dilapidated sedan about three hundred yards back.

Rapp plugged his phone into his headset and dialed Kennedy.

"I understand the truck's been located," she said by way of greeting.

"Yeah. Southeast of Monterrey, Mexico, so he's going for one of the East Texas crossings. We're two and a half hours from the border by car. That can't be more than a few minutes out by jet. Get one over here."

"I'm afraid we're not going to be able to do that."

"Bullshit, Irene. This is a perfect scenario for us. He's a sitting duck and there's no one else close. We can slag that thing with zero civilian casualties and get our plane back across the border before the Mexicans even—"

"It's not the president, Mitch. He's authorized the strike."

"Then what are we waiting for?"

"I've had a number of demolitions experts and biologists looking at this. No one knows how much frozen food is in that truck or what kind. We also don't know what the false chamber those people are in is made of. That makes it impossible to be one hundred percent sure we can incinerate the trailer and its contents with no chance of flinging infected tissue away from the blast site. According to the notes we've retrieved from Gabriel Bertrand's university computer account, this disease likely started in Yemeni bats. That means we don't know if wild animals in Mexico could be infected and—"

"Have you run this by Gary?"

"Yes and he agrees. Letting the truck cross the border is still our best chance for containment."

"Shit," Rapp muttered, but it was lost in the drone of the chopper. Gary Statham was the best in the world at what he did. Questioning his knowledge of biological threats was like questioning Stan Hurley's knowledge of Southeast Asian hookers.

"Fine," he said. "I'm out."

"Wait, Mitch. There's something else."

"You've got to be kidding. What now?"

"I just got a call from a Mexican intelligence executive who I have a back channel to. His bosses have been asking about the possibility that the CIA is carrying out an illegal operation there. It seems that someone high up in the U.S. government has been calling and asking questions."

"What the *fuck*, Irene? You know where these leaks are coming from as well as I do. Shut them down or I'll fly to Washington and do it for you."

"Right now, you need to focus on that truck. My concern is that these inquiries could get to someone being paid by Halabi. If that's the case, things could become very unpredictable very quickly. We can revisit the subject of what to do about the leaks later." She paused for a moment. "If there is a later."

CHAPTER 50

EAST OF MONTERREY
MEXICO

THE highway below Rapp was split now, with two lanes running in each direction and a broad dirt median between. Low, scrubby trees extended to the horizon and traffic remained light. The truck driven by Muhammad Attia was little more than a dot in his binocular lenses. Joe Maslick and Charlie Wicker were in separate vehicles about one mile and one and a half miles in front of it, respectively. Bruno McGraw was bringing up the rear, hanging back about three-quarters of a mile.

For one of the first times in his career, things seemed to be going too smoothly. The truck's last turn had put it on a highway that made only one border crossing practical. Gary Statham was currently loading his team on a transport and he'd guaranteed that they'd be ready when Attia arrived.

"Is he still holding his speed, Fred?"

"Yup. Two kilometers an hour under the limit. Slow and steady."

As expected. Attia didn't need to hurry. He just needed to avoid attracting attention.

"Scott. Give me an updated ETA."

"Some of those hills back there slowed him down a little. We're around an hour forty-five to Texas. Our guys at the border crossing are reporting light traffic and they're not anticipating any change to that."

Rapp glanced down at his phone. No messages. "Maybe we should have brought beer."

The former SEAL grinned. "Wanna bet? Your Charger would look good in my garage."

Rapp didn't respond, sweeping his binoculars east in an attempt to find a threat and again coming up empty.

The wisdom of not accepting Coleman's bet became clear nineteen minutes later when Claudia's voice came over the chopper's comm.

"The rumors spreading around the Mexican government have finally made the press, Mitch. A story just appeared online about the U.S. tracking an anthrax shipment across Mexico without the government's knowledge."

Rapp swore under his breath and glanced at his watch. The truck's time to the border had just gone under the hour-and-a-half mark.

"No need to panic yet," Claudia said. "It's one very speculative story on a pretty sensational Spanish-language site. All anonymous sources."

"Halabi's people aren't just going to be monitoring CNN," Rapp said. "And I'm pretty sure they know how to use Google Translate. If we found it, he's not going to be far behind."

"You're probably right," she admitted. "The question is when and what's he going to do with the information?"

"Mas," Rapp said. "Slow down. I want eyes on that truck. Wick and Bruno. Maintain your position."

"Roger that," Joe Maslick said. "But if I can see him, he's going to be able to see me. I won't be able to match his speed for long without making him suspicious."

Coleman turned his laptop toward Rapp and tapped a blue dot

on the screen. It represented a vehicle their people had stashed in the trees just off the main road.

"Copy. We've got a car about twelve miles ahead of your position. You can pull off and make a switch. Bruno, when he does, you can close in and take over surveillance. From now until the border I want one of you close. Claudia, you're going to have to coordinate personnel and vehicle changes along the route."

"I'm already working on it."

"Mitch," their pilot cut in. "I'm seeing brake lights on the target."

"Is there an obstacle?"

"Not that I can see. Looks wide-open. Wait . . . He's turning into the median."

Rapp put the binoculars to his eyes as Fred Mason banked in an effort to keep their interval. All that was visible was a dust cloud. When the truck emerged, it had reversed course.

"The target has crossed the median and is accelerating back west," Rapp said. "I repeat, the target is now westbound. Bruno, cross over and get in front of him. Stay out of sight. Wick and Mas, cross over and get behind. Wick, close the gap and get eyes on him. Mas, you stay back far enough to keep out of sight. Claudia, patch in Irene."

A moment later, Kennedy's voice came on the line. "Go ahead."

"Looks like Halabi reads the news. Attia's jumped the median and he's headed toward Monterrey."

She started to speak, but Wick drowned her out. "I've got him in sight and he's hauling ass. Eighty-nine miles an hour by my speedo."

"Mitch," Kennedy said when she came back on. "Monterrey is an urban center with over a million people. Based on the satellite image I'm looking at, he can make it to the outskirts in less than thirty minutes. If he has a way to offload those people, they'll scatter and we'll never find them. Letting him reach Monterrey isn't an option."

Rapp considered her words for a moment. "We've got an RPG. We could go for the cab and crash it."

"That just puts us back in the situation that we talked about earlier. The scattering of Attia's potentially contaminated body parts. The chance of infecting animals. Possible damage to the trailer, blood, police, Good Samaritans . . ." Her voice faded for a moment. "The plan hasn't changed. We need to get that truck over the border and into the hands of Gary's team."

"From where I'm sitting, that's easier said than done, Irene."

"I'm going to call the president and see if there's anything he can do. But I'm not hopeful. Time is against us and his counterpart in Mexico is—"

"A scumbag with the IQ of a head of lettuce?" Rapp offered.

"I'm afraid so. I'll get back to you as soon as I can. In the meantime do *not* let that truck reach Monterrey."

She disconnected and Coleman spoke up. "He's got the hills in front of him. The first time he went over them, he was barely able to hold twenty-five miles an hour."

"Yeah, but we have the same problems at twenty-five miles an hour that we do at eighty-nine."

"We've got the chopper, a few guys, and some weapons," the former SEAL said. "If we disable the truck and take him out inside the cab, we could keep the cops and any bystanders back for a while. Maybe long enough for Alexander to explain the situation to the Mexicans?"

Rapp shook his head. It left too much to chance. The only thing more unpredictable than viruses was politics.

"Fred," Rapp said to their pilot. "Get us over those hills ahead. Let's see if we can find something."

Mason pushed the chopper to its less-than-impressive top speed while Rapp examined a tractor-trailer hauling pipes on the road below. Less than a minute later, they buzzed another semi, this one pulling a trailer emblazoned with the logo of a fast-food company.

"You got something?" Coleman said, recognizing his expression from years of working together.

Rapp remained silent, craning his neck to keep eyes on Attia's truck as it disappeared behind a rise.

"That one's not going to work," Rapp said, watching a tractor-trailer make its way up the steep slope they were hovering over. It was already more than a hundred yards into the climb and had barely slowed. Likely empty.

"We've still got the two we saw earlier," Coleman said. "Fast food and pipes."

Rapp nodded. "How's our fuel, Fred?"

"We've got another forty minutes in the air. Thirty if you count the time it'll take to get to our closest fuel stash."

The semi with POLLO FELIZ painted on the trailer reached the bottom of the hill and immediately started losing speed. "That's the one. Scott, what's Attia's ETA?"

"Call it just under five minutes."

"And we're still out of sight?"

"Yeah," Mason said. "As long as we stay low, he won't be able to see us until he crests that last rise."

"Okay, then let's do it."

Mason dove toward the truck, coming to a stable hover about five feet off the ground and thirty feet in front of it. The driver reacted immediately, slamming on his brakes and sounding the horn. The steep grade combined with the weight of his trailer allowed him to bring the vehicle to a full stop in seconds.

Mason dropped the chopper to within a couple feet of the asphalt and Rapp jumped out. The driver watched what was happening through his dusty windshield, not even bothering to lock himself inside the cab as Rapp ran toward it. He undoubtedly assumed this was a cartel operation and figured that complete cooperation was his only hope for survival. No point in dying over a bunch of frozen chicken.

Rapp yanked the door open and dragged the man out before taking his place behind the wheel. He'd never driven a truck exactly like it, but had extensive experience piloting similar rigs in Iraq and Afghanistan. Finding first gear wasn't as easy as he'd hoped, but once he did he was able to start the slow process of getting the loaded semi back up to speed. Mason climbed again and the truck's driver retreated to the side of the road with his cell phone already against his ear. Not that it mattered. One way or another, this thing was going public.

In his side-view mirror, Rapp saw an off-road pickup rolling up fast behind him. It moved into the left lane and slowed, coming alongside. Bruno McGraw leaned over the empty passenger seat and shouted through his open window. "You okay, boss?"

"Yeah. Go forward. Find me a place to turn around."

McGraw sped off as Rapp continued to push the semi's motor to its limit. He was almost to fifteen miles an hour when he saw Attia barreling toward the base of the hill. He hit the slope at almost ninety miles an hour, but the effect of gravity became immediately evident. His speed began to plummet as he closed the distance to the trailer Rapp was towing. When there was about a hundred yards between them Attia pulled into the left lane to pass, probably still traveling ten miles an hour faster than Rapp. By the time he'd made it to within twenty yards, that speed differential was almost cut in half.

Rapp kept his eyes glued to his side mirror, waiting for Attia to close to with ten feet before swerving in front of him and hitting the brakes.

Contact was almost instantaneous. Rapp was thrown back in his seat but managed to keep his hands on the wheel and his eyes on the mirror. Attia, now aware of what was happening, tried to swerve back into the right lane, but Rapp followed the move, gearing down and feathering the brakes.

They swerved along the road for another ten seconds, slowing to four miles an hour before the pressure on the back of Rapp's truck disappeared. Attia had applied his own brakes and disconnected from him.

An assault rifle appeared through the terrorist's open window and Rapp's side-view mirror exploded, spraying him with shattered glass. Attia continued to fire short bursts as he drifted left, managing to get a few rounds into Rapp's cab and punch holes in the windshield.

Rapp had had about enough of their slow-motion car chase, so he twisted the wheel, bringing his truck to a halt across the road. Attia was forced to stop but now had a better angle. He took full advantage, forcing the CIA man to the floorboards as he emptied his magazine into the driver's-side door. Somewhere beneath the roar of the assault rifle, though, a deep thump became audible.

The sound of gunfire continued, but the ring of rounds hitting metal stopped. Rapp rose from the floorboard and spotted Coleman hanging out of the side of the chopper squeezing off careful individual shots in Attia's direction. The terrorist reloaded and trained his fire on the former SEAL. A moment later a smoke plume sprouted from the back of the aircraft. Mason lost control and the helicopter started to spin, slipping away from the truck.

Rapp escaped through the passenger door and landed shoulder-first on the running board before dragging himself behind the truck's front wheel. He barely made cover before Attia began spraying the cab again.

Rapp hadn't had time to take the truck out of gear and it idled slowly toward the steep slope on the west side of the road. He pulled his Glock and paced the front wheel, dropping to the ground when the cab started to go over the edge. Dust kicked into the air as the trailer was jacked upward and dragged down the precipice. Attia lost sight of his target and stopped shooting. Rapp took his time, bracing the pistol with both hands from his location on the ground.

When the trailer finally cleared his position and began tumbling down the slope, he spotted the side of Attia's face around the front bumper of his vehicle. It was all Rapp needed.

A gentle squeeze of the trigger jerked the terrorist's head back and dropped him to the asphalt. He still had hold of the assault rifle and Rapp sprinted toward him, getting a foot on the weapon before he could lift it again. The bullet had grazed his cheekbone, leaving a deep wound that was bleeding profusely but not serious enough to rob him of consciousness. A sound that came out somewhere between a shout and a scream erupted from his throat when he recognized Rapp.

The CIA man pointed his pistol toward Attia's forehead, but then readjusted his aim to the man's chest before firing a single round. He'd already made too much of a mess as it was.

Rapp glanced down the slope and saw Mason trying to control his descent with mixed results. Wicker and Maslick were approaching from the east but Rapp waved them back. Attia was dead but maybe more dangerous now than he had been when he was alive. Despite the fact that his heart was no longer pumping, the wound in his face continued to pour blood—likely infected with YARS—onto the asphalt.

He leaned over the body, hesitating for a moment before grabbing it under the arms and dragging it back to the cab of the truck. By the time he got it inside, he was so covered in blood that he looked like an extra in a low-budget zombie flick.

"Wick!" Rapp said into his throat mike. "There's a shitload of blood on the road. You need to clean it up."

"Clean it up? With what?"

"How the fuck would I know? Maybe punch a hole in your fuel tank and use that. Call Gary and ask him what'll work."

"Roger that," came the unenthusiastic reply.

"Bruno," Rapp said, starting Attia's truck and putting it in gear. "Did you find me a turnaround?"

"About two hundred yards over the top of the hill. It's going to be about a ten-point turn, but we'll get it done."

"All right. Once I turn around, we're heading full-gas for the border. Bruno and Mas, you're blocking for me. Try not to kill any civilians or cops, but if you don't have any choice, do it. I'll take the heat for any casualties. Wick. Once you're done with that blood, head out into the desert and lay low until someone from Statham's team can pick you up."

He crested the hill and saw McGraw's truck parked sideways across the road, blocking oncoming traffic. Someone got out and motioned angrily at him but then thought better of it when McGraw pulled an HK416 assault rifle from the backseat and fired into the air.

"Scott!" Rapp said into his radio. "You dead?"

"Not yet, asshole. But we're down. Fred swears he can fix it. He says thirty minutes."

"You have fifteen. I want that fucking chopper in the air, do you understand me?"

"Roger that, Mitch."

The music that had been playing over the truck's radio suddenly went silent and a panicked Arabic voice came on.

"Muhammad? What's happening? Did we hit something? Was that shooting we heard?"

Rapp reached into his shirt pocket and retrieved a few antibiotic pills from a box soaked through with Attia's blood. He tossed them in his mouth, breaking them apart with his teeth and savoring the bitterness.

"Muhammad! Answer! Was that shooting?"

Of course that asshole Gary Statham would lecture him on how antibiotics didn't work against viruses, but screw it. The taste made him feel better. It was like soft body armor when the rifles came out. Sure, it wouldn't save you, but there was something strangely comforting about the weight.

CHAPTER 51

NORTHERN MEXICO

"WE'RE looking good," Joe Maslick said over Rapp's earpiece. "Road's pretty open and still no cops. ETA to the border at our current speed is approximately one hour, three minutes."

"Roger that," Rapp said, leaning forward over the truck's steering wheel and scanning the terrain surrounding the highway. Empty.

His speedometer was reading one kilometer an hour under the speed limit and he was keeping the vehicle steady despite increasingly powerful gusts coming from the south. Maslick was a couple of miles in front of him, completely out of sight. Bruno McGraw was visible in his side-view mirror.

The CIA had dedicated no fewer than three dozen native-level Spanish speakers to interfering with the police in the region. They were calling in false reports, scrambling communications, and impersonating officers in an effort to create confusion. It was a house of cards for sure, but one that only had to last for a little longer.

"We're back in the air," Scott Coleman said over a spotty connection. "Sorry it's a little late. The damage was worse than it looked.

If Fred's jury-rigging holds together, we should be able to get to you in thirty. If not, it's going to be another exciting landing."

"Copy," Rapp said.

A shrill ring filled the cab and Rapp glanced at the bloody sat phone lying next to Muhammad Attia's body. He leaned down to reject the call like he had four times before but then Claudia's voice came on the comm.

"Mitch. The NSA says Attia's phone's ringing again. They think they can trace the call. You need to pick up."

He rolled the window down a couple of inches before complying.

"Muhammad! Are you there?"

Even on speakerphone and mixed with the wind, Sayid Halabi's voice was unmistakable. Rapp had only heard it a few times, but the sound of it was indelibly burned into his mind.

He downshifted, increasing the engine noise and then shouting over it. "I'm here!"

"I can barely hear you. What's your status?"

It was exactly the question he wanted to hear—one that proved Halabi didn't know what was happening. Attia hadn't had time to get a call out and if the ISIS leader was tracking the truck via GPS, the slight detour toward Monterrey had been chalked up to a signal anomaly.

The Agency had been concerned that the people trapped in the trailer might be able to communicate out, but the risk turned out to be low. A couple of the CIA's tech geeks had physically closed themselves up in the back of a truck full of frozen food and confirmed that getting cell or satellite signal was virtually impossible.

"All is well," Rapp said in Arabic. "I'm about an hour from the border crossing."

"Why haven't you been answering my calls?"

Rapp found himself mesmerized by the man's voice—as though it were emanating from beyond the grave. He'd dropped an entire cave system on the ISIS leader and still he'd managed to survive. Would the NSA be able to locate him? And would Rapp live long enough to look into his eyes before putting a bullet between them?

"This is the first call I've received. It's possible that the cell coverage isn't as good as we anticipated."

There was a brief silence as Halabi processed what he'd heard.

"Very well. God be with you. Contact me when you're across."

It was incredible how much you could get away with in the modern world by using bad cell coverage as an excuse.

"God be with you," Rapp responded, though it seemed that Halabi had already disconnected. A moment later Claudia came back on.

"Mitch, do you copy?"

"Yeah. Was that long enough? Did they get him?"

"I'll try to find out, but in the meantime I have Gary Statham on the line. Can you talk to him?"

"Yeah, put him on," he said, rolling the window back up.

"Mitch? How're you holding up?"

"I'm covered in blood, I've got a corpse jammed under the dash, and I forgot my driver's license. Other than that, fine."

"Understood. We're at the border quietly setting up. We don't want to tip off the Mexicans that it's not business as usual. The border's still open and operating normally. Still not too much activity and the Mexicans aren't stopping anyone leaving their side. When you get here, you'll just be waved through. Once you're on the U.S. side, stop. And whatever you do, don't get out of the truck."

"Roger that."

"Then we'll see you in about fifty-three minutes. Good luck."

"Mitch," Coleman said over the comm. "You've got a cop coming at you on the opposite side of the highway. ETA is about two minutes, but he doesn't look like he's in a hurry. Likely he'll just pass on by."

"Good to have you back. How's the chopper? Is it going to hold together?"

"Fred says fifty-fifty. But we're due a little luck, right."

Just over a half an hour to the border and everything was going as smoothly as could be hoped for. Gauges all looked good and the only vehicle visible was Bruno McGraw in his mirror.

"Cop just went by me," Joe Maslick said. "Still normal speeds."

The police cruiser appeared in the distance and Rapp followed it with his eyes as it passed and began to recede in his mirror. Then, after about a hundred yards, taillights flashed.

"Are you seeing this?" Rapp said.

"Yeah," McGraw responded as the police car crossed the median and began coming up behind them with siren wailing.

"Then deal with it."

His man drifted into the right lane in what appeared to be an effort to let the cop pass. But when it came even with the pickup, McGraw swerved left. The unexpected impact was enough to send the cruiser back into the median, where it flipped three times before coming to a rest on its roof.

"Claudia," Rapp said. "A cop just came after us and McGraw took him out."

"Copy that. We haven't heard anything over the police radios about you. Did you do anything to get his attention?"

"Negative."

"Then they may be communicating by cell phone, which is probably not a good sign."

"Looks like the Mexicans have finally decided to join the party," Coleman broke in. "You've got two more cruisers coming in on you from the east. They're still about five miles out but their lights are on and they're hauling ass. Hold on . . . Looks like they're slowing down. Yeah. They're crossing the median and setting up a roadblock. And you've got another cop coming up behind you. A ways back though and he's struggling to close the gap. You'll have a visual on him before you get to the roadblock, but I don't think he'll be on top of you yet."

Rapp glanced at his speedometer. Eighty-seven miles an hour. It was about all he was going to get out of the truck on this road. "Can I get around it?"

"That's a negative. They picked a place with rocky terrain and trees on either side."

"Mas!"

"I'm on it, Mitch."

When the roadblock finally came into view, it was chaos. Maslick had his pickup sideways in the road and was firing his assault rifle across the hood at the cruiser blocking the right lane. From that distance, Rapp couldn't tell what the cops were doing in response and at this point he didn't care.

"What the fuck?" he said over the comm. "I'm less than a minute out and I'm not planning on slowing down. *Get me through*."

Twenty seconds later, he still didn't have a lane, but Maslick's rifle had been replaced with an RPG. There was a puff of smoke and then the cruiser on the left flew into the air on a pillar of flame. Rapp eased into that lane and maintained his speed as the dry brush in the median caught fire.

The cruiser was still hanging out into the asphalt, making it a tight squeeze. There was a deafening crash when his left fender caught the edge of the police vehicle's bumper, but he managed to hold the wheel steady.

"I'm clear," Rapp said. "ETA's coming down fast. Is Gary ready?"

"He says yes," Claudia replied over the comm. "But they're seeing some increased activity on the Mexican side of the border. Not sure what they're up to yet, but it's clear they know something's going on."

"Roger that. It's not much farther. We just have to hold this shit show together for a few more minutes."

He ignored McGraw as he passed, focusing instead on the police car that had appeared through the smoke and was overtaking him from behind. A moment later, though, Coleman's chopper became visible and the former SEAL opened up on the vehicle from above. It skidded off the tarmac and began spinning through the dirt, coming to a stop and staying that way. Whether it was damaged or whether the driver had decided he'd had enough was impossible to tell. Either way, he was out of the game.

The traffic started getting heavier and buildings began springing up on both sides of the road. He slowed, matching the speed limit. Cross streets started to split off the main thoroughfare and the increasing density of buildings made it impossible to see if anyone was going to pull out.

"So far, no stop signs, but if we run into any, someone's going to have to get control of the intersection so I can roll through. I can't risk a cra—"

Rapp fell silent when a light bar came on fifty yards ahead. The border patrol vehicle turned sideways in the road, blocking it at a choke point between two buildings. Rapp didn't even have time to give an order before McGraw swerved toward it. His brush guard connected hard with the cruiser's front quarter panel, spinning it completely around and through the front window of a shop to the left.

Unfortunately, it had a similar effect on McGraw's pickup. Rapp saw the air bags go off as the top-heavy vehicle teetered on two wheels before finally landing on its side. McGraw seemed unaffected, climbing out the open driver's-side window and firing his assault rifle in the air. The locals scattered, clearing a path.

Rapp shifted gears and slammed the accelerator to the floor. "We've lost Bruno. Mas, come around me. It's time to start breaking shit."

"Copy that."

Rapp had the semi up to almost fifty again when Maslick's supercharged Jeep Grand Cherokee passed and took a position twenty yards in front. He lay on his horn, and when that wasn't enough to clear the road, a nudge from his brush guard did the trick.

"I've got eyes on you!" came Gary Statham's excited voice over the comm. "There's a lot of activity on the Mexican side, but it's still disorganized. Just keep coming my way and don't—I repeat, *do not* crash that truck."

"Keep them off me, Scott."

"On it."

The chopper passed overhead with Coleman leaning through the open door firing at pretty much anything that moved. The border crossing was now visible and Maslick was driving like he was in a demolition derby. On the U.S. side, all the barriers had been lifted and what little backed-up traffic that existed was being waved through.

As Rapp approached, two Mexican border security vehicles started to pull out of their spaces to block him. Maslick sideswiped the front of both and then threw his vehicle in reverse, pulling it back and forth as they tried desperately to get around him.

Rapp swerved into a lane reserved for commercial trucks, aiming for the open gate that marked the border. Once through, he slammed on the brakes and downshifted, forcing the rig to a stop. A moment later, vehicles had pulled in front and behind, blocking him in. A few particularly stupid civilians were filming with their phones instead of fleeing, but a little automatic fire ran them off.

Men in hazmat suits appeared from nowhere, surrounding the truck with their weapons trained on him. One spoke into a microphone attached to a speaker on his hip.

"Do not exit the truck. Do you understand me, Mitch? *Stay in* the truck."

Rapp leaned his forehead on the steering wheel as people

swarmed the vehicle, adding chocks to the wheels and disabling its electrical system. The AC went off and he was suddenly aware of the sun pounding through the windows.

"Mitch?" Claudia said over his earpiece. "Are you all right?"

He didn't answer, instead fishing the last two antibiotic pills from his pocket and tossing them in his mouth.

CHAPTER 52

WEST OF TALEH
SOMALIA

THE truck's headlights created a circle of illumination that quickly faded into the blackness around them. Some three hundred meters ahead, Sayid Halabi could see two similar rings of illumination and he knew there were others behind. They had been on the road now for almost forty-eight hours, traveling by night and taking cover by day.

The landscape was wide-open and the skies had been clearer than forecasted, making their situation even more precarious. It was the reason he'd allowed his men to disperse and surrounded himself instead with local jihadists. The goal was to lose himself in the chaotic rhythms of a country that the Americans didn't understand.

He'd made the grave error of calling Muhammad Attia during the operation. And when the man hadn't answered, he'd compounded that error by calling again. And again. Finally he'd connected and spoken on a connection so filled with noise that the conversation was nearly unintelligible.

It was clear now that the garbled voice on the other end of that call hadn't belonged to his loyal disciple. It had belonged to Mitch Rapp.

Halabi looked through his open window at the star-filled sky, searching for any sign of the Americans. They were out there somewhere. Watching, collecting data, calculating probabilities. Waiting to strike.

Only God could protect him now, but he wasn't sure that protection would be forthcoming. The YARS operation had expended every resource and burned every bridge in order to ultimately accomplish nothing. The truck containing his people had been stopped just across the U.S. border, sealed in plastic, and airlifted to an undisclosed location.

Irene Kennedy had skillfully disseminated the story that the trailer was filled with the radioactive components for a dirty bomb. It was a narrative that made locking down the area child's play. No one from the outside had any interest in approaching a contaminated zone, while the ones inside had every incentive to stay. The radiation source was gone and the government was promising testing and treatment for anyone exposed. In the unlikely event the virus had escaped the truck, it was containable.

Halabi glanced over at his Somali driver before staring off again into the darkness. Attia was dead. ISIS forces had been scattered and were now transforming into isolated criminal gangs. The highly trained group of men he'd surrounded himself with would spend the rest of their short lives being hunted by the world's intelligence agencies.

The other major threat to America, Christine Barnett, also seemed to be fading. Her attacks on America's intelligence agencies had been badly undermined by the heroism and competence displayed by the DEA, CIA, and army. For the first time in her political career, she was adrift.

Halabi closed his eyes for a moment, hiding from the reality of what he had done. He hadn't just failed to destroy the United States, he'd provided it with a tangible, terrifying external threat. The country that had been busy tearing itself apart would now turn away from imaginary dangers and focus on real ones. He had unwittingly provided the American people with the truths that their politicians and media had worked so hard to obscure.

Halabi retrieved a new phone from the floorboard, removing it from its packaging before just letting it fall from his hand. There was no one left to call. Nothing left to be learned. Details, strategies, and elaborate plans meant nothing. He knew that now. Mitch Rapp wasn't just the enemy of Islam. He was more than that. The forces of evil had chosen him. And now they were supporting him. Giving him strength.

Until he was dead, God's will could not be done.

Halabi understood that he was aging and injured. That he and his network would become the targets of a manhunt unprecedented in world history. He would never again have an opportunity like the one that he'd just allowed to wither. But he wasn't without resources. He still had benefactors and millions of dollars hidden in bank accounts throughout the world. He still had thousands of followers willing to die on his command.

There was no question that he was soon for the grave, but with his last breath he would drag Mitch Rapp in with him.

The poorly maintained roadbed became strewn with rocks and his driver was forced to slow, swerving through the obstacles. All sense of progress—already nearly nonexistent in Halabi's new reality—seemed to disappear.

A flash appeared ahead in the darkness, unmistakable but impossible to pinpoint exactly. A split second later, a bullet penetrated the windshield and slammed his driver back in his seat.

Halabi grabbed the handle and threw himself against the door but found it blocked. A barely visible figure leaned closer to the open window, his features gaining detail in the hazy artificial light.

Not a Somali bandit. His face was streaked with paint and his hair was covered with a sand-colored cap. What he couldn't hide, though, were his Caucasian features and bright blue eyes.

A pistol appeared and Halabi jerked back, raising an arm protectively as the man spoke.

"Mitch Rapp sends his compliments, motherfucker."

CHAPTER 53

FORT DETRICK
MARYLAND
USA

RAPP lifted the remote control with difficulty, using it to increase the volume of the television bolted to the wall.

Senator Christine Barnett was jogging up the Capitol steps, besieged by reporters shouting questions, aiming cameras, and jostling each other with outstretched microphones. The press that she'd manipulated for so long suddenly seemed completely beyond her control.

". . . leak exposed a counterterrorist operation and allowed a serious threat to cross the border," someone shouted. "Is your committee going to investigate?"

"Of course," she said, looking haggard and uncertain. "This is an extremely important matter and it'll be fully vetted."

The authoritative rhythm of her speech was gone now. Her responses seemed canned. Fake.

"Now, if you'll excuse me," she continued, trying to pick up her pace without looking like she was breaking into a full run, "I have a meeting."

The screen faded back to an interview with a governor who was running a distant second to Barnett in her party's presidential primary. Rapp had met him on a number of occasions and in the scheme of things he wasn't that bad. A former army captain whose brain hadn't yet been completely scrambled by Washington.

"Your thoughts?" the host said.

"Obviously, there are a lot of questions here. About the leaks. About the senator's attacks on the CIA and DEA operatives putting their lives on the line to protect America. It's my understanding that the man who captured the ISIS truck and delivered it to the army may not survive. I wonder if she would have done the same for her country?"

"And the reports that her campaign manager Kevin Gray has resigned and is being interviewed by the FBI?"

"More questions," the man agreed. "If Senator Barnett intends to lead our party in the next presidential election, they're going to need to be answered."

They cut to a clip that Rapp had seen before and he hit the pause button to freeze Barnett's face in a deer-in-the-headlights expression that bordered on fear. It was his favorite shot of her.

He sank back into the pillows and focused on a ceiling that had become a little too familiar over the past couple of weeks. The room he was imprisoned in was about twenty feet square, constructed mostly of stainless steel and glass. Mysterious medical machines hummed around him, displaying vital signs and other information that confirmed he was still alive. As though the cracking headache and constant labor of getting air in and out weren't enough.

The illness had hit him thirty-six hours after he'd been quarantined. It started with a single, innocuous cough and then progressed to a temperature north of 104, a respirator, and finally unconsciousness.

He heard a familiar hiss to his left and let his head loll over to watch Gary Statham come through the air lock in full biohazard gear.

"How're you feeling?" he asked while he checked the machines.

"Great."

"Happy to hear it. I didn't think you were going to make it."

"What're you talking about?" Rapp managed to get out. "You've been telling me I was going to be fine since I got here."

"I was lying. But today I come bearing good tidings. Your lungs and kidneys look good and we're not seeing any permanent damage. It's going to take a little time but you're going to make a full recovery."

"Is that straight? Or another lie?"

"That's straight," Statham said, turning toward the bed. He was a little hard to hear through the space suit. "You'll be back shooting people in the face before you know it."

"Outstanding," Rapp said, already a little out of breath from the conversation. It was hard to imagine even being able to get out of bed. Combat seemed a million miles away.

"Believe it or not, there are some people here who seem anxious to see you. Are you up for a five-minute visit?"

"Sure."

Statham clipped a microphone to Rapp's shirt and then disappeared back through the air lock. A few moments later, Claudia and Anna appeared on the other side of a long window to his right.

"They tell me you're going to be fine," Claudia said, sounding relieved, but still looking worried beneath the harsh fluorescent lights.

"Mom says you got the flu," Anna said, straining to get eye level with the bottom of the viewing window. "My teacher says they have shots for that."

Every time he came home from an operation the worse for wear, they had to come up with a cover story. And every time, his invented carelessness met with the girl's disapproval. Car accidents earned him admonishments about seat belts. Falls down stairs brought on scolding about proper lighting and sensible shoes. Now he was going to get the vaccine lecture.

"Maybe I need to start going to class with you," he said, thankful that the microphone made his voice sound stronger than it really was.

"You're older than my teacher! Can you play a game, Mitch? We brought an Xbox and they said they'd hook it up, but it might take a few days because of the Internet and stuff."

"Sure."

"What do you want to play?"

"How about one of those zombie games?"

"You always want to play the shooters because you always win!"

"This could be your year."

Her eyes narrowed.

"Let's not badger Mitch, okay, sweetie? He isn't feeling well and he's always nice to you when you're sick."

"Okay," she said, sounding a little guilty. Her eyes disappeared as she dropped from her tiptoes, leaving only the top of her head visible.

A long silence stretched out as Claudia stared through the glass. She'd never seen him like this and it appeared to terrify her. He'd have said something to reassure her but he was still recovering from his extended conversation with Anna.

"Scott's here to see you. Should I tell him no? That you need to rest?"

Rapp shook his head. "I'm okay."

"Irene said she'd come tomorrow, when you're feeling a little stronger. She's working on a project she says you're going to like." Claudia patted her daughter's head. "Say good-bye."

"Bye, Mitch! I'll tell them to hurry with that Xbox!"

They disappeared and were quickly replaced by the slightly sunburned face of Scott Coleman. He'd been in a similar hospital bed after his run-in with Grisha Azarov and he seemed to be enjoying the tables being turned.

"You look like shit."

"Fuck you. How are the guys?"

"Good. Wick's just down the hall bouncing off the walls. He didn't catch it, but they want to keep him for another week to make sure. Mas made it over the border and he's home with a broken hand and a dislocated shoulder. Bruno's still in Mexican prison, but the diplomats say they'll spring him in the next couple of days. Doesn't really matter. The head of the most powerful gang there died in a freak drowning accident involving a toilet and Bruno's hands around his throat. Word is he's pretty much running the place."

Rapp just nodded as a broad grin spread across Coleman's face.

"He was there, you know."

"Who was where?"

"We tracked those calls from Halabi to somewhere near Hargeisa. They'd been holed up in a cave system there. By the time we found it they'd already taken off, but we had heavy overhead coverage and the Agency guys were able to run the timeline backward and piece together their movements from satellite photos. It wasn't easy. The weather was crap and the convoy kept breaking up and reforming."

"Is this story going somewhere?"

Coleman's grin widened further and he slapped a color eight-by-ten against the glass. The lighting was garish, a powerful flash in the darkness that illuminated a bearded man with part of his head missing. Rapp lifted himself off the pillows, forgetting the lines attached to him and locking on the image of Sayid Halabi.

"Don't worry," Coleman said. "I told him it was from you."

EPILOGUE

ARLINGTON
VIRGINIA
USA

CHRISTINE Barnett used a key to unlock the office she kept in the southern wing of her Georgetown home. It was her private sanctum—a place that even her husband was prohibited from entering on the rare occasion he was in town. And now she needed it more than ever.

Barnett had barely slept in weeks, instead lying in bed hovering somewhere between dream and reality. Endless scenarios, dangers, and opportunities raced through her mind. The faces of allies and enemies floated in the darkness. She had lost control of her universe for the first time in her career and didn't know how to get it back.

Over the past weeks her poll numbers had plummeted enough to put her in a dead heat with her nearest primary challenger. Dramatic video of Mitch Rapp fighting his way across the border and then being surrounded by the army was still on every channel. The homeland security agencies she'd spent so much time railing against were now being deified by the American public.

Suddenly heroism and patriotism were generating better ratings than personal attacks and partisanship. The rage and negativity that she'd used to fuel her rise through the political ranks was faltering. The American people were looking for something new.

But what?

Kevin Gray wasn't returning her calls, and without him, her campaign's damage control strategy had never fully formed. More important, though, were his meetings with the FBI. She still hadn't been able to find out why he'd been interviewed or what had been discussed. It seemed unimaginable that he would have said anything about the leaks. He was smart enough to know that punishments for such things tended to be doled out to people on his level, not hers. But could she be sure of that?

No.

Her quest to become president was no longer about her thirst for power or the immortality that would accompany being America's first female president. It was about survival. She needed the full support of her party, the White House's ability to manipulate the press, and the authority to remove Irene Kennedy and her loyalists. Once ensconced in the Oval Office she would be untouchable. Until then she was vulnerable.

An increasingly familiar sense of fury and helplessness began to rise in her. She tried to swallow it, knowing that she wouldn't sleep at all that night if it hit full force. Six hours of staring into the darkness wasn't something she could afford. Her day started at 5 a.m. and wouldn't end until after midnight. During that time, she couldn't put a single foot wrong. One ill-considered word, one awkward pause, one unguarded facial expression . . . That's all it would take to put the White House forever out of her reach.

She sat down behind her desk and flipped on the lamp, squinting against the glare to take in the opulent room. As her eyes adjusted, they were drawn to something unusual in a rocking chair near the wall.

"Late night," Mitch Rapp observed.

Her body tensed and she drew in a breath to scream, but it

got caught in her chest. His hair was close cropped and his normally full beard was short and neatly trimmed. The dark eyes were sunken and bloodshot, but still carried the intensity she'd grown to hate over the years. For some reason, though, it wasn't his stare that made the bile rise in her throat. It was the surgical gloves covering his hands.

She swallowed and finally managed to get out a panicked shout. "Help! Come up here now!"

The pounding footsteps of Secret Service agents on the stairs didn't materialize. All she could hear was her own breathing and the creak of the antique chair Rapp was rocking in.

"I didn't slip by them," he said. "They let me in."

Barnett remained frozen. This couldn't be happening. Even Mitch Rapp wouldn't dare. He wouldn't kill one of the front-runners in the U.S. presidential election.

"What do you want?" she heard herself say. "The directorship of the CIA? Homeland Security?"

He just rocked.

"Secretary of defense? Just tell me."

"I know you leaked the anthrax story that almost got me killed."

"That's not true! Who told you that?"

There was no way Rapp had proof. Even if Gray had talked, it would just be his word against hers. The laptop he'd used was brand-new and was now in pieces at the bottom of a landfill. The open-source operating system it ran had been confirmed secure by her husband's top people—some of whom he'd hired away from the NSA.

"There've been a lot of leaks over the years," Rapp continued. "And it's been hard not to notice that quite a few have helped you and hurt your opponents."

"Those have all been investigated and no one has ever even *suggested* that I was involved," Barnett said, starting to overcome her initial shock. She had to think clearly. Her life might depend on it.

Rapp smiled, but in a way that was so devoid of humor that it came off as more of a baring of teeth. Barnett went motionless as though she were faced with a wild animal.

"You had us going for a while," Rapp admitted. "The NSA threw everything at those leaks and no one could trace them."

"Getting to the bottom of this will be one of my administration's top priorities," Barnett said. "There's nothing more important than the safety of this country and the men and women who ensure that safety."

This time his smile was even wider, causing Barnett to silently curse herself. She'd been a politician so long that she couldn't shut it off. The platitudes that were so popular with her millions of followers would be a joke to someone like Rapp.

"Do you want to know where you went wrong, Senator?"

"I have no idea what you're talking about."

"Kevin Gray. Brilliant guy, but a creature of habit. He always gets those new laptops at the same place. The Best Buy a few miles from his house. For the last two years, he's been buying ones custom built by us."

Barnett's mind began to spin as she tried to make the calculations she was famous for. How many leaks had she ordered over that time frame? How many had been carried out by Gray? Why hadn't Kennedy released this information long ago? Was it possible that Rapp was bluffing? Or had Kennedy been squirreling away the evidence to be used if Barnett ever reached the White House?

"I don't believe it," she said. "I don't believe Kevin would do that."

The only plausible way out was to shift the blame. To assert that Gray had acted alone. He already had the reputation as one of the most ruthless and ambitious campaign strategists in Washington. She could use that to create a portrait of a man who would do anything to win.

"If you provide my committee the evidence you have against

him, we'll give it a full, bipartisan vetting. And if we find out he's leaked classified information, I'll be the first one to recommend prosecution."

Rapp reached into his jacket and Barnett's bladder almost let go. When his hand reappeared, though, it wasn't holding the infamous Glock, but instead a mobile phone.

"Like I said, a brilliant guy," he said, tapping the screen. "Brilliant enough to know you'd throw him under the bus."

"Ma'am, Rapp's dead and—" she heard Gray's recorded voice say over the phone's speaker.

"He's not dead! That son of a bitch has more lives than an alley cat. He's alive and they're not telling us. That means he's out there, still working on this operation. Waiting."

"Waiting? Waiting for what?"

"For me to win the primary. Then, at just the right moment, he's going to reappear and save the day. Alexander and Kennedy will be heroes and I'll be standing there looking like a fool."

"Senator, the idea that Mitch Rapp is involving himself in some kind of complex political game is—"

"He sees me as a threat. Just like Kennedy. They're going to use this to come after me. We have to find out what's happening in Mexico. We have to get ahead of it."

"We have no way of finding out what's happening. No one's going to tell us anything, and if we try to twist arms at the intelligence agencies, it's going to go public and blow up in our faces."

"Not the American government. We can use our contacts in the Mexican government. They want us to get off their backs regarding immigrants and drugs, right? Well, as president, I can make that happen. And all I ask in return is a little cooperation and information."

"Now hold on, Senator. If Rapp's alive, it's possible that he's actually still on the trail of ISIS. We—"

"I'm not going to sit on my hands and see that son of a bitch shooting it out with terrorists on television!"

He fast-forwarded the recording.

"Call them, Kevin. Call the Mexicans. Quietly. Find out what's going on. We can still head this off. If there really is something happening down there, we might be able to get the Mexican authorities to deal with it and keep Rapp and Kennedy from getting the win. If it works out, we might even be able to take some credit. Show the American people that I can stop threats before they make it to the United States."

By the time Rapp turned off the recording, enough blood had drained from Barnett's head that she had to steady herself against the desk. She wasn't just going to lose the primary. She was going to be held up as a traitor. She was going to be marched into court in handcuffs and convicted of treason. The fear she used to keep her enemies and allies in line would disappear. For the first time in her career the blood in the water would be hers.

Rapp stood and reached into his jacket again, this time retrieving a bottle of pills that he threw to her. She caught it and looked down at the label. Painkillers backdated to a minor surgery she'd had two years ago.

"That's a present from Irene Kennedy. It's the easy way out. For you and the country."

He went to the door but paused with his gloved hand on the knob. "Take the gift, Senator. Because if you don't, we're going to do it my way."

And then he was gone.

Barnett stared down at the bottle for a long time. Finally, she opened it and reached for a bottle of water near the desk lamp. She gagged on the first pill, terror causing her throat to constrict. After that, it was easy.

Turn the page for a sneak peek at the latest
Mitch Rapp thriller by Kyle Mills, *Enemy at the Gates* . . .

SOUTHWESTERN UGANDA

"WE'RE taking fire," a voice said over Rapp's headphones. "Permission to return it."

"Only if it's focused and absolutely necessary," Rapp responded. "We have friendlies on the ground, and we don't know exactly where they are."

Their entire complement of choppers was in the air, skimming the trees over the search area and occasionally lowering lines to the ground. The idea was to make it impossible for Gideon Auma's men to discern the real rescue from the decoys. Not a perfect plan, but the best they could do under the circumstances.

Fred Mason was keeping their aircraft well above the canopy and out of range of any potential small arms fire. They had coordinates for their target, but the chances of actually setting down were low. Apparently, David Chism was hunkered down in a shallow cave halfway up one of the seemingly endless mountains in the area.

"I think I see it," Mason said over the comm. "Three prominent rocky bands, just like you said." As they passed overhead, a human form appeared from a curtain of foliage hanging from a cliff face. He gazed up at them, waving his arms over his head a couple of times before disappearing again.

"How are we looking?" Rapp asked.

“I think the description was even more optimistic than we thought. Forget landing, I can’t even get close enough to drop you down without putting my rotors into the cliff.”

“I’m not interested in problems, Fred. Give me solutions.”

“We can toss a rope out. If you rappel about forty feet down it, I can probably swing you onto the ledge. When you hit, though, you’ll have to disengage fast as hell. Otherwise, you’ll get dragged back off.”

Rapp looked down at the loose, rocky slope that was his potential landing zone. “That’s a lot of ‘abouts’ and ‘probablys’, Fred.”

“Relax. There’s definitely a non-zero chance you won’t die.”

“Great. Fine. Swing around again. Let’s do this before someone starts shooting at us.”

Rapp slung a tired looking AK-47 over his shoulder before connecting a rope to the belay device on his harness. Mason’s copilot came back to help him put on a ragged backpack and then used a Magic Marker to blacken part of the rope.

“That’s about forty feet,” she said, slapping him encouragingly on the back before returning to the cockpit.

Rapp stared into the blinding sunlight for a few seconds, then put his boots on the edge of the open door and rappelled to the designated mark. After that, there wasn’t much he could do but hang there helplessly as the chopper continued its collision course with the cliff. Fred Mason was unquestionably the best in the business. Hopefully, it would be enough.

When it seemed certain they were going to crash, the chopper reared back, sending Rapp swinging out from beneath it. He hit the ground harder than anticipated, dazing him badly enough that his fingers were incapable of disengaging the rappel device on his waist. He finally managed to release the brake but continued to be dragged toward the drop-off by the friction of the rope passing through the device. It cracked like a whip when it finally cleared, the end contacting Rapp’s forearm and leaving a deep gash.

“Stop rolling!” he heard Mason shout over his earpiece. “Stop fucking rolling, Mitch!”

Clear of the line, he changed his focus to trying to follow his pilot's advice. Most of the rocks he grabbed were too small and loose to have much of an effect, but he eventually managed to aim for one that looked solid. And it was. He slammed into it shoulder first, coming to an abrupt halt three feet from the cliff.

"Mitch! You all right? Say something!"

"Son of a bitch..." he managed to get out, blood drooling from his mouth as he spoke.

"Oh, man!" Mason said. "I'd have bet my life savings on that not working! Am I good or what?"

Rapp just lay there as the chopper disappeared over the mountain. Nothing felt broken or torn. At least nothing important.

He finally struggled to his feet and stumbled toward the tangle of foliage that Chism had built to camouflage the cave entrance. By the time he passed through it, his mind was more or less clear.

"Jeez... That was crazy. Are you okay?"

By way of response, Rapp slapped Chism in the side of the head hard enough to almost drop him.

"Shit, man! That hurt!" he said, stumbling back. An Asian woman watched from the rear of the cave where she was hovering over a man lying in a bed of fronds.

Rapp pointed. "Is he still breathing?"

"Yeah."

"You're sure?"

"I'm a fucking doctor, man."

Rapp stepped forward and slapped him in the side of the head again.

"Ow! Stop it! I couldn't risk that you'd just leave them. They wouldn't be in this mess if it weren't for me."

"And that's the only reason I didn't just collect my paycheck and go home," Rapp said, walking back toward the cave entrance. The dull hum of helicopters was audible outside, punctuated by the occasional burst of automatic fire.

"Fred," he said into his throat mike. "I'm going to need the stretcher. Can you get it in here?"

"Apparently I can do anything!"

"Focus."

"Sorry, Mitch. Yeah. Basically the same drill. But you're going to have to catch it."

"Understood. ETA?"

"Two minutes."

"Roger that. Two minutes out."

He turned and pointed to Matteo Ricci. "Drag him out. We're not going to have a lot of time."

They broke into the sunlight just as Mason came overhead. The litter was already dangling beneath the aircraft as he banked and bore down on them. When he pulled up, the fiberglass stretcher came at Rapp like a projectile. In this instance, Mason's aim was a little too good—forcing Rapp to dive to one side. The litter skidded past and smashed into the rock wall, resting there for a moment as Mason's copilot let the cable reel spin free. Then the weight of the line started dragging it back. Rapp grabbed hold of the litter as it slid by but didn't have enough body weight to arrest its momentum. It looked like his bike-racing diet was going to get him pulled over the cliff.

He was about to release it when David Chism dove onto the other side. They continued to be dragged through the rocks but managed to get control in time.

They pulled it behind the boulder that had stopped Rapp and wedged it in place. Not a long-term solution, but it didn't have to be. The Asian woman whose name Rapp couldn't remember was dragging Ricci downslope toward them.

Dust and pebbles from the rotor wash hammered him as he put the Italian inside. The first strap was barely cinched down over Ricci's chest when automatic fire erupted from the jungle below.

"Bad news," Mason said over the comm. "Those guys are shooting at *us*. They're still a little out of range but I can see them coming up the slope."

"Shit," Rapp muttered as Mason's copilot began firing controlled bursts from the chopper's open door. This was going to turn into a complete clusterfuck if he didn't get them out of there fast.

"We're inbound," he heard Bruno McGraw say. "Approximately one and a half minutes out."

"Not sure we have that long," Mason said. "We're a stationary target here."

"Everybody in," Rapp said.

"What?" Chism was a little wide-eyed.

"You heard me. Get in on top of him."

"Will this thing even hold three people's weight?"

"We're about to find out," Rapp said, shoving him down on top of Ricci. The Asian woman was both more cooperative and quite a bit smaller. She ended up with her face between Ricci's feet and her knees in Chism's side as Rapp threw the rest of the straps over them.

Another burst of automatic fire became audible, this time accompanied by the sound of rounds finding their target. As expected, Mason kept his hover steady. He didn't seem happy when he came back on the comm, though.

"We just took a couple, Mitch. Did you stop for coffee down there?"

Rapp finished with the last buckle and dragged the litter out from behind the boulder. "They're all in! Go!"

Mason didn't need to be told twice. The overfilled litter slid toward the cliff and then went over it, swinging wildly as its occupants screamed in terror. The chopper had gained maybe fifty feet of altitude when a contrail appeared from the jungle.

"Rocket!" Rapp shouted reflexively as Mason took evasive action. The projectile missed by a good fifty yards and the aircraft continued to climb as another—this one containing Bruno McGraw—came into view. They'd retrofitted his rig with a chain gun, and he began firing from the open door, hosing down the area where the rocket had originated. Accuracy wasn't great, but it was hard to blame the marksman. The chopper wasn't designed for the recoil and it was getting pushed all over the place.

Mason's erratic climb had set the litter to spinning out of control, but it was high enough now that Rapp had to squint to make out detail. Another contrail appeared, missing by a good five hundred yards before arcing back into the jungle and failing to detonate. If the black-market SAMs Auma's army used had ever had guidance systems, they'd rusted away long ago.

McGraw redirected his fire on the second rocket's launch point just as a series of rounds stitched the rock wall ten feet over Rapp's head.

"It's too hot for me to go down," he said over his throat mike. "I'm gonna have to climb up and over. I'll contact you when I get to a viable extraction point."